# Understanding Neural Development

# Understanding Neural Development

Edited by Stella Osborne

hayle medical

New York

Hayle Medical,
750 Third Avenue, 9th Floor,
New York, NY 10017, USA

Visit us on the World Wide Web at:
www.haylemedical.com

ISBN: 978-1-63241-687-2

**Cataloging-in-Publication Data**

Understanding neural development / edited by Stella Osborne.
      p. cm.
Includes bibliographical references and index.
ISBN 978-1-63241-687-2
1. Nervous system--Growth. 2. Developmental neurobiology. 3. Neurology.
4. Nervous system--Diseases. 5. Neurosciences. I. Osborne, Stella.
RC341 .U54 2019
612.8--dc23

# Table of Contents

# Preface

This book has been an outcome of determined endeavour from a group of educationists in the field. The primary objective was to involve a broad spectrum of professionals from diverse cultural background involved in the field for developing new researches. The book not only targets students but also scholars pursuing higher research for further enhancement of the theoretical and practical applications of the subject.

Neural development is an amalgamation of the studies of neuroscience and developmental biology. It describes the cellular and molecular mechanisms responsible for the emergence and development of complex nervous systems during embryonic development which continues throughout life. During the embryonic stage, the development of the nervous system entails the processes of neurulation, the formation of the brain and the spinal cord. Neurons travel from their points of origin to the final positions in the brain in a process termed as neuronal migration which can occur through the processes of radial migration, tangential migration and axophilic migration. The study of neurogenesis and neurodevelopment in the adult brain is an area of significant research. Such studies as well as the studies focused on neurotrophic factors that regulate and promote neuronal survival in the developing nervous system are the mainstay of research in neural development. This book brings forth some of the most innovative concepts and elucidates the unexplored aspects of neural development. Different approaches, evaluations, methodologies and advanced studies have been included in this book. It is a resource guide for experts as well as students.

It was an honour to edit such a profound book and also a challenging task to compile and examine all the relevant data for accuracy and originality. I wish to acknowledge the efforts of the contributors for submitting such brilliant and diverse chapters in the field and for endlessly working for the completion of the book. Last, but not the least; I thank my family for being a constant source of support in all my research endeavours.

**Editor**

# Microtubule-associated protein 1b is required for shaping the neural tube

Pradeepa Jayachandran[1†], Valerie N. Olmo[1†], Stephanie P. Sanchez[1†], Rebecca J. McFarland[1], Eudorah Vital[1], Jonathan M. Werner[1], Elim Hong[1,2], Neus Sanchez-Alberola[1], Aleksey Molodstov[1] and Rachel M. Brewster[1*]

## Abstract

**Background:** Shaping of the neural tube, the precursor of the brain and spinal cord, involves narrowing and elongation of the neural tissue, concomitantly with other morphogenetic changes that contribue to this process. In zebrafish, medial displacement of neural cells (neural convergence or NC), which drives the infolding and narrowing of the neural ectoderm, is mediated by polarized migration and cell elongation towards the dorsal midline. Failure to undergo proper NC results in severe neural tube defects, yet the molecular underpinnings of this process remain poorly understood.

**Results:** We investigated here the role of the microtubule (MT) cytoskeleton in mediating NC in zebrafish embryos using the MT destabilizing and hyperstabilizing drugs nocodazole and paclitaxel respectively. We found that MTs undergo major changes in organization and stability during neurulation and are required for the timely completion of NC by promoting cell elongation and polarity. We next examined the role of Microtubule-associated protein 1B (Map1b), previously shown to promote MT dynamicity in axons. *map1b* is expressed earlier than previously reported, in the developing neural tube and underlying mesoderm. Loss of Map1b function using morpholinos (MOs) or δMap1b (encoding a truncated Map1b protein product) resulted in delayed NC and duplication of the neural tube, a defect associated with impaired NC. We observed a loss of stable MTs in these embryos that is likely to contribute to the NC defect. Lastly, we found that Map1b mediates cell elongation in a cell autonomous manner and polarized protrusive activity, two cell behaviors that underlie NC and are MT-dependent.

**Conclusions:** Together, these data highlight the importance of MTs in the early morphogenetic movements that shape the neural tube and reveal a novel role for the MT regulator Map1b in mediating cell elongation and polarized cell movement in neural progenitor cells.

## Background

The neural tube, the precursor of the central nervous system, derives from the neurectoderm through a process known as neurulation. In anterior regions of mouse, chick and *Xenopus* embryos, conserved aspects of this process entail thickening of the neural ectoderm to shape the neural plate, elevation of the edges of the neural plate to form neural folds and convergent extension of the neural plate that narrows and elongates the neural ectoderm [1–4] and contributes to neural groove formation. The neural folds on either side of the neural plate eventually fuse at the dorsal midline and separate from the overlying non-neural ectoderm to shape the neural tube [5]. Mechanisms of teleost neurulation are often thought to diverge from primary neurulation due to the initial formation of a solid rod (and hence absence of a neural groove), which only later cavitates to give rise to a neural tube [6]. A common misconception is that the neural rod is assembled from the coalescence of neurectodermal cells that exhibit mesenchymal properties (reviewed in [3]), akin to secondary neurulation in mammals. However, closer examination of this process in zebrafish revealed that the neural tube derives in fact from a bilayered neural plate, albeit incompletely epithelialized, that infolds as a continuous sheet. The two sides of the neural plate are closely juxtaposed during infolding, explaining the absence of a neural groove. Thus, medio-

* Correspondence: brewster@umbc.edu
†Equal contributors
[1]Department of Biological Sciences, University of Maryland Baltimore County, Baltimore, MD, USA
Full list of author information is available at the end of the article

lateral positions of cells in the deep layer of the neural plate correlate with dorso-ventral positions in the neural tube [7, 8]. In this regard, neural tube formation in zebrafish is similar to primary neurulation in mammals, which also entails the folding of an epithelialized neural plate.

As in other vertebrates [9-11], the zebrafish neural plate undergoes neural convergence and extension. However, in zebrafish, narrowing and elongation of the neural anlage is not limited to the neural plate stage, since convergence also drives infolding of the neural plate to shape the neural rod and extension occurs concomitantly with this event. This later convergence event (referred to henceforth as NC, for neural convergence) is driven by polarized migration towards the dorsal midline and cell elongation along the medio-lateral (prospective apico-basal) axis. Failure to undergo proper NC, as a consequence of disruption of the planar cell polarity (PCP) pathway, results in severe neural tube defects in zebrafish [12], highlighting the importance of this early stage of neural tube formation.

The cellular mechanisms underlying NC were first revealed in *Xenopus* and zebrafish, owing to early access and transparency (zebrafish) of the embryo. In *Xenopus*, explant assays have revealed that migration of deep neural cells in the medial neural plate is mediated by monopolar protrusions (filopodia and lamellipodia) directed towards the midline [11, 13, 14]. We have previously demonstrated that cells in the zebrafish neural plate also extend medially-oriented protrusions and elongate as they converge towards the midline [8]. Narrowing of the neural plate in mice involves cell elongation [15] and cellular rearrangements [10, 16] that are driven by polarized apical boundary rearrangement and bipolar protrusive activity at the basal pole of cells [9]. Thus, the ability of neuroepithelial cells to form polarized protrusions appears to be an essential and conserved aspect of neural tube morphogenesis, the molecular underpinnings of which remain poorly understood.

Many inroads have been made in understanding how the microtubule (MT) network contributes to cell polarity during migration [17]. MTs are dynamic heteropolymers of $\alpha$- and $\beta$-tubulin, existing in alternating states of active polymerization and depolymerization known as dynamic instability [18, 19]. These cytoskeletal elements establish the position of cortical polarity (manifested as actin-rich lamellipodia in migrating cells) via multiple pathways [20, 21]. Key to MT-mediated establishment of cellular asymmetry is the polarized (radial) organization of these structures, with slow-growing minus-ends anchored at the centrosome and the faster growing plus-ends clustered at the leading edge, adjacent to the cell cortex [22]. In addition to their role in cell migration, dynamic MTs play an active role in cell elongation and maintenance of

homeostatic length [23]. The role of stable MTs in cellular dynamics is less well established.

MT stability and dynamics are regulated in part by microtubule-associated proteins (MAPs). Members of the MAP1 family bind along the entire MT lattice. MAP1B, a founding member of this family, is posttranslationally cleaved into a heavy chain (HC) and a light chain (LC1) [24]. The heavy chain contains domains for actin, MTs and LC1 binding [25–27] and can therefore crosslink MTs and microfilaments [28, 29]. The light chain also binds MTs and actin and regulates the cytoskeleton [30, 31]. MAP1B proteins were first identified based on their MT-stabilizing properties [31–33]. However, unlike tau, MAP1B preferably associates with dynamic (tyrosinated) MTs, helping to maintain a pool of dynamic MTs required for axonal elongation [34, 35]. This activity of MAP1B is controlled by several kinases, including Glycogen synthase kinase-3$\beta$ (GSK-3$\beta$), which increases MAP1B MT binding and dynamicity [36]. The poor MT stabilizing properties of MAP1B combined with its ability to promote MT dynamics, suggest MAP1B function differs from the other MAPs [35]. *MAP1B* is also expressed prior to other members of this family in the nervous system [37–40], as it is observed in neuronal progenitors prior to their last mitotic division [41]. Despite this early expression and function in promoting MT dynamics, MAP1B has not been implicated in early stages of neural tube development.

We investigate here whether zebrafish Map1b plays a role in the polarized cell movements that shape the neural rod during NC. Our studies reveal that MTs undergo major changes during neural tube formation, as they become progressively more stable and elongated. The perturbation of cell elongation and polarized migration following nocodazole and paclitaxel treatments suggests that the regulation of MT stability during NC is essential for proper completion of this process. To gain insight into underlying mechanism, we characterized the function of Map1b, previously shown to promote MT dynamicity in axons. *map1b* is expressed earlier than previously reported, in the developing neural tube and underlying mesoderm. Loss of Map1b function using morpholinos (MOs) or $\delta$Map1b, encoding a truncated Map1b protein product, resulted in delayed NC and duplication of the neural tube, a defect previously observed in PCP mutants in which NC is also defective [12]. We observed a loss of stable MTs in these embryos that is likely to contribute to the NC defect. Lastly, we reveal that Map1b mediates cell elongation in a cell autonomous manner and polarized protrusive activity, two cell behaviors that underlie NC and are MT-dependent. Together, these data highlight the importance of MTs in the early morphogenetic movements that shape the neural tube and reveal a novel role for the MT regulator Map1b in mediating cell elongation and polarized cell movement in neural progenitor cells.

## Results

### Microtubules undergo dramatic changes during neurulation

During early stages of neurulation, MTs appear to undergo global morphological changes. Immunolabeling with anti-β–tubulin (anti-β-tub, a marker for the total MT population) revealed that at the neural plate stage (tb-1 som), when neural cells extend polarized protrusions towards the midline, MTs are distributed throughout the cytosol (Fig. 1a, a'), consistent with the radial organization we previously reported [42]. In contrast, at the neural keel stage (so named because of the keel shape adopted by the neural tissue as it transition from a neural plate to a neural rod, 4–5 som) and neural rod (12–13 som) stage, MTs organize into long linear arrays (bundles), which align along the future apico-basal axis of neural cells, coincident with epithelialization that occurs following NC (Fig. 1b–c') [43].

The organizational changes observed in MTs suggest that they become increasingly stable as neurulation

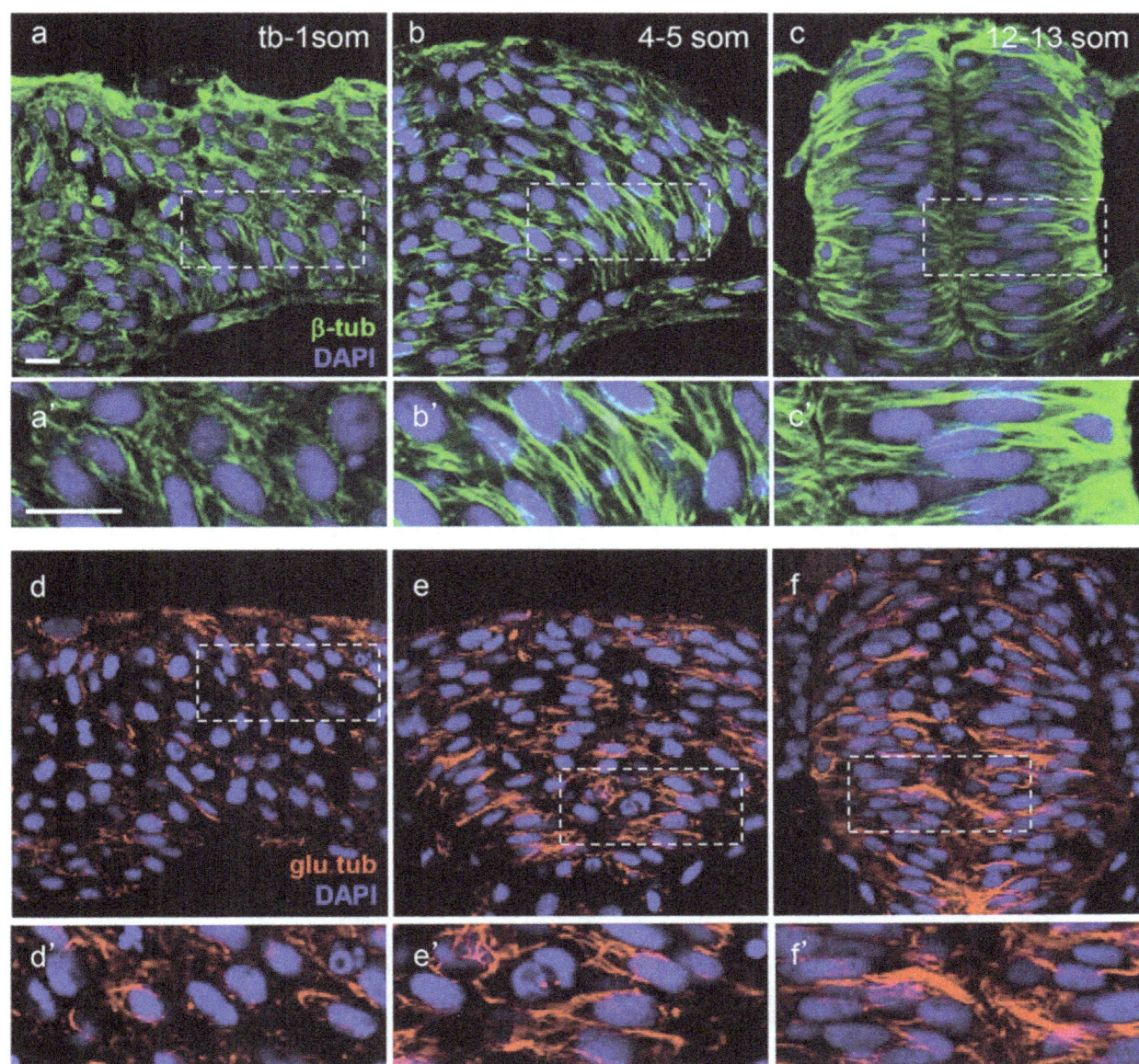

**Fig. 1** Microtubules become increasingly stabilized during neurulation. Hindbrain sections of embryos at the neural plate (tb-1 som) (**a**, a', **d**, d'), neural keel (4–5 som) (**b**, b', **e**, e') and neural rod (12–13 som) (**c**, c', **f**, f') stages immunolabeled with anti-β-tub (total MTs) in green (**a**–c') and anti-glu-tub (detyrosinated MTs) in red (**d**–f'). (a'–c') and (d'–f') Higher magnification of boxed areas in (**a**–c) and (**d**–f), respectively. Scale bars: 10 μm

progresses. In order to investigate the distribution of stable MTs at different stages of neurulation, embryos were immunolabeled with anti-detyrosinated-tubulin (glu-tub). Glu-tub antibodies recognize stable, detyrosinated MTs by binding to the exposed carboxy-terminal glutamic acid of α-tubulin (α-tub) in MT polymers [44, 45]. At the neural plate stage, glu-tub labeling is diffuse and more punctate than β-tub (Fig. 1d, d'). However, by the neural keel stage (Fig. 1e, e') detyrosinated MTs organize into linear structures, which become more accentuated at the neural rod stage (Fig. 1f, f'). The distribution of glu-tub labeling thus implies that detyrosination of MTs occurs initially in discrete foci along the MT polymers that subsequently expand to include the entire polymer. These observations suggest that stable MTs increase over time, reaching elevated levels in the epithelialized neural tube. To quantify the relative abundance of stable

MTs, we analyzed the ratio of glu-tub (stable MTs) to α-tub (total MTs) at the neural plate (tb), neural keel and neural rod stages and found this ratio to be highest at the neural rod stage (Additional File 1: Figure S1).

We next analyzed the distribution of dynamic MTs using an antibody that specifically recognizes the tyrosinated form of α-tubulin (anti-tyr-tub) [46]. In contrast to the spotty distribution of glu-tub at the neural plate and neural keel stages, tyr-tub was abundant and appeared to near fully overlap with the bulk of MTs labeled with α β-tub (Fig. 2a1–a3, b1–b3), with the exception of discrete puncta of α tyr-tub labeling that may correspond to depolymerized tyrosinated tubulin (Fig. 2b3). At the neural rod stage, the overlap remained extensive but some segments of MT bundles were more intensely labeled with anti- β-tub than with anti- tyr-tub (Fig. 2c3, c3'). These regions may coincide with areas of MT

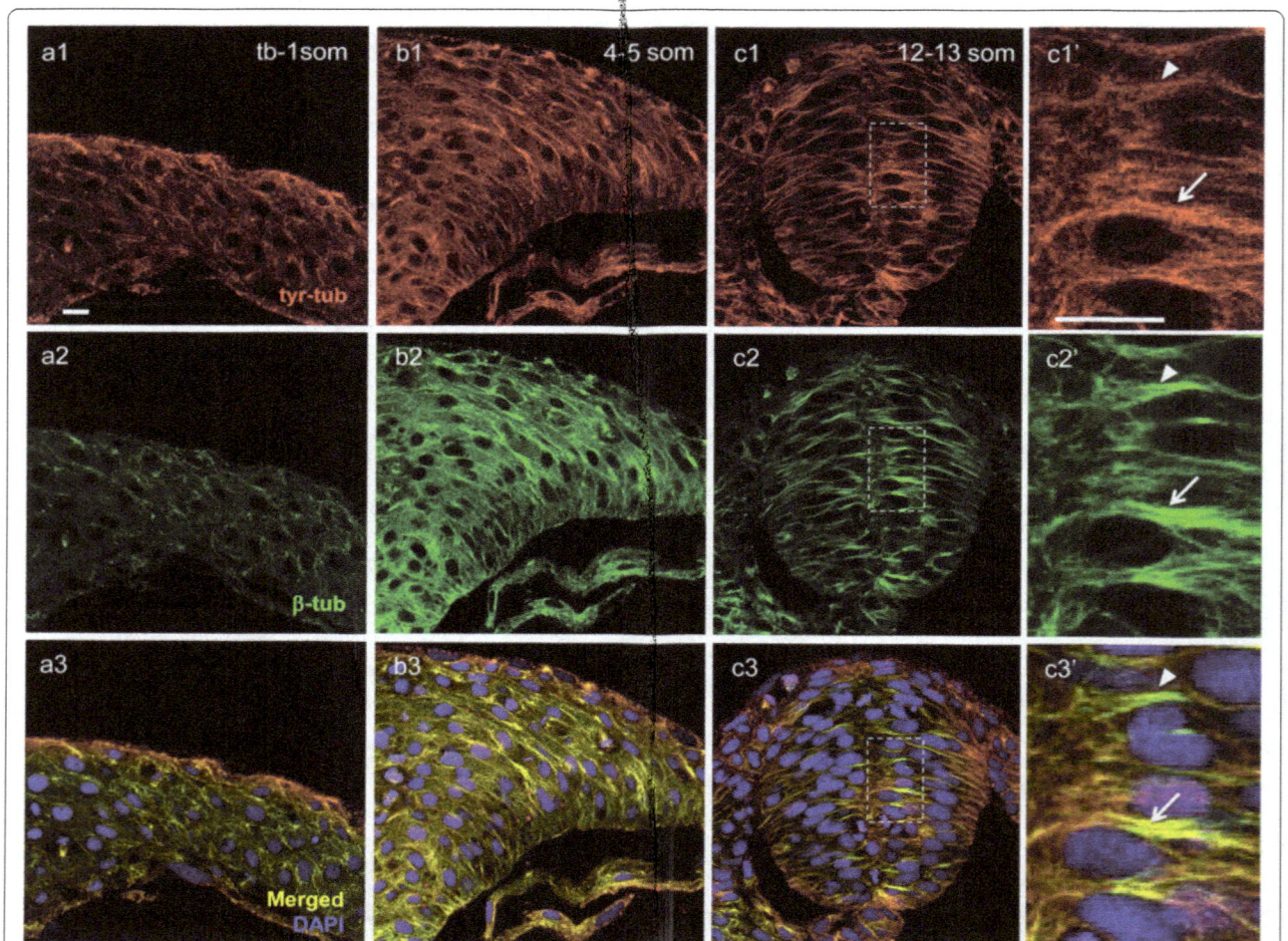

**Fig. 2** Distribution of dynamic microtubules during neurulation. Hindbrain sections of embryos at the neural plate (tb-1 som) (**a1**–**a3**), neural keel (4–5 som) (**b1**–**b3**) and neural rod (12–13 som) (**c1**–*c3'*) stages immunolabeled with anti-tyr-tub (dynamic MTs) in red (**a1**, **b1**, **c1**, *c1'*), anti-β-tub (total MTs) in green (**a2**, **b2**, **c2**, *c2'*). (**a3**, **b3**, **c3**, *c3'*) Red-Green overlay (yellow) of images in (**a1**-*c2'*) with nuclei labeled in blue using DAPI. (*c1'*-*c3'*) Higher magnification of boxed areas in (**c1**–**c3**). Arrows indicate high overlap between anti-tyr-tub and anti-β-tub; arrowheads indicate area of reduced overlap between these two markers. Scale bars: 10 μm

stabilization (arrowhead in Fig. 2c3'). Thus, dynamic MTs represent the bulk of the MT population during NC, while stable MTs steadily increase over time.

### Microtubules are required for NC

The striking increase in the levels of detyrosinated MTs suggests that the stability of these cytoskeletal elements is regulated during neural tube development and likely to be important for neural tube morphogenesis. To test this, we treated early neural stage (2–3 som) embryos with nocodazole (17 and 32 μM) or paclitaxel (50 μM), which destabilize and hyperstabilize MTs respectively, and analyzed the effect of these drugs on cell behaviors at the neural keel stage (4–5 som). The efficacy of these drugs was first confirmed by immunolabeling with anti-β-tub, which revealed that the linear organization of MTs was disrupted following both treatments (Additional file 2: Figure S2).

To analyze the effect of altering MT stability on NC following nocodazole or paclitaxel treatments, the width of the neural plate was assessed using $dlx3$, a gene expressed at the border of the neural and non neural ectoderm. While untreated embryos displayed no NC defects, the neural plates of nocodazole and paclitaxel-treated embryos were abnormally wide (A,B) (untreated embryos: 194 μm ± 31 μm, $n$= 38 embryos; nocodazole-treated (17μM): 276 μm ± 47 μm, $n$ = 34 embryos; paclitaxel-treated (50 μM): 279 μm ± 47 μm, $n$ = 42 embryos). In order to investigate the underlying cellular cause for the NC defects, embryos mosaically expressing cell-surface Green Fluorescent Protein (mGFP) were exposed to nocodazole (17 and 32 μM) or paclitaxel (50 μM) and imaged in the hindbrain region at the neural keel (4–5 som) stage. Cells were significantly shortened following treatment with nocodazole and paclitaxel (Fig. 3c), as determined by length-to-width (LWR) ratio measurements (LWR of untreated cells: 4.48 ± 0.3, $n$ = 26 cells from 7 embryos; LWR of nocodazole-treated cells 1.9 ± 0.19, $n$ = 18 cells from 4 embryos; LWR of paclitaxel-treated cells: 3.0 ± 0.24, $n$ = 30 cells from 7 embryos) (Fig. 3D), indicating sensitivity to perturbations of the MT network that either destabilize or hyperstabilize MTs.

In order to investigate whether MTs play a role in polarized cell migration, time-lapse confocal imaging was carried out at the neural plate (tb-1 som) stage using control and nocodazole-treated embryos mosaically expressing mGFP. Cells from untreated embryos exhibit an elongated appearance with protrusions oriented medially, as previously described [8]. In contrast, cells from nocodazole-treated embryos were rounded in shape and failed to migrate in a directional manner, as a result of randomized membrane protrusions (Additional files 3 and 4). This observation suggests that MTs are not required for

the formation of protrusions but are rather implicated in the proper polarization of these extensions.

Together these findings identify MTs as key mediators of cell elongation and polarized cell movement during NC. They further suggest that regulation of MT stability is tightly controlled during early development, pointing to a potential role for microtubule-associated proteins (MAPs) in this process.

### Zebrafish map1b is expressed in the developing neural tube

Mammalian MAP1B is one of the earliest MAPs to be expressed in the developing nervous system and hence a good candidate for mediating early morphogenetic movements during neural tube formation. Gene ontology analysis revealed a high level of sequence similarity between zebrafish Map1b and its orthologues in chick, mouse, rat and human. The regions of highest conservation (98 % identity) comprise a stretch of 550 amino acids in the N-terminus and 120 amino acids in the C-terminus [31]. Mammalian MAP1B contains two MT-binding domains, each composed of multiple repeats of KKEE or KKEI/V motifs [26, 30]. Domain analysis of zebrafish Map1b revealed the presence of the conserved KKE signature repeats at the N-terminus, in the region encoding the heavy chain. Furthermore, synteny analysis showed that zebrafish map1b is located in a conserved region of the genome.

In order to determine whether zebrafish map1b is expressed during neurulation, we performed whole-mount in situ hybridization. We observed that map1b is broadly distributed at the neural plate (tb-1som), neural keel (4–5 som) and neural rod (8–10 som) stages (Fig. 4a–c). Its expression appears to be in a gradient that is highest in the mesoderm at the neural plate stage (Fig. 4a). By the neural keel and rod stages the level of map1b increases and expression expands dorsally, as map1b is present throughout the developing neural tube (Fig. 4b, c). To confirm that the signal observed at these developmental stages is specific, in situ hybridization using a sense riboprobe was also performed. No labeling was observed with the latter (Fig. 4a'–c').

These observations indicate that map1b is expressed earlier than previously reported, in undifferentiated neural progenitor cells undergoing NC.

### Depletion of Map1b causes NC defects

We next tested whether map1b is required for NC by performing functional studies using two splice-blocking MOs (map1b MO1 and map1b MO2, Additional file 5: Figure S3). RT-PCR analysis confirmed that these MOs block map1b mRNA splicing (Additional file 5: Figure S3). We observed that the neural plate of map1b MO1 (10 ng)- and map1b MO2 (4 and 10 ng)-injected

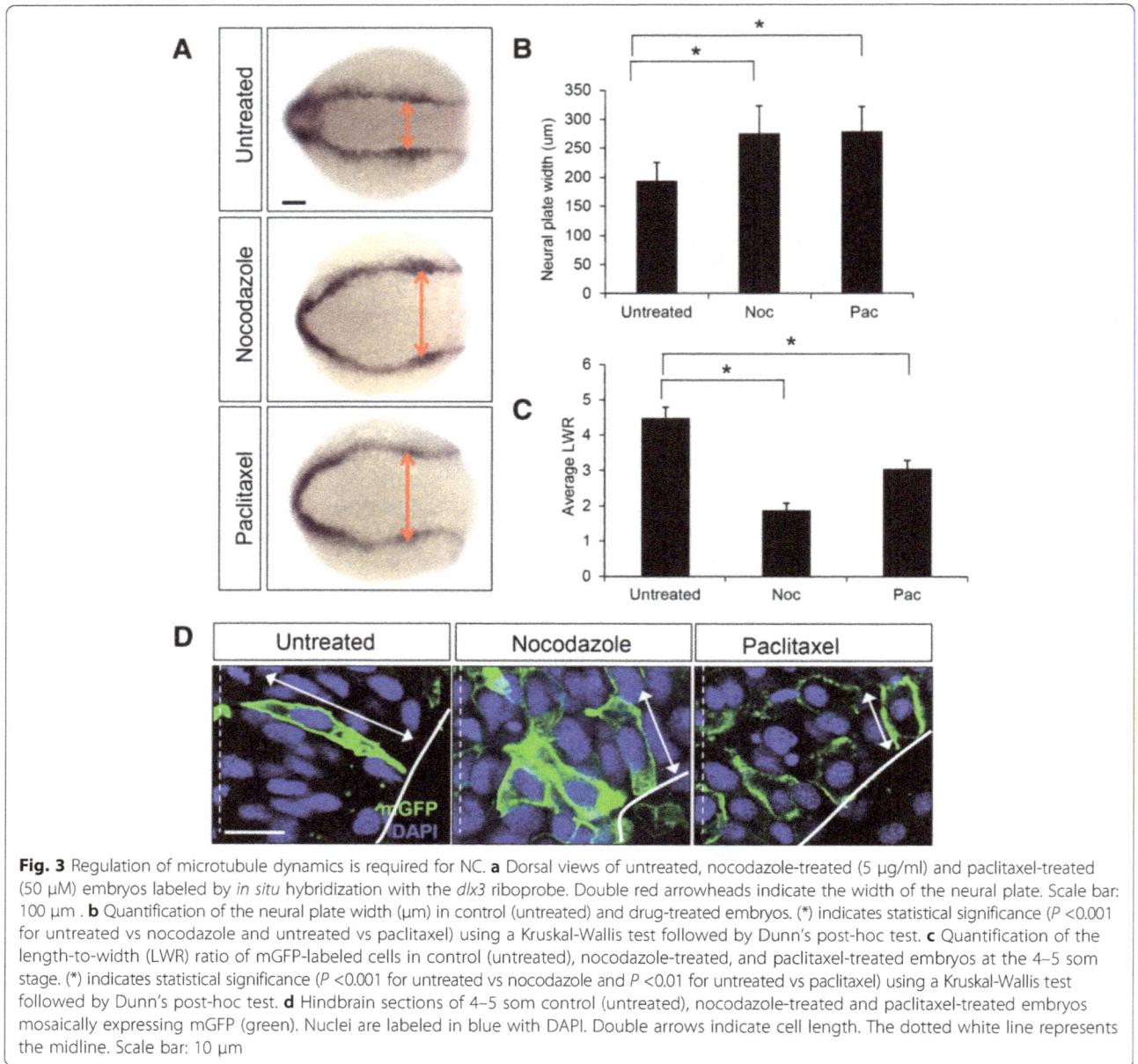

**Fig. 3** Regulation of microtubule dynamics is required for NC. **a** Dorsal views of untreated, nocodazole-treated (5 μg/ml) and paclitaxel-treated (50 μM) embryos labeled by *in situ* hybridization with the *dlx3* riboprobe. Double red arrowheads indicate the width of the neural plate. Scale bar: 100 μm . **b** Quantification of the neural plate width (μm) in control (untreated) and drug-treated embryos. (*) indicates statistical significance ($P < 0.001$ for untreated vs nocodazole and untreated vs paclitaxel) using a Kruskal-Wallis test followed by Dunn's post-hoc test. **c** Quantification of the length-to-width (LWR) ratio of mGFP-labeled cells in control (untreated), nocodazole-treated, and paclitaxel-treated embryos at the 4–5 som stage. (*) indicates statistical significance ($P < 0.001$ for untreated vs nocodazole and $P < 0.01$ for untreated vs paclitaxel) using a Kruskal-Wallis test followed by Dunn's post-hoc test. **d** Hindbrain sections of 4–5 som control (untreated), nocodazole-treated and paclitaxel-treated embryos mosaically expressing mGFP (green). Nuclei are labeled in blue with DAPI. Double arrows indicate cell length. The dotted white line represents the midline. Scale bar: 10 μm

embryos were significantly wider than those of uninjected and standard control MO (4 ng)-injected embryos (uninjected: 272 μm ± 11 μm, $n$ = 58 embryos; standard MO: 220 μm ± 7 μm, $n$ = 29 embryos; *map1b* MO1: 332 μm ± 15 μm, $n$ = 8 embryos; *map1b* MO2: 319 μm ± 10 μm, $n$ = 68 embryo; Fig. 5a), suggesting that *map1b* is required for NC. A MO targeting *pard3* (10 ng), a gene implicated in later aspects of neural tube development [42, 47], was used as an additional negative control and confirmed to not cause an NC defect (*pard3*-MO: 200 ± 15 μm, $n$= 14 embryos; Fig. 5a). To further confirm these results, a translation-blocking *map1b* MO (MO3) was designed, but

was found to be less effective than the splice-blocking MO1 at producing a widened neural plate phenotype. However, co-injection of MO3 (10 ng) with lower concentrations of *map1b* MO1 (4 ng) resulted in a wider neural plate, which was not observed in embryos injected with *map1b* MO1 alone at the suboptimal concentration (uninjected embryos: 165 ± 21 μm, $n$ = 10 embryos; *map1b* MO1 (4 ng): 145 ± 24 μm, $n$ = 13 embryos; *map1b* MO3 (10 ng): 212 ± 23 μm, $n$ = 26 embryos; *map1b* MO1 (4 ng) + MO3 (10 ng); 291 ± 29 μm, $n$ = 24 embryos) (Additional file 5: Figure S3). Therefore, we conclude that the neural plate widening we observe is most

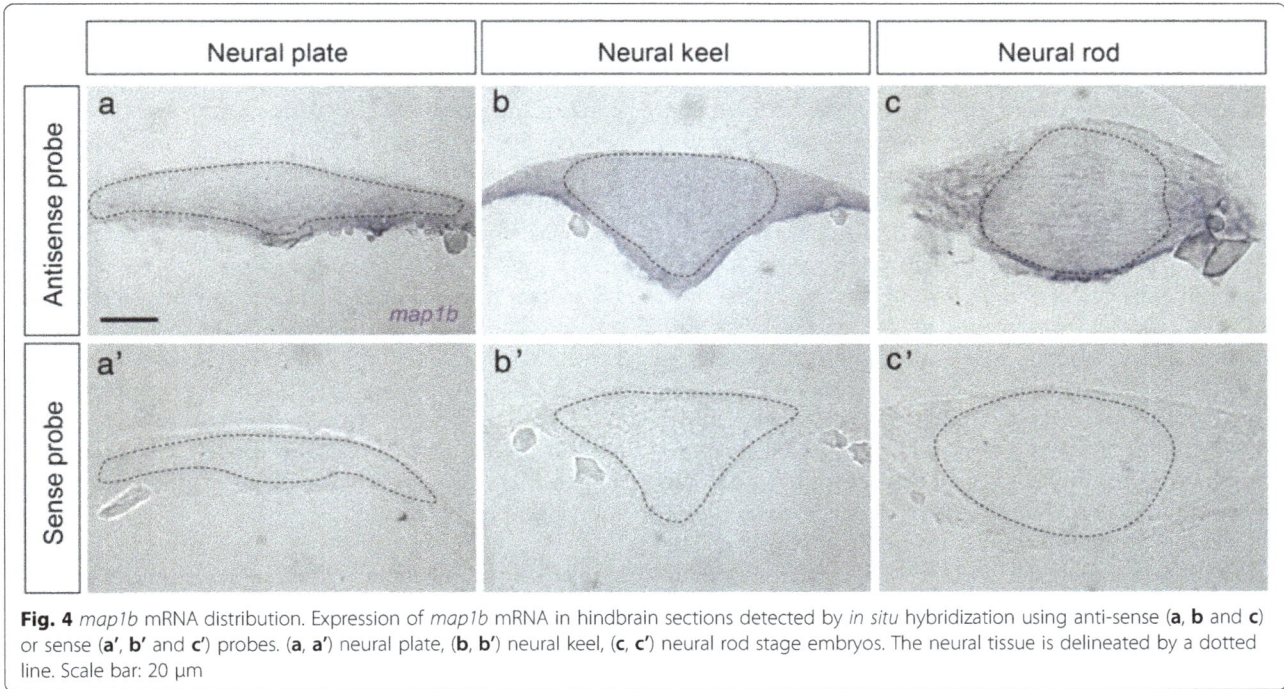

**Fig. 4** *map1b* mRNA distribution. Expression of *map1b* mRNA in hindbrain sections detected by *in situ* hybridization using anti-sense (**a**, **b** and **c**) or sense (**a'**, **b'** and **c'**) probes. (**a**, **a'**) neural plate, (**b**, **b'**) neural keel, (**c**, **c'**) neural rod stage embryos. The neural tissue is delineated by a dotted line. Scale bar: 20 μm

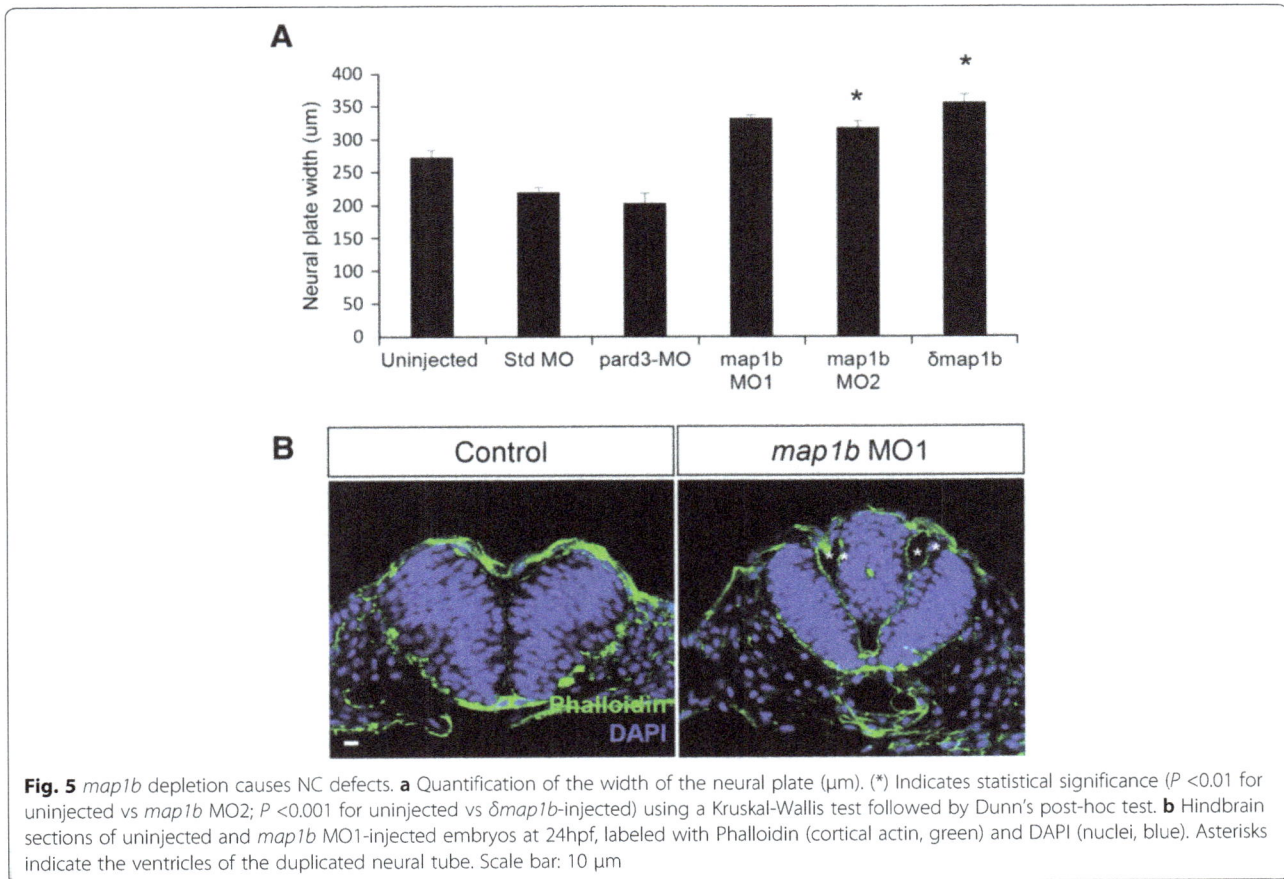

**Fig. 5** *map1b* depletion causes NC defects. **a** Quantification of the width of the neural plate (μm). (*) Indicates statistical significance ($P < 0.01$ for uninjected vs *map1b* MO; $P < 0.001$ for uninjected vs δ*map1b*-injected) using a Kruskal-Wallis test followed by Dunn's post-hoc test. **b** Hindbrain sections of uninjected and *map1b* MO1-injected embryos at 24hpf, labeled with Phalloidin (cortical actin, green) and DAPI (nuclei, blue). Asterisks indicate the ventricles of the duplicated neural tube. Scale bar: 10 μm

likely due to loss of *map1b* rather than an off-target effect of the MOs.

The MT-binding affinity and activity of Map1b is known to be modulated by several kinases, including Gsk3β [48–50]. Consistent with this model, we observed a widened neural plate in embryos in which Gsk3β was disrupted with a translation-blocking MO and a synergistic interaction between Gsk3β and *map1b* (data not shown).

To evaluate whether *map1b* disruption results in later developmental defects, *map1b* MO1 and MO2 (10 ng)-injected embryos were imaged at 24 hpf. We observed a disorganization of the hindbrain region in these embryos, characterized by absence of morphological landmarks (Additional file 5: Figure S3) that were more pronounced with MO1 than MO2. Sectioning through the hindbrain of MO1-injected embryos revealed that the disorganization was caused by a partial ($n$ = 4 out of 10 embryos) or full ($n$ = 1 out of 10 embryos) duplication of the neural tube (Fig. 5b). This striking phenotype was first observed in PCP mutants [12] and is thought to be a consequence of delayed NC [47, 51]. In addition to the disorganized hindbrain, we observed a shortened body axis (Additional file 5: Figure S3), a phenotype often associated with impaired convergent extension in the axial mesoderm [52].

### Truncated Map1b lacking the MT-binding-domain causes delayed NC

In order to confirm the role of Map1b in mediating NC using a MO-independent method, we designed a construct based on a mouse mutation thought to function as a dominant-negative allele [31, 53, 54]. The zebrafish mutant construct, δ*map1b*, encodes the first 571 aa of Map1b, which includes the Map1b light chain (LC1) binding domain (in the heavy chain region) but not the MT-binding domain (6A). Mice that are heterozygous for this mutation have a spectrum of phenotypes including slow growth rates and small eyes, while their homozygous siblings die during embryogenesis [53]. Interestingly, zebrafish embryos injected with δ*map1b* RNA (25, 50, 75 and 100 ng/μl) exhibit an increasingly severe reduction in body and eye size with higher concentrations of RNA (Additional file 6: Figure S4B), suggesting that the truncated Map1b protein functions in a similar manner in both species.

To test whether δMap1b disrupts NC, we injected an intermediate concentration of δ*map1b* RNA (50 ng/μl) and performed the previously described convergence assay. As was reported for *map1b* MO1 and MO2-injected embryos, we observed delays in NC in δ*map1b*-injected relative to controls (Fig. 5a) (uninjected: 272 μm ± 11 μm, $n$ = 58 embryos vs δ*map1b*: 355 μm ± 13 μm, $n$ = 45 embryos).

The more severe phenotype in δ*map1b*-injected embryos compared to *map1b* MO-injected embryos suggests that δMap1b functions in a dominant-negative manner. Given that δ Map1b retains the ability to bind to LC1 [31], which is implicated in the regulation of MT stability and other MT-independent processes [31, 55], it is likely that depletion of this peptide accounts for some of the pronounced defects observed in injected embryos. In addition, the unbound endogenous heavy chain in δ*map1b*-injected embryos may also play a contributing role.

Together these findings reveal a previously unknown role for Map1b in mediating NC in the neural ectoderm. The fully or partially duplicated neural tube observed in *map1b* MO-injected embryos is consistent impaired NC. Furthermore, the fact that a neural tube, albeit abnormal, forms in Map1b-depleted embryos indicates that Map1b is required for the timely progression rather than completion of neurulation.

### Loss of Map1b results in the loss of stable microtubules

Previous studies indicate that Map1b maintains a dynamic population of MTs that promotes axonal growth [48, 56]. If Map1b plays a similar role in the neuroectoderm, its loss-of-function should result in increased MT stability. To test this prediction, neural keel (4–5 som) stage uninjected, standard MO-injected, *map1b* MO2-injected and δ*map1b*-injected embryos were sectioned and labeled with anti-β-tub (total MTs), anti-glu-tub (stable, detyrosinated MTs) and DAPI (nuclei) and imaged at the hindbrain level. Unlike the dramatic perturbation of the MT network observed following treatments with nocodazole and paclitaxel (Additional file 2: Figure S2), the overall organization of MTs visualized with β-tub labeling in *map1b* MO2- and δ*map1b*-injected embryos appeared similar to controls (Fig. 6a), although in some samples (insets in Fig. 6a *b1*, *c1*) the β-tub-labeled bundles were less well defined than those of uninjected (inset in Fig. 6a *a1*) and standard MO (data not shown).

Enhanced MT stability is often manifested in either an increase in MT bundle length or the average number of MT bundles/cell. Quantification of the length of glu-tub- and β-tub-positive bundles in the different treatment groups did not reveal any differences (data not shown). However, the average number of stable, glu-tub-positive bundles per cell (nucleus) revealed an unexpected decrease in *map1b* MO2- and δ*map1b*-injected embryos relative to uninjected embryos (Fig. 6b) (uninjected embryos: 3.2 ± 0.23, $n$ = 13 embryos; standard MO-injected embryos: 2.8 ± 0.69, $n$ = 3 embryos; *map1b* MO2-injected embryos: 2.18 ± 0.23, $n$ = 6 embryos; δ*map1b*-injected embryos: 2.19 ± 0.27, $n$ = 9 embryos). Although a decrease in bundle number in experimental groups relative to standard MO-injected embryos was also observed, this number was not statistically significant,

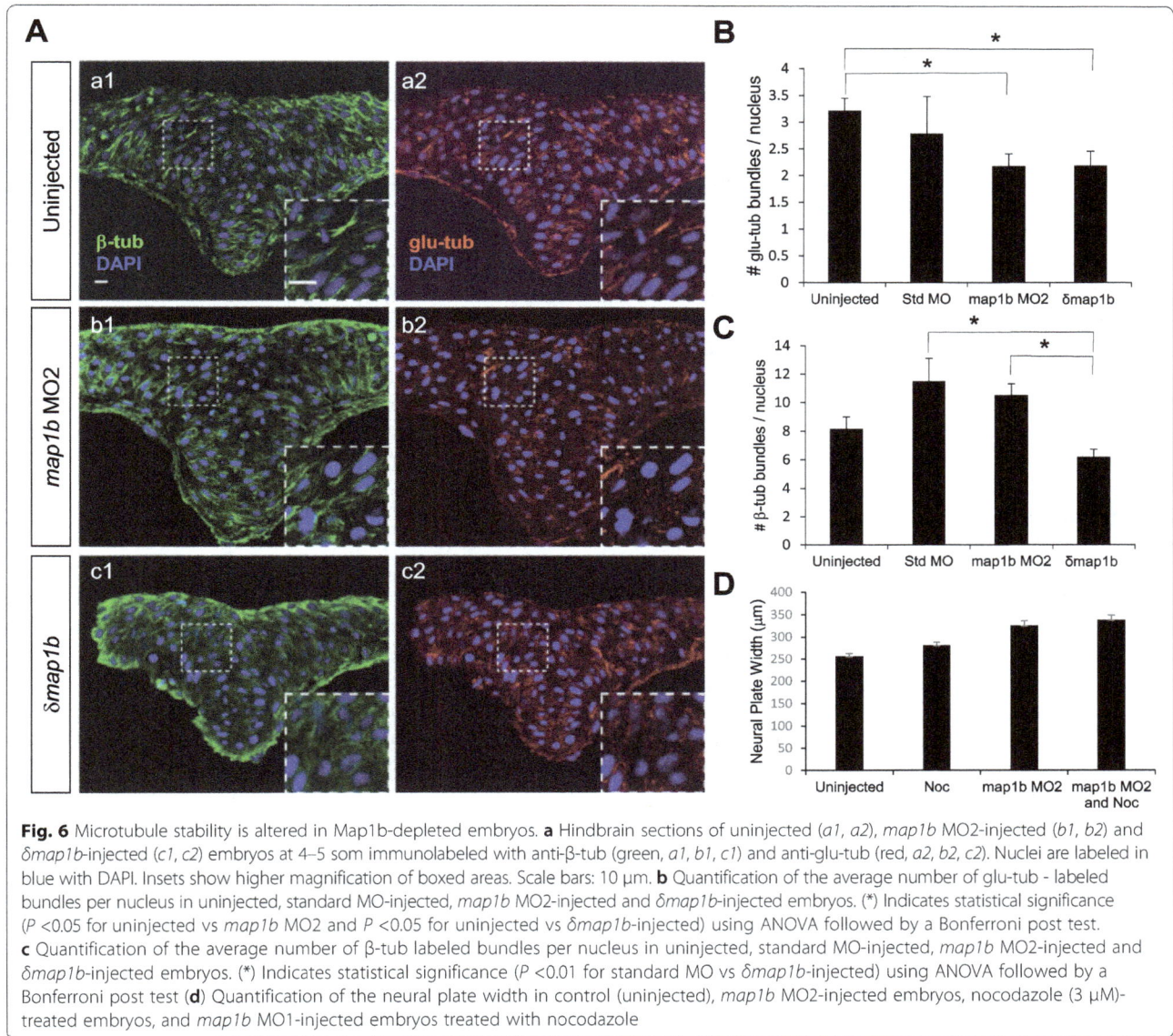

**Fig. 6** Microtubule stability is altered in Map1b-depleted embryos. **a** Hindbrain sections of uninjected (*a1*, *a2*), *map1b* MO2-injected (*b1*, *b2*) and *δmap1b*-injected (*c1*, *c2*) embryos at 4–5 som immunolabeled with anti-β-tub (green, *a1*, *b1*, *c1*) and anti-glu-tub (red, *a2*, *b2*, *c2*). Nuclei are labeled in blue with DAPI. Insets show higher magnification of boxed areas. Scale bars: 10 μm. **b** Quantification of the average number of glu-tub - labeled bundles per nucleus in uninjected, standard MO-injected, *map1b* MO2-injected and *δmap1b*-injected embryos. (*) Indicates statistical significance (*P* <0.05 for uninjected vs *map1b* MO2 and *P* <0.05 for uninjected vs *δmap1b*-injected) using ANOVA followed by a Bonferroni post test. **c** Quantification of the average number of β-tub labeled bundles per nucleus in uninjected, standard MO-injected, *map1b* MO2-injected and *δmap1b*-injected embryos. (*) Indicates statistical significance (*P* <0.01 for standard MO vs *δmap1b*-injected) using ANOVA followed by a Bonferroni post test (**d**) Quantification of the neural plate width in control (uninjected), *map1b* MO2-injected embryos, nocodazole (3 μM)-treated embryos, and *map1b* MO1-injected embryos treated with nocodazole

most likely due to the smaller sample size of the latter (Fig. 6b). These observations suggest that in the context of NC, Map1b functions to stabilize MTs rather than promote MT dynamics.

A decrease in total bundle number per cell was also observed with β-tub labeling, but only in *δmap1b*-injected embryos (uninjected embryos: 8.16 ± 0.85, *n* = 14 embryos; standard MO-injected embryos: 11.5 ± 1.6, *n* = 5 embryos; *δmap1b*-injected embryos: 6.18 ± 0.54, *n* = 9 embryos) (Fig. 6c). This reduction is unlikely to reflect the loss of stable MTs from the total MT population given that a decrease in total MTs was not observed in *map1b* MO2-injected embryos. Thus, δMap1b may disrupt total MTs (dynamic and stable) whereas *map1b*-MO2 alters stable MTs specifically. However, a more likely explanation, is that

the apparent loss of total MT bundles in *δmap1b*-injected embryos reflects subtle changes in the organization of the MT cytoskeleton (bundles that are less well defined) that make the automated quantification method less accurate.

To more directly tease apart the role of Map1b in regulating stable versus dynamic MTs, we also analyzed the levels and distribution of tyrosinated α-tub (dynamic MTs) in *map1b*-MO2- and *δmap1b*-injected embryos. We did not observed an obvious difference in the number and organization of tyr-tub MTs in these embryos (*map1b* MO2-injected embryos: *n*= 4 embryos; *δmap1b*-injected embryos: *n*= 3 embryos) relative to controls (uninjected embryos: *n* = 5 embryos). We did however notice an increase in the number of puncta labeled with anti tyr-tub (arrowheads in Additional File 7: Figure S5).

Since re-tyrosination has been reported to occur on the non-assembled tubulin dimer pool [57], these puncta may correspond to depolymerized tubulin. Overall these observations suggest that loss of Map1b does not impact dynamic MTs.

To further test whether Map1b is implicated in MT stabilization, we performed a nocodazole sensitization test in *map1b* MO2-injected (4 ng) embryos. However, treatment of these embryos with a low dose of nocodazole (1 μg/ml) did not worsen NC defects (Fig. 5d). This may be due to intrinsic differences in the mechanisms by which these molecules alter MT properties. Alternatively, Map1b may function via additional MT-independent mechanisms to promote NC.

### Map1b functions cell-autonomously to regulate cell elongation

In order to identify the cellular mechanisms underlying delayed NC in Map1b-deficient embryos, we analyzed the morphology of hindbrain cells mosaically expressing mGFP at the neural keel (4–5 som) stage. We observed that in contrast to control (uninjected) cells (Fig 6a *a–a'*), cells in *map1b* MO1 (data not shown), *map1b* MO2- and *δmap1b*-injected embryos failed to elongate (Fig. 7a *b – b', c-c'*), as was observed with drug-treated embryos (Fig. 3c, d). LWR measurements of control and Map1b-deficient cells revealed a significant difference in cell shape (LWR of uninjected cells = 3.70 ± 0.1, *n* = 111 cells from 7 embryos; LWR of cells from embryos injected with *map1b* MO2 = 2.78 ± 0.2, *n* = 43 cells from 5 embryos; LWR of cells from embryos injected with *δmap1b* = 2.41 ± 0.1, *n* = 135 cells from 9 embryos) (Fig. 7b). Thus, Map1b is required for cell elongation during NC and its ability to regulate MTs may underlie this process.

Since *map1b* is expressed in the mesoderm and neuroectoderm (Fig. 4), it is possible that the widened neural plate of Map1b-deficient embryos is an indirect consequence of defective convergent extension movements in the mesoderm [52]. If Map1b functions in a cell-autonomous manner in the neuroectoderm to regulate cell elongation, then Map1b-deficient cells isochronically transplanted into WT hosts are expected to be rounded. Conversely, isochronic transplantation of control (WT) cells into Map1b-deficient embryos should not impact the ability of these donor cells to adopt their correct elongated morphology.

To perform the first isochronic transplantation experiment, donor embryos were injected with RNA encoding mRFP with or without *map1b* MO1 (10 ng) and host embryos were injected with *mGFP* DNA (which is mosaically expressed). Cell shapes of both donor (red) and host (green) cells were analyzed in hindbrain sections of host embryos fixed at the neural keel stage

(4–5 som). We observed that transplanted control cells were similar in shape to WT host cells (LWR of control cells = 3.37 ± 0.5, *n* = 100 cells from 18 embryos; LWR of host cells = 3.52 ± 0.69, *n* = 88 cells from 14 embryos; Fig. 7c, d *a–a'*), whereas transplanted Map1b-deficient cells consistently appeared rounder than WT host cells (LWR of *map1b* MO1-injected cells = 1.51 ± 0.27, *n* = 135 cells from 14 embryos; LWR of WT host cells = 3.63 ± 0.52, *n* = 92 cells from 14 embryos; Fig. 7c, d *b–b.2'*). There was no apparent bias to the location of transplanted cells in the neural tube of their hosts, eliminating position as a contributing factor to differences in cell shape. These data reveal that Map1b functions cell autonomously to regulate cell elongation in the neural ectoderm.

The reciprocal isochronic transplantation could not be completed as the Map1b-deficient hosts did not survive the transplantation.

### Map1b is required for polarized migration during NC

To test whether Map1b plays a role in polarized cell migration during NC, mGFP-labeled cells in control (uninjected) and *map1b* MO1(10 ng)-injected embryos were imaged using time-lapse microscopy (Fig. 8a and Additional files 8 and 9). Cell tracing revealed that control cells (from uninjected embryos) were initially rounded and gradually elongated as they approached the midline. In contrast, cells in *map1b* MO1-injected embryos took longer to elongate, consistent with the LWR measurements of cells in fixed preparations. In addition, their migration towards the midline was delayed (Fig. 8b; *n* = 3 embryos; 6–9 cells/embryo).

In order to determine whether delayed migration in *map1b* MO1-injected embryos was caused by defective protrusive activity, as observed in drug-treated embryos, the angular distribution of plasma membrane extensions was quantified and ploted. At the neural plate (tb-1 som) and neural keel (4–5 som) stages, membrane protrusions of control cells were biased towards the medio-lateral axis, whereas the membrane protrusions in Map1b-deficient cells were less polarized and failed to align with the medio-lateral axis (Fig. 8c). Together these findings suggest that Map1b mediates both cell elongation and the polarized orientation of protrusive activity, two cell behaviors that are MT-dependent.

### Discussion
#### MTs are required for NC
Cellular dynamics during convergent extension movements in vertebrates are powered by actin polymerization, cell-cell adhesion and cell-extracellular matrix (ECM) interactions [52]. Since MTs play a prominent role in cell migration [17, 22], it seems intuitive that they would also be implicated in the mechanics of cellular rearrangements

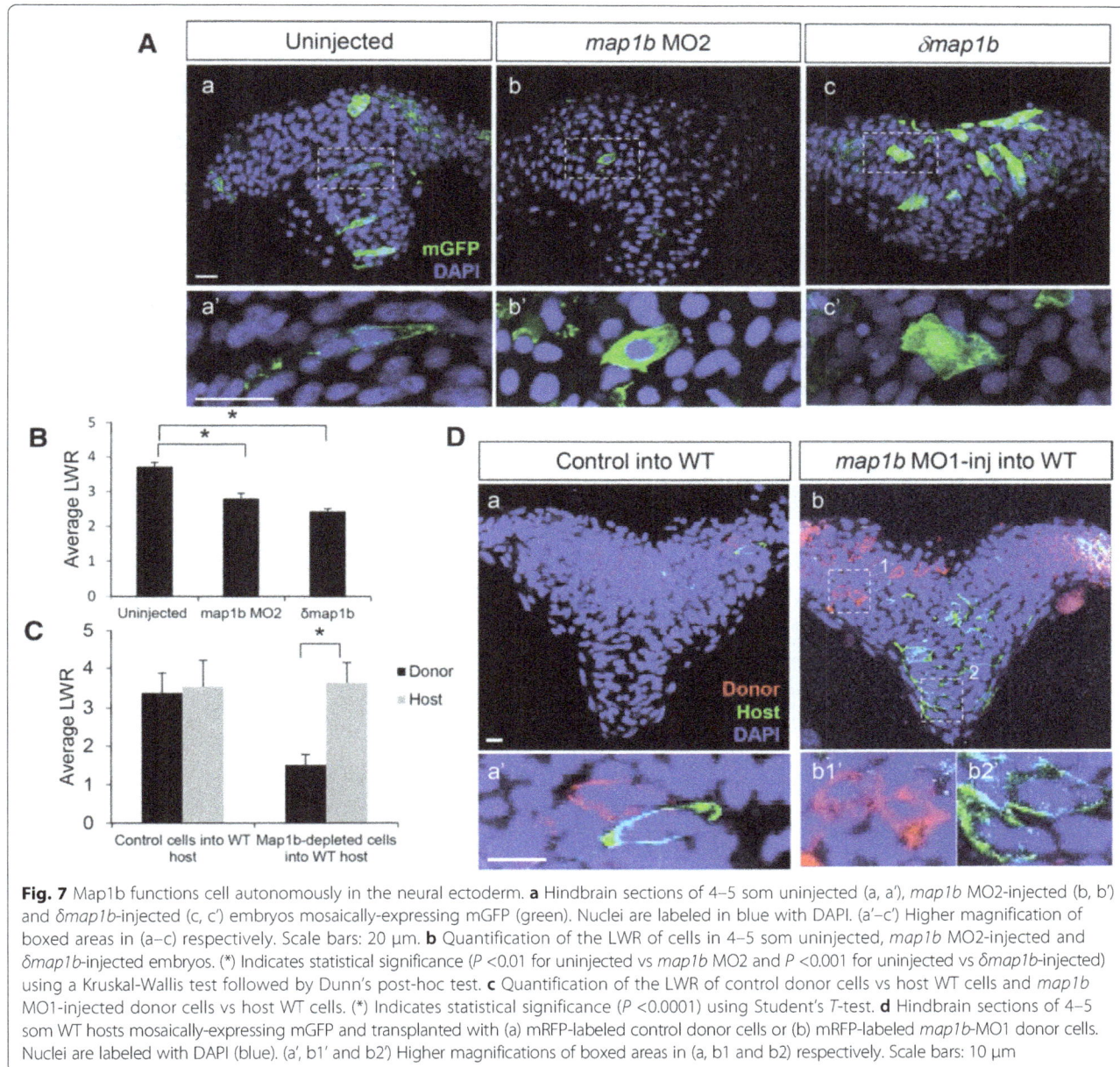

**Fig. 7** Map1b functions cell autonomously in the neural ectoderm. **a** Hindbrain sections of 4–5 som uninjected (a, a'), *map1b* MO2-injected (b, b') and δ*map1b*-injected (c, c') embryos mosaically-expressing mGFP (green). Nuclei are labeled in blue with DAPI. (a'–c') Higher magnification of boxed areas in (a–c) respectively. Scale bars: 20 μm. **b** Quantification of the LWR of cells in 4–5 som uninjected, *map1b* MO2-injected and δ*map1b*-injected embryos. (*) Indicates statistical significance ($P < 0.01$ for uninjected vs *map1b* MO2 and $P < 0.001$ for uninjected vs δ*map1b*-injected) using a Kruskal-Wallis test followed by Dunn's post-hoc test. **c** Quantification of the LWR of control donor cells vs host WT cells and *map1b* MO1-injected donor cells vs host WT cells. (*) Indicates statistical significance ($P < 0.0001$) using Student's *T*-test. **d** Hindbrain sections of 4–5 som WT hosts mosaically-expressing mGFP and transplanted with (a) mRFP-labeled control donor cells or (b) mRFP-labeled *map1b*-MO1 donor cells. Nuclei are labeled with DAPI (blue). (a', b1' and b2') Higher magnifications of boxed areas in (a, b1 and b2) respectively. Scale bars: 10 μm

during convergent extension in the mesoderm and neurectoderm. There is some experimental evidence supporting MT-mediated cellular rearrangement in the mesoderm, however, there is a dearth of data on the involvement of MTs during NC. With respect to the mesoderm, disruption with nocodazole in early gastrula *Xenopus* embryos prevents mediolateral intercalation, involution and convergent extension of the marginal zone (the precursor of the mesoderm) [58]. Kwan and Kirschner further demonstrated that treatment of *Xenopus* dorsal marginal zone explants with nocodazole but not taxol prevents lamellipodia formation, indicating that the bulk of polymerized tubulin rather than MT dynamics (which

would be altered by both drug treatments) is important for convergent extension [59]. In zebrafish embryos, MTs are known to mediate cell-cell contacts and initiation of planar polarity, by localizing PCP pathway component Prickle in a polarized manner during mesodermal convergent extension [60].

In amniotes, narrowing of the neural plate is brought about by a combination of cell elongation and intercalation. In chick embryos, treatment of the neural plate with nocodazole prevents cell lengthening along the apico-basal axis, resulting in a wider neural plate [61]. While it is currently unknown whether MTs also power cell intercalation in amniotes, the medio-lateral oriented

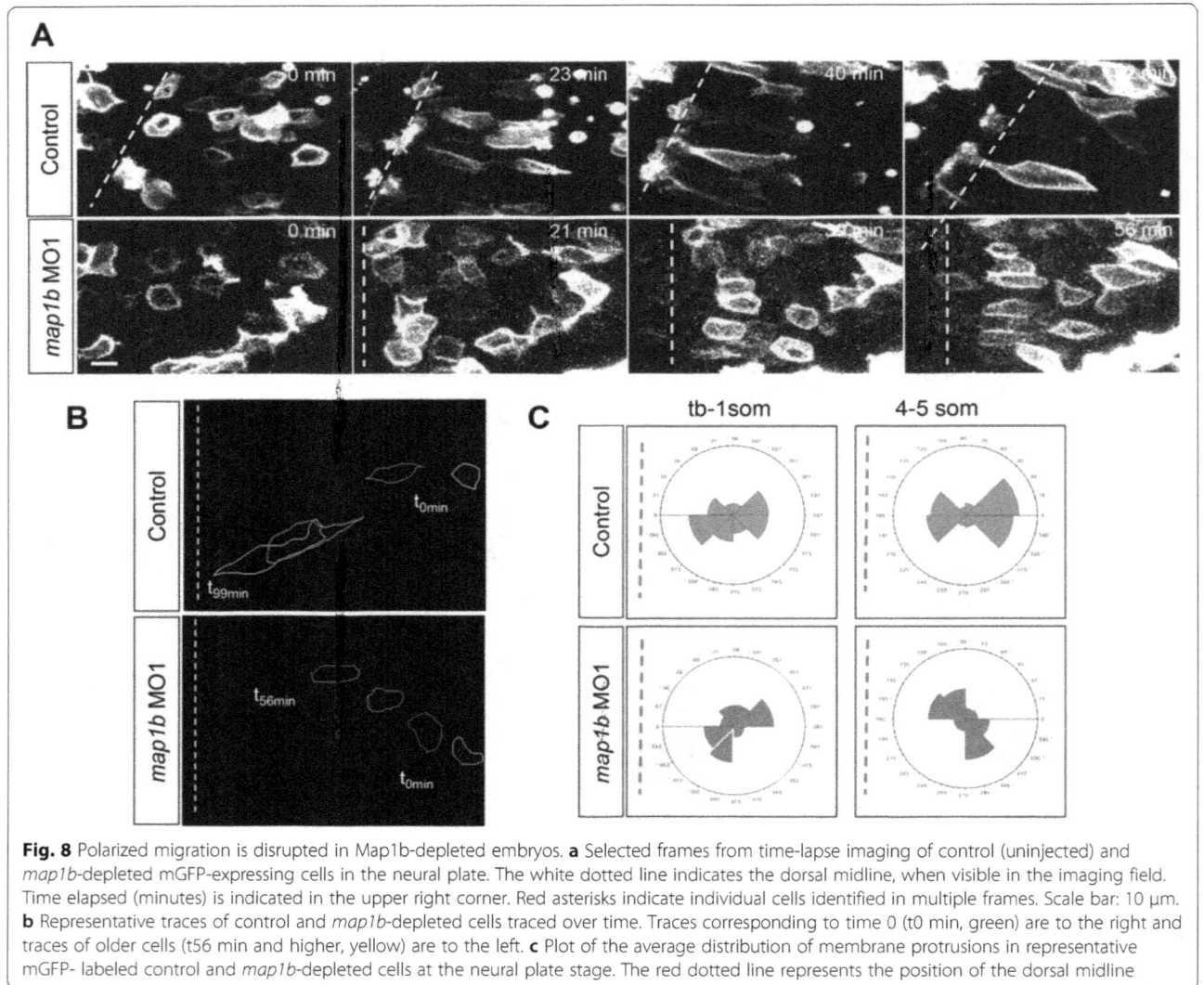

**Fig. 8** Polarized migration is disrupted in Map1b-depleted embryos. **a** Selected frames from time-lapse imaging of control (uninjected) and *map1b*-depleted mGFP-expressing cells in the neural plate. The white dotted line indicates the dorsal midline, when visible in the imaging field. Time elapsed (minutes) is indicated in the upper right corner. Red asterisks indicate individual cells identified in multiple frames. Scale bar: 10 μm. **b** Representative traces of control and *map1b*-depleted cells traced over time. Traces corresponding to time 0 (t0 min, green) are to the right and traces of older cells (t56 min and higher, yellow) are to the left. **c** Plot of the average distribution of membrane protrusions in representative mGFP- labeled control and *map1b*-depleted cells at the neural plate stage. The red dotted line represents the position of the dorsal midline

basal protrusions that drive cellular rearrangement in the mouse epithelialized neural plate [9] are reminiscent of MT-dependent polarized basal protrusions in *C. elegans* epithelial cells undergoing dorsal closure [62], raising the possibility that MT-based mechanisms may also be employed to narrow the neural in chick and mouse embryos.

We have previously shown that MTs in neural plate cells have a radial organization, which is characteristic of migratory cells. Following NC, MTs become linear, an architecture often observed in epithelial cells [42]. We report here that the levels of stable MTs steadily increase as neurulation proceeds. Our functional analysis using MT-disrupting drugs further suggests that proper regulation of MT stability is essential for both cell elongation and polarized migration during NC. In addition, the fact that protrusive activity is still observed (albeit random) in nocodazole-treated embryos, indicates that MTs are

required for polarization but not the formation of these membrane extensions.

Thus, despite the more prominent mesenchymal properties of zebrafish neural plate cells relative to their amniote counterparts, evidence suggests that MTs and their regulators play a central role in driving NC in vertebrates.

### Map1b promotes stable microtubules

The prominent changes in MT stability during neurulation are likely to be regulated by microtubule associated proteins. We show here that stable/detyrosinated MTs are lost in Map1b-deficient embryos. The apparent selective reduction in detyrosinated MTs (observed in *map1b* MO2-injected embryos) argues against a role for Map1b as a general MT stabilizing factor. Rather, Map1b may protect stable MTs or promote the α-tub detyrosination event that is revealed by glu-tub labeling.

Despite the focus on MTs in this study, it is likely that Map1b also influences the actin cytoskeleton. In this regard, Map1b is known to bind actin in addition to MTs [25, 63], thereby crosslinking the two cytoskeletons. Furthermore, Rac1 and Cdc42 are downstream effectors of Map1b [64] that are both implicated in the crosstalk between actin and MTs [65].

### Map1b regulates distinct cell behaviors during NC

We have previously shown that, during NC, cells elongate as they migrate towards the dorsal midline. These cellular dynamics are accompanied by extensive protrusive activity polarized along the medio-lateral axis [8]. Since perturbation of MT dynamics with nocodazole or paclitaxel prevents cell elongation and polarized migration in the zebrafish neural plate (this study) and other contexts [23, 66-71], we investigated whether these cell behaviors are also altered in Map1b-depleted embryos.

We found that despite the broad distribution of mRNA in mesodermal and ectodermal cells, Map1b is required cell autonomously for cell elongation in the neural tissue. A recent study has shown that a polarized population of dynamic MTs is required for cell length maintenance in the zebrafish neural tube [23]. While our studies reveal a role for Map1b in promoting stable MTs rather than MT dynamicity, it is likely that both MT populations contribute to cell elongation.

In addition to cell elongation, directional migration is also defective in Map1b-depleted embryos. Impaired migration may also be attributable to abnormal MTs, as stable MTs, anchored at the cell cortex, are thought to function as tracks to deliver regulators of actin polymerization to the leading edge [17]. Whether the same population of Map1b-regulated MTs mediates cell elongation and migration in the zebrafish neural tube is unclear.

Analysis of protrusive activity in Map1b-depleted embryos revealed a lack of biased orientation along the medio-lateral axis and ectopic persistent protrusions on the anterior and posterior pole of neural cells. This abnormal protrusive activity may underlie the delay in cell elongation and migration. It is unclear how Map1b biases protrusive activity medially. However, the recent finding that Map1b binds and sequesters EB3 in the cytosol of developing neuronal cells [72] raises an interesting possibility. EB3 is a MT-plus end binding protein that is enriched in growth cones and has been shown to coordinate the interaction between F-actin (required for protrusive activity) and dynamic MTs during neuritogenesis [73]. Furthermore, EB3-capped MT plus ends orient towards the leading edge in migrating cells, possibly in response to an extracellular signal [17]. In this context, Map1b may regulate polarized protrusive activity by controlling the levels of EB3 available to associate with MT plus ends. In the absence of Map1b, increased binding of EB3 to MTs plus ends could cause the formation of ectopic F-actin nucleation.

Despite the significant increase in neural plate width in *map1b* MO-injected embryos, the neural tube eventually forms (albeit abnormally), indicative of a delay rather than blockage of NC. A similar outcome was also observed following depletion of PCP pathway components, suggesting compensatory mechanisms that ensure proper completion of neural development.

Whether *map1b* function during NC is conserved remains to be determined, as neural tube defects have not been reported in mouse *map1b* knockouts [74], possibly due to functional redundancy among MAP family members [75, 76] or distinct cellular mechanisms underlying the narrowing of the neural plate. Despite these differences, loss of Map1b function in mice also causes a delay rather than a blockage in neural development [34].

## Conclusions

We show that MTs become progressively more stable as neurulation progresses. Drug treatments that either destabilize or hyperstabilize MTs impair NC by disrupting cell elongation and polarization, indicating that the regulation of MT stability is a key event during neural tube development. We demonstrate that the microtubule-associated protein Map1b is broadly expressed during neurulation and promotes stable MTs. Furthermore, loss of Map1b function causes a delay in NC, cell autonomous disruption of cell elongation, impaired directional migration and polarized protrusive activity. Based on these findings, we propose that Map1b enables NC at least in part by maintaining a population of stable MTs.

Collectively, these studies identify *map1b* as a key regulator of early morphogenetic movements in the neural tube. It will be interesting in the future to identify the signaling pathways that function upstream of Map1b to control the MT cytoskeleton during NC.

## Methods

### Zebrafish strains

Studies were performed using wildtype (AB) strains. All experiments were approved by the University of Maryland, Baltimore County's Institutional Animal Care and Use Committee (IACUC) and were performed according to national regulatory standards.

### Embryo staging

Staging was done according to [77]. Stages of neurulation were defined as previously described [8].

### Cloning of zebrafish *map1b*

RNA was extracted from 24 hpf AB embryos using TRIzol (Invitrogen, cat no. 15596–026). cDNA was synthesized with RETROscript (Invitrogen, cat no. AM1710) and oligodT primers. Primers were designed to amplify a conserved, 302 bp region of zebrafish *map1b* corresponding to exon 5 (accession # XM_003198629):

Forward primer: 5'-AGCACCGTACATCCAGCCAACA-3'
Reverse primer: 5'-GCAAACAATGCAGAGTCACCCC GT-3'

PCR was performed using PfuUltra (Agilent Technologies, cat no. 600385) and products were cloned into PCR II-TOPO vector (Invitrogen, cat no. K4600-01).

The δ*map1b* construct, a codon optimized sequence encoding the first 571 aa of zebrafish Map1b, was synthesized by Genewiz based on the published zebrafish *map1b* sequence (accession # XM_003198629). δ*map1b* was subsequently subcloned into the pCS2+ vector.

### Nucleic acid and morpholino injections
DNA encoding membrane-targeted Green Fluorescent Protein (mGFP) (Richard Harland, University of California, Berkeley, CA, USA) and Red Fluorescent Protein (mRFP) [78] for mosaic expression were prepared using a midiprep kit (Macherey-Nagel, cat. no. 740410.10) and injected (50–200 pg) into one- to eight-cell stage embryos.

For RNA injections, *mGFP or mRFP* expressing plasmids were linearized with NotI and transcribed using SP6 mMESSAGE mMACHINE kit (Ambion, cat. no. AM1340). 50 pg of RNA was injected into one- to four-cell stage embryos.

MOs were synthesized by GeneTools (Philomath, Oregon, USA) and injected into one- to four-cell stage embryos: *map1b* splice-blocking MO1 (4 or 10 ng), *map1b* splice-blocking MO2 (4 or 10 ng), *map1b* translation (ATG)-blocking MO3 (10 ng) and, as negative controls, *pard3* (10 ng) and a standard negative control MO recommended by GeneTools that targets a human betaglobin intron, causing little change in phenotype in any known test system (10 ng).

*map1b* MO1: 5'-CCAAGAAAAACAGTC ACTTACCTCT- 3'
*map1b* MO2: 5'-AATTTGACTTACAGA TTGGAGAGCT- 3'
*map1b* MO3: 5'-CCGCAGTATCAACCAGC GTCGCCAT- 3'
*pard3* MO: 5' TCAAAGGCTCCCGTGCTC TGGTGTC 3' [79]
*Gsk3β* MO: 5'-GTTCTGGGCCGACCGGAC ATTTTTC-3' [80]
Standard MO: 5'-CCTCTTACCTCAGTTAC AATTTATA- 3' [81]

Microinjections were performed using a PCI-100 microinjector (Harvard Apparatus, Holliston, MA, USA).

### Cell transplantation
Transplantation was performed as described in [82] 50–100 cells from donors were transplanted isochronically into the animal pole of host embryos at the sphere to dome stage.

### Drug treatments
Early neural keel stage (2–3 som) embryos mosaically expressing mGFP were manually dechorionated and exposed to nocodazole (concentrations ranging from 3 to 32 μM) (Sigma, cat. no. M1404) or paclitaxel (50 μM) (Sigma, cat. no. T7191) until embryos reached 4–5 som stage (~30 min) at 28 °C. The embryos were immediately fixed overnight in 4 % paraformaldehyde (PFA) diluted in PBS at 4°C.

### Time-lapse confocal microscopy
Time-lapse microscopy was performed as previously described [83]. Embryos were imaged using a Leica confocal microscope (Leica SP5 TCS 4D) at 30 s-1 min intervals. Images were analyzed using the Leica LAS software, Image J (NIH) and Adobe PhotoShop.

### Labeling and imaging of fixed preparations
For immunolabeling, embryos were fixed for 3 h with 4 % PFA diluted in MAB buffer (80mM KPIPES, 5mM EGTA, 1mM MgCl2, 0.2 % Triton-X, pH 6.4) at room temperature. Embryos were then sectioned (40μm, 1500 Sectioning System) and immunolabeling on floating sections was carried out as in [84].

Antibodies used: mouse anti-β-tubulin (Sigma, Clone: TUB 2.1) at 1:500; rabbit anti-α-tubulin (Genetex, Clone: GTX108784) at 1:500; rabbit anti-tyrosinated tubulin (Millipore, ABT171) at 1:1000; rabbit anti-glu-tubulin (Millipore, Clone: AB201) at 1:1000 and rabbit anti-GFP (Invitrogen, cat. no. A11122) at 1:1000. Secondary antibodies conjugated to Alexa 488, Alexa 594, or Cy3 (Molecular Probes, cat. nos A11001 and A11008; Molecular Probes cat. A21442; Invitrogen cat. no. A10520) were used at a 1:500 dilution. Alexa Fluor 488-conjugated Phalloidin (Invitrogen, cat. no. A12379) at 1:75 and DAPI (Invitrogen, cat. No. D1306) were used according to manufacturer's instructions.

For cell shape analysis, *mGFP* or *mRFP* RNA/DNA injected embryos were sectioned and either imaged directly (mRFP) or immunolabeled with anti-GFP prior to imaging. All fluorescently labeled sections were imaged using an SP5 confocal microscope (Leica SP5 TCS 4D).

### Wholemount *in situ* hybridization
ISH was conducted as described [85]. Plasmid containing *dlx3* (obtained from Igor Dawid, NIH) was linearized with *NotI* and T7 polymerase was used to generate anti-sense probe. *map1b* (in pCRII-TOPO vector) was

linearized using *NotI* and *KpnI* for sense and anti-sense probes, respectively. T7 and SP6 polymerases were used to generate anti-sense and sense probes respectively. ISH labeled embryos were sectioned and imaged using a Zeiss Axioscope2 microscope.

### Whole cell lysis and Western blotting

~200 embryos were collected, dechorionated, and batch deyolked as described elsewhere [86] with the following modifications. After deyolking, cells were vortexed for one minute in lysis buffer (100 mM PIPES, 0.5 % Nonidet P-40, 1 mM $MgCl_2$, 2 mM EDTA, 1 mM dithiotheitrol, 1:100 dilution of Sigma protease inhibitor cocktail, cat. No. P8340) and centrifuged for 5 min at high speed. Supernatant was boiled for 5 min in 2x SDS-loading buffer, run on a 4-20 % Tris-glycine polyacrylamide gel (BioRad, cat. no. 456–1085) and transferred onto a nitrocellulose membrane (Pall Corporation, cat. no. S30209). Blots were blocked in 5 % dry milk dissolved in PBST (1X PBS, 0.5 % Tween) for 30 min, then incubated with 1:1000 anti-α-tub (Millipore, clone DM1A) or 1:500 anti-glu-tub (Millipore, Clone: AB201). Blots were then incubated with 1:1000 anti-mouse or anti-rabbit HRP-conjugated secondary antibodies (Santa Cruz, cat. nos. SC-2005 and SC-2004). Blots were developed using an enhanced chemiluminescence kit (Thermo Scientific, cat. no. 34079).

### Measurements and statistical analysis
#### Length-to-Width ratios
LWRs were calculated as previously described [8].

### Tracing and quantification of cell behaviors
Cell tracing of single cells over multiple time frames was performed using Metamorph (MolecularDevices).

### Protrusion analysis
Stacks of images from time-lapse microscopy were flattened to a single frame per time point using Volocity v5.5 (Perkin-Elmer) and exported as tifs. Interphase cells that stayed in frame for the extent of the movie were selected. Using a plugin created for imageJ (NIH), individual cells were threshholded and the outline traced. Each cell was then divided into 8 segments based on the centroid and the orientation to the midline. Finally individual frames were overlaid and any new membrane extensions were counted for each frame. The percent protrusions for each section was then calculated and plotted in Mathematica v9 (Wolfram).

### Synteny analysis
Performed using synteny (http://cinteny.cchmc.org/).

### Statistical analysis
InStat (GraphPad) was used to run statistical analysis on data sets. Student's *T*-test, ANOVA followed by Bonferroni or Kruskal-Wallis test followed by Dunn's post-hoc test were used to analyze data groups as appropriate.

### Quantification of Western band intensity
Band intensity was determined using digital scans followed by analysis with ImageJ (NIH). The area used to measure was constant for all experiments.

### Quantification of MTs
Measurements of MT bundle length and number of MT bundles/nuclei were done using Volocity (Perkin-Elmer). A maximum intensity projection of the total confocal sections (40 μm) imaged using the Leica SP5 was generated. The neural keel was cropped to quantify only MT signal within the neural tissue. Filters that identified nuclei (DAPI), stable MTs (glu-tub) and total MTs (β-tub) based on the standard deviation of intensity was used. To compensate for objects close together, an automated algorithm that separates object was run as part of the filter. The measurements were automatically collected and analyzed in excel

## Additional files

**Additional file 1: Figure S1.** Microtubule stability increases during neurulation. (A) Western blot of whole cell lysates blotted for glu-tub (stable MTs) and α-tub (total MTs) at neural plate (tb-1 som), neural keel (4–5 som) and neural rod (12 som) stages. Two bands (1) and (2) are observed for glu-tub. (B) Ratio of stable:total MTs at neural plate (tb-1 som), neural keel (4–5 som) and neural rod (12 som) stages, calculated using glu-tub bands 1 and 2 (A). (PDF 83 kb)

**Additional file 2: Figure S2.** Nocodazole and paclitaxol disrupt microtubule organization. (a-c') Hindbrain sections of 4–5 som control (a, a'), nocodazole-treated (b, b') and paclitaxel-treated (c, c') embryos immunolabeled with anti-β-tub. (a'-c') Higher magnifications of boxed areas in panels (a,b and c) respectively. Scale bars: 20 μm. (PDF 8922 kb)

**Additional file 3: Time lapse imaging of cell behaviors during NC in a WT embryo (high magnification).** Time-lapse movie (1 min intervals) of a control, mGFP-labeled embryo imaged from a dorsal view, anterior towards the top, beginning approximately at the 2–3 som stage and extending to the 6–7 som stage. (MOV 48 kb)

**Additional file 4: Time lapse imaging of cell behaviors during NC in a nocodazole-treated embryo (high magnification).** Time-lapse movie (1 min intervals) of a nocodazole-treated embryo, mosaically expressing mGFP, imaged from a dorsal view, anterior towards the top, beginning approximately at the 2–3 som stage. (MOV 163 kb)

**Additional file 5: Figure S3.** Efficacy of *map1b* MOs. (A) Schematic representation of zebrafish *map1b*, showing *map1b* MO1 binding site at the exon 4- intron 4 splice junction (red line and lettering), *map1b* MO2 binding site at the intron 4- exon 5 splice junction (blue line and lettering) and *map1b* MO3 at the translational start site (green line and lettering). Exons are represented by black boxes with corresponding numbers on top. (B) RT-PCR analysis of the region targeted by splice MOs . The upper (750bp) and lower (300bp) bands correspond to unspliced and spliced product respectively. (C) Quantification of the width of the neural plate (tb- 1 som) of control embryos and embryos injected with *map1b* MO1 (4 ng), *map1b* MO3 (10 ng) and *map1b* MO1 (4 ng) + *map1b* MO3 (10 ng).

* Indicates statistical significance using a Kruskal-Wallis test followed by Dunn's post-hoc test ($P < 0.05$ compared to the rest of the groups). (D) Side views of 24 hpf uninjected, map1b MO1-injected (10 ng) and map1b MO2-injected (10 ng) embryos. Black line indicates morphological defects in the hindbrain region. Anterior is to the left, dorsal is up. Scale bar: 250 μm. (PDF 4983 kb)

**Additional file 6: Figure S4.** δmap1b construct and RNA titration. Representation of zebrafish full length Map1b and δMap1b protein indicating percent amino acid similarity to human ortholog. Black represents the highest level of homology and white, the lowest. Hatch marks indicate the MT-binding domain (MTBD). (B) Titration analysis of δmap1b RNA. Percent of embryos with WT, mild, moderate, severe and very severe phenotypes are indicated in the table for each concentration of RNA. (C) 24 hpf embryos correspond to the phenotypic categories in the table (a: WT, b: mild, c: moderate, d: severe e: very severe). Black arrowhead indicates missing eye. (PDF 2953 kb)

**Additional file 7: Figure S5.** Dynamic microtubules appear normal in Map1b-depleted embryos. Hindbrain sections of embryos at the neural keel (4–5 som) stage immunolabeled with anti-tyr-tub (dynamic MTs) in red (a2, b2, c2) anti-β-tub (total MTs) in green (a3, b3, c3). (a1, b1, c1) Red-Green overlay (yellow) with nuclei labeled in blue using DAPI. Boxed areas are shown in higher magnification in (a2-c3). Arrowheads indicate puncta exclusively labeled with anti-tyr-tub. Scale bars: 10 μm. (PDF 9616 kb)

**Additional file 8: Time lapse imaging of NC in a WT embryo.** Time-lapse movie (1 min intervals) of a control, mGFP-labeled embryo imaged from a dorsal view, anterior towards the top, beginning approximately at the 2–3 som stage and extending to the 6–7 som stage.] (MOV 581 kb)

**Additional file 9: Time lapse imaging of NC in a map1b MO1-injected embryo.** Time-lapse movie (1 min intervals) of a map1b MO1 (10 ng)-injected embryo mosaically expressing mGFP, imaged from a dorsal view, anterior towards the top, beginning approximately at the 2–3 som stage and extending to the 6–7 som stage. (MOV 538 kb)

## Abbreviations
Hpf: Hours-post-fertilization; Map1b: Microtubule associated protein 1 b; MT: Microtubule; MO: Morpholino; NC: Neural convergence; Som: Somites.

## Competing interests
The author(s) declare that they have no competing interests.

## Authors' contributions
PJ, VO and SS: performed the majority of the experiments and contributed to data analysis and manuscript preparation. EH: carried out the analysis of dynamic changes in MT organization in WT embryos and the initial studies on the effect of MT-disrupting drugs on cell elongation and migration. EV and JW worked with SS to perform Map1b loss of function studies using primarily δmap1b but also map1b MO2 and performed data quantification for multiple experiments. RJM performed the analysis and quantification of the protrusive activity, assisted in the quantification of MT stability, carried out the statitiscal analyses for most experiments and helped to assemble figures. NSA designed δMap1b and assisted with the molecular work on this construct. AM characterized the function of Gsk3β. RMB supervised the research and data analysis and wrote the manuscript. All authors read and approved the final manuscript.

## Acknowledgements
We thank the following people for their technical assistance: Robyn Goodman (cell transplantation experiments), Jeff Leips (statistical analysis), Lakshmi Goli (cell tracing) and Tim Ford (figure preparation). We appreciate the comments of Michelle Starz-Gaiano and Mark Van Doren on the manuscript. The Leica SP5 confocal microscope was purchased with funds from the National Science Foundation, grant # DBI-0722569. The research was supported by NIH/NIGMS grants # GM085290-02S1 to V. Olmo and # GM085290 to R. Brewster. E. Vital was supported in part by a grant to UMBC from the Howard Hughes Medical Institute through the Precollege and Undergraduate Science Education Program, grant # 52008090.

## Author details
[1]Department of Biological Sciences, University of Maryland Baltimore County, Baltimore, MD, USA. [2]Institut de Biologie Paris Seine-Laboratoire Neuroscience Paris Seine INSERM UMRS 1130, CNRS UMR 8246, UPMC UM 118 Université Pierre et Marie Curie, Paris, France.

## References
1. Davidson LA, Keller RE. Neural tube closure in Xenopus laevis involves medial migration, directed protrusive activity, cell intercalation and convergent extension. Development. 1999;126(20):4547–56.
2. Morriss-Kay G, Wood H, Chen WH. Normal neurulation in mammals. Ciba Found Symp. 1994;181:51–63. discussion 63–59.
3. Lowery LA, Sive H. Strategies of vertebrate neurulation and a re-evaluation of teleost neural tube formation. Mech Dev. 2004;121(10):1189–97.
4. Smith JL, Schoenwolf GC. Further evidence of extrinsic forces in bending of the neural plate. J Comp Neurol. 1991;307(2):225–36.
5. Colas JF, Schoenwolf GC. Towards a cellular and molecular understanding of neurulation. Dev Dyn. 2001;221(2):117–45.
6. Reichenbach A, Schaaf P, Schneider H. Primary neurulation in teleosts–evidence for epithelial genesis of central nervous tissue as in other vertebrates. J Hirnforsch. 1990;31(2):153–8.
7. Papan C, Campos-Ortega JA. On the formation of the neural keel and neural tube in the zebrafish Danio (Brachydanio) rerio. Roux's Arch Dev Biol. 1994;203:178–86.
8. Hong E, Brewster R. N-cadherin is required for the polarized cell behaviors that drive neurulation in the zebrafish. Development. 2006;133(19):3895–905.
9. Williams M, Yen W, Lu X, Sutherland A. Distinct apical and basolateral mechanisms drive planar cell polarity-dependent convergent extension of the mouse neural plate. Dev Cell. 2014;29(1):34–46.
10. Ybot-Gonzalez P, Savery D, Gerrelli D, Signore M, Mitchell CE, Faux CH, et al. Convergent extension, planar-cell-polarity signalling and initiation of mouse neural tube closure. Development. 2007;134(4):789–99.
11. Keller R, Shih J, Sater A. The cellular basis of the convergence and extension of the Xenopus neural plate. Dev Dyn. 1992;193(3):199–217.
12. Ciruna B, Jenny A, Lee D, Mlodzik M, Schier AF. Planar cell polarity signalling couples cell division and morphogenesis during neurulation. Nature. 2006; 439(7073):220–4.
13. Elul T, Keller R. Monopolar protrusive activity: a new morphogenic cell behavior in the neural plate dependent on vertical interactions with the mesoderm in Xenopus. Dev Biol. 2000;224(1):3–19.
14. Elul T, Koehl MA, Keller R. Cellular mechanism underlying neural convergent extension in Xenopus laevis embryos. Dev Biol. 1997;191(2):243–58.
15. Sausedo RA, Smith JL, Schoenwolf GC. Role of nonrandomly oriented cell division in shaping and bending of the neural plate. J Comp Neurol. 1997; 381(4):473–88.
16. Wang J, Hamblet NS, Mark S, Dickinson ME, Brinkman BC, Segil N, et al. Dishevelled genes mediate a conserved mammalian PCP pathway to regulate convergent extension during neurulation. Development. 2006; 133(9):1767–78.
17. Siegrist SE, Doe CQ. Microtubule-induced cortical cell polarity. Genes Dev. 2007;21(5):483–96.
18. Mitchison T, Kirschner M. Dynamic instability of microtubule growth. Nature. 1984;312(5991):237–42.
19. Desai A, Mitchison TJ. Microtubule polymerization dynamics. Annu Rev Cell Dev Biol. 1997;13:83–117.
20. Waterman-Storer CM, Worthylake RA, Liu BP, Burridge K, Salmon ED. Microtubule growth activates Rac1 to promote lamellipodial protrusion in fibroblasts. Nat Cell Biol. 1999;1(1):45–50.
21. Brandt DT, Grosse R. Get to grips: steering local actin dynamics with IQGAPs. EMBO Rep. 2007;8(11):1019–23.
22. Kaverina I, Straube A. Regulation of cell migration by dynamic microtubules. Semin Cell Dev Biol. 2011;22(9):968–74.
23. Picone R, Ren X, Ivanovitch KD, Clarke JD, McKendry RA, Baum B. A polarised population of dynamic microtubules mediates homeostatic length control in animal cells. PLoS Biol. 2010;8(11):e1000542.
24. Hammarback JA, Obar RA, Hughes SM, Vallee RB. MAP1B is encoded as a polyprotein that is processed to form a complex N-terminal microtubule-binding domain. Neuron. 1991;7(1):129–39.

25. Cueille N, Blanc CT, Popa-Nita S, Kasas S, Catsicas S, Dietler G, et al. Characterization of MAP1B heavy chain interaction with actin. Brain Res Bull. 2007;71(6):610–8.

25. Noble M, Lewis SA, Cowan NJ. The microtubule binding domain of microtubule-associated protein MAP1B contains a repeated sequence motif unrelated to that of MAP2 and tau. J Cell Biol. 1989;109(6 Pt 2):3367–76.

27. Schoenfeld TA, McKerracher L, Obar R, Vallee RB. MAP 1A and MAP 1B are structurally related microtubule associated proteins with distinct developmental patterns in the CNS. J Neurosci. 1989;9(5):1712–30.

28. Hirokawa N, Bloom GS, Vallee RB. Cytoskeletal architecture and immunocytochemical localization of microtubule-associated proteins in regions of axons associated with rapid axonal transport: the beta, beta'-iminodipropionitrile-intoxicated axon as a model system. J Cell Biol. 1985; 101(1):227–39.

29. Sato-Yoshitake R, Shiomura Y, Miyasaka H, Hirokawa N. Microtubule-associated protein 1B: molecular structure, localization, and phosphorylation-dependent expression in developing neurons. Neuron. 1989;3(2):229–38.

30. Zauner W, Kratz J, Staunton J, Feick P, Wiche G. Identification of two distinct microtubule binding domains on recombinant rat MAP 1B. Eur J Cell Biol. 1992;57(1):66–74.

31. Togel M, Wiche G, Propst F. Novel features of the light chain of microtubule-associated protein MAP1B: microtubule stabilization, self interaction, actin filament binding, and regulation by the heavy chain. J Cell Biol. 1998;143(3):695–707.

32. Takemura R, Okabe S, Umeyama T, Kanai Y, Cowan NJ, Hirokawa N. Increased microtubule stability and alpha tubulin acetylation in cells transfected with microtubule-associated proteins MAP1B, MAP2 or tau. J Cell Sci. 1992;103(Pt 4):953–64.

33. Vandecandelaere A, Pedrotti B, Utton MA, Calvert RA, Bayley PM. Differences in the regulation of microtubule dynamics by microtubule-associated proteins MAP1B and MAP2. Cell Motil Cytoskeleton. 1996;35(2):134–46.

34. Gonzalez-Billault C, Avila J, Caceres A. Evidence for the role of MAP1B in axon formation. Mol Biol Cell. 2001;12(7):2087–98.

35. Tymanskyj SR, Scales TM, Gordon-Weeks PR. MAP1B enhances microtubule assembly rates and axon extension rates in developing neurons. Mol Cell Neurosci. 2012;49(2):110–9.

36. DiTella MC, Feiguin F, Carri N, Kosik KS, Caceres A. MAP-1B/TAU functional redundancy during laminin-enhanced axonal growth. J Cell Sci. 1996; 109(Pt 2):467–77.

37. Gordon-Weeks PR, Fischer I. MAP1B expression and microtubule stability in growing and regenerating axons. Microsc Res Tech. 2000;48(2):63–74.

38. Garner CC, Garner A, Huber G, Kozak C, Matus A. Molecular cloning of microtubule-associated protein 1 (MAP1A) and microtubule-associated protein 5 (MAP1B): identification of distinct genes and their differential expression in developing brain. J Neurochem. 1990;55(1):146–54.

39. Calvert R, Anderton BH. A microtubule-associated protein (MAP1) which is expressed at elevated levels during development of the rat cerebellum. EMBO J. 1985;4(5):1171–6.

40. Tucker RP, Garner CC, Matus A. In situ localization of microtubule-associated protein mRNA in the developing and adult rat brain. Neuron. 1989;2(3):1245–56.

41. Cheng A, Krueger BK, Bambrick LL. MAP5 expression in proliferating neuroblasts. Brain Res Dev Brain Res. 1999;113(1–2):107–13.

42. Hong E, Jayachandran P, Brewster R. The polarity protein Pard3 is required for centrosome positioning during neurulation. Dev Biol. 2010;341(2):335–45.

43. Musch A. Microtubule organization and function in epithelial cells. Traffic. 2004;5(1):1–9.

44. Wen Y, Eng CH, Schmoranzer J, Cabrera-Poch N, Morris EJ, Chen M, et al. EB1 and APC bind to mDia to stabilize microtubules downstream of Rho and promote cell migration. Nat Cell Biol. 2004;6(9):820–30.

45. Westermann S, Weber K. Post-translational modifications regulate microtubule function. Nat Rev Mol Cell Biol. 2003;4(12):938–47.

46. Gundersen GG, Kalnoski MH, Bulinski JC. Distinct populations of microtubules: tyrosinated and nontyrosinated alpha tubulin are distributed differently in vivo. Cell. 1984;38(3):779–89.

47. Tawk M, Araya C, Lyons DA, Reugels AM, Girdler GC, Bayley PR, et al. A mirror-symmetric cell division that orchestrates neuroepithelial morphogenesis. Nature. 2007;446(7137):797–800.

48. Goold RG, Owen R, Gordon-Weeks PR. Glycogen synthase kinase 3beta phosphorylation of microtubule-associated protein 1B regulates the stability of microtubules in growth cones. J Cell Sci. 1999;112(Pt 19):3373–84.

49. Owen R, Gordon-Weeks PR. Inhibition of glycogen synthase kinase 3beta in sensory neurons in culture alters filopodia dynamics and microtubule distribution in growth cones. Mol Cell Neurosci. 2003;23(4):626–37.

50. Hall AC, Brennan A, Goold RG, Cleverley K, Lucas FR, Gordon-Weeks PR, et al. Valproate regulates GSK-3-mediated axonal remodeling and synapsin I clustering in developing neurons. Mol Cell Neurosci. 2002;20(2):257–70.

51. Clarke J. Role of polarized cell divisions in zebrafish neural tube formation. Curr Opin Neurobiol. 2009;19(2):134–8.

52. Roszko I, Sawada A, Solnica-Krezel L. Regulation of convergence and extension movements during vertebrate gastrulation by the Wnt/PCP pathway. Semin Cell Dev Biol. 2009;20(8):986–97.

53. Edelmann W, Zervas M, Costello P, Roback L, Fischer I, Hammarback JA, et al. Neuronal abnormalities in microtubule-associated protein 1B mutant mice. Proc Natl Acad Sci U S A. 1996;93(3):1270–5.

54. Takei Y, Kondo S, Harada A, Inomata S, Noda T, Hirokawa N. Delayed development of nervous system in mice homozygous for disrupted microtubule-associated protein 1B (MAP1B) gene. J Cell Biol. 1997; 137(7):1615–26.

55. Mei X, Sweatt AJ, Hammarback JA. Regulation of microtubule-associated protein 1B (MAP1B) subunit composition. J Neurosci Res. 2000;62(1):56–64.

56. Trivedi N, Marsh P, Goold RG, Wood-Kaczmar A, Gordon-Weeks PR. Glycogen synthase kinase-3beta phosphorylation of MAP1B at Ser1260 and Thr1265 is spatially restricted to growing axons. J Cell Sci. 2005;118(Pt 5): 993–1005.

57. Beltramo DM, Arce CA, Barra HS. Tubulin, but not microtubules, is the substrate for tubulin:tyrosine ligase in mature avian erythrocytes. J Biol Chem. 1987;262(32):15673–7.

58. Lane MC, Keller R. Microtubule disruption reveals that Spemann's organizer is subdivided into two domains by the vegetal alignment zone. Development. 1997;124(4):895–906.

59. Kwan KM, Kirschner MW. A microtubule-binding Rho-GEF controls cell morphology during convergent extension of Xenopus laevis. Development. 2005;132(20):4599–610.

60. Sepich DS, Usmani M, Pawlicki S, Solnica-Krezel L. Wnt/PCP signaling controls intracellular position of MTOCs during gastrulation convergence and extension movements. Development. 2011;138(3):543–52.

61. Schoenwolf GC, Powers ML. Shaping of the chick neuroepithelium during primary and secondary neurulation: role of cell elongation. Anat Rec. 1987; 218(2):182–95.

62. Williams-Masson EM, Heid PJ, Lavin CA, Hardin J. The cellular mechanism of epithelial rearrangement during morphogenesis of the Caenorhabditis elegans dorsal hypodermis. Dev Biol. 1998;204(1):263–76.

63. Pedrotti B, Islam K. Dephosphorylated but not phosphorylated microtubule associated protein MAP1B binds to microfilaments. FEBS Lett. 1996;388(2–3): 131–3.

64. Montenegro-Venegas C, Tortosa E, Rosso S, Peretti D, Bollati F, Bisbal M, et al. MAP1B regulates axonal development by modulating Rho-GTPase Rac1 activity. Mol Biol Cell. 2010;21(20):3518–28.

65. Wittmann T, Waterman-Storer CM. Cell motility: can Rho GTPases and microtubules point the way? J Cell Sci. 2001;114(Pt 21):3795–803.

66. Bershadsky AD, Vaisberg EA, Vasiliev JM. Pseudopodial activity at the active edge of migrating fibroblast is decreased after drug-induced microtubule depolymerization. Cell Motil Cytoskeleton. 1991;19(3):152–8.

67. Liao G, Nagasaki T, Gundersen GG. Low concentrations of nocodazole interfere with fibroblast locomotion without significantly affecting microtubule level: implications for the role of dynamic microtubules in cell locomotion. J Cell Sci. 1995;108(Pt 11):3473–83.

68. Tanaka E, Ho T, Kirschner MW. The role of microtubule dynamics in growth cone motility and axonal growth. J Cell Biol. 1995;128(1–2):139–55.

69. Grigoriev IS, Chernobelskaya AA, Vorobjev IA. Nocodazole, vinblastine and taxol at low concentrations affect fibroblast locomotion and saltatory movements of organelles. Membrane Cell Biol. 1999;13(1):23–48.

70. Stone MC, Nguyen MM, Tao J, Allender DL, Rolls MM. Global up-regulation of microtubule dynamics and polarity reversal during regeneration of an axon from a dendrite. Mol Biol Cell. 2010;21(5):767–77.

71. Yang H, Ganguly A, Cabral F. Inhibition of cell migration and cell division correlates with distinct effects of microtubule inhibiting drugs. J Biol Chem. 2010;285(42):32242–50.

72. Tortosa E, Galjart N, Avila J, Sayas CL. MAP1B regulates microtubule dynamics by sequestering EB1/3 in the cytosol of developing neuronal cells. EMBO J. 2013;32(9):1293–306.

73. Geraldo S, Khanzada UK, Parsons M, Chilton JK, Gordon-Weeks PR. Targeting of the F-actin-binding protein drebrin by the microtubule plus-tip protein EB3 is required for neuritogenesis. Nat Cell Biol. 2008;10(10):1181–9.

74. Meixner A, Haverkamp S, Wassle H, Fuhrer S, Thalhammer J, Kropf N, et al. MAP1B is required for axon guidance and Is involved in the development of the central and peripheral nervous system. J Cell Biol. 2000;151(6):1169–78.

75. Takei Y, Teng J, Harada A, Hirokawa N. Defects in axonal elongation and neuronal migration in mice with disrupted tau and map1b genes. J Cell Biol. 2000;150(5):989–1000.

76. Teng J, Takei Y, Harada A, Nakata T, Chen J, Hirokawa N. Synergistic effects of MAP2 and MAP1B knockout in neuronal migration, dendritic outgrowth, and microtubule organization. J Cell Biol. 2001;155(1):65–76.

77. Kimmel CB, Ballard WW, Kimmel SR, Ullmann B, Schilling TF. Stages of embryonic development of the zebrafish. Dev Dyn. 1995;203(3):253–310.

78. Megason SG, Fraser SE. Digitizing life at the level of the cell: high-performance laser-scanning microscopy and image analysis for in toto imaging of development. Mech Dev. 2003;120(11):1407–20.

79. Wei X, Cheng Y, Luo Y, Shi X, Nelson S, Hyde DR. The zebrafish Pard3 ortholog is required for separation of the eye fields and retinal lamination. Dev Biol. 2004;269(1):286–301.

80. Lee HC, Tsai JN, Liao PY, Tsai WY, Lin KY, Chuang CC, et al. Glycogen synthase kinase 3 alpha and 3 beta have distinct functions during cardiogenesis of zebrafish embryo. BMC Dev Biol. 2007;7:93.

81. Eisen JS, Smith JC. Controlling morpholino experiments: don't stop making antisense. Development. 2008;135(10):1735–43.

82. Kemp HA, Carmany-Rampey A, Moens C. Generating chimeric zebrafish embryos by transplantation. J Vis Exp. 2009;29.

83. Jayachandran PHE, Brewster R. Labeling and imaging cells in the zebrafish hindbrain. J Vis Exp. 2010.

84. Westerfield M. The zebrafish book. A guide for the laboratory use of zebrafish (Danio rerio). 4th ed. Eugene: University of Oregon Press; 2000.

85. Thisse C, Thisse B, Schilling TF, Postlethwait JH. Structure of the zebrafish snail1 gene and its expression in wild-type, spadetail and no tail mutant embryos. Development. 1993;119(4):1203–15.

86. Link V, Shevchenko A, Heisenberg CP. Proteomics of early zebrafish embryos. BMC Dev Biol. 2006;6:1.

# 2

# FGF signaling controls Shh-dependent oligodendroglial fate specification in the ventral spinal cord

Marie-Amélie Farreny, Eric Agius, Sophie Bel-Vialar, Nathalie Escalas, Nagham Khouri-Farah, Chadi Soukkarieh, Cathy Danesin, Fabienne Pituello, Philippe Cochard and Cathy Soula* (iD)

## Abstract

**Background:** Most oligodendrocytes of the spinal cord originate from ventral progenitor cells of the pMN domain, characterized by expression of the transcription factor Olig2. A minority of oligodendrocytes is also recognized to emerge from dorsal progenitors during fetal development. The prevailing view is that generation of ventral oligodendrocytes depends on Sonic hedgehog (Shh) while dorsal oligodendrocytes develop under the influence of Fibroblast Growth Factors (FGFs).

**Results:** Using the well-established model of the chicken embryo, we show that ventral spinal progenitor cells activate FGF signaling at the onset of oligodendrocyte precursor cell (OPC) generation. Inhibition of FGF receptors at that time appears sufficient to prevent generation of ventral OPCs, highlighting that, in addition to Shh, FGF signaling is required also for generation of ventral OPCs. We further reveal an unsuspected interplay between Shh and FGF signaling by showing that FGFs serve dual essential functions in ventral OPC specification. FGFs are responsible for timely induction of a secondary Shh signaling center, the lateral floor plate, a crucial step to create the burst of Shh required for OPC specification. At the same time, FGFs prevent down-regulation of Olig2 in pMN progenitor cells as these cells receive higher threshold of the Shh signal. Finally, we bring arguments favoring a key role of newly differentiated neurons acting as providers of the FGF signal required to trigger OPC generation in the ventral spinal cord.

**Conclusion:** Altogether our data reveal that the FGF signaling pathway is activated and required for OPC commitment in the ventral spinal cord. More generally, our data may prove important in defining strategies to produce large populations of determined oligodendrocyte precursor cells from undetermined neural progenitors, including stem cells. In the long run, these new data could be useful in attempts to stimulate the oligodendrocyte fate in residing neural stem cells.

**Keywords:** Oligodendrogenesis, Spinal cord, Sonic hedgehog, Fibroblast growth factors

## Background

Oligodendrocytes, the myelin-forming cells of the vertebrate central nervous system (CNS), differentiate from oligodendrocyte precursor cells (OPCs) generated during development. OPCs are specified at embryonic stages and are known to originate from multiple progenitor domains of the ventricular zone [69]. In the developing spinal cord, two spatially and temporally distinct sources of OPCs have been evidenced. An initial ventral source, producing most OPCs of the spinal cord, emanates from a subset of ventral neural progenitors populating the so called pMN domain [68]. A later dorsal source that produces a minority of OPCs, starting at fetal stages, takes place in more dorsal progenitor domains [13, 27, 80]. The importance of extracellular signaling factors in defining both the dorso-ventral position of OPC sources and the precise timing of OPC specification are widely recognized. Induction of ventral OPCs depends on the morphogenetic activity of Sonic Hedgehog (Shh)

* Correspondence: catherine.soula@univ-tlse3.fr
Centre de Biologie du Développement (CBD) CNRS/UPS, Centre de Biologie Intégrative (CBI), Université de Toulouse, F-31062 Toulouse, France

produced by ventral medial cells of the developing spinal cord [19]. During this first wave of production, the restriction of OPC generation to ventral progenitors is also controlled by the repressive activity of the dorsalizing factors BMPs and Wnts which at that time prevent OPC generation from dorsally located neural progenitor cells [48, 50]. In contrast, the second phase of OPC generation from dorsal progenitor cells occurs independently of Shh and has been proposed instead to depend on Fibroblast growth factors (FGFs) that have been proposed to act by counteracting BMP signaling [9, 14, 40, 80]. Therefore, it is currently assumed that commitment of ventral and dorsal spinal cord OPCs depends on Shh and FGFs, respectively. Similarly, multiple spatial and temporal waves of OPC generation have been reported to occur in the developing brain. The first wave of OPCs occurs in the ventral forebrain and requires Shh activity [5, 54, 73, 77]. However, evidences has further emerged that generation of ventral OPCs in the mouse forebrain also depends on the FGF signaling pathway [30]. A similar observation has been made in the zebrafish ventral rhombencephalon where FGF signaling has been shown to cooperate with Shh to control expression of Olig2 [26]. Therefore, contrasting with the proposed model for the spinal cord, ventral OPC generation in the developing brain depends on a Shh and FGF interplay, whose precise mechanism remains, however, to be elucidated.

Although a number of studies established a framework for understanding mechanisms controlling Shh-dependent OPC induction in the ventral spinal cord, a number of questions remain. A prerequisite for ventral OPC generation is establishment of the pMN domain characterized by expression of Olig2, an obligatory transcription factor for oligodendrocyte development. This domain initially forms in the ventral neural tube in response to Shh secreted from the notochord and medial floor plate (MFP) cells [21]. Once established, the pMN domain produces motor neurons (MNs) and start generating OPCs only after completion of MN generation [8]. Shh is still necessary at these late stages for OPC induction [3, 57, 60, 72]. Significantly, Olig2 progenitor cells must not only receive Shh but must be submitted to a high threshold Shh signal to change their fate and generate OPCs [20, 72]. Accordingly, a temporal rise of Shh signaling occurs in the ventral spinal cord at the time of OPC specification [4, 20, 78]. This results in up-regulation of the homeodomain protein Nkx2.2 within Olig2-expressing progenitor cells that finally ends up with establishment of a new domain, named the p* domain, populated by Nkx2.2 and Olig2-coexpressing cells (Fig. 1a) [3, 28, 66, 78, 83]. During patterning process of the neural tube, activation of Nkx2.2 in ventral-most progenitor cells is known to repress Olig2 expression, an essential function allowing formation of the two distinct p3 (Nkx2.2) and pMN (Olig2) domains [22, 37, 74]. However, at the time of OPC specification, activation of Nkx2.2 in pMN cells no longer represses Olig2 and their coexpression drives progenitor cells to the OPC fate [75, 83]. Thus, the Shh signal must not only remain active over development but must also be temporally strengthened to modify the transcriptional status of Olig2 progenitor cells. Changes in both Shh source cell identity and position, that undergo significant transformations over time, have been proposed to underlie timely activation of Shh signaling [4, 19]. In particular, a secondary source of Shh, named the lateral floor plate (LFP), forms shortly before OPC induction by up-regulation of Shh expression in progenitor cells of the p3 domain, thereby bringing a source of Shh in closer proximity to the pMN domain (Fig. 1a) [4, 15, 38, 71]. However, how LFP induction is controlled over time and why Nkx2.2 activation no more represses Olig2 expression in cells of the pMN domain at initiation of OPC generation are still open questions.

In this study, we bring answers to these issues by highlighting the key role of FGF signaling in controlling OPC induction also in the ventral spinal cord. Using chicken as a well-established model of OPC development, we provide evidence for a dual role of FGF signaling acting upstream of Shh to promote induction of the LFP but also together with Shh to ensure maintenance of Olig2 expression in pMN progenitor cells as they activate Nkx2.2 in response to high threshold Shh signal.

## Methods
Fertilized White Leghorn chicken eggs, obtained from a commercial source, were incubated at 38 °C until they reached the appropriate stages [33].

### Isolation and culture of spinal cord explants
Flat-mount preparations of spinal cord explants were cultivated using an organotypic culture system previously described [2]. Briefly, embryonic day 4 (E4) spinal cord explants, isolated from surrounding tissues, were opened along the dorsal midline and flattened on a nitrocellulose membrane (Sartorius) with the neural progenitor cells up and grown as organotypic cultures in DMEM (Invitrogen) supplemented with 10% FCS (Sigma). When indicated, the FGFR inhibitors SU5402 [52] and PD166866 [59], two cell-permeable ATP-competitive inhibitors of the tyrosine kinase activity of FGFRs, or the Shh signaling inhibitor cyclopamine [35] were added to the culture medium at the time of plating or after 24 h in culture. The working concentrations of inhibitors were as follows: SU5402 20 µM (Calbiochem); PD166866 2,5 µM (Calbiochem); cyclopamin 5 mM (Enzo life

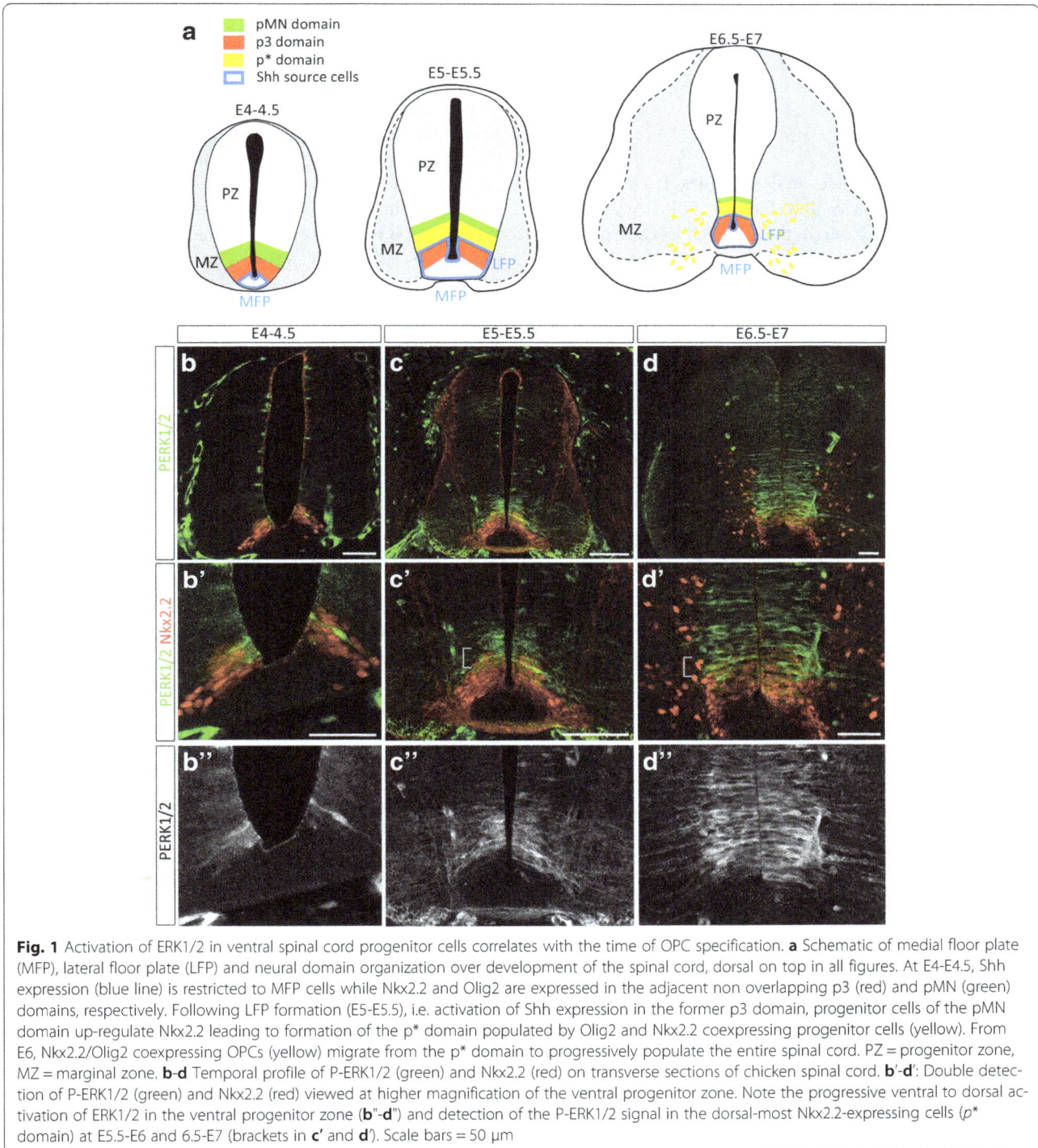

**Fig. 1** Activation of ERK1/2 in ventral spinal cord progenitor cells correlates with the time of OPC specification. **a** Schematic of medial floor plate (MFP), lateral floor plate (LFP) and neural domain organization over development of the spinal cord, dorsal on top in all figures. At E4-E4.5, Shh expression (blue line) is restricted to MFP cells while Nkx2.2 and Olig2 are expressed in the adjacent non overlapping p3 (red) and pMN (green) domains, respectively. Following LFP formation (E5-E5.5), i.e. activation of Shh expression in the former p3 domain, progenitor cells of the pMN domain up-regulate Nkx2.2 leading to formation of the p* domain populated by Olig2 and Nkx2.2 coexpressing progenitor cells (yellow). From E6, Nkx2.2/Olig2 coexpressing OPCs (yellow) migrate from the p* domain to progressively populate the entire spinal cord. PZ = progenitor zone, MZ = marginal zone. **b-d** Temporal profile of P-ERK1/2 (green) and Nkx2.2 (red) on transverse sections of chicken spinal cord. **b'-d'**: Double detection of P-ERK1/2 (green) and Nkx2.2 (red) viewed at higher magnification of the ventral progenitor zone. Note the progressive ventral to dorsal activation of ERK1/2 in the ventral progenitor zone (**b''-d''**) and detection of the P-ERK1/2 signal in the dorsal-most Nkx2.2-expressing cells (p* domain) at E5.5-E6 and 6.5-E7 (brackets in **c'** and **d'**). Scale bars = 50 μm

Sciences). Inhibitors were solubilized and diluted in DMSO that was added to control cultures. Flat-mounted explants were fixed at appropriate intervals in 3.7% formaldehyde/PBS, sectioned at 60–80 μm using a vibratome (Microm) and processed for immunostaining or in situ hybridization.

**Tissue preparation**

Chicken embryos or flat-mounted explants were fixed in 4% paraformaldehyde (PFA) in PBS. Embryos and explants were fixed overnight at 4 °C or 1 h at room temperature, respectively, for immunodetection analysis. When intended to in situ hybridization, an overnight fixation (4 °C) was performed followed by dehydratation and storage in 100% ethanol (– 20 °C). Tissues were then sectioned at 60–80 μm using a vibratome (Microm). In all experiments, sections were performed at the brachial level.

## Immunostaining

For immunofluorescence analysis, chicken tissues were processed as previously described [3, 20]. Primary antibodies were applied overnight at 4 °C. Secondary antibodies were applied at room temperature for 1 h. The antibodies used were as follows: rabbit anti Phospho-p44/42 MAPK (PERK) 1/200 (Cell Signaling); rabbit anti-Olig2 1/500 (Chemicon); mouse monoclonal O4 antibody (O4 mAb), 1/4 (culture supernatant obtained from O4 hybridoma cells, a gift from R. Bansal); mouse anti-Nkx2.2 1/4 (DSHN) [25]; rabbit anti-clived Caspase 3 1/400 (Cell Signaling), mouse anti-BrdU 1/2000 (DHSB). Alexa 488, 555 or 647 goat anti-rabbit and goat anti-mouse (1/500) were from Molecular Probes. For BrdU staining, spinal cord explants were incubated for 2 h with BrdU (0.15 μg/μl, Sigma), 24, 32 or 48 h after plating. Tissues were then fixed for 4 h and processed for BrdU immunostaining.

## In situ hybridization

In situ hybridization (ISH) was performed on vibratome sections of chicken embryos and spinal cord explants either by hand or automatically (InsituPro, Intavis) using the whole-mount ISH protocol previously described [10, 20]. Digoxigenin (DIG)-labeled sense and antisense RNA probes were synthesized using T3 and T7 polymerases. RNA labeled probes were detected by an alkaline-phosphatase coupled antibody (Roche Diagnostics) and NBT/BCIP (nitroblue tetrazolium/5-bromo-4-chloro-3-indolyl phosphate) was used as a chromogenic substrate for alkaline phosphatase (Boehringer, Mannheim). The following RNA probes were used: *spry1 and spry2, fgfr1, fgfr2* and *fgfr4* (provided by K. Storey); *mkp3* and *fgf8* (provided S Martinez), *Shh* (provided by C. Tabin). Counterstaining of Nkx2.2 was performed after color development following a post-fixation step in 4% PFA for 1 h.

## Electroporation

Expression constructs were cloned into either the pCAG-IRES-GFP (Addgene) for the truncated FGF receptor (dnFGFR), containing intact extracellular and transmembrane domains but completely lacking the intracellular tyrosine kinase domain [6] or the pCMV vector for the chimeric protein FGF8b-GFP [61]. To allow cell body detection of electroporated cells, the pCMV FGF8b-GFP vector was co-electroporated with the empty pCIG vector (a gift from A. McMahon) used

at 0.5 μg/μl. In ovo electroporation in E1.5 neural tube was performed as described previously [36]. Briefly, the FGF8 and/or Shh constructs were injected at 1 μg/μl in the rostral neural tube using a glass pipette. Electrodes (Nepa Gene Corporation) were positioned on each side of the neural tube and four pulses of 20 V (Intracel TSS10) were applied to trigger unilateral entry of the DNA into the neural tube, the non-transfected half constituting an internal control. Electroporation of E4 spinal cord was performed ex ovo. The dnFGFR expression vector was used at 1 μg/μl. Controls were performed with pCAG-IRES-GFP vector alone. Embryos were harvested and isolated in a Petri dish with the dorsal side up, and DNA solution was injected into the lumen of the spinal cord as previously described [20, 78]. Electrodes were positioned on each side of the brachial region of the spinal cord, the positive electrode being placed more ventrally than the negative one, allowing satisfactory electroporation of ventral regions. Ten pulses of 25 V were applied and spinal cord was further dissected and grown in organotypic culture as above.

## Experimental design and statistical analysis

Fluorescence photomicrographs were collected with Leica SP5 and Zeiss 710 confocal microscopes. Images of ISHs were collected with Nikon digital camera DXM1200C and a Nikon eclipse 80i microscope. Images were processed using Adobe Photoshop CS2. Unless otherwise stated in figure legends, provided data are the average of three embryos or explants (*n*) per condition from at least two independent experiments. Cell counting was performed on at least 5 tissue slices per chicken explant. For each tissue slice (60–80 μm), at least 4 optical sections were acquired at 6 μm intervals and cells were counted in each optical section. Quantifications are expressed as the mean number of cells (mean ± s.e.m) in an optical section of hemi-explants. Statistical analyses were performed using the Mann–Whitney U test. Significance was determined at $p < 0.05$. $p$ values are indicated in figure legends or in text when quantifications are not included in figures.

## Results

### MAPK signaling is activated at initiation of OPC commitment in the ventral spinal cord

Previous studies have reported that FGFs can induce production of OPCs from dorsal spinal cord and cerebral cortex progenitor cells [1, 9, 13, 14, 31, 40, 53]. This inductive property has been attributed to robust activation of the MAPK signaling pathway [9, 14, 40]. As a first step to define possible involvement of FGFs also in generation of ventral OPCs, we examined activation of the canonical MAPK pathway at the time of ventral OPC specification in chicken, i.e. between 5.5 and 6 days of development (E5.5/E6) [72, 83]. For this, we analyzed expression of the active form of the signal-regulated protein kinase ERK1/2 (P-ERK1/2) together with that of Nkx2.2 on transverse spinal cord sections starting at E4 up to E7. At E4-E4.5, cells expressing P-ERK1/2 were detected in the ventral-most region of the ventricular zone (Fig. 1b). From E5, both intensity and dorso-ventral extent of the P-ERK1/2 immunostaining significantly increased (Fig. 1c, d), indicating temporal activation of the MAPK signaling pathway in ventral progenitor cells. Positioning of P-ERK1/2 positive cells with respect to Nkx2.2 showed that activation of ERK1/2 was initially restricted to Nkx2.2-expressing cells of the ventral-most p3 domain (Fig. 1b). At E5-E5.5, Nkx2.2 expression extended dorsally compared to earlier stages. P-ERK1/2 staining was then mostly detected in the dorsal-most Nkx2.2-expressing cells (Fig. 1c), indicating activation of the MAPK pathway in cells of the p* domain that has already being established at this stage [3, 28, 78, 83]. Similar patterns were observed at E6.5-E7 although the P-ERK1/2 signal extended more dorsally at these later stages (Fig. 1d).

Our data, showing activation of ERK1/2 in the ventral spinal cord at stages of OPC specification, indicate that, in addition to Shh, ventral progenitor cells perceived growth factor signals. Furthermore, the progression of ERK1/2 activation over time, starting in the p3 domain (prospective LFP cells) and further extending to dorsally-located progenitor cells (p* domain), was suggestive of a role of the MAPK signaling pathway both in LFP induction and OPC commitment.

**Ventral neural progenitors activate FGFR signaling at the time of OPC specification**

We next sought to define whether ventral progenitor cells of the spinal cord are indeed targets for FGFs focusing on expression of FGFR and FGF target gene expression at stages of OPC specification. To date, four high affinity receptors for FGF (FGFRs1−4) have been identified. FGFRs 1−3 are known to be expressed in regions of the ventral embryonic forebrain that give rise to OPCs [7]. In the spinal cord, solely FGFR3 expression has been studied and it is preferentially expressed in progenitor domains dedicated to generate astrocytes but not OPCs [3, 63]. We thus sought to establish expression patterns of FGFR1, 2 and 4. From E4-E4.5 until E6, mRNAs encoding for the three receptors were all detected in ventral progenitor cells with no gross change in their expression patterns over time (Fig. 2a-f). While *fgfr1* was uniformly and broadly expressed in progenitor cells (Fig. 2a, d), distinct expression levels for *fgfr2* and *fgfr4* were observed along the ventral to dorsal axis of the progenitor zone. *Fgfr2* mRNA was detected at higher level in a restricted domain of the ventral region, in a

position very reminiscent to the source of OPCs (Fig. 2e). To confirm this, we performed double detection experiments using antibodies directed against Olig2 and Nkx2.2. Our data showed that Olig2-expressing cells as well as the dorsal-most Nkx2.2 positive cells were indeed included in the domain of high *fgfr2* expression (Fig. 2g, i). *Fgfr4* was detected in the entire ventral progenitor zone at E4-E4.5. However, at E5.5-E6, expression of this gene decreased in the ventral-most cells. Comparison with Olig2 and Nkx2.2 indicated that *fgfr4* expression overlapped the Olig2 domain as well as the dorsal-most region of the Nkx2.2 domain but was down-regulated in the ventral-most Nkx2.2-expressing domain (Fig. 2h, j) populated at this stage by LFP cells [4]. Together, these data indicate that ventral progenitor cells of both the p3 and pMN/p* domains can sense FGF signals at developmental stages of OPC specification.

We then assessed activation of the FGFR signaling pathway by analyzing expression of the FGF target genes, *mkp3* [23, 24, 39] and *sprouty1/2* (*spry1/2*) [41, 51]. Before OPC specification (E4/E4.5), we detected *mkp3* expression in pools of ventral neurons but not in progenitor cells (Fig. 2k). At this stage, low level of *spry1* expression was detected in a very ventral domain of the progenitor zone, adjacent to the MFP, while *spry2* mRNA extended in a broader domain of the ventral progenitor zone (Fig. 2l, m). At E5.5-E6, expression of *mkp3* became apparent in cells of the ventral progenitor zone (Fig. 2n), indicating activation of FGFR signaling at stages of OPC specification. Accordingly, we detected higher level of *spry1/2* expression in ventral progenitor cells (Fig. 2o, p). Double detection of *spry1/2* and Olig2 or Nkx2.2 indicated preferential expression of these genes in Nkx2.2- and Olig2-expressing progenitor cells with higher levels of *spry1* and *spry2* expression in Nkx2.2 and Olig2 positive cells, respectively (Fig. 2q-t), suggesting domain specific responses to FGFR activation in the ventral progenitor zone.

Together, our data, showing that ventral progenitor cells of the p3 and p* domains both express FGFRs and up-regulate FGF target genes at stages of OPC specification, support the view that FGF signaling pathway might play a role in controlling generation of ventral spinal OPCs.

**FGFR activity is required for OPC specification in the ventral spinal cord**

To test the role of FGFs in ventral OPC specification, we turned to organotypic culture of chicken spinal cord explants that allows interfering with cell signaling precisely at the time of OPC induction [2, 3, 20, 78]. In this paradigm, brachial spinal cord explants are isolated prior to OPC specification (E4-E4.5) and plated in culture as an opened-book (Fig. 3a). With this system, the temporal

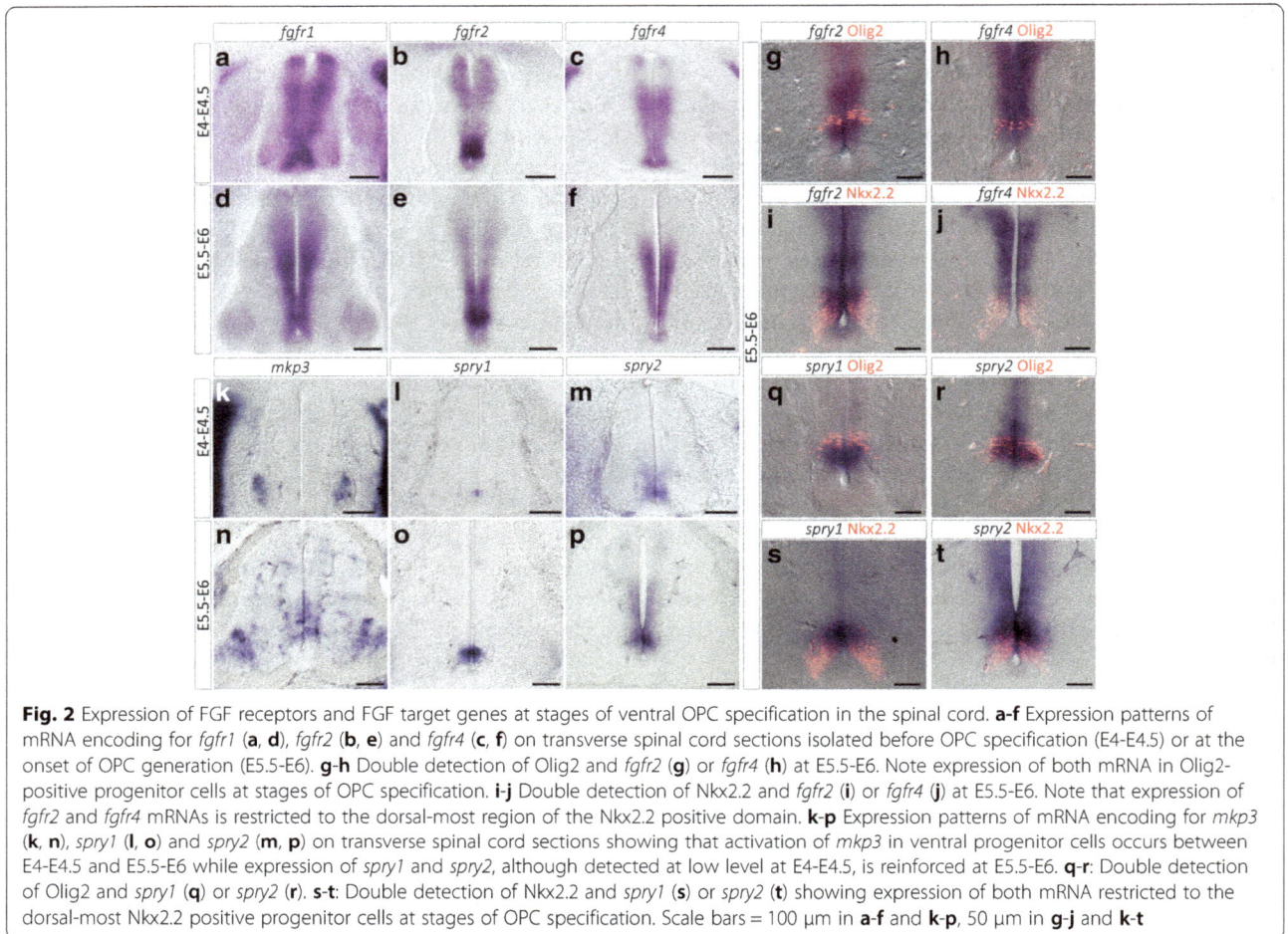

**Fig. 2** Expression of FGF receptors and FGF target genes at stages of ventral OPC specification in the spinal cord. **a-f** Expression patterns of mRNA encoding for *fgfr1* (**a**, **d**), *fgfr2* (**b**, **e**) and *fgfr4* (**c**, **f**) on transverse spinal cord sections isolated before OPC specification (E4-E4.5) or at the onset of OPC generation (E5.5-E6). **g-h** Double detection of Olig2 and *fgfr2* (**g**) or *fgfr4* (**h**) at E5.5-E6. Note expression of both mRNA in Olig2-positive progenitor cells at stages of OPC specification. **i-j** Double detection of Nkx2.2 and *fgfr2* (**i**) or *fgfr4* (**j**) at E5.5-E6. Note that expression of *fgfr2* and *fgfr4* mRNAs is restricted to the dorsal-most region of the Nkx2.2 positive domain. **k-p** Expression patterns of mRNA encoding for *mkp3* (**k**, **n**), *spry1* (**l**, **o**) and *spry2* (**m**, **p**) on transverse spinal cord sections showing that activation of *mkp3* in ventral progenitor cells occurs between E4-E4.5 and E5.5-E6 while expression of *spry1* and *spry2*, although detected at low level at E4-E4.5, is reinforced at E5.5-E6. **q-r**: Double detection of Olig2 and *spry1* (**q**) or *spry2* (**r**). **s-t**: Double detection of Nkx2.2 and *spry1* (**s**) or *spry2* (**t**) showing expression of both mRNA restricted to the dorsal-most Nkx2.2 positive progenitor cells at stages of OPC specification. Scale bars = 100 μm in **a-f** and **k-p**, 50 μm in **g-j** and **k-t**

fate of Olig2 progenitor cells is maintained and OPC migration in the mantle zone can be observed after 2 days in culture, a stage equivalent to E6-E6.5 in vivo [3, 20, 78]. To address the requirement of FGF activity for ventral OPC generation, we inactivated FGF receptors (FGFRs) prior to OPC commitment (E4-E4.5) and analyzed OPC production after 2 days in culture. FGFR inactivation was performed either incubating explants with the FGFR inhibitors SU5402 and PD166866 [52, 59] or by overexpressing of a dominant-negative form of FGFRs (dnFGFR) that completely lacks the intracellular tyrosine kinase domain [6] using the electroporation method. As a first step, we controlled efficient inactivation of FGFRs. SU5402 or PD166866 were added to the culture medium at the time of plating and expression of P-ERK1/2 and *spry1/2* were analyzed 2 days later. In control explants, P-ERK1/2 and *spry1/2* expressions were detected in ventral progenitor cells (Fig. 3a, c, e), identifying cells with patterns very similar to those observed on transverse spinal cord sections at E6. After treatment with FGFR inhibitors, we found that both P-ERK1/2 immunostaining

and *spry1/2* expression were nearly abolished (Fig. 3c, e, g and data not shown). Similarly, electroporation of the dnFGFR expression vector, performed just prior to spinal cord explantation, prevented both ERK1/2 activation and *spry1/2* expression while electroporation of a control vector had no effect (Fig. 3h-k). These results, beyond validating the approach, support the view that FGFRs are indeed responsible for stimulation of MAPK activity and *spry1/2* expression in the ventral spinal cord.

We next examined OPC generation after FGFR inactivation. In the chicken embryonic spinal cord, co-expression of Olig2 and Nkx2.2 has been reported to specifically identify OPCs [3, 4, 20, 28, 78, 83]. Triple immunostaining of Olig2, Nkx2.2 and O4, also a specific and early marker of OPCs in chicken [49, 56, 72], performed on explants cultivated for 2 days allowed identifying the same cell population, i.e. newly committed OPCs still located in the progenitor zone as well as OPCs that have already emigrated from the progenitor zone to populate the mantle zone (Fig. 4b). Double immunostainings of Olig2 and Nkx2.2 were further performed on explants treated with FGFR inhibitors or

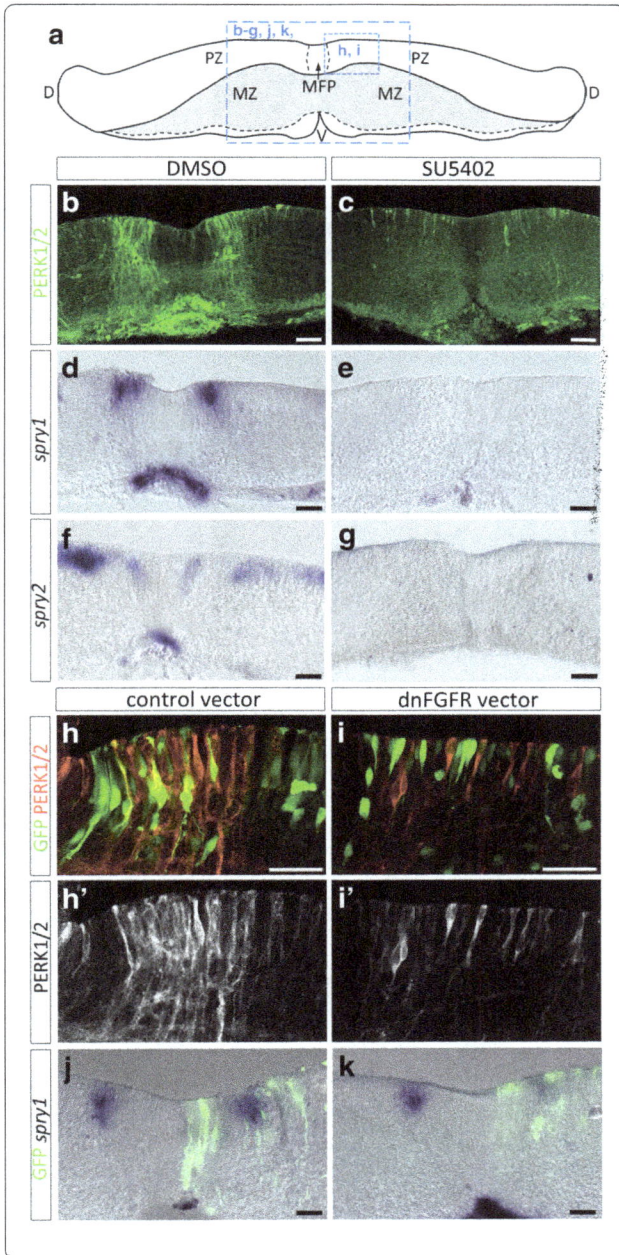

**Fig. 3** Inactivation of FGFRs results in defective activation of ERK1/2 and in down-regulation of *spry1/2* expression in spinal cord explants. **a** Scheme of a transverse section through spinal cord explant cultivated as opened-book showing the progenitor zone (PZ) on top and the mantle zone (MZ) at the bottom of the explant. The former dorsal region of the spinal cord (D) lies on each side of the explant while the ventral region (V) is in the middle. The dashed blue panels outline the areas shown in images below. **b-c** Immunodetection of P-ERK1/2 on transverse sections of spinal cord explants isolated at E4.5 and cultivated as opened-book explants (progenitor cell layer on top) for 2 days in control condition (**a**) or in presence of SU5402 (**b**). **d-g** Detection of *spry1* (**d, e**) and *spry2* (**f, g**) in control condition (**d, f**) or in presence of SU5402 (**f, g**). **h-i** Higher magnification of the ventral progenitor zone (floor plate cells are on the left) showing immunodetection of P-ERK1/2 (red in **h** and **i**, **h',i'**) after electroporation of the control vector (green in **h**) or the dnFGFR vector (green in **i**). **j-k** Detection of *spry1* mRNA after electroporation of the control vector (green in **j**) or the dnFGFR vector (green in **k**). MFP = medial floor plate. Scale bars = 50 μm

explants overexpressing dnFGFR. After 2 days in culture, only few Nkx2.2/Olig2-coexpressing cells were detected in the mantle zone of explants incubated with SU5402 or PD166866 (Fig. 4b and data not shown). Cell counting of Olig2 positive cells in the mantle zone indicated that their number was reduced by more than 80% in presence of inhibitors compared to control explants (for SU5402 see Fig. 4i; for PD166866, mean number of OPCs was $1.72 \pm 0.47$ versus $12.63 \pm 0.62$ in control explants, $p \leq 0.01$). Similarly, overexpression of the dnFGFR led to a greater than 5-fold reduction in the number of Olig2 positive cell in the mantle zone of the electroporated side of the explants compared to the non-electroporated side or to explants electroporated with a control vector (Fig. 4g, h, k, l). Together, our data, showing that inactivation of FGFRs is sufficient to inhibit OPC development, indicate that FGFR signaling is required for proper generation of OPCs in the ventral spinal cord.

We next asked whether the deficient OPC generation observed after inactivation of FGFR resulted from a failure in the initial commitment of Olig2 progenitors towards the OPC fate. To address this question, we focused on the progenitor zone in which formation of the p* domain, i.e. dorsal extension of Nkx2.2 expression within the Olig2-expressing domain, reflects active process of OPC commitment [3, 4, 20, 28, 78, 83]. After 2 days in culture, Nkx2.2/Olig2-coexpressing cells were detected in the progenitor zone forming the p* domain in control explants, indicating ongoing generation of OPCs from Olig2-expressing progenitor cells (Fig. 4e). Examination of the progenitor zone of explants treated with FGFR inhibitors showed that, while position and size of the Olig2 expression domain were not affected, the dorsal extent of the Nkx2.2-expressing domain was reduced compared to control explants (Fig. 4f). Cell

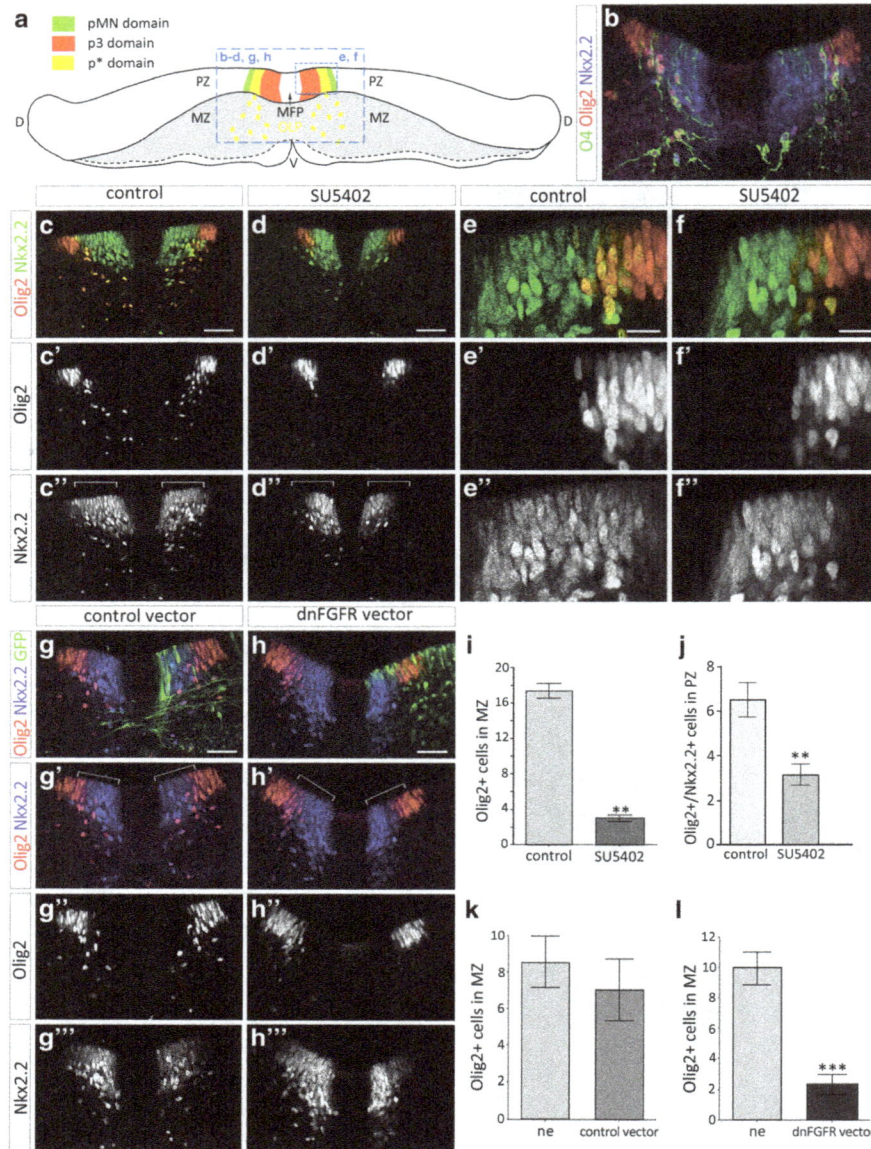

**Fig. 4** Inactivation of FGFRs impairs OPC specification. **a** Scheme of a transverse section through spinal cord explant cultivated as opened-book showing ventral progenitor domains. The dashed blue panels outline the areas shown in images below. **b** Immunodetection of O4 (green), Olig2 (red) and Nkx2.2 (blue) on transverse section of spinal cord explant cultivated for 2 days in control condition. Note overlapping of the three markers both in the p* domain and in cells emigrating ventrally in the mantle zone. **c-d** Immunodetection of Olig2 (red in **c** and **d**, **c'**, **d'**) and Nkx2.2 (green in **c** and **d**, **c"**, **d"**) on transverse sections of spinal cord explants cultivated for 2 days in control condition (**c**) or in presence of SU5402 (**d**). Note that while Nkx2.2/Olig2-positive OPCs have already invaded the mantle zone in control explants, very few develop in presence of the inhibitor. Note also reduced dorsal extent of the Nkx2.2-positive domain (brackets) in SU5402 treated explant (**d"**) compared to control explant (**c"**). **e-f** Higher magnification of the progenitor zone showing reduced number of Olig2/Nkx2.2-positive cells in the progenitor zone of explant treated with SU5402 (**f**, **f'**, **f"**) compared to control explant (**e**, **e'**, **e"**). **g-h** Immunodetection of Olig2 (red in **g**, **g'**, **h** and **h'**, **g"**, **h"**) and Nkx2.2 (blue in **g**, **h**, **g'** and **h'**, **g'''**, **h'''**) after electroporation of control (green in **g**) or dnFGFR (green in **h**) vectors. Note reduction of the dorsal extent of the Nkx2.2 positive domain on the side of explant electroporated with the dnFGFR vector compared to the non electroporated side of the explant or with explant electroporated with the control vector (brackets in **g'** and **h'**). Note also that migrating Olig2/Nkx2.2 double-labeled cells are not detected on the side of explant electroporated with the dnFGFR vector. **i** Quantification of Olig2-positive cells in the mantle zone in control conditions ($n = 7$) or in presence of the FGFR inhibitor SU5402 ($n = 8$). **j** Quantification of Nkx2.2/Olig2-positive cells in the progenitor zone (PZ) of explants cultivated in control conditions ($n = 7$) or in presence of SU5402 ($n = 8$). **k-l** Quantification of Olig2-positive cells migrating in the mantle zone on each side of the explants after electroporation of control ($n = 4$, **k**) or dnFGFR ($n = 9$, **l**) vectors. Results are presented as mean number of cells ± sem (**$p \leq 0.01$; ***$p \leq 0.001$). ne: non-electroporated side of explants. PZ = progenitor zone, MZ = mantle zone, MFP = medial floor plate, V = ventral, D = dorsal. Scale bars = 50 μm in **b-d**, **g**, **h** and 25 μm in **e**, **f**

counting performed in explants treated with SU5402 or PD166866 showed a significant decrease in the number of Olig2/Nkx2.2-coexpressing progenitor cells compared to control explants (for SU5402 see Fig. 4j; for PD166866, mean number of Olig2/Nkx2.2-positive progenitor cells was $4.1 \pm 0.31$ versus $8.33 \pm 0.34$ in control explants, $p \leq 0.01$), indicating defective generation of the p* domain in the presence of FGFR inhibitors. Similar results were obtained when FGFR inhibition was performed using dnFGFR overexpression in ventral progenitor cells (Fig. 4g, h). Importantly, cell proliferation studies showed that overall BrdU incorporation in progenitor cells in the presence of SU5402 was not significantly different from controls (Fig. 5c-e). Similarly, cell survival, assessed by detection of the activated form of Caspase 3, was not affected by treatment with the inhibitor (Fig. 5a, b, e).

These data, showing that inhibition of FGFR signaling activity is sufficient to prevent formation of the p* domain and that this function does not rely on the control of cell proliferation or cell survival, highlight the key role of FGFRs in controlling specification of OPCs in the ventral spinal cord.

### Formation of the lateral floor plate requires activation of FGFR signaling

We know from our previous work that formation of the LFP, characterized by up-regulation of *shh* expression in Nkx2.2-expressing cells of the p3 domain, is temporally correlated with time commitment of Olig2 progenitor cells to the OPC fate [4, 19]. However, whether LFP formation contributes to create the burst of Shh signaling activity required for OPC specification remains elusive. Based on our present data, showing that Nkx2.2-expressing cells of the p3 domain express FGFRs and activate P-ERK1/2 prior to LFP induction (E4/E4.5, Figs. 2 and 3), we hypothesized that FGFs might contribute to induce OPCs indirectly, by stimulating Shh expression within prospective LFP cells. To test this, we analyzed the effects of FGFR inactivation on Shh expression using the spinal cord explant paradigm. As a first step, we asked whether LFP forms properly in explanted spinal cords. At E4, corresponding to the stage of spinal cord explantation, *shh* mRNA expression was restricted to MFP cells (Fig. 6a). After 9 h in culture, the time required for explant attachment to the substratum, detection of *shh* mRNA was still limited to ventral medial cells of the MFP (Fig. 6b). By contrast, 1 day after plating, equivalent to E5-E5.5 in vivo, *shh* expression extended in dorsal direction, i.e. laterally in opened-book explants (Fig. 6c). Comparison with Nkx2.2 expression at an equivalent culture time indicated that *shh* expression encompassed the Nkx2.2 positive p3 domain (Fig. 6c, e). After 2 days in vitro, *shh* mRNA was still

detected in LFP cells and, expectedly, the domain of *shh* expression did not span the dorsal-most part of Nkx2.2 positive domain corresponding, at that time, to the p* domain (Fig. 6d, f). Therefore, LFP develops properly in spinal cord explants and its induction occurs within the first day of culture, in agreement with its period of formation in vivo [4]. Strikingly, SU5402 treatment, while not modifying *shh* expression in MFP cells, nearly abolished extension of *shh* expression in cells of the p3/LFP domain at either 1 or 2 days in culture (Fig. 6g, h). Confirming these data, overexpression of the dnFGFR in cells of the p3 domain appeared sufficient to prevent activation of *shh* expression in these cells (Fig. 6o). We next limited SU5402 treatment to the first day of culture, i.e. prior to LFP induction, or to the second day of culture, after LFP formation, and analyzed, in either case, *shh* expression at day 2. We found that inhibition of FGFR was sufficient to prevent up-regulation of *shh* when performed prior to LFP induction (Fig. 6i) but had no influence on *shh* expression after the time of LFP induction (Fig. 6j). Therefore, FGFR activation is required for induction but not for maintenance of LFP cells. We next asked whether LFP induction, as reported for induction of the MFP [70], resulted from concerted activities of FGFs and Shh which is still secreted by MFP cells at the time of LFP formation. We then incubated spinal cord explants with cyclopamine, a potent inhibitor of the Shh signaling pathway [16, 35] and analyzed LFP formation. As previously reported [3], after 2 days in culture, cyclopamine treatment inhibited expression of Olig2, known to require Shh activity to be maintained, but also prevented dorsal extension of Nkx2.2 expression (Fig. 6k, l). By contrast, this treatment had no effect on *shh* expression, indicating that LFP forms properly in cyclopamine treated explants (Fig. 6m, n). Therefore, induction of the LFP is independent of Shh but depends on FGFR signaling. These data are in agreement with our data showing that cells of the p3 domain express activated forms of ERK1/2 as well as FGF target genes (see Figs 1 and 2) and down-regulate the Shh receptor Patched over time [78]. We next took advantage of this paradigm to assess the requirement of LFP formation for OPC induction. For this, we inactivated FGFRs in prospective LFP cells by targeting electroporation of the dnFGFR vector to the p3 domain. We then analyzed OPC generation in these explants using Olig2 and Nkx2.2 double immunostaining. We found that inactivation of FGFR signaling in cells of the p3 domain was sufficient to prevent OPC generation (Fig. 6p-r). Of note, inactivation of FGFRs in the p3 domain prevented dorsal extension of the Nkx2.2-expressing domain but did not impair Olig2 expression that was still detected in cells of the adjacent pMN domain (Fig. 6q). These data demonstrate that

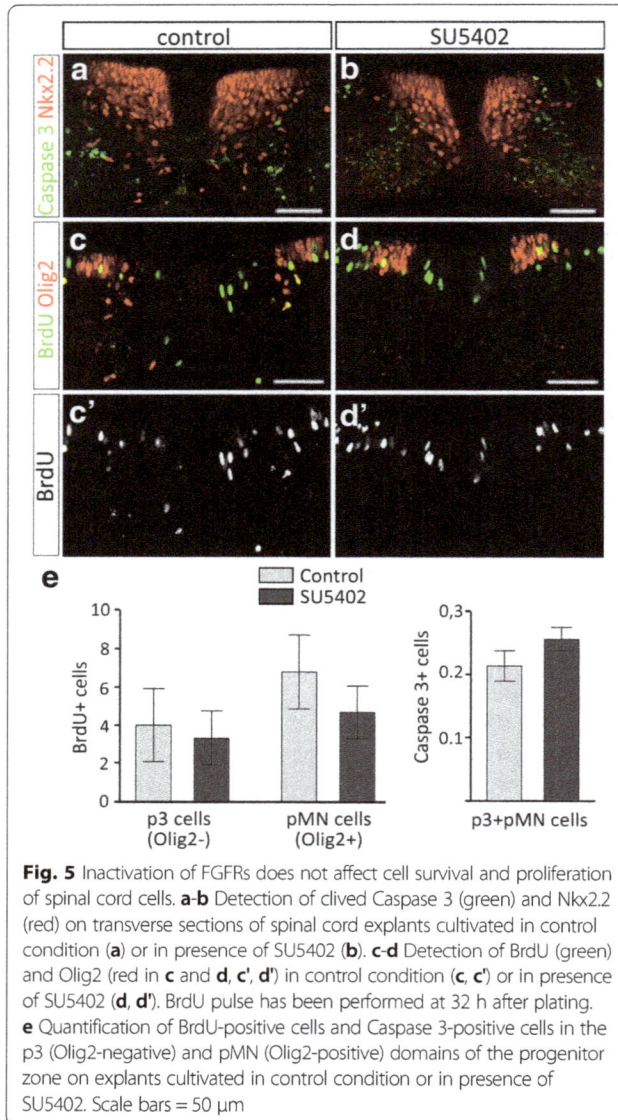

**Fig. 5** Inactivation of FGFRs does not affect cell survival and proliferation of spinal cord cells. **a-b** Detection of clived Caspase 3 (green) and Nkx2.2 (red) on transverse sections of spinal cord explants cultivated in control condition (**a**) or in presence of SU5402 (**b**). **c-d** Detection of BrdU (green) and Olig2 (red in **c** and **d**, **c'**, **d'**) in control condition (**c**, **c'**) or in presence of SU5402 (**d**, **d'**). BrdU pulse has been performed at 32 h after plating. **e** Quantification of BrdU-positive cells and Caspase 3-positive cells in the p3 (Olig2-negative) and pMN (Olig2-positive) domains of the progenitor zone on explants cultivated in control condition or in presence of SU5402. Scale bars = 50 μm

as they start generating OPCs, we hypothesized that FGFRs might also control OPC commitment, acting cell-autonomously on these cells. To test this, we selected explants in which Olig2 progenitor cells, but not the more ventrally located Nkx2.2-expressing ones, had been targeted by electroporation of the dnFGFR expression vector. Accordingly, after 2 days in culture, we observed equivalent ventral to dorsal extension of Nkx2.2 expression domain either in dnFGFR electroporated side of explants, non electroporated explants or in explants electroporated with the control vector (Fig. 7a, b). Despite this, overexpression of dnFGFR in Olig2 progenitor cells reduced the population of Nkx2.2./Olig2-coexpressing OPCs emigrating in the mantle layer (Fig. 7b). Noticeably, in the dnFGFR electroporated side of these explants, we observed a marked reduction in the expression of Olig2 while Nkx2.2 expression was unaffected. More specifically, the number of cells expressing high level of Olig2 appeared reduced when the dnFGFR expression vector, instead of the control vector, was used (Fig. 7c), suggesting that FGFR activity on Olig2-expressing cells contribute to maintain high level of Olig2 expression at stages of OPC commitment, a necessary condition for triggering progenitor cells to follow an OPC fate [45, 55, 65].

Together, these data, showing that inactivation of FGFR specifically on Olig2 progenitors is sufficient to impair OPC production, highlighted a cell autonomous role of FGFR on Olig2-expressing progenitor cells and point to a role of FGFRs in maintaining Olig2 expression.

### FGF8 and Shh work together on neural progenitor cells to promote co-expression of Olig2 and Nkx2.2

Olig2 expression is known to depend on low doses of Shh for its induction [46, 82]. It is also known to be repressed by high levels of Shh signaling at early stages of neural tube patterning, a process mediated by the activation of Nkx2.2 [22, 37, 43, 44, 55, 74]. As mentioned above, the situation is quite different at stages of p* domain formation since up-regulation of Nkx2.2 no more represses Olig2 expression. The lowered intensity of the Olig2 signal observed in dnFGFR overexpressing pMN cells at the time of OPC specification therefore led us to consider the possibility that FGFR activation might be a key determinant for providing a cell context allowing maintenance of Olig2 expression as Shh signaling rises in the ventral spinal cord. To test whether FGFs might influence Olig2 expression in a context of high Shh signaling activity, we turned to the early neural tube and monitored expression of Olig2 and Nkx2.2 after in vivo electroporation of constructs, used alone or in combination, that encode for Shh or for FGF8, a ligand known to bind and activate FGFR1–4 in vertebrates [47]. When

establishment of the LFP is required to trigger OPC generation and indicate that the prime function of LFP cells is to activate Nkx2.2 expression to form the p* domain but not to maintain Olig2 expression in pMN progenitor cells, the latter function being probably assumed by Shh still provided by MFP cells in this experimental context.

Together, our data highlight a key and indirect function for FGFR signaling in triggering ventral OPC specification, through the induction of a secondary source of Shh required for formation of the p* domain.

### FGFR activation on Olig2 progenitors is required for OPC generation

As Olig2 progenitor cells of the pMN domain also express FGFRs and activate expression of FGF target genes

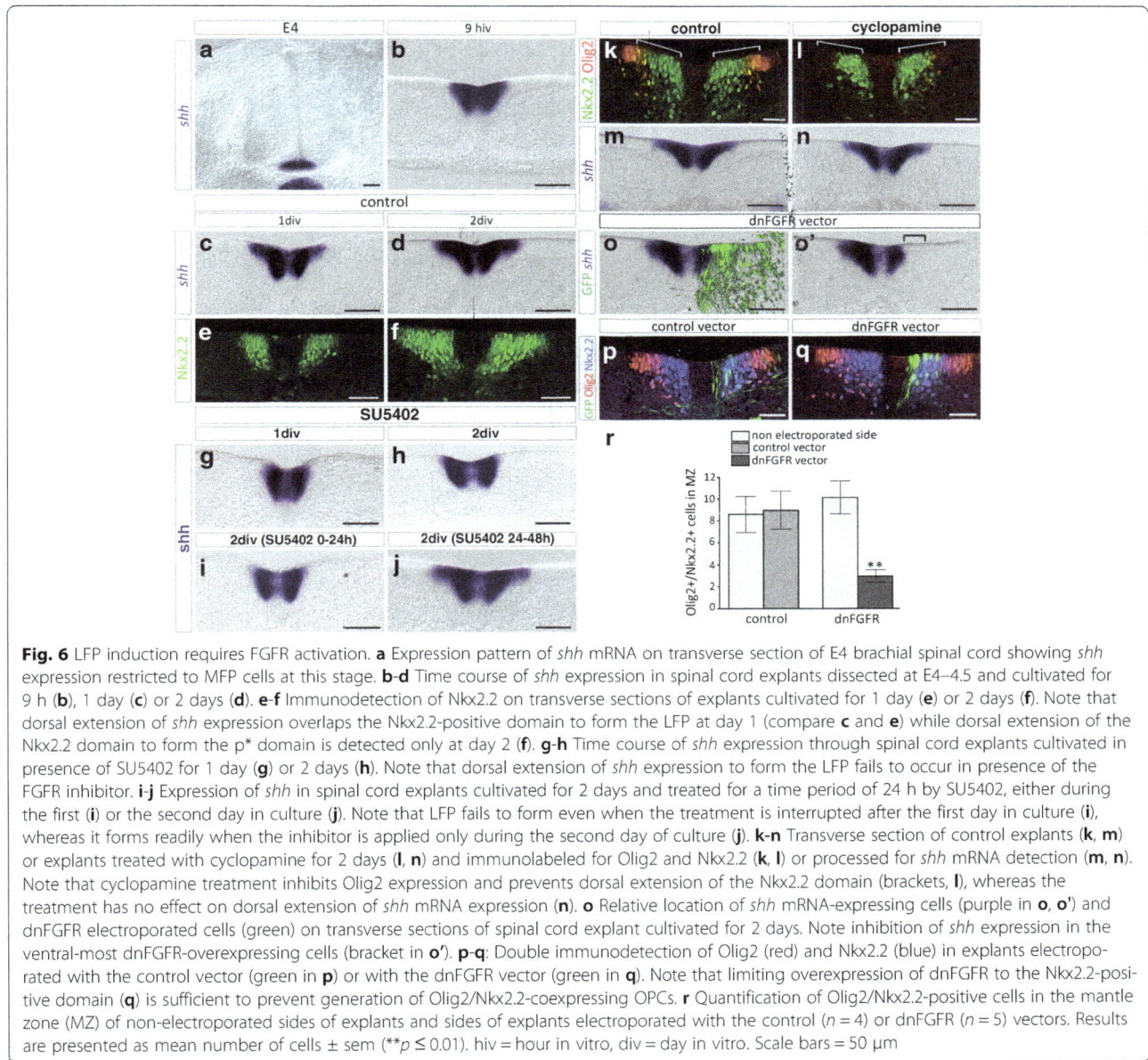

**Fig. 6** LFP induction requires FGFR activation. **a** Expression pattern of *shh* mRNA on transverse section of E4 brachial spinal cord showing *shh* expression restricted to MFP cells at this stage. **b-d** Time course of *shh* expression in spinal cord explants dissected at E4–4.5 and cultivated for 9 h (**b**), 1 day (**c**) or 2 days (**d**). **e-f** Immunodetection of Nkx2.2 on transverse sections of explants cultivated for 1 day (**e**) or 2 days (**f**). Note that dorsal extension of *shh* expression overlaps the Nkx2.2-positive domain to form the LFP at day 1 (compare **c** and **e**) while dorsal extension of the Nkx2.2 domain to form the p* domain is detected only at day 2 (**f**). **g-h** Time course of *shh* expression through spinal cord explants cultivated in presence of SU5402 for 1 day (**g**) or 2 days (**h**). Note that dorsal extension of *shh* expression to form the LFP fails to occur in presence of the FGFR inhibitor. **i-j** Expression of *shh* in spinal cord explants cultivated for 2 days and treated for a time period of 24 h by SU5402, either during the first (**i**) or the second day in culture (**j**). Note that LFP fails to form even when the treatment is interrupted after the first day in culture (**i**), whereas it forms readily when the inhibitor is applied only during the second day of culture (**j**). **k-n** Transverse section of control explants (**k, m**) or explants treated with cyclopamine for 2 days (**l, n**) and immunolabeled for Olig2 and Nkx2.2 (**k, l**) or processed for *shh* mRNA detection (**m, n**). Note that cyclopamine treatment inhibits Olig2 expression and prevents dorsal extension of the Nkx2.2 domain (brackets, **l**), whereas the treatment has no effect on dorsal extension of *shh* mRNA expression (**n**). **o** Relative location of *shh* mRNA-expressing cells (purple in **o, o'**) and dnFGFR electroporated cells (green) on transverse sections of spinal cord explant cultivated for 2 days. Note inhibition of *shh* expression in the ventral-most dnFGFR-overexpressing cells (bracket in **o'**). **p-q**: Double immunodetection of Olig2 (red) and Nkx2.2 (blue) in explants electroporated with the control vector (green in **p**) or with the dnFGFR vector (green in **q**). Note that limiting overexpression of dnFGFR to the Nkx2.2-positive domain (**q**) is sufficient to prevent generation of Olig2/Nkx2.2-coexpressing OPCs. **r** Quantification of Olig2/Nkx2.2-positive cells in the mantle zone (MZ) of non-electroporated sides of explants and sides of explants electroporated with the control (*n* = 4) or dnFGFR (*n* = 5) vectors. Results are presented as mean number of cells ± sem (**p ≤ 0.01). hiv = hour in vitro, div = day in vitro. Scale bars = 50 μm

the FGF8 expression vector was electroporated alone, expression of Nkx2.2 or Olig2 was not obviously altered and we did not detect ectopic expression of either protein in the dorsal neural tube (Fig. 8a, d). As expected, misexpression of Shh alone induced ectopic expression of Nkx2.2 and Olig2 in progenitor cells of the dorsal neural tube (Fig. 8b, e). Most of these ectopic cells expressed either Olig2 or Nkx2.2, likely reflecting cell exposure to distinct levels of Shh, and only very few of them co-expressed Nkx2.2 and Olig2 (Fig. 8e). By contrast, when both FGF8 and Shh were misexpressed in the neural tube, most if not all induced cells co-expressed Olig2 and Nkx2.2 (Fig. 8c, f). Thus, joint

exposure of progenitor cells to FGF8 and high levels of Shh promotes induction of Olig2 and Nkx2.2 coexpressing cells, supporting the idea that FGFR activation contributes to maintain Olig2 expression in progenitor cells as they activate Nkx2.2 in response to high threshold Shh signaling.

We then postulated that, according to this conclusion, overexpression of FGF8 might be sufficient to promote Olig2/Nkx2.2 coexpression in ventral progenitor cells at the time of LFP formation, i.e. when Shh signaling activity rises in the ventral spinal cord. To test this, we overexpressed FGF8 at E4-E4.5 and analyzed expression of Olig2 and Nkx2.2 after 2 days in culture to cover the

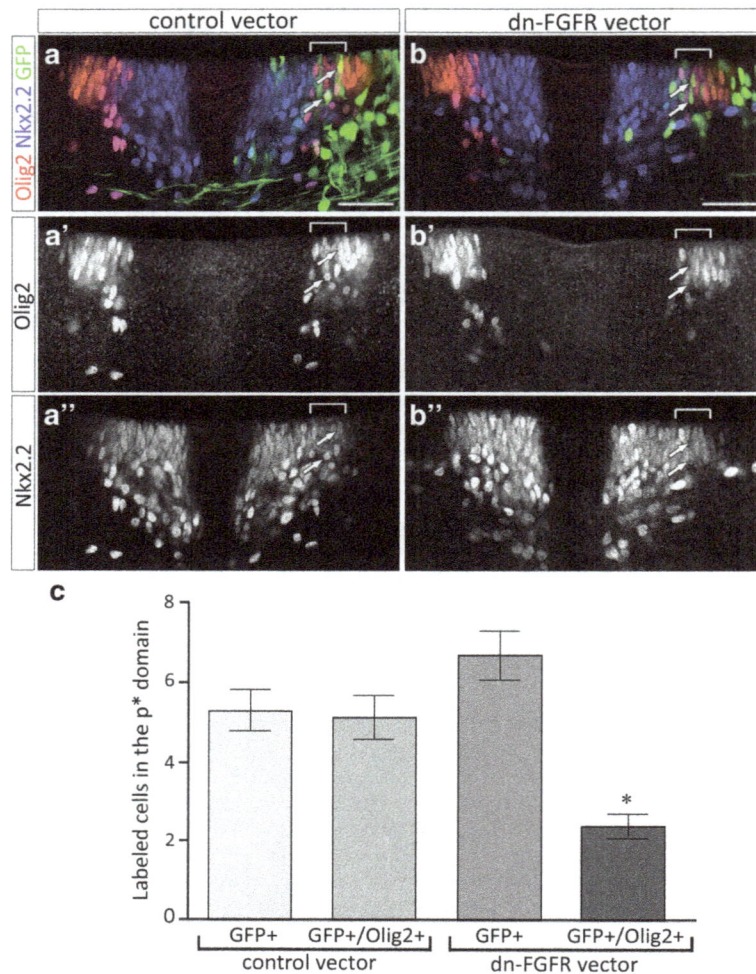

**Fig. 7** Cell autonomous activation of FGFRs on pMN progenitor cells is required to maintain Olig2 expression at the time of OPC specification. **a-b** Immunodetection of Olig2 (red in **a** and **b**, **a'**, **b'**) and Nkx2.2 (blue in **a** and **b**, **a"**, **b"**) on transverse sections of explants electroporated with the control vector (green in **a**) or with the dnFGFR vector (green in **b**) and cultivated for 2 days. Note the reduced number of Olig2/Nkx2.2-positive cells generated in the dnFGFR electroporated side of explant in (**b**). Note also diminished level of Olig2 expression in progenitor cells electroporated with the dnFGFR vector (arrows in **b**) compared to those electroporated with the control vector (arrows in **a**). **c** Quantification of GFP-positive and GFP/Olig2-positive cells in the $p*$ domain (brackets in **a**, **a'**, **a"**, **b**, **b'**, **b"**) in control ($n = 3$) and dnFGFR electroporated ($n = 4$) explants. Results are presented as mean number of cells $\pm$ sem (* $p \leq 0.03$). Scale bars = 50 μm

time period of Shh signaling activation. Contrasting with data got in the earlier neural tube, we found that electroporation of the FGF8 expression vector in these later stages, invariably promoted induction of Olig2 and Nkx2.2 coexpression in ventral progenitor cells compared to explants electroporated with control vector (Fig. 9a, b). To define whether the inductive activity of FGF8 at these later stages depends of Shh, we performed similar experiments incubating explants with cyclopamine. In agreement with previous report [3], we found that, after 2 days in culture in explants electroporated with the control vector, cyclopamine treatment downregulated Olig2 expression in pMN progenitor cells and prevented dorsal extension of the Nkx2.2 domain thus

totally abolishing OPC production (Fig. 9c). Similar experiments were then performed in explants electroporated with the FGF8 vector. In this context, the Olig2 progenitor domain as such was still not detectable either in FGF8 electroporated or non electroporated sides of explants and very few Olig2/Nkx2.2 coexpressing cells were found emigrating in the mantle layer in the electroporated side of explants (Fig. 9d). Therefore, FGF8 overexpression, although able to rescue generation of very few Nkx2.2/Olig2-coexpressing cells, was not sufficient to prevent cyclopamine-dependent down-regulation of Olig2 in progenitor cells.

Together, these data provide additional support to the view that commitment of ventral spinal OPCs depends

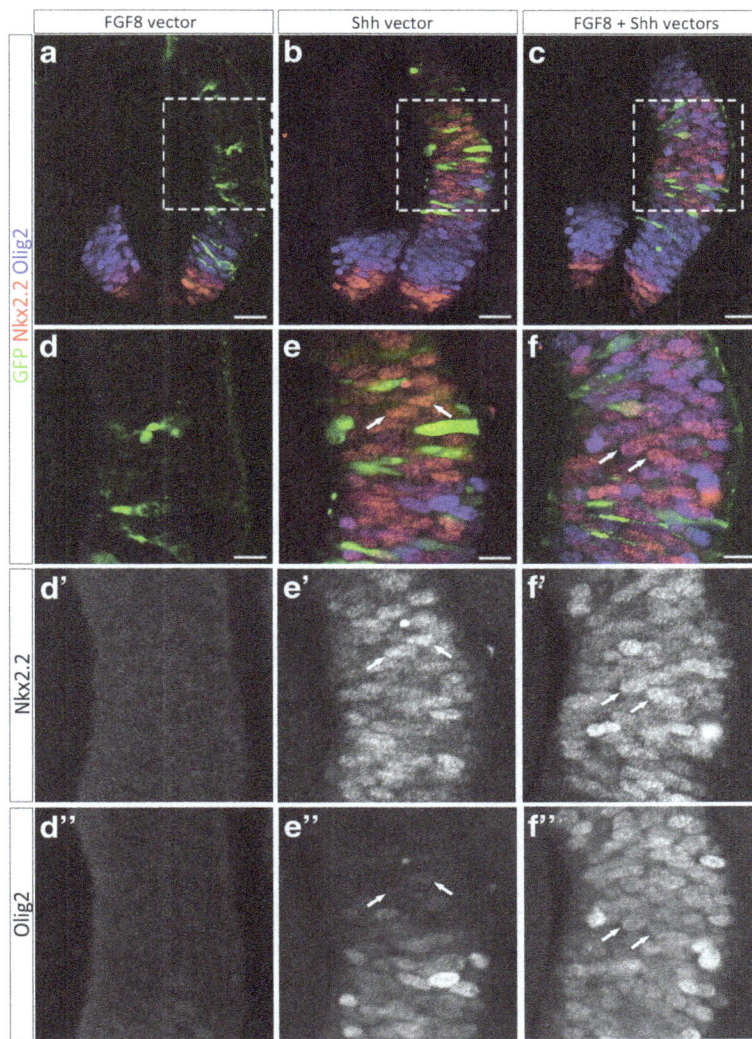

**Fig. 8** Coexposure of neural progenitor cells to FGF8 and Shh signals favors co-expression of Olig2 and Nkx2.2. **a-f**: Immunodetection of Olig2 (blue) and Nkx2.2 (red) on transverse E2.5 neural tube sections after electroporation at E1.5 with FGF8 (**a**, **d**), Shh (**b**, **e**) or both FGF8 and Shh expression vectors (**c**, **f**). **d**, **e** and **f** show higher magnification of the areas framed in (**a**, **b**) and (**c**), respectively. Note that Olig2 expression is detected in most of the Nkx2.2 positive cells induced by overexpression of both FGF8 and Shh (arrows in **f**, **f'** and **f"**) but not in Nkx2.2 positive cell induced by overexpression of Shh alone (arrows in **e**, **e'** and **e"**). Scale bars = 50 μm in **a-c**, 25 μm in **d-f**

on combined activation of FGF and Shh signaling, a cell context favoring Olig2 and Nkx2.2 coexpression.

### FGF8 is a good candidate for triggering induction of ventral OPCs in vivo

Our results raise the question of which cell subtype delivers FGF(s) signal(s) to initiate OPC commitment. FGF8 being efficient in its ability to induce OPCs, we analyzed its expression over spinal cord development. At E2.5, during ongoing generation of neurons, we did not find *fgf8* expression in the spinal cord (Fig. 10a). By contrast, from E4, high levels of *fgf8* expression were detected in sub-set of neurons located at the lateral edge of the progenitor zone. These neurons were at first restricted to intermediate regions of the developing spinal cord but they further shifted ventrally to position themselves in the vicinity of the p3 and pMN domains (Fig. 10b, c). Comparison with the expression pattern of Pax2, a specific marker of interneurons in the ventral spinal cord [11], was supportive of *fgf8* being expressed in ventral interneuron sub-types (Fig. 10d-f). Activation of FGF8 in a subset of ventral neurons at the right time and place makes this ligand a good candidate to cooperate with Shh for OPC induction in the ventral spinal cord. Unexpectedly, these data also open the possibility that ventral interneurons might be players of Olig2 progenitor decision to engage in OPC generation.

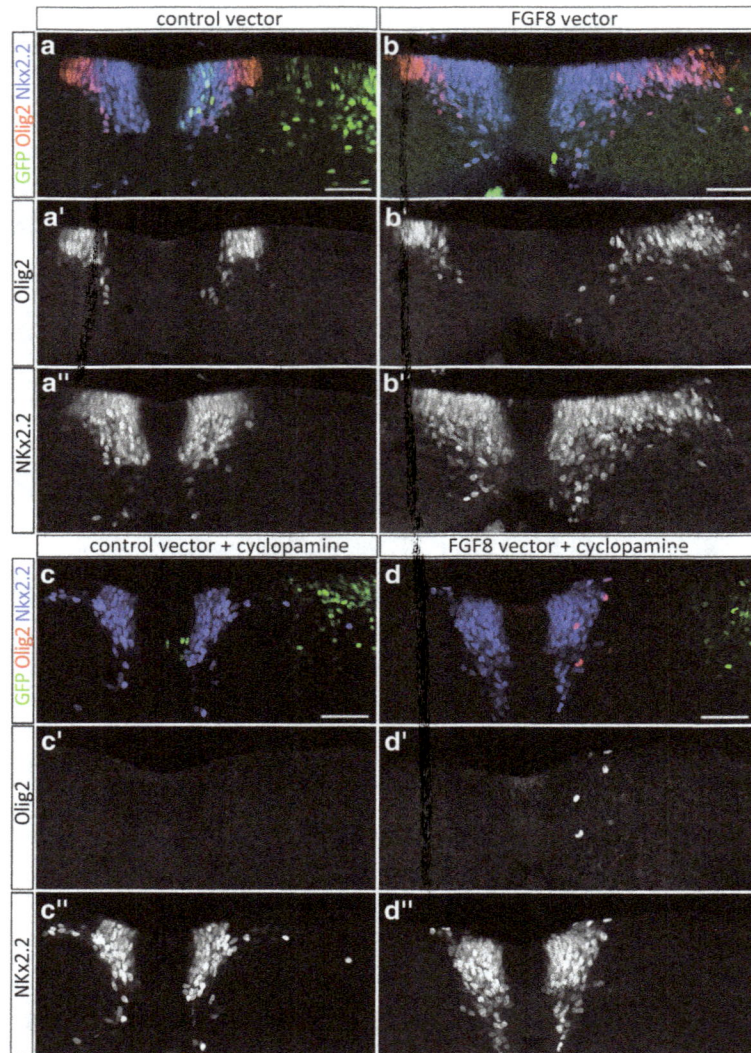

**Fig. 9** FGF8 promotes OPC specification following a Shh-dependent process. **a-b** Immunodetection of Olig2 (red in **a** and **b**, **a'**, **b'**) and Nkx2.2 (blue in **a** and **b**, **a"**, **b"**) on transverse sections of spinal cord explants cultivated for 2 days after electroporation of the control vector (green in **a**) or the FGF8 vector (green in **b**) at E4-E4.5. **c-d** Immunodetection of Olig2 (red in **c** and **d**, **c'**, **d'**) and Nkx2.2 (blue in **c** and **d**, **c"**, **d"**) on transverse sections of spinal cord explants electroporated with the control vector (green in **c**) or the FGF8 vector (green in **d**) and cultivated for 2 days in presence of cyclopamine. Scale bars = 50 μm

## Discussion

Olig2 progenitor cells of the ventral spinal cord stop generating MNs and start producing OPCs in response to timely activation of Shh signaling. Here, we report that FGFs are key regulators of Shh-mediated fate change in Olig2 progenitor cells, acting both upstream of Shh and together with Shh to ensure specification of ventral OPCs (Fig. 11). Our results support a model whereby newly differentiated ventral interneurons, that become providers of FGFs at the right time and place, might be initiators of the neuronal to oligodendroglial fate change in the ventral spinal cord.

Shh-mediated signaling has long been recognized as essential for the ventral phase of oligodendrogenesis in the spinal cord. Because of its ability to promote OPC generation in the neural tube, Shh was also considered for some time to be sufficient to induce OPC commitment from neural progenitor cells [20, 57, 62, 64, 72, 79]. The present study, by revealing that ventral OPC specification also needs FGFR signaling activation challenges this conclusion. Inactivation of FGFR signaling just prior to OPC specification proved to be as efficient to prevent generation of ventral OPCs as Shh signaling inhibition. The requirement of FGFR signaling for ventral spinal OPC specification is consistent with studies performed in various regions of the developing brain. Like in the spinal cord, the first wave of OPC production in the brain occurs in the ventral progenitor zone and requires Shh signaling

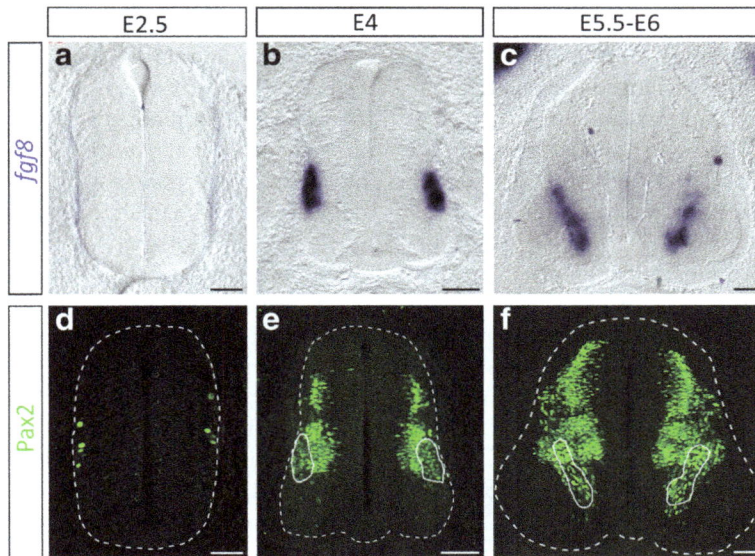

**Fig. 10** FGF8 expression is activated in ventral neurons at the time of OPC specification. **a-c** Time course of *fgf8* expression on transverse sections of brachial spinal cords isolated at E2.5 (**a**), E4 (**b**) and E5.5-E6 (**c**). **d-f** Immunodetection of Pax2 depicting spinal cord interneurons at E2.5 (**d**), E4 (**c**) and E5.5-E6 (**d**). Note that *fgf8* expressing cells correspond to a subpopulation of Pax2-positive cells (circled in **e**, **f**). Scale bars = 50 μm in **a**, **d** and 100 μm in **b**, **c**, **e**, **f**

activity [5, 29, 54, 73, 77]. However, evidence further emerged that lack of FGFR1/2 or FGFR inactivation in mouse and zebrafish result in failure of ventrally-derived brain OPCs to form properly [26, 30]. Requirement of FGFR signaling for generation of ventral OPCs therefore comes up as a conserved process in the central nervous system. In agreement with Furusho and collaborators [30], we found that FGFR signaling does not play a role in the regulation of cell proliferation or survival at stages of OPC generation but, instead, is part of the mechanism that triggers fate change of progenitor cells. Whether inactivation of FGFR signaling might trigger neural progenitors to follow a distinct neural fate, i.e. production of either neurons or astrocytes remains an opened question. We here highlight that FGFRs play a key role in changing the transcriptional identity of ventral progenitor cells over time, a change that ends up with induction of progenitor cells marked by Nkx2.2 and Olig2 coexpression. Activation of Nkx2.2 within Olig2 progenitor cells is well recognized to assign an OPC identity to these cells in chicken and zebrafish [3, 4, 42, 72, 83]. Combined expression of Olig2 and Nkx2.2 is also efficient in triggering OPC specification

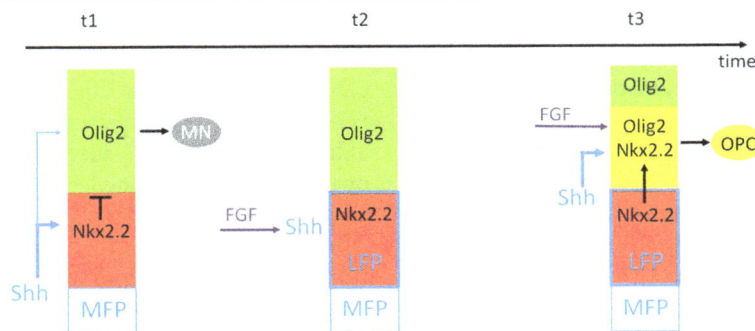

**Fig. 11** Model for FGF functions in OPC specification. At stage of ongoing neuronal generation (t1), the Olig2 (pMN, green) and Nkx2.2 (p3, red) progenitor domains do not overlap due to the repressive activity of Nkx2.2 on Olig2 expression. Olig2 progenitor cells generate motor neurons while Shh secreted by MFP cells activates low level of intracellular signaling (blue) to maintain expression of Olig2. As development proceeds (t2), Nkx2.2 progenitor cells become exposed to FGFs, possibly provided by ventral neurons. These cells subsequently up-regulate Shh expression to form the LFP. Soon after (t3), Olig2 progenitors, because they are submitted to higher Shh signaling activity, up-regulate Nkx2.2. At that time, Olig2 expression is no more repressed by Nkx2.2 thanks to joint exposure of these cells to FGFs. Olig2 and Nkx2.2 coexpressing progenitor cells, included in the p* domain (yellow), then start generating OPCs

from human embryonic stem cells [34]. Although the role of Nkx2.2 in OPC specification is still uncertain in mouse, Nkx2.2 has been reported to be up-regulated in Olig2 progenitor cells at the time OPC specification also in this species [38, 76, 78] and this transcription factor, which is maintained in migratory OPCs, controls the timing of their differentiation [12, 28, 32, 66, 76, 84]. Up-regulation of Nkx2.2 in Olig2 progenitor cells is known to depend on time activation of Shh signaling that occurs in the ventral spinal cord immediately prior to OPC specification [4, 19, 20, 78]. In agreement, Nkx2.2 is a direct but also high threshold Shh responsive gene [43, 44, 67, 81]. Our study, while not calling into question the role Shh in assigning an Nkx2.2 identity to Olig2 progenitor cells, reveals essential roles of FGFs in this process.

The present study unravels a complex interplay between Shh and FGFR signaling for ventral OPC induction. First, FGFR signaling, by inducing LFP formation, establishes a novel Shh signaling center in close proximity to Olig2 progenitor cells. FGFs therefore emerge as positive regulators of Shh expression in the ventral spinal cord. FGFs have already been involved in induction of Shh source cells, namely MFP cells [70]. However, mechanisms involved in induction of MFP and LFP are quite different. While FGFs regulate the competence of prospective MFP cells to respond to the Shh inductive signal [70], we found that LFP induction in response to FGFR activation occurs independently of Shh. Importantly, failure of LFP induction, that occurs when FGFR are inactivated in LFP prospective cells of the p3 domain, is sufficient to prevent OPC specification. Therefore, Shh provided by MFP cells is not able to compensate the deficient production of Shh caused by lack of LFP formation. This is in agreement with our previous work showing that the extracellular enzyme Sulf1 contributes to induce OPCs by favoring provision of active forms of the morphogen by LFP cells but not by MFP cells [4, 78]. Thus, the present study not only directly demonstrates that LFP induction is an obligatory step to turn Olig2 progenitor cells to the OPC fate but also reveals the essential function of FGFs, acting upstream of Shh, in the induction of ventral OPCs.

In addition to their role in LFP induction, FGFRs proved to assume a second essential function in the control of OPC specification: they act cell-autonomously on progenitor cells of the pMN domain to ensure high level of Olig2 expression as these cells up-regulate Nkx2.2. Previous reports have convincingly shown that dorsal spinal progenitor cells in culture up-regulate Olig2 expression in response to FGFs [1, 9, 13, 14, 31, 40]. However, different underlying molecular mechanisms, dependent of Shh [31, 40] or independent of Shh [1, 9, 13, 14] have

been proposed. The data presented here indicate that FGFR activation in spinal cord progenitor cells is not efficient in inducing Olig2 expression in progenitor cells in their endogenous context of the neural tube or when Shh signaling activity is impaired. Therefore, in the developing spinal cord, FGFR signaling regulates Olig2 expression at least in part through a Shh-dependent mechanism. Furthermore, at the time of OPC specification, attenuation of Olig2 expression by FGFR inactivation is noticed only when the LFP can form properly in ventral spinal cord explants. Olig2 expression in progenitor cells indeed appeared unaffected in experimental contexts where LFP formation has been prevented, i.e. when FGFRs were inactivated in both the p3 and pMN domains using FGFR inhibitors or when FGFR inactivation was limited to cells of the p3 domain by targeted overexpression of the dnFGFR. We therefore conclude that the cell-autonomous FGFR activation is needed to ensure maintenance of Olig2 expression only when these cells are submitted to high Shh signaling activity, i.e. when they activate Nkx2.2 expression. Reinforcing this conclusion, FGFR activation in the neural tube becomes a potent activator of Olig2 and Nkx2.2 coexpression when combined with Shh overproduction. Although the underlying mechanisms remains to be elucidated, this observation introduces FGF signaling as a way to prevent the Nkx2.2-dependent Olig2 repression in cells of the prospective p* domain as these cells upregulate Nkx2.2 in response to elevation of Shh signaling.

Two distinct models to account for FGF and Shh interplay in induction of ventral brain OPCs have been proposed. Esain and collaborators [26] proposed a model in which Shh first establishes a progenitor cell domain competent to express Olig2 and then, FGFR signaling permits Olig2 gene transcription. By contrast, Furusho and collaborators [30] proposed that FGFRs function downstream of Shh in the induction of ventrally derived OPCs. Our study by highlighting dual functions for FGFRs, acting both upstream of Shh and together with Shh to control OPC specification in the spinal cord might, somehow reconciles these apparently contradictory models. However, whether time activation of Shh signaling activity underlies initiation of OPC commitment in the developing brain remains to be established.

Our work opens the question of the source of FGFR ligands responsible for ventral OPC specification. Of the FGF members, FGF8, known to bind all four FGFRs and to control neural progenitor cell patterning in the embryonic brain [17, 18, 58], represents a good candidate. Populations of ventral spinal neurons, which progressively locate in close proximity to Olig2 progenitor cells, indeed up-regulate FGF8 at the right time to account for

OPC induction. The interesting idea behind is that ventral spinal neurons, that are generated before OPC specification, might represent key initiators of oligodendrogenesis, an area that has yet to be explored.

## Conclusions

In conclusion, our study evidence that the coordination of Olig2 progenitor cell fate transition in the ventral spinal cord is primarily controlled by FGF signaling. This study furthermore elucidate an intimate interplay between FGFs and Shh in this process where FGFs are responsible for provision of higher threshold Shh signal while ensuring appropriate response to this signal in Shh receiving cells.

### Abbreviations
FGF: Fibroblast growth factor; FGFR: Fibroblast growth factor receptor; FP: Floor plate; LFP: Lateral floor plate; MN: Motor neuron; OPC: Oligodendrocyte precursor cell; Shh: Sonic hedgehog

### Acknowledgements
We acknowledge J. Guimera, S. Martinez, K. Storey, C. Tabin and R. Bansal who kindly provided us with valuable reagents. We are grateful to colleagues in the CBD for help, encouragement and advice. We thank the Toulouse Regional Imaging Platform (TRI) for technical assistance in confocal microscopy. We acknowledge the Developmental Studies Hybridoma Bank, developed under the auspice of NICHD and maintained by the University of Iowa, Department of Biological Sciences, Iowa City, IA, for supplying monoclonal antibodies.

### Funding
This work was supported by the Agence Nationale de la Recherche (ANR); the Fondation pour l'Aide à la Recherche sur la Sclérose En Plaques (ARSEP); the Centre National de la.
Recherche Scientifique (CNRS) and the University of Toulouse. M-A.F. was supported by grant from French Ministry of National Education, Research, and Technology.

### Authors' contributions
M-AF and EA planned, performed and analyzed experiments. SB-V., NE, NK-F. and ChS performed experiments. CD and PC analyzed experiments and participated in writing the manuscript. FP provided scientific input on the project and revised the manuscript. CS supervised the project, planned the experiments, analyzed the data and wrote the manuscript. All authors read and approved the final manuscript.

### Competing interests
The authors declare that they have no competing interests.

### References
1. Abematsu M, Kagawa T, Fukuda S, Inoue T, Takebayashi H, Komiya S, Taga T. Basic fibroblast growth factor endows dorsal telencephalic neural progenitors with the ability to differentiate into oligodendrocytes but not gamma-aminobutyric acidergic neurons. J Neurosci Res. 2006;83:731–43.
2. Agius E, Decker Y, Soukkarieh C, Soula C, Cochard P. Role of BMPs in controlling the spatial and temporal origin of GFAP astrocytes in the embryonic spinal cord. Dev Biol. 2010;344:611–20.
3. Agius E, Soukkarieh C, Danesin C, Kan P, Takebayashi H, Soula C, Cochard P. Converse control of oligodendrocyte and astrocyte lineage development by sonic hedgehog in the chick spinal cord. Dev Biol. 2004;270:308–21.
4. Al Oustah A, Danesin C, Khouri-Farah N, Farreny MA, Escalas N, Cochard P, Glise B, Soula C. Dynamics of sonic hedgehog signaling in the ventral spinal cord are controlled by intrinsic changes in source cells requiring sulfatase 1. Development. 2014;141:1392–403.
5. Alberta JA, Park SK, Mora J, Yuk D, Pawlitzky I, Iannarelli P, Vartanian T, Stiles CD, Rowitch DH. Sonic hedgehog is required during an early phase of oligodendrocyte development in mammalian brain. Mol Cell Neurosci. 2001; 18:434–41.
6. Amaya E, Musci TJ, Kirschner MW. Expression of a dominant negative mutant of the FGF receptor disrupts mesoderm formation in Xenopus embryos. Cell. 1991;66:257–70.
7. Bansal R, Lakhina V, Remedios R, Tole S. Expression of FGF receptors 1, 2, 3 in the embryonic and postnatal mouse brain compared with Pdgfralpha, Olig2 and Plp/dm20: implications for oligodendrocyte development. Dev Neurosci. 2003;25:83–95.
8. Bergles DE, Richardson WD. Oligodendrocyte development and plasticity. Cold Spring Harb Perspect Biol. 2015;8:a020453.
9. Bilican B, Fiore-Heriche C, Compston A, Allen ND, Chandran S. Induction of Olig2 precursors by FGF involves BMP signalling blockade at the Smad level. PLoS One. 2008;3:e2863.
10. Braquart-Varnier C, Danesin C, Clouscard-Martinato C, Agius E, Escalas N, Benazeraf B, Ai X, Emerson C, Cochard P, Soula C. A subtractive approach to characterize genes with regionalized expression in the gliogenic ventral neuroepithelium: identification of chick sulfatase 1 as a new oligodendrocyte lineage gene. Mol Cell Neurosci. 2004;25:612–28.
11. Burrill JD, Moran L, Goulding MD, Saueressig H. PAX2 is expressed in multiple spinal cord interneurons, including a population of EN1+ interneurons that require PAX6 for their development. Development. 1997; 124:4493–503.
12. Cai J, Zhu Q, Zheng K, Li H, Qi Y, Cao Q, Qiu M. Co-localization of Nkx6.2 and Nkx2.2 homeodomain proteins in differentiated myelinating oligodendrocytes. Glia. 2010;58:458–68.
13. Cai J, Qi Y, Hu X, Tan M, Liu Z, Zhang J, Li Q, Sander M, Qiu M. Generation of oligodendrocyte precursor cells from mouse dorsal spinal cord independent of Nkx6 regulation and Shh signaling. Neuron. 2005;45:41–53.
14. Chandran S, Kato H, Gerreli D, Compston A, Svendsen CN, Allen ND. FGF-dependent generation of oligodendrocytes by a hedgehog-independent pathway. Development. 2003;130:6599–609.
15. Charrier JB, Lapointe F, Le Douarin NM, Teillet MA. Dual origin of the floor plate in the avian embryo. Development. 2002;129:4785–96.
16. Cooper MK, Porter JA, Young KE, Beachy PA. Teratogen-mediated inhibition of target tissue response to Shh signaling. Science. 1998;280:1603–7.
17. Crossley PH, Martin GR. The mouse Fgf8 gene encodes a family of polypeptides and is expressed in regions that direct outgrowth and patterning in the developing embryo. Development. 1995;121:439–51.
18. Crossley PH, Martinez S, Martin GR. Midbrain development induced by FGF8 in the chick embryo. Nature. 1996;380:66–8.
19. Danesin C, Soula C. Moving the Shh source over time: what impact on neural cell diversification in the developing spinal cord? J Dev Bio. 2017;5(2):4.
20. Danesin C, Agius E, Escalas N, Ai X, Emerson C, Cochard P, Soula C. Ventral neural progenitors switch toward an oligodendroglial fate in response to increased sonic hedgehog (Shh) activity: involvement of sulfatase 1 in modulating Shh signaling in the ventral spinal cord. J Neurosci. 2006;26:5037–48.
21. Dessaud E, McMahon AP, Briscoe J. Pattern formation in the vertebrate neural tube: a sonic hedgehog morphogen-regulated transcriptional network. Development. 2008;135:2489–503.

22. Dessaud E, Yang LL, Hill K, Cox B, Ulloa F, Ribeiro A, Mynett A, Novitch BG, Briscoe J. Interpretation of the sonic hedgehog morphogen gradient by a temporal adaptation mechanism. Nature. 2007;450:717–20.

23. Eblaghie MC, Lunn JS, Dickinson RJ, Münsterberg AE, Sanz-Ezquerro JJ, Farrell ER, Mathers J, Keyse SM, Storey K, Tickle C. Negative feedback regulation of FGF signaling levels by Pyst1/MKP3 in chick embryos. Curr Biol. 2003;13:1009–18.

24. Echevarria D, Martinez S, Marques S, Lucas-Teixeira V, Belo JA. Mkp3 is a negative feedback modulator of Fgf8 signaling in the mammalian isthmic organizer. Dev Biol. 2005;277:114–28.

25. Ericson J, Morton S, Kawakami A, Roelink H, Jessell TM. Two critical periods of sonic hedgehog signaling required for the specification of motor neuron identity. Cell. 1996;87:661–73.

26. Esain V, Postlethwait JH, Charnay P, Ghislain J. FGF-receptor signalling controls neural cell diversity in the zebrafish hindbrain by regulating olig2 and sox9. Development. 2010;137:33–42.

27. Fogarty M, Richardson WD, Kessaris N. A subset of oligodendrocytes generated from radial glia in the dorsal spinal cord. Development. 2005;132: 1951–9.

28. Fu H, Qi Y, Tan M, Cai J, Takebayashi H, Nakafuku M, Richardson W, Qiu M. Dual origin of spinal oligodendrocyte progenitors and evidence for the cooperative role of Olig2 and Nkx2.2 in the control of oligodendrocyte differentiation. Development. 2002;129:681–93.

29. Fuccillo M, Rallu M, McMahon AP, Fishell G. Temporal requirement for hedgehog signaling in ventral telencephalic patterning. Development. 2004; 131:5031–40.

30. Furusho M, Kaga Y, Ishii A, Hébert JM, Bansal R. Fibroblast growth factor signaling is required for the generation of oligodendrocyte progenitors from the embryonic forebrain. J Neurosci. 2011;31:5055–66.

31. Gabay L, Lowell S, Rubin LL, Anderson DJ. Deregulation of dorsoventral patterning by FGF confers trilineage differentiation capacity on CNS stem cells in vitro. Neuron. 2003;40:485–99.

32. Gokhan S, Marin-Husstege M, Yung SY, Fontanez D, Casaccia-Bonnefil P, Mehler MF. Combinatorial profiles of oligodendrocyte-selective classes of transcriptional regulators differentially modulate myelin basic protein gene expression. J Neurosci. 2005;25:8311–21.

33. Hamburger V, Hamilton HL. A series of normal stages in the development of the chick embryo. 1951. Dev Dyn. 1992;195:231–72.

34. Hu BY, Du ZW, Li XJ, Ayala M, Zhang SC. Human oligodendrocytes from embryonic stem cells: conserved SHH signaling networks and divergent FGF effects. Development. 2009;136:1443–52.

35. Incardona JP, Gaffield W, Kapur RP, Roelink H. The teratogenic Veratrum alkaloid cyclopamine inhibits sonic hedgehog signal transduction. Development. 1998;125:3553–62.

36. Itasaki N, Bel-Vialar S, Krumlauf R. 'Shocking' developments in chick embryology: electroporation and in ovo gene expression. Nat Cell Biol. 1999;1:E203–7.

37. Jeong J, McMahon AP. Growth and pattern of the mammalian neural tube are governed by partially overlapping feedback activities of the hedgehog antagonists patched 1 and Hhip1. Development. 2005;132:143–54.

38. Jiang W, Ishino Y, Hashimoto H, Keino-Masu K, Masu M, Uchimura K, Kadomatsu K, Yoshimura T, Ikenaka K. Sulfatase 2 modulates fate change from motor neurons to oligodendrocyte precursor cells through coordinated regulation of Shh signaling with sulfatase 1. Dev Neurosci. 2017;39(5):361–74.

39. Kawakami Y, Rodríguez-León J, Koth CM, Büscher D, Itoh T, Raya A, Ng JK, Esteban CR, Takahashi S, Henrique D, Schwarz MF, Asahara H, Izpisúa Belmonte JC. MKP3 mediates the cellular response to FGF8 signalling in the vertebrate limb. Nat Cell Biol. 2003;5:513–9.

40. Kessaris N, Jamen F, Rubin LL, Richardson WD. Cooperation between sonic hedgehog and fibroblast growth factor/MAPK signalling pathways in neocortical precursors. Development. 2004;131:1289–98.

41. Kim HJ, Bar-Sagi D. Modulation of signalling by Sprouty: a developing story. Nat Rev Mol Cell Biol. 2004;5:441–50.

42. Kucenas S, Snell H, Appel B. nkx2.2a promotes specification and differentiation of a myelinating subset of oligodendrocyte lineage cells in zebrafish. Neuron Glia Biol. 2008;4:71–81.

43. Lei Q, Jeong Y, Misra K, Li S, Zelman AK, Epstein DJ, Matise MP. Wnt signaling inhibitors regulate the transcriptional response to morphogenetic Shh-Gli signaling in the neural tube. Dev Cell. 2006;11: 325–37.

44. Lek M, Dias JM, Marklund U, Uhde CW, Kurdija S, Lei Q, Sussel L, Rubenstein JL, Matise MP, Arnold HH, Jessell TM, Ericson J. A homeodomain feedback circuit underlies step-function interpretation of a Shh morphogen gradient during ventral neural patterning. Development. 2010;137:4051–60.

45. Liu Z, Hu X, Cai J, Liu B, Peng X, Wegner M, Qiu M. Induction of oligodendrocyte differentiation by Olig2 and Sox10: evidence for reciprocal interactions and dosage-dependent mechanisms. Dev Biol. 2007;302:683–93.

46. Lu QR, Yuk D, Alberta JA, Zhu Z, Pawlitzky I, Chan J, McMahon AP, Stiles CD, Rowitch DH. Sonic hedgehog–regulated oligodendrocyte lineage genes encoding bHLH proteins in the mammalian central nervous system. Neuron. 2000;25:317–29.

47. Mason I. Initiation to end point: the multiple roles of fibroblast growth factors in neural development. Nat Rev Neurosci. 2007;8:583–96.

48. Mekki-Dauriac S, Agius E, Kan P, Cochard P. Bone morphogenetic proteins negatively control oligodendrocyte precursor specification in the chick spinal cord. Development. 2002;129:5117–30.

49. Miller RH, Payne J, Milner L, Zhang H, Orentas DM. Spinal cord oligodendrocytes develop from a limited number of migratory highly proliferative precursors. J Neurosci Res. 1997;50:157–68.

50. Miller RH, Dinsio K, Wang R, Geertman R, Maier CE, Hall AK. Patterning of spinal cord oligodendrocyte development by dorsally derived BMP4. J Neurosci Res. 2004;76:9–19.

51. Minowada G, Jarvis LA, Chi CL, Neubüser A, Sun X, Hacohen N, Krasnow MA, Martin GR. Vertebrate Sprouty genes are induced by FGF signaling and can cause chondrodysplasia when overexpressed. Development. 1999;126:4465–75.

52. Mohammadi M, McMahon G, Sun L, Tang C, Hirth P, Yeh BK, Hubbard SR, Schlessinger J. Structures of the tyrosine kinase domain of fibroblast growth factor receptor in complex with inhibitors. Science. 1997;276:955–60.

53. Naruse M, Nakahira E, Miyata T, Hitoshi S, Ikenaka K, Bansal R. Induction of oligodendrocyte progenitors in dorsal forebrain by intraventricular microinjection of FGF-2. Dev Biol. 2006;297:262–73.

54. Nery S, Wichterle H, Fishell G. Sonic hedgehog contributes to oligodendrocyte specification in the mammalian forebrain. Development. 2001;128:527–40.

55. Novitch BG, Chen AI, Jessell TM. Coordinate regulation of motor neuron subtype identity and pan-neuronal properties by the bHLH repressor Olig2. Neuron. 2001;31:773–89.

56. Ono K, Bansal R, Payne J, Rutishauser U, Miller RH. Early development and dispersal of oligodendrocyte precursors in the embryonic chick spinal cord. Development. 1995;121:1743–54.

57. Orentas DM, Hayes JE, Dyer KL, Miller RH. Sonic hedgehog signaling is required during the appearance of spinal cord oligodendrocyte precursors. Development. 1999;126:2419–29.

58. Ornitz DM, Xu J, Colvin JS, McEwen DG, MacArthur CA, Coulier F, Gao G, Goldfarb M. Receptor specificity of the fibroblast growth factor family. J Biol Chem. 1996;271:15292–7.

59. Panek RL, Lu GH, Dahring TK, Batley BL, Connolly C, Hamby JM, Brown KJ. In vitro biological characterization and antiangiogenic effects of PD 166866, a selective inhibitor of the FGF-1 receptor tyrosine kinase. J Pharmacol Exp Ther. 1998;286:569–77.

60. Park HC, Shin J, Appel B. Spatial and temporal regulation of ventral spinal cord precursor specification by hedgehog signaling. Development. 2004; 131:5959–69.

61. Pombero A, Bueno C, Saglietti L, Rodenas M, Guimera J, Bulfone A, Martinez S. Pallial origin of basal forebrain cholinergic neurons in the nucleus basalis of Meynert and horizontal limb of the diagonal band nucleus. Development. 2011;138:4315–26.

62. Poncet C, Soula C, Trousse F, Kan P, Hirsinger E, Pourquié O, Duprat AM, Cochard P. Induction of oligodendrocyte progenitors in the trunk neural tube by ventralizing signals: effects of notochord and floor plate grafts, and of sonic hedgehog. Mech Dev. 1996;60:13–32.

63. Pringle NP, Yu WP, Howell M, Colvin JS, Ornitz DM, Richardson WD. Fgfr3 expression by astrocytes and their precursors: evidence that astrocytes and oligodendrocytes originate in distinct neuroepithelial domains. Development. 2003;130:93–102.

64. Pringle NP, Yu WP, Guthrie S, Roelink H, Lumsden A, Peterson AC, Richardson WD. Determination of neuroepithelial cell fate: induction of the oligodendrocyte lineage by ventral midline cells and sonic hedgehog. Dev Biol. 1996;177:30–42.

65. Qi Y, Tan M, Hui CC, Qiu M. Gli2 is required for normal Shh signaling and oligodendrocyte development in the spinal cord. Mol Cell Neurosci. 2003; 23:440–50.

66. Qi Y, Cai J, Wu Y, Wu R, Lee J, Fu H, Rao M, Sussel L, Rubenstein J, Qiu M. Control of oligodendrocyte differentiation by the Nkx2.2 homeodomain transcription factor. Development. 2001;128:2723–33.

67. Ribes V, Balaskas N, Sasai N, Cruz C, Dessaud E, Cayuso J, Tozer S, Yang LL, Novitch B, Marti E, Briscoe J. Distinct sonic hedgehog signaling dynamics specify floor plate and ventral neuronal progenitors in the vertebrate neural tube. Genes Dev. 2010;24:1186–200.

68. Rowitch DH. Glial specification in the vertebrate neural tube. Nat Rev Neurosci. 2004;5:409–19.

69. Rowitch DH, Kriegstein AR. Developmental genetics of vertebrate glial-cell specification. Nature. 2010;468:214–22.

70. Sasai N, Kutejova E, Briscoe J. Integration of signals along orthogonal axes of the vertebrate neural tube controls progenitor competence and increases cell diversity. PLoS Biol. 2014;12:e1001907.

71. Schäfer M, Kinzel D, Winkler C. Discontinuous organization and specification of the lateral floor plate in zebrafish. Dev Biol. 2007;301:117–29.

72. Soula C, Danesin C, Kan P, Grob M, Poncet C, Cochard P. Distinct sites of origin of oligodendrocytes and somatic motoneurons in the chick spinal cord: oligodendrocytes arise from Nkx2.2-expressing progenitors by a Shh-dependent mechanism. Development. 2001;128:1369–79.

73. Spassky N, Heydon K, Mangatal A, Jankovski A, Olivier C, Queraud-Lesaux F, Goujet-Zalc C, Thomas JL, Zalc B. Sonic hedgehog-dependent emergence of oligodendrocytes in the telencephalon: evidence for a source of oligodendrocytes in the olfactory bulb that is independent of PDGFRalpha signaling. Development. 2001;128:4993–5004.

74. Stamataki D, Ulloa F, Tsoni SV, Mynett A, Briscoe J. A gradient of Gli activity mediates graded sonic hedgehog signaling in the neural tube. Genes Dev. 2005;19:626–41.

75. Sun T, Dong H, Wu L, Kane M, Rowitch DH, Stiles CD. Cross-repressive interaction of the Olig2 and Nkx2.2 transcription factors in developing neural tube associated with formation of a specific physical complex. J Neurosci. 2003;23:9547–56.

76. Sun T, Echelard Y, Lu R, Yuk DI, Kaing S, Stiles CD, Rowitch DH. Olig bHLH proteins interact with homeodomain proteins to regulate cell fate acquisition in progenitors of the ventral neural tube. Curr Biol. 2001;11:1413–20.

77. Tekki-Kessaris N, Woodruff R, Hall AC, Gaffield W, Kimura S, Stiles CD, Rowitch DH, Richardson WD. Hedgehog-dependent oligodendrocyte lineage specification in the telencephalon. Development. 2001a;128:2545–54.

78. Touahri Y, Escalas N, Benazeraf B, Cochard P, Danesin C, Soula C. Sulfatase 1 promotes the motor neuron-to-oligodendrocyte fate switch by activating Shh signaling in Olig2 progenitors of the embryonic ventral spinal cord. J Neurosci. 2012;32:18018–34.

79. Trousse F, Giess MC, Soula C, Ghandour S, Duprat AM, Cochard P. Notochord and floor plate stimulate oligodendrocyte differentiation in cultures of the chick dorsal neural tube. J Neurosci Res. 1995;41:552–60.

80. Vallstedt A, Klos JM, Ericson J. Multiple dorsoventral origins of oligodendrocyte generation in the spinal cord and hindbrain. Neuron. 2005;45:55–67.

81. Vokes SA, Ji H, McCuine S, Tenzen T, Giles S, Zhong S, Longabaugh WJ, Davidson EH, Wong WH, McMahon AP. Genomic characterization of Gli-activator targets in sonic hedgehog-mediated neural patterning. Development. 2007;134:1977–89.

82. Zhou Q, Wang S, Anderson DJ. Identification of a novel family of oligodendrocyte lineage-specific basic helix-loop-helix transcription factors. Neuron. 2000;25:331–43.

83. Zhou Q, Choi G, Anderson DJ. The bHLH transcription factor Olig2 promotes oligodendrocyte differentiation in collaboration with Nkx2.2. Neuron. 2001;31:791–807.

84. Zhu Q, Zhao X, Zheng K, Li H, Huang H, Zhang Z, Mastracci T, Wegner M, Chen Y, Sussel L, Qiu M. Genetic evidence that Nkx2.2 and Pdgfra are major determinants of the timing of oligodendrocyte differentiation in the developing CNS. Development. 2014;141:548–55.

# 3

# Fragile X mental retardation protein knockdown in the developing *Xenopus* tadpole optic tectum results in enhanced feedforward inhibition and behavioral deficits

Torrey L. S. Truszkowski[1], Eric J. James[1], Mashfiq Hasan[1], Tyler J. Wishard[2], Zhenyu Liu[3], Kara G. Pratt[3], Hollis T. Cline[2] and Carlos D. Aizenman[1]*

**Abstract**

**Background:** Fragile X Syndrome is the leading monogenetic cause of autism and most common form of intellectual disability. Previous studies have implicated changes in dendritic spine architecture as the primary result of loss of Fragile X Mental Retardation Protein (FMRP), but recent work has shown that neural proliferation is decreased and cell death is increased with either loss of FMRP or overexpression of FMRP. The purpose of this study was to investigate the effects of loss of FMRP on behavior and cellular activity.

**Methods:** We knocked down FMRP expression using morpholino oligos in the optic tectum of *Xenopus laevis* tadpoles and performed a series of behavioral and electrophysiological assays. We investigated visually guided collision avoidance, schooling, and seizure propensity. Using single cell electrophysiology, we assessed intrinsic excitability and synaptic connectivity of tectal neurons.

**Results:** We found that FMRP knockdown results in decreased swimming speed, reduced schooling behavior and decreased seizure severity. In single cells, we found increased inhibition relative to excitation in response to sensory input.

**Conclusions:** Our results indicate that the electrophysiological development of single cells in the absence of FMRP is largely unaffected despite the large neural proliferation defect. The changes in behavior are consistent with an increase in inhibition, which could be due to either changes in cell number or altered inhibitory drive, and indicate that FMRP can play a significant role in neural development much earlier than previously thought.

**Keywords:** Fragile X syndrome, Fragile X Mental Retardation Protein, inhibition, *Xenopus laevis*, FMRP

## Background

Fragile X Syndrome (FXS) is the leading monogenetic cause of autism and most common form of inherited intellectual disability [1–3]. FXS is typically caused by the expansion of a trinucleotide (CGG) repeat in the 5′ untranslated region of the Fragile X mental retardation 1 (FMR1) gene [4, 5]. The mutation prevents expression of

Fragile X Mental Retardation Protein (FMRP) throughout development. The most well understood neuroanatomical marker in FXS is the presence of immature dendritic spines in the cortex [6, 7]. This is thought to occur because FMRP is a RNA binding protein that inhibits protein synthesis downstream of group 1 metabotropic glutamate receptor activation [8], and therefore prevents normal plasticity and synaptic maturation. However, FMRP disruption prior to synapse formation results in abnormalities that may lead to neurodevelopmental deficits [9], indicating a possible role for FMRP much earlier than initially known.

---

* Correspondence: carlos_aizenman@brown.edu
[1]Department of Neuroscience, Brown University, Box G-LN60 Olive St., 02912 Providence, RI, USA
Full list of author information is available at the end of the article

Previous work from Faulkner et al. [10] identified a cell proliferation defect associated with excessive and decreased levels of FMRP. In this study, *Xenopus laevis* tadpoles were used to assess the early effects of FMRP upregulation and knockdown in the optic tectum. Tadpoles express FMRP throughout central nervous system (CNS) development [11, 12], and thus are ideally placed for studying the effects of FMR1 gene disruption during early development. Since tadpole development occurs in the absence of a womb, this experimental animal provides easy access to developmental stages that occur in utero in mammals [13]. The tadpole optic tectum is homologous to the mammalian superior colliculus and is the main sensory processing area in the tadpole [13]. The optic tectum receives direct visual input via retinal ganglion cells and generates outputs that directly inform behavior, and thus can be used to assay the emergence of functional properties of neural circuits during development.

Faulkner et al. [10] showed that FMR1 is expressed in neural progenitor cells that line the brain ventricle and neurons located lateral to the progenitor cells, as well as in puncta throughout the optic tectum. Both knockdown and overexpression of FMRP reduced cell proliferation in the tectum and increased cell death, providing evidence that FMRP is required at tightly controlled levels. Furthermore, Faulkner et al. [10] showed that FMRP regulates neuronal differentiation and dendritic morphology, with both overexpression and knockdown of FMRP levels resulting in abnormal numbers of neural progenitor cells and reduced dendritic arborization of tectal neurons. These results indicate a critical role for FMRP in early development, both in the generation of new neurons and in the wiring of the proper neural circuit. These data also suggest a clear role for FMRP prior to synapse formation. However, this study did not investigate the consequences of abnormal proliferation and arborization on the functional properties of tectal circuits. Furthermore, it is not clear how the cells that do survive are affected by knockdown of FMRP.

Here we investigate the behavioral and cellular changes induced by FMRP knockdown in the optic tectum. We use translation-blocking antisense morpholino oligonucleotides to decrease FMRP expression in the optic tectum during a key developmental period. We measured behavior using several assays that measure swimming speed, escape responses, social aggregation, and seizure susceptibility. We also investigated the electrophysiological properties of cells in the optic tectum. Our results show that FMRP knockdown results in decreased swimming speed, reduced schooling behavior and decreased seizure severity. However, FMRP knockdown does not perturb intrinsic properties of tectal neurons, but rather results in enhanced synaptic inhibition. This circuit abnormality is consistent with the behavioral results and shows that the early effects seen for FMRP knockdown have important functional consequences.

## Methods

All animal experiments were performed in accordance with and approved by Brown University Institutional Animal Care and Use Committee standards.

### Experimental animals

Tadpoles were raised in Steinberg's rearing media on a 12 h light/dark cycle at 18–21 °C for 7–8 d, until they reached developmental stage 46 [10, 14]. They were then electroporated with the FMR1 or scrambled control morpholino and reared until they reached developmental stages of either 47 or 49, depending on the experiment (see below). Developmental stages of tadpoles were determined according to [14]. The rearing medium was renewed every 3 d. Tadpoles that were used for acoustic startle, schooling, or seizure protocols were not used again for other experiments, whereas after visual avoidance experiments, tadpoles were in some cases also used in startle and schooling experiments after having 24 h of rest in the rearing solution. At least two different clutches of tadpoles from different husbandry were used for every set of behavioral experiments. Animals of either sex were used because at these developmental stages tadpoles of either sex are phenotypically indistinguishable.

### Morpholinos

As described and validated in a prior study [10], a Xenopus laevis homolog of FMR1, fmr1a, was knocked down using a 3′ lissamine-tagged translation-blocking antisense morpholino oligonucleotide (GeneTools) with the sequence 5′-AGCTCCTC<u>CAT</u>GTTGCGTCCGCACA-3′ (start codon underlined), referred to as fmr1a MO to generate FMRP knockdown (FMRP KD). Control lissamine-tagged oligonucleotides had the sequences 5′-TAACTCGCATCGTAGATTGACTAAA-3′ or 5′-CCTCTTACCTCAGTTACAATTTATA-3′, referred to as control. Morpholinos were dissolved in water. Morpholinos were injected into the brain ventricle, then platinum electrodes were placed on each side of the midbrain and voltage pulses were applied across the midbrain to electroporate optic tectum cells in stage 46 tadpoles.

### Behavioral experiments

#### Seizures

For seizure experiments, stage 47 tadpoles were transferred into individual wells in a six-well plate (Corning), each filled with 7 ml of 5 mM pentylenetetrazol (PTZ) solution in Steinberg's rearing media. The plate was diffusely illuminated from below and imaged from above with a SCB 2001 color camera (Samsung) at 30 frames/s.

Tadpole positions were tracked in Noldus EthoVision XT (Noldus Information Technology) and processed offline in a custom MATLAB program (MathWorks). Onset of regular seizures happened on average $3.9 \pm 1.3$ min into the recording; seizure events were defined as periods of rapid and irregular movement, interrupted by periods of immobility [15], and were detected automatically using swimming speed thresholding at a level of half of the maximal swimming speed. Frequency of seizures and length of seizure events were measured across 5 min intervals of a 20-min-long recording.

### Collision avoidance

Stage 49 tadpoles were placed in a clear plastic Petri dish (8.5 cm in diameter) filled to an approximate depth of 1 cm with Steinberg's solution at 18 °C. The dish was put on top of a CRT monitor screen (maximum luminance, 57 $cd/m^2$ and minimum luminance, 0.3 $cd/m^2$; Dell Ultrascan 1600 SH Series; Dell Computer Company) and screened from all sides with an opaque black cloth. Stimuli were generated by a custom-written MATLAB program using the Psychophysics Toolbox [16, 17]. A black circle of a radius of 0.3 cm was projected in the center of the dish. Every 30 s, this circle was sent toward the tadpole at a speed of 1.4 cm/s. Only collisions in which the animal was swimming within 1 s before the encounter with the circle were included in the dataset. Experiments were performed in the morning (from 9:00 A.M. to 1:00 P.M.), because animals seemed to be less responsive in the afternoon; each testing session lasted for 5 min. Videos were acquired in EthoVision; both the tadpole and the stimulus were manually tracked offline, and trajectories were exported for additional automated analysis in MATLAB. Avoidance response initiation points were identified as points of peak acceleration immediately after an encounter with a visual stimulus; escape speed was averaged over a 17 ms window (five frames) around the swimming velocity peak.

### Schooling

Fifteen to twenty tadpoles at developmental stage 49 were transferred to a glass bowl 17 cm in diameter (for each batch, control tadpoles matched FMRP KD tadpoles in number). A still image of tadpole distribution in the bowl was made every 5 min using Yawcam software (Magnus Lundvall, Yawcam) for 1 h (13 images per experiment). A strong acoustic stimulus was delivered 2.5 min after each photo was taken to elicit a startle response and force tadpoles to redistribute [18]. Coordinates of tadpole heads and tails were tracked manually in NIH ImageJ and exported for additional processing in MATLAB. We defined neighboring tadpoles through point set triangulation and used a Kolmogorov–Smirnov test to compare distributions of inter-tadpole distances between FMRP KD tadpoles and matched controls. For all pairs of "neighboring tadpoles" that were located closer than 5.7 cm to each other (two-thirds of the bowl radius), we also estimated the angle between their orientations in the bowl [19, 20].

### Statistics and presentation of behavior data

For behavioral data, averages and SDs are presented. When the Mann–Whitney test was used to compare values between the groups, significance values were reported as $P_{MW}$, whereas for Kolmogorov–Smirnov test, $p$ values are reported as $P_{KS}$. Sample sizes are reported as $n = x$, $N = y$, where lowercase n stands for the number of measurements and capital N stands for the number of animals.

### Electrophysiology experiments

For whole-brain recordings, tadpole brains were prepared as described by [21] and [22]. In brief, tadpoles were anesthetized in 0.02 % tricainemethane sulfonate (MS-222). To access the ventral surface of the tectum, brains were filleted along the dorsal midline and dissected in HEPES-buffered extracellular saline [in mM: 115 NaCl, 2 KCl, 3 $CaCl_2$, 3 $MgCl_2$, 5 HEPES, 10 glucose, and 0.1 picrotoxin, pH 7.2 (osmolarity 255 mOsm)]. Brains were then pinned to a submerged block of Sylgard in a recording chamber and maintained at room temperature (24 °C). To access tectal cells, the ventricular membrane surrounding the tectum was carefully removed using a broken glass pipette. For evoked synaptic response experiments, a bipolar stimulating electrode (FHC) was placed on the optic chiasm to activate retinal ganglion cell (RGC) axons.

Whole-cell voltage-clamp and current-clamp recordings were performed using glass micropipettes (8–12 M$\Omega$) filled with K-gluconate intracellular saline [in mM: 100 K-gluconate, 8 KCl, 5 NaCl, 1.5 MgCl2, 20 HEPES, 10 EGTA, 2 ATP, and 0.3 GTP, pH 7.2 (osmolarity 255 mOsm)]. Recordings were restricted consistently to retinorecipient neurons in the middle one-third of the tectum, thus avoiding any developmental variability existing along the rostrocaudal axis [21, 23, 24]. Electrical signals were measured with a Multiclamp 700B amplifier (Molecular Devices), digitized at 10 kHz using a Digidata 1440A analog-to-digital board, and acquired using pClamp 10 software. Leak subtraction was done in real time using the acquisition software. Membrane potential in the figures was not adjusted to compensate for a predicted 12 mV liquid junction potential. Data were analyzed using AxographX software. The $GABA_A$ antagonist picrotoxin (100 μM) was added to the external saline in a subset of experiments. Spontaneous synaptic events were collected and quantified using a variable amplitude template [25]. Spontaneous excitatory post-synaptic currents (sEPSCs) were recorded at −60 mV in the presence of picrotoxin, whereas spontaneous inhibitory post-synaptic currents (sIPSCs) were collected in control media at 5 mV (the reversal for glutamatergic currents). For each cell, 60 s of spontaneous activity was recorded. For evoked synaptic response experiments, a bipolar stimulating electrode (FHC) was placed on the optic chiasm to activate RGC axons. Synaptic stimulation experiments were conducted by collecting EPSCs evoked by stimulating the optic chiasm at a stimulus intensity that consistently evoked maximal amplitude EPSCs. Evoked responses at $-45$ mV (excitation) and 5 mV (inhibition) were used to calculate the excitation/inhibition (E/I) ratio. Excitation and inhibition were calculated as a measure of area under the curve for a 250 ms time window beginning at the onset of the synaptic response. Evoked monosynaptic events (at a stimulus intensity that does not evoke polysynaptic activity, typically 30–60 % of the maximum) were used to collect AMPA/NMDA ratios. Peak current amplitude at $-65$ mV (1 ms window at peak; 10–15 trials per cell) was used to calculate AMPAR-mediated currents, and average current amplitude collected at 55 mV (10 ms window 20 ms after peak AMPA; 5–15 trials per cell) was used to calculate NMDAR-mediated currents. Experiments to measure polysynaptic network activity were performed by collecting EPSCs evoked by stimulating the optic chiasm at a stimulus intensity that evoked the maximal amplitude EPSC. Quantification of polysynaptic activity was calculated by measuring the total change in current over 100 ms time bins beginning at the onset of the evoked response. A spontaneous barrage was defined as a change in holding current of 10 or 20 pA intervals for a period of >200 ms. To quantify intrinsic cell excitability, cells were presented with a series of depolarizing steps (20 pA intervals) in current clamp, starting from $-65$ mV. The number of spikes elicited by current injection was quantified using the following criteria: to qualify as a spike, the height of the spike had to be at least half the height of its preceding spike and no wider than three times the width of the first original spike [26]. Voltage-gated $Na^+$ and $K^+$ current–voltage ($I$–$V$) curves were calculated as in the study by [22], by measuring the early $Na^+$ peak current and the steady-state $K^+$ current. All data were tested for normality; parametric statistical tests were completed on normally distributed data and nonparametric Mann–Whitney $U$ tests were completed on nonnormal data. Graphs show mean and standard deviation as error bars, and data in the text show means and standard deviations, unless otherwise indicated.

## Results

Behavioral and electrophysiological experiments were performed on stage 49 tadpoles in which FMRP expression was knocked down using a morpholino-antisense oligomer [10] during critical neural proliferation and circuit wiring time periods, referred to as FMRP KD tadpoles throughout. Tadpoles were compared with a control group which was transfected with a scrambled version of the morpholino. Our results show behavioral and electrophysiological deficits that implicate impaired inhibitory circuitry as the primary change resulting from knockdown of FMRP.

We performed a series of behavioral experiments designed to test various functional aspects of neural circuit development [20]. Visual avoidance behavior is a test useful for assaying basic swimming ability as well as overall visual system function by measuring escape responses in response to a virtual object [13]. The collision avoidance response is a conserved behavior in *Xenopus laevis* tadpoles, and across species that relies heavily on the optic tectum for sensory integration and perception. Organisms engage in this behavior to maneuver away from impending predators or objects. We observed that FMRP KD tadpoles have significantly decreased background swimming speed prior to stimulus presentation (Fig. 1a, $P_t = 0.049$, 0.91 cm/s $\pm 0.65$, $N = 6$, $n = 31$ for control tadpoles; 0.61 cm $\pm 0.48$, $N = 6$, $n = 27$ for FMRP KD tadpoles), indicating an overall decrease in activity levels. However, we found that FMRP KD tadpole collision escape responses were not significantly different from controls in measures of escape speed (Fig. 1b $P_t >$ 0.089; 6.7 $\pm$ 3.5 cm/s, for control tadpoles; 5.1 $\pm$ 3.4 cm/s for FMRP KD tadpoles) and collision escape distance (Fig. 1c, $P_{MW} = 0.777$, 1.46 $\pm$ 0.4 cm for control tadpoles; 1.57 $\pm$ 0.8 cm for FMRP KD tadpoles). These data indicate that while FMRP KD tadpoles are overall slower swimmers, the basic visual function and escape responses are largely unchanged by FMRP KD.

Without major effects to the basic escape behavior, we wanted to identify if behaviors particularly relevant to FXS were affected in our FMRP KD tadpoles. A common behavioral marker of FXS and autism spectrum disorders (ASDs) is social interaction deficits. Tadpoles normally engage in a social aggregation behavior, called schooling [19]. Schooling is defined as structured aquatic animal aggregation marked by coordinated unidirectional group swimming behavior [27]. Recent work in our lab found that control tadpoles that are in schools normally swim parallel to each other (with an inter-tadpole body-axis angle less than 45°) and within at least two-thirds of the bowl's radius to each other [20]. This schooling behavior requires integration of various sensory cues, including visual, auditory and olfactory. Here, we observed abnormal schooling patterns in FMRP KD tadpoles (Fig. 1d–e). Comparing the distributions of angles and distances of 2035 control and 2054 FMRP KD sample measurements in 51 experimental runs, we found that FMRP KD tadpoles showed a significantly different distribution of inter-tadpole distances (Fig. 1d, $P_{KS} < 0.05$; $N = 51$ for FMRP and control tadpoles; see Fig. 1e inset), with decreased short and long inter-tadpole distances and increased intermediate distances,

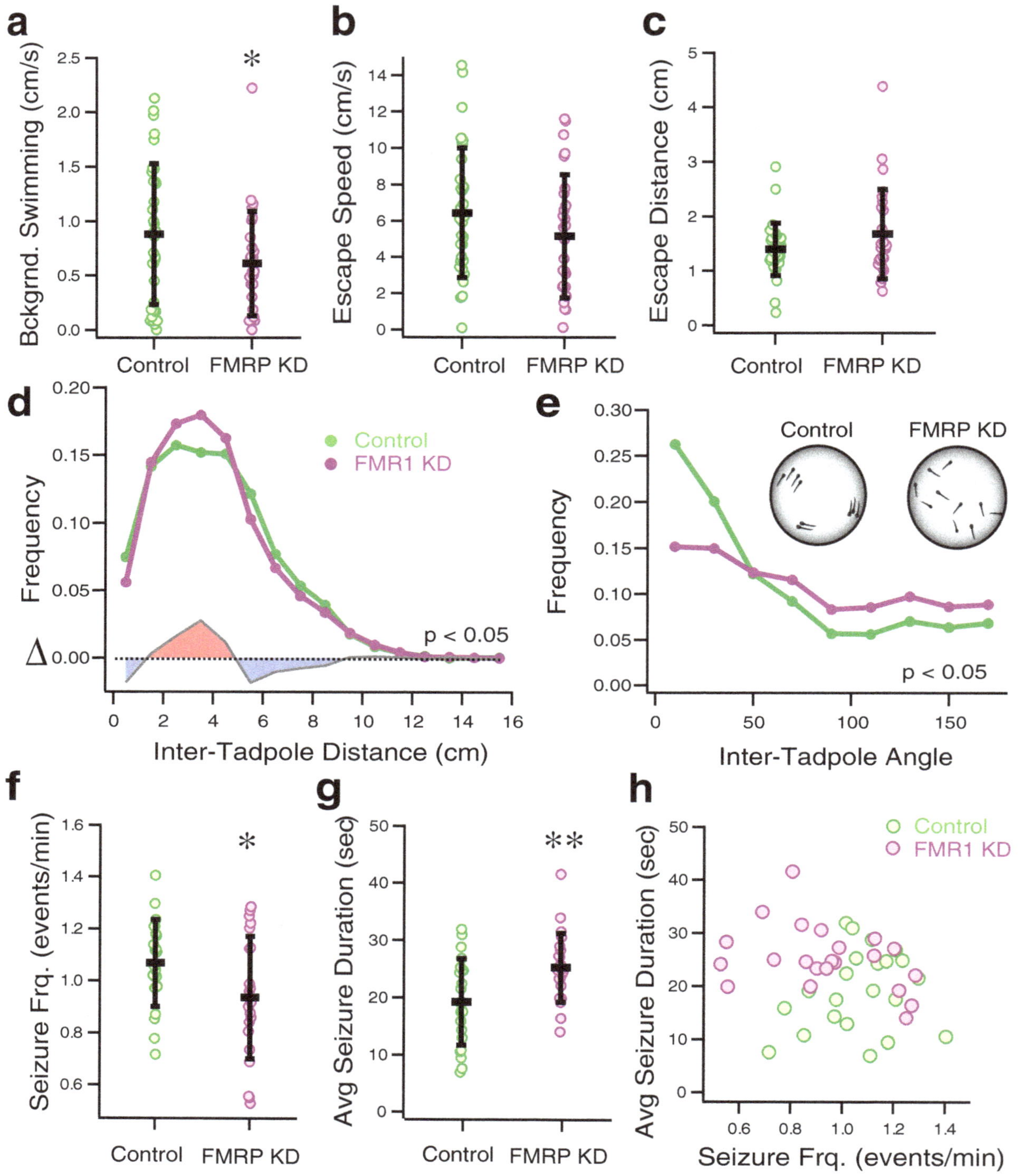

**Fig. 1** (See legend on next page.)

(See figure on previous page.)

**Fig. 1** Background swimming speeds, schooling behavior and seizure severity are affected by FMRP KD. **a** Background swimming is decreased in FMRP KD tadpoles ($P_t < 0.05$). **b–c** Visual avoidance behavior is unaffected. Collision-escape velocity (**b**, the velocity of the tadpole after collision with virtual object) and escape distance (**c**, the distance between the tadpole and the virtual object when the tadpole initiates avoidance response) are unaffected ($P_t > 0.05$ for controls and FMRP KD tadpoles in **b**, **c**). **d–e** FMRP KD tadpoles show reduced schooling. **d** FMRP KD tadpoles have fewer long and short distances and more medium distances between neighboring tadpoles, indicating more dispersed swimming and decreased aggregation ($P_{KS} < 0.05$). **e** Control tadpoles have a higher frequency of less than 90° angles for co-orientation whereas FMRP KD tadpoles have no preference for alignment ($P_{KS} < 10^{-20}$), inset. Diagram explaining schooling behavior, with small clusters of tadpoles with more short (inter-cluster) and long (intra-cluster) distances in controls, and more medium distances in FMRP KD tadpoles. Tadpoles are also co oriented with their nearest neighbor. **f–h** FMRP KD tadpoles seize significantly less frequently and for longer than controls, indicating decreased seizure susceptibility. **f** FMRP KD tadpoles seize with significantly reduced frequency compared to control MO tadpoles ($P_t < 0.01$), **g** FMRP KD tadpoles have significantly longer seizures ($P_t < 0.005$), **h** Seizure length plotted against seizure frequency indicates a negative correlation between the two, and separation between experimental groups

indicating more disperse swimming and less aggregation in FMRP KD tadpoles. Consistently, FMRP KD tadpoles also had fewer neighboring tadpoles that swam in the same direction (angle < 45°) and more tadpoles that swam perpendicular and opposite (90° and 180°, respectively) to their neighboring tadpoles (Fig. 1e, $P_{KS} < 10^{-20}$; $N = 51$ for both FMRP KD and control tadpoles). Both of these measures indicate that FMRP KD tadpoles show decreased schooling behavior.

Next we tested for seizure susceptibility. When presented with a convulsant, tadpoles develop seizures within 20 min [15]. Prior work has shown that abnormalities in excitatory connectivity, or in local inhibition can strongly affect the severity and length of these seizures. Seizures were induced pharmacologically with 5 mM pentylenetetrazol (PTZ) applied to the rearing media [20]. Under control conditions, increasing the concentration of PTZ results in an increase in seizure frequency and a decrease in seizure length. We found that FMRP KD tadpoles had less frequent (Fig. 1f, $P_t = 0.038$ $1.06 \pm 0.16$ events per minute for controls and $0.94 \pm 0.23$ events per minute for FMRP; $N = 22$ for controls and FMRP KD tadpoles) and significantly longer seizures (Fig. 1g, $P_t < 0.005$, length of seizure $19.24 \pm 7.37$ s for controls and $25.28 \pm 5.86$ s for FMRP). The decreased seizure frequency and increased seizure length (Fig. 1h) are consistent with decreased seizure severity, indicating that FMRP KD tadpoles show decreased seizure susceptibility.

Disrupted schooling behavior indicates abnormal integration of multisensory input potentially resulting from abnormal neural circuit development, and decreased seizure susceptibility and lower baseline swimming could indicate decreased overall excitation or enhanced inhibition in the brain. Together with the prior observation that FMRP KD tadpoles show changes in tectal neuron proliferation and arborization [10], these findings lead us to perform electrophysiological recordings to assess whether there was a corresponding alterations in tectal excitability or network function. We explored three potential mechanisms to account for decreased tectal activity, including lowered intrinsic excitability of tectal

neurons, abnormal development of excitatory synaptic transmission and increased synaptic inhibition.

To begin to examine the underlying causes of the behavioral phenotypes, we first investigated the intrinsic properties of the tectal neurons [28]. We found no difference in membrane capacitance or action potential threshold, but membrane resistance was significantly lower in FMRP KD cells (Table 1). We also measured voltage-gated sodium (Fig. 2a, b, $P_t = 0.86$, Peak current: $-333.1 \pm 39.0$ pA, $n = 25$ for controls, $-331.4 \pm 38.5$ pA, $n = 26$ for FMRP KD) and potassium currents (Fig. 2a, b, $P_t = 0.054$, Max current: $664.5 \pm 59.2$ pA, $n = 25$ for controls, $889.3 \pm 114.5$ pA, $n = 26$ for FMRP KD), and found no significant difference. We also did not find any significant differences in spike output evoked by direct depolarization over a range of current injections (Fig. 2c–e) and the maximum spike count (Fig. 2d, $4.3 \pm 3.2$ spikes, $n = 29$ for controls, $3.9 \pm 3.1$ spikes, $n = 29$ for FMRP KD). These results indicate that despite altered arborization, FMRP KD does not affect normal development of intrinsic excitability in tectal neurons.

We next examined the connectivity of the tectal network. Given the known cell proliferation defect [10], we know that there are fewer cells in the tectum. Therefore, the network properties could be altered. However, we found no difference in the spontaneous synaptic activity of tectal cells (Fig. 3a, b). Between groups, spontaneous excitatory post-synaptic currents (sEPSC) had similar frequency (Fig. 3c, $P_{MW} > 0.67$, $4.73 \pm 2.95$ events per

**Table 1** Cell size, action potential threshold, and membrane resistance in control and FMR1 KD tadpoles

|  | Control | FMR1 KD |
|---|---|---|
| Membrane Capacitance | $10.82 \pm 4.90$ pF, $n = 31$ | $11.28 \pm 2.90$ pF, $n = 33$ |
| Membrane resistance* | $2.419 \pm 1.93$ mΩ, $n = 31$ | $1.387 \pm 0.638$ mΩ, $n = 33$ |
| Action potential threshold | $-22.90 \pm 4.55$ mV, $n = 29$ | $-20.93 \pm 3.80$ mV, $n = 29$ |

*Membrane resistance is significantly different in FMR1 KD tadpoles ($p = 0.0261$, Mann–Whitney U-test). Mean ± standard deviation reported for each group

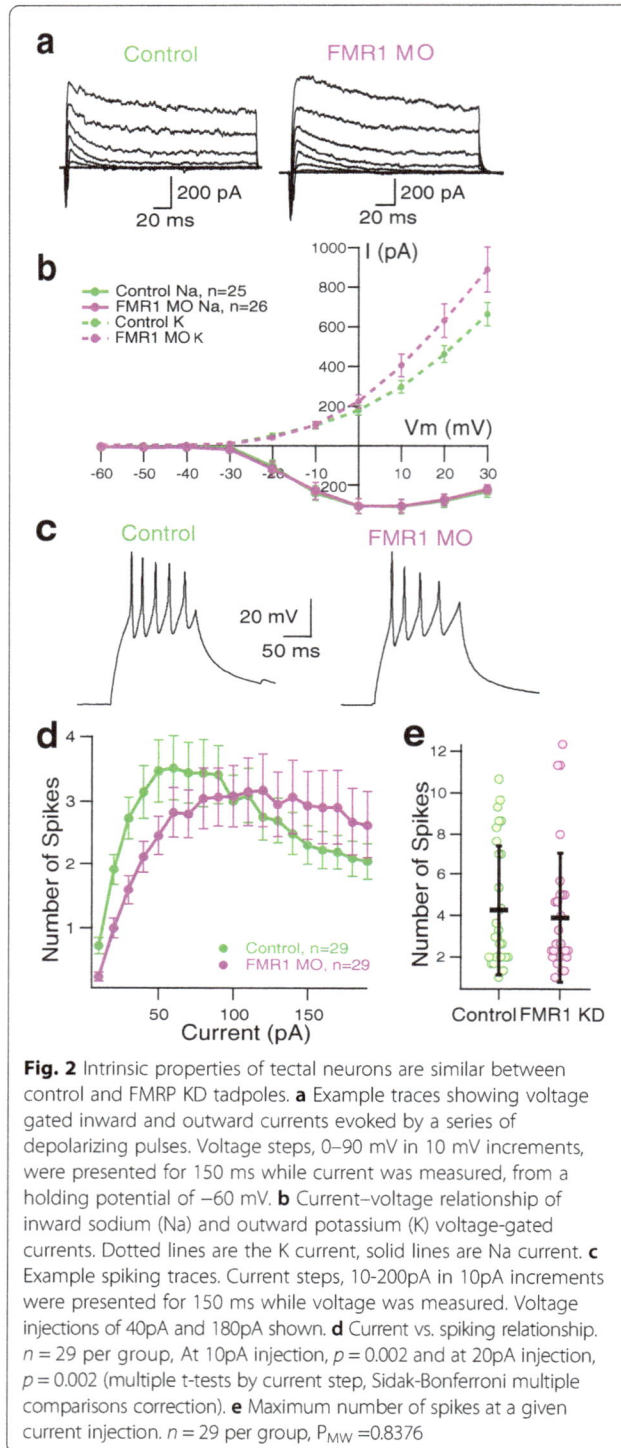

**Fig. 2** Intrinsic properties of tectal neurons are similar between control and FMRP KD tadpoles. **a** Example traces showing voltage gated inward and outward currents evoked by a series of depolarizing pulses. Voltage steps, 0–90 mV in 10 mV increments, were presented for 150 ms while current was measured, from a holding potential of −60 mV. **b** Current–voltage relationship of inward sodium (Na) and outward potassium (K) voltage-gated currents. Dotted lines are the K current, solid lines are Na current. **c** Example spiking traces. Current steps, 10-200pA in 10pA increments were presented for 150 ms while voltage was measured. Voltage injections of 40pA and 180pA shown. **d** Current vs. spiking relationship. $n = 29$ per group, At 10pA injection, $p = 0.002$ and at 20pA injection, $p = 0.002$ (multiple t-tests by current step, Sidak-Bonferroni multiple comparisons correction). **e** Maximum number of spikes at a given current injection. $n = 29$ per group, $P_{MW} = 0.8376$

second, $n = 28$ for controls, $5.18 \pm 3.24$ events per second, $n = 28$ for FMRP KD) and amplitude (Fig. 3d, $P_{MW} > 0.11$, $7.50 \pm 2.23$ pA, $n = 28$ for controls, $6.73 \pm 2.23$ pA, $n = 28$ for FMRP KD), as did the inhibitory post-synaptic currents (sIPSC) (Fig. 3e, frequency: $P_t = 0.13$, $3.16 \pm 2.12$ events per second, $n = 18$ for controls,

$2.23 \pm 1.88$ events per second, $n = 27$ for FMRP KD; Fig. 3f, amplitude: $P_t = 0.63$, $7.51 \pm 4.56$ pA, $n = 18$ for controls, $6.90 \pm 3.89$ pA, $n = 27$ for FMRP KD). Spontaneous recurrent activity is measured as the occurrence of barrages of activity of at least 200 ms duration with a 10 pA change in holding current and indicates the amount of recurrent circuitry present in the network. It is a measure of how interconnected the tectal network is. We found no difference in the frequency of spontaneous recurrent activity (Fig. 3g, excitatory: $P_t = 0.48$, $1.28 \pm 1.65$ events per minute, $n = 29$ for controls, $1.57 \pm 1.50$ events per minute, $n = 28$ for FMRP KD; Fig 3h, inhibitory: $P_t = 0.33$, $2.11 \pm 2.95$ events per minute, $n = 18$ for controls, $1.39 \pm 1.99$ events per minute, $n = 28$ for FMRP KD). These results indicate that the synaptic connectivity of the cells present in the network appears similar, and that a given cell has roughly the same number, frequency and type of synapses.

While spontaneous synaptic transmission might be indicative of the total input a tectal neuron receives, it does not tell us anything specific about the state of visual inputs to the tectum. To that end, we investigated responses to evoked visual stimulation. Evoked synaptic activity provides a measure of synaptic strength and network connectivity. First, we assayed basic synaptic properties. The AMPA to NMDA ratio is a measure of synaptic maturation, as cells incorporate additional AMPA receptors as they mature; therefore more mature cells have a larger AMPA:NMDA ratio [21]. We found no difference in the AMPA:NMDA ratios, indicating that FMRP KD does not affect synaptic maturation (Fig 4a, b, $P_t = 0.78$, $2.3 \pm 1.0$, $n = 13$ for controls, $3.4 \pm 2.2$, $n = 8$ for FMRP KD). Furthermore, paired pulse facilitation, a presynaptic measure of synaptic efficacy [29], was not affected by FMRP KD (Fig 4c, d, $P_t > 0.22$, $1.68 \pm 0.60$, $n = 12$ for control, $2.10 \pm 0.86$, $n = 9$ for FMRP KD). In the tectum, afferent visual input recruits a large amount of recurrent excitation [30, 31]. First, we measured recurrent activity in response to visual pathway stimulation to assess network connectivity and monosynaptic responses to assess direct synaptic connections. There was no difference in the response size of excitatory monosynaptic or recurrent activity as measured by calculating the total charge during the response (Fig. 4e, f, 0-50 ms: $P_t = 0.84$, $1620.9 \pm 1342.9$ pA.ms, $n = 18$ for controls, $1716.7 \pm 1395.7$ pA.ms, $n = 15$ for FMRP KD; 0-300 ms: $P_t = 0.91$, $7126.6 \pm 6365.6$ pA.ms, $n = 18$ for controls, $7339.9 \pm 4784.7$ pA.ms, $n = 15$ for FMRP KD), indicating an overall normal network level responses to visual inputs. We also measured the ratio of charge evoked by the monosynaptic afferent input, to the total amount of network activity. This provides us with a measure which we term monosynapticity index, which is a measure of how much network activity is evoked by visual input [28]. We found no difference in monosynapticity

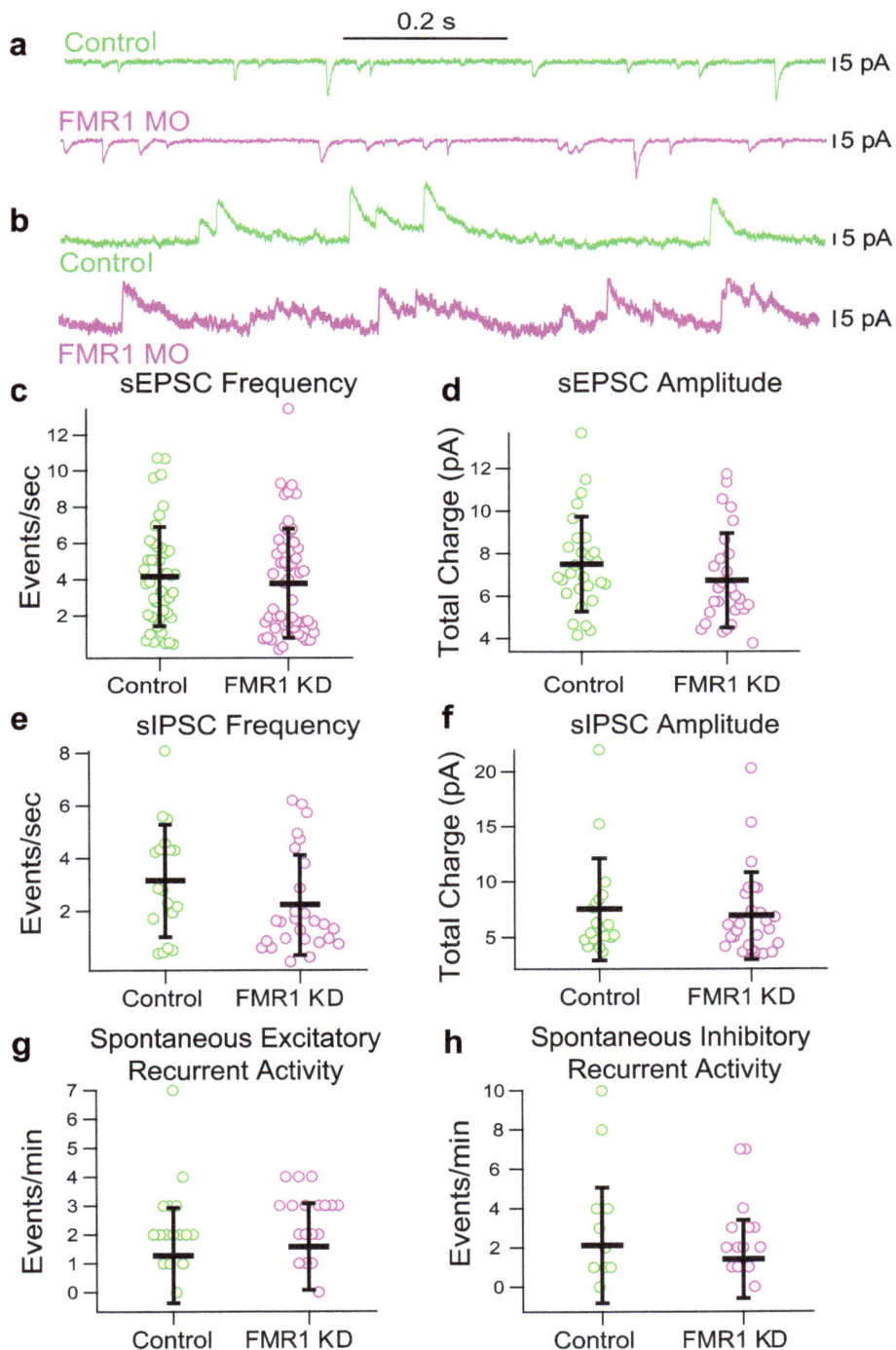

**Fig. 3** Spontaneous synaptic activity in tectal neurons is similar between control and FMRP KD tadpoles. **a** Example spontaneous EPSCs recorded at -60 mV in the presence of GABA$_A$ receptor blocker, picrotoxin. **b** Example spontaneous IPSCs recorded at +5 mV, the reversal potential for excitatory currents. **c** Frequency of sEPSCs. $n = 28$ for each group, $P_{MW} = 0.6784$. **d** Amplitude of sEPSCs. $n = 28$ for each group, $P_{MW} = 0.1069$. **e** Frequency of sIPSCs. $n = 18$ control, $n = 27$ FMRP KD, $P_{MW} = 0.1789$. **f** Amplitude of sIPSCs. $n = 18$ control, $n = 27$ FMRP KD, $P_{MW} = 0.5740$. **g** Excitatory recurrent activity, defined as the presence of a barrage of activity at least 200 ms in duration with a change in holding current of at least 10pA. $n = 28$ for each group, $P_{MW} = 0.3136$. **h** Inhibitory recurrent activity, defined as the presence of a barrage of activity at least 200 ms in duration with a change in holding current of at least 10pA. $n = 18$ control, $n = 27$ FMRP KD, $P_{MW} = 0.5101$

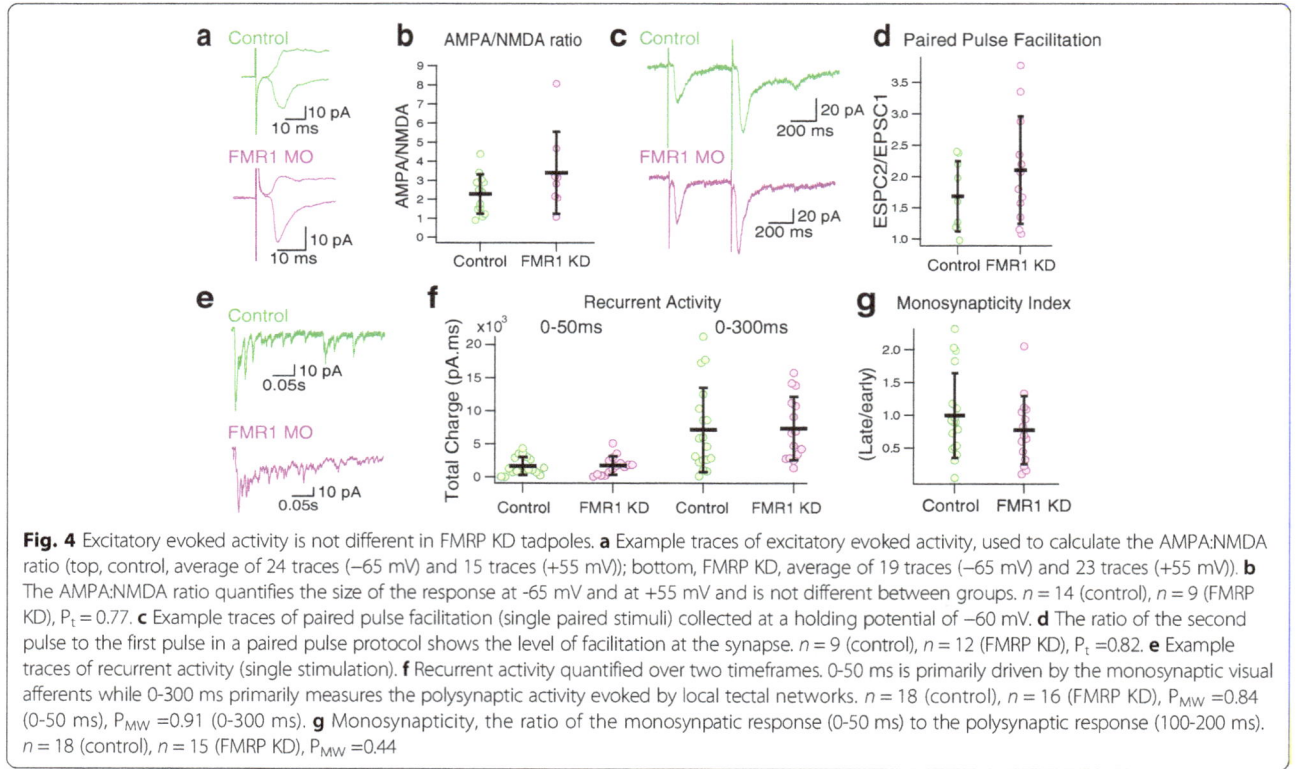

**Fig. 4** Excitatory evoked activity is not different in FMRP KD tadpoles. **a** Example traces of excitatory evoked activity, used to calculate the AMPA:NMDA ratio (top, control, average of 24 traces (−65 mV) and 15 traces (+55 mV)); bottom, FMRP KD, average of 19 traces (−65 mV) and 23 traces (+55 mV)). **b** The AMPA:NMDA ratio quantifies the size of the response at -65 mV and at +55 mV and is not different between groups. $n = 14$ (control), $n = 9$ (FMRP KD), $P_t = 0.77$. **c** Example traces of paired pulse facilitation (single paired stimuli) collected at a holding potential of −60 mV. **d** The ratio of the second pulse to the first pulse in a paired pulse protocol shows the level of facilitation at the synapse. $n = 9$ (control), $n = 12$ (FMRP KD), $P_t = 0.82$. **e** Example traces of recurrent activity (single stimulation). **f** Recurrent activity quantified over two timeframes. 0-50 ms is primarily driven by the monosynaptic visual afferents while 0-300 ms primarily measures the polysynaptic activity evoked by local tectal networks. $n = 18$ (control), $n = 16$ (FMRP KD), $P_{MW} = 0.84$ (0-50 ms), $P_{MW} = 0.91$ (0-300 ms). **g** Monosynapticity, the ratio of the monosynpatic response (0-50 ms) to the polysynaptic response (100-200 ms). $n = 18$ (control), $n = 15$ (FMRP KD), $P_{MW} = 0.44$

between experimental groups (Fig. 4g, $P_{MW} = 0.44$, $1.0 \pm 0.64$, $n = 18$ for controls, $0.77 \pm 0.51$, $n = 15$ for FMRP KD), indicating that excitatory network connectivity is unaffected. Together, these data show that excitatory synaptic activity and recurrent excitation are not changed by FMRP knockdown by FMR1 morpholino despite decreased proliferation and dendritic arborization.

It has been noted in other studies that a discoordination of excitation and inhibition may underlie many neurodevelopmental disorders [32, 33]. To that end, we investigated evoked inhibitory recurrent synaptic activity. We found that evoked inhibitory currents were significantly greater in FMRP KD tadpoles (Fig. 5a, b, $P_{MW} = 0.048$, $1714 \pm 1363$ pA.ms, $n = 11$ for controls, $3421 \pm 2490$ pA.ms, $n = 17$ for FMRP KD). However, the excitation is not affected by FMRP KD (Fig. 5c, $P_{MW} > 0.88$, $1789 \pm 817.5$ pA.ms, $n = 11$ for control, $1845 \pm 1029$ pA.ms, $n = 17$ for FMRP KD), which yields a significantly smaller excitation to inhibition ratio in FMRP KD tadpoles (Fig. 5d, $P_t = 0.009$, $1.64 \pm 1.17$, $n = 11$ for controls, $0.73 \pm 0.50$, $n = 17$ for FMRP KD). We also looked at the overall time course of recurrent inhibition, and found that inhibitory activity remained elevated for a longer time following synaptic stimulation in the FMRP KD tadpoles (Fig. 5a, e, 0-100 ms: $824.6 \pm 128.6$ pA.ms for controls, $1313.1 \pm 222.3$ pA.ms for FMRP KD; 100-200 ms: $651.0 \pm 191.5$ pA.ms for controls, $1279.9 \pm 255.8$ pA.ms for FMRP KD; 200-300 ms: $599.1 \pm 176.8$ pA.ms for controls, $833.4 \pm 163.0$ pA.ms for FMRP KD;

$n = 11$ for controls, $n = 17$ for FMRP KD), indicating altered dynamics of inhibitory circuits.

## Discussion

Our findings indicate that FMRP knockdown by FMR1 morpholino in the developing optic tectum has behavioral and electrophysiological consequences. Behaviorally, FMRP KD animals showed slightly reduced baseline swimming activity, decreased schooling behavior and decreased seizure susceptibility, but normal visual avoidance. These behavioral findings are consistent with decreased excitation within the tectum. Electrophysiologically we confirmed that neuronal intrinsic excitability and development of synaptic connectivity appear to be normal, however we found a significantly larger amount and longer lasting evoked network inhibition within the tectum, suggesting that this imbalance in the excitation to inhibition ratio may be responsible for the behavioral phenotypes.

These findings are unexpected since Faulkner et al. [10] identified a clear proliferative defect and abnormal tectal cell dendritic branching. Our experiments here show that despite these deficits individual cells develop normal excitability profiles and that excitatory and inhibitory synapses show normal maturation in the absence of FMRP. Nevertheless our findings also confirm that there is abnormal network connectivity since there is an increase in evoked inhibitory currents. Since we did not observe any differences in spontaneous inhibitory transmission, our

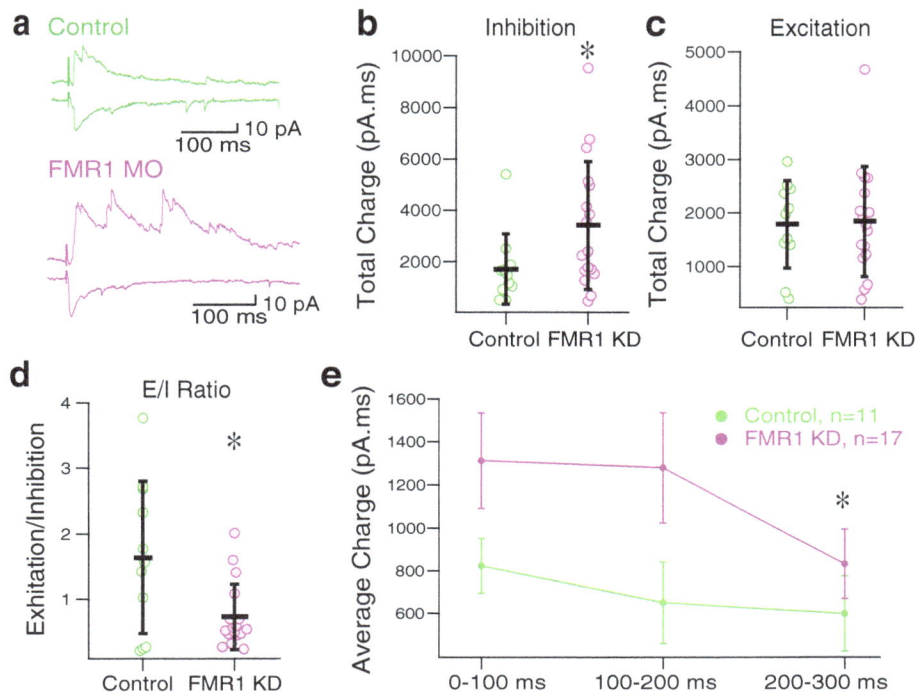

**Fig. 5** FMRP KD tadpole cells show increased evoked inhibitory activity. **a** Example traces of inhibitory evoked activity (recorded at +5 mv), and excitatory (recorded at −45 mv) used to calculate the excitation-inhibition balance (top, control; bottom, FMRP KD). **b** Evoked inhibitory recurrent activity at +5 mV, $P_{MW} = 0.048$, $n = 11$ (control), $n = 17$ (FMRP KD). **c** Evoked excitatory recurrent activity at -45 mV, $n = 11$ (control), $n = 17$ (FMRP KD). **d** Excitation to inhibition ratio, $P_t = 0.009$, $n = 11$ (control), $n = 17$ (FMRP KD). **e** Average charge of inhibitory responses calculated over bins of 100 msec following stimulus show altered time course of inhibitory responses in FMRP KD group

findings suggest that the effects observed are likely occurring in cells other than the principal deep layer cells that we recorded from in this study. For example one could speculate that a change in intrinsic excitability of inhibitory interneurons, or increased excitatory drive to interneurons may explain our findings. It could also be that there are a greater number of inhibitory cells present in the tecta of FMRP KD tadpoles, or elevated numbers of excitatory interneurons driving inhibition. These changes could link our findings to the abnormal neuronal proliferation described previously using the same experimental manipulation. Furthermore, our findings that excitatory synapse maturation is unaffected, together with previous findings that neuronal proliferation is disrupted, are consistent with the view that FMRP deficits can have effects much earlier in development than previously thought. Development of normal brain connectivity requires a careful interplay between cell proliferation, migration and differentiation, and altering this interplay could result in abnormal neural circuit formation and behavioral deficits, even if individual neurons still appear to develop normally [34].

Disruptions in the normal balance of excitation and inhibition during development have been implicated in a number of neurodevelopmental disorders, ranging from schizophrenia to autism [33, 35–37]. Thus our findings

are consistent with this view, and consistent with findings in other models of autism in which increased levels of inhibition are observed [38]. Other studies, in contrast, have also associated autism and Fragile X syndrome with alterations that result in decreased inhibition over excitation, resulting in increased seizure susceptibility [39–42]. For example in the rodent cortex, knockout of the FMR1 gene results in decreased synaptic drive to inhibitory interneurons and increased intrinsic excitability of excitatory cortical neurons, which result in prolonged evoked "up states" [43, 44]. In the amygdala, FMR1 knockouts have overall decreased tonic inhibition, leading to altered E/I balance and hyper excitability (Martin 2014). Interestingly, in the amygdala during development (p14) the FMR1 knockouts show a transient period of enhanced inhibition, which they ascribe to a homeostatic adaptation that ultimately fails in adult animals [41]. It is also worth noting that the seizures associated with Fragile X syndrome tend to be relatively mild and occur in only 10–20 % of individuals. This suggests that there could be a compensatory mechanism to counteract increased excitability, and perhaps this mechanism is more strongly evident in our brain structure and model organism. The effects of FMRP knockout also seem to be brain region specific and may manifest differently in the midbrain. However, the basic principle that small disruptions in network connectivity can lead to imbalances in information processing, which can then cascade into visible behavioral phenotypes, seems to be a common factor conserved across different brain regions, species and disorders.

To follow up on this study, it will be important to investigate the network properties of the optic tectum. The interaction of the decreased neural proliferation found by Faulkner et al. [10] and the increased evoked inhibition at the single cell level may manifest itself as a change in how the neural network interacts and interprets visual information to generate behavioral output. These studies could be carried out via in vivo Ca++ imaging of ensemble neuronal activity within the tectum [45]. It will also be important to identify whether the increased evoked inhibition is due to a larger proportion of GABAergic interneurons, or to alterations in interneuron physiology.

## Conclusions

Fragile X Syndrome and other neurodevelopmental disorders affect people in many ways, but have proven difficult to treat clinically. With our work, we have shown an explanation of why that may occur. It is clear that one particular insult does not result in a single, robust phenotype. Our research shows the opposite: small changes at the cellular level, combined with a neural proliferation defect, gives rise to the behavioral phenotype.

### Abbreviations
ASD, autism spectrum disorders; CNS, central nervous system; FMR1, fragile X mental retardation 1 gene; FMRP, fragile X mental retardation protein; FXS, Fragile X Syndrome; K, Potassium; KD, knock down; MO, morpholino; Na, sodium; Pks, P value for Kolmogorov-Smirnov test; Pmw, P value for Man-Whitney $u$-test; Pt, P value for $t$-test; PTZ, pentylenetetrazol; RGC, retinal ganglion cell; RNA, ribonucleic acid; sEPSC, spontaneous excitatory post-synaptic current; sIPSC, spontaneous inhibitory post-synaptic current

### Acknowledgements
We thank Mimi Oupravanh for animal care and experimental support and Carolina Ramirez Vizcarrondo for critical help and training in the behavioral protocols.

### Funding
T.L.S.T is supported by NIH F31 NS09379001. E.J.J. is supported by NSF GFRP, T.J.W. by NIH T34GM087193. M.H. supported by Brown University UTRA Fellowship. This research was supported by funds from Brown University and NSF IOS (to C.D.A), NIH grants EY011261 to H.T.C.), an endowment from the Hahn Family Foundation (to H.T.C.), the Department of Defense (Grant W81XWH-12-1-0207 to H.T.C.) and NIH P30-GM-32128 (to K.G.P. and Z.L.). The funding bodies had no role in the design of the study and collection, analysis, and interpretation of data and in writing the manuscript.

### Authors' contributions
TLST and CDA wrote the manuscript. TLST, EJJ, ZL and KGP conducted, analyzed and interpreted the electrophysiology experiments. MH and TW conducted, analyzed and interpreted behavior experiments. The project was conceived and designed by CDA and HTC. All authors had a role in revising and approving the final version of the manuscript and made substantial contributions to the conception and experimental design of the study.

### Competing interests
The authors declare that they have no competing interests.

### Author details
[1]Department of Neuroscience, Brown University, Box G-LN60 Olive St., 02912 Providence, RI, USA. [2]Department of Molecular and Cellular Neuroscience, Scripps Research Institute, 10550 North Torrey Pines Road, 92037 La Jolla, CA, USA. [3]Department of Zoology and Physiology, University of Wyoming, 82071 Laramie, WY, USA.

### References
1.  Bhakar AL, Dölen G, Bear MF. The Pathophysiology of Fragile X (and What It Teaches Us about Synapses). Annu Rev Neurosci. 2012;35:417–43.
2.  Santoro MR, Bray SM, Warren ST. Molecular Mechanisms of Fragile X Syndrome: A Twenty-Year Perspective. Annu Rev Pathol Mech Dis. 2012;7:219–45.
3.  Wijetunge LS, Chattarji S, Wyllie DJA, Kind PC. Fragile X syndrome: From targets to treatments. Neuropharmacology. 2013;68:83–96. Neurodevelopmental Disorders.
4.  Fu Y-H, Kuhl DPA, Pizzuti A, Pieretti M, Sutcliffe JS, Richards S, Verkert AJMH, Holden JJA, Fenwick Jr RG, Warren ST, Oostra BA, Nelson DL, Caskey CT. Variation of the CGG repeat at the fragile X site results in genetic instability: Resolution of the Sherman paradox. Cell. 1991;67:1047–58.
5.  Verkerk AJMH, Pieretti M, Sutcliffe JS, Fu Y-H, Kuhl DPA, Pizzuti A, Reiner O, Richards S, Victoria MF, Zhang F, Eussen BE, van Ommen G-JB, Bloncen LAJ, Riggins GJ, Chastain JL, Kunst CB, Galjaard H, Thomas Caskey C, Nelson DL, Oostra BA, Warren ST. Identification of a gene (FMR-1) containing a CGG repeat coincident with a breakpoint cluster region exhibiting length variation in fragile X syndrome. Cell. 1991;65:905–14.
6.  He CX, Portera-Cailliau C. The trouble with spines in fragile X syndrome: density, maturity and plasticity. Neuroscience. 2013;251:120–8. Dendritic Spine Plasticity in Brain Disorders.
7.  Irwin SA, Galvez R, Greenough WT. Dendritic Spine Structural Anomalies in Fragile-X Mental Retardation Syndrome. Cereb Cortex. 2000;10:1038–44.
8.  Waung MW, Huber KM. Protein translation in synaptic plasticity: mGluR-LTD, Fragile X. Curr Opin Neurobiol. 2009;19:319–26. Signalling Mechanisms.
9.  Li Y, Zhao X. Concise Review: Fragile X Proteins in Stem Cell Maintenance and Differentiation. STEM CELLS. 2014;32:1724–33.
10. Faulkner RL, Wishard TJ, Thompson CK, Liu H-H, Cline HT. FMRP regulates neurogenesis in vivo in Xenopus laevis tadpoles. eNeuro. 2015;2, e0055.
11. Gessert S, Bugner V, Tecza A, Pinker M, Kühl M. FMR1/FXR1 and the miRNA pathway are required for eye and neural crest development. Dev Biol. 2010; 341:222–35. Special Section: Morphogenesis.
12. Lim JH, Luo T, Sargent TD, Fallon JR. Developmental expression of Xenopus Fragile X mental retardation-1 gene. Int J Dev Biol. 2005;49:981–4.
13. Pratt KG, Khakhalin AS. Modeling human neurodevelopmental disorders in the Xenopus tadpole: from mechanisms to therapeutic targets. Dis Model Mech. 2013;6:1057–65.
14. Nieuwkoop P, Faber J. Normal Table of Xenopus Laevis (Daudin); a Systematical and Chronological Survey of the Development from the Fertilized Egg till the End of Metamorphosis. Amsterdam: North-Holland Pub. Co.; 1956.
15. Bell MR, Belarde JA, Johnson HF, Aizenman CD. A neuroprotective role for polyamines in a Xenopus tadpole model of epilepsy. Nat Neurosci. 2011;14:505–12.
16. Brainard DH. The Psychophysics Toolbox. Spat Vis. 1997;10:433–6.

17. Wu G-Y, Zou D-J, Koothan T, Cline HT. Infection of frog neurons with vaccinia virus permits in vivo expression of foreign proteins. Neuron. 1995;14:681–4.

18. Katz LC, Potel MJ, Wassersug RJ. Structure and mechanisms of schooling intadpoles of the clawed frog, Xenopus laevis. Anim Behav. 1981;29:20–33.

19. Wassersug R, Hessler CM. Tadpole behaviour: Aggregation in larval Xenopus laevis. Anim Behav. 1971;19:386–9.

20. James EJ, Gu J, Ramirez-Vizcarrondo CM, Hasan M, Truszkowski TLS, Tan Y, Oupravanh PM, Khakhalin AS, Aizenman CD. Valproate-Induced Neurodevelopmental Deficits in Xenopus laevis Tadpoles. J Neurosci Off J Soc Neurosci. 2015;35:3218–29.

21. Wu G-Y, Malinow R, Cline HT. Maturation of a Central Glutamatergic Synapse. Science. 1996;274:972–6.

22. Aizenman CD, Akerman CJ, Jensen KR, Cline HT. Visually Driven Regulation of Intrinsic Neuronal Excitability Improves Stimulus Detection In Vivo. Neuron. 2003;39:831–42.

23. Hamodi AS, Pratt KG. The horizontal brain slice preparation: a novel approach for visualizing and recording from all layers of the tadpole tectum. J Neurophysiol. 2014;113(1):400–7. jn.00672.2014.

24. Khakhalin AS, Aizenman CD. GABAergic Transmission and Chloride Equilibrium Potential Are Not Modulated by Pyruvate in the Developing Optic Tectum of Xenopus laevis Tadpoles. PLoS One. 2012;7:e34446.

25. Clements JD, Bekkers JM. Detection of spontaneous synaptic events with an optimally scaled template. Biophys J. 1997;73:220–9.

26. Pratt KG, Aizenman CD. Homeostatic Regulation of Intrinsic Excitability and Synaptic Transmission in a Developing Visual Circuit. J Neurosci. 2007;27: 8268–77.

27. Shaw E. Schooling Fishes: The school, a truly egalitarian form of organization in which all members of the group are alike in influence, offers substantial benefits to its participants. Am Sci. 1978;66:166–75.

28. Ciarleglio CM, Khakhalin AS, Wang AF, Constantino AC, Yip SP, Aizenman CD. Multivariate analysis of electrophysiological diversity of Xenopus visual neurons during development and plasticity. eLife. 2015;4:e11351.

29. Aizenman CD, Cline HT. Enhanced Visual Activity In Vivo Forms Nascent Synapses in the Developing Retinotectal Projection. J Neurophysiol. 2007;97:2949–57.

30. Liu Z, Ciarleglio CM, Hamodi AS, Aizenman CD, Pratt KG. A population of gap junction-coupled neurons drives recurrent network activity in a developing visual circuit. J Neurophysiol. 2016;115:1477–86.

31. Pratt KG, Wei D, Aizenman CD. Development and spike timing–dependent plasticity of recurrent excitation in the Xenopus optic tectum. Nat Neurosci. 2008;11:467–75.

32. Akerman CJ, Cline HT. Depolarizing GABAergic Conductances Regulate the Balance of Excitation to Inhibition in the Developing Retinotectal Circuit In Vivo. J Neurosci. 2006;26:5117–30.

33. Fenton AA. Excitation-Inhibition Discoordination in Rodent Models of Mental Disorders. Biol Psychiatry. 2015;77:1079–88. Cortical Oscillations for Cognitive/Circuit Dysfunction in Psychiatric Disorders.

34. Rice D, Barone S. Critical periods of vulnerability for the developing nervous system: evidence from humans and animal models. Environ Health Perspect. 2000;108 Suppl 3:511–33.

35. Lewis DA, Hashimoto T, Volk DW. Cortical inhibitory neurons and schizophrenia. Nat Rev Neurosci. 2005;6:312–24.

36. Di Cristo G. Development of cortical GABAergic circuits and its implications for neurodevelopmental disorders. Clin Genet. 2007;72:1–8.

37. Cea-Del Rio CA, Huntsman MM. The contribution of inhibitory interneurons to circuit dysfunction in Fragile X Syndrome. Front Cell Neurosci. 2014;8:245.

38. Dani VS, Chang Q, Maffei A, Turrigiano GG, Jaenisch R, Nelson SB. Reduced cortical activity due to a shift in the balance between excitation and inhibition in a mouse model of Rett Syndrome. Proc Natl Acad Sci U S A. 2005;102:12560–5.

39. Belmonte MK, Cook EH, Anderson GM, Rubenstein JLR, Greenough WT, Beckel-Mitchener A, Courchesne E, Boulanger LM, Powell SB, Levitt PR, Perry EK, Jiang YH, DeLorey TM, Tierney E. Autism as a disorder of neural information processing: directions for research and targets for therapy*. Mol Psychiatry. 2004;9:646–63.

40. Hagerman PJ, Stafstrom CE. Origins of epilepsy in fragile X syndrome. Epilepsy Curr Am Epilepsy Soc. 2009;9:108–12.

41. Vislay RL, Martin BS, Olmos-Serrano JL, Kratovac S, Nelson DL, Corbin JG, Huntsman MM. Homeostatic Responses Fail to Correct Defective Amygdala Inhibitory Circuit Maturation in Fragile X Syndrome. J Neurosci. 2013;33: 7548–58.

42. Martin BS, Corbin JG, Huntsman MM. Deficient tonic GABAergic conductance and synaptic balance in the fragile X syndrome amygdala. J Neurophysiol. 2014;112:890–902.

43. Gibson JR, Bartley AF, Hays SA, Huber KM. Imbalance of Neocortical Excitation and Inhibition and Altered UP States Reflect Network Hyperexcitability in the Mouse Model of Fragile X Syndrome. J Neurophysiol. 2008;100:2615–26.

44. Paluszkiewicz SM, Martin BS, Huntsman MM. Fragile X Syndrome: The GABAergic System and Circuit Dysfunction. Dev Neurosci. 2011;33:349–64.

45. Xu H, Khakhalin AS, Nurmikko AV, Aizenman CD. Visual Experience-Dependent Maturation of Correlated Neuronal Activity Patterns in a Developing Visual System. J Neurosci. 2011;31:8025–36.

# 4

# The microtubule plus-end-tracking protein TACC3 promotes persistent axon outgrowth and mediates responses to axon guidance signals during development

Burcu Erdogan, Garrett M. Cammarata, Eric J. Lee, Benjamin C. Pratt, Andrew F. Francl, Erin L. Rutherford and Laura Anne Lowery*

## Abstract

**Background:** Formation of precise neuronal connections requires proper axon guidance. Microtubules (MTs) of the growth cone provide a critical driving force during navigation of the growing ends of axons. Pioneer MTs and their plus-end tracking proteins (+TIPs) are thought to play integrative roles during this navigation. TACC3 is a + TIP that we have previously implicated in regulating MT dynamics within axons. However, the role of TACC3 in axon guidance has not been previously explored.

**Results:** Here, we show that TACC3 is required to promote persistent axon outgrowth and prevent spontaneous axon retractions in embryonic *Xenopus laevis* neurons. We also show that overexpressing TACC3 can counteract the depolymerizing effect of low doses of nocodazole, and that TACC3 interacts with MT polymerase XMAP215 to promote axon outgrowth. Moreover, we demonstrate that manipulation of TACC3 levels interferes with the growth cone response to the axon guidance cue Slit2 ex vivo, and that ablation of TACC3 causes pathfinding defects in axons of developing spinal neurons in vivo.

**Conclusion:** Together, our results suggest that by mediating MT dynamics, the + TIP TACC3 is involved in axon outgrowth and pathfinding decisions of neurons during embryonic development.

**Keywords:** Microtubule, +TIPs, TACC3, XMAP215, *Xenopus laevis*, Neuronal development, Growth cone, Axon guidance

## Background

Plus-end tracking proteins (+TIPs) selectively bind to the dynamic plus-ends of microtubules (MTs), which extend into the distal part of the axon and growth cone [1]. This enables + TIPs to come into close contact with the cell cortex, where guidance cue receptors reside. These receptors transduce asymmetrically-distributed guidance signals down to intracellular effectors, which then regulate MT dynamics in a spatially-restricted manner that likely plays a key role in growth cone turning events [2, 3]. Thus, +TIPs deserve attention for their potential function in regulating MT dynamics during axon guidance. One of the first + TIPs to be discovered

for its role in axon guidance was CLASP [4]. Genetic studies in *Drosophila* demonstrated that *CLASP* is a downstream target of Abelson tyrosine kinase (Abl) in the Slit/Robo guidance pathway during central nervous system midline crossing [4]. Moreover, the + TIP and MT polymerase, *msps* (fly ortholog of XMAP215/ch-TOG) interacts with *CLASP* antagonistically during this guidance decision in an Abl-dependent manner [5]. In addition to its role in *Drosophila*, XMAP215 has been implicated in promoting axon outgrowth in vertebrates [6]. We have recently shown that the XMAP215-interactor, TACC3, is also a + TIP that regulates MT dynamics in vertebrate growth cones and is essential for normal axonal outgrowth [7]. However, how TACC3 specifically affects axon outgrowth and

* Correspondence: Laura.lowery@bc.edu
Department of Biology, Boston College, Chestnut Hill, MA 02467, USA

whether TACC3 plays a role during axon guidance remain to be explored.

In this study, we examine the role of TACC3 in axon outgrowth and pathfinding in vivo within the developing nervous system of *Xenopus laevis* which is a great model for studying cytoskeletal dynamics during axon outgrowth and guidance [8, 9]. Using time-lapse live imaging, we demonstrate that TACC3 is required for persistent axon outgrowth in *Xenopus laevis*, and that both the N- and C- terminal conserved domains of TACC3 are necessary for enhanced axon outgrowth. Moreover, TACC3-overexpressing growth cones can mitigate the reductive impacts of the MT-depolymerizing agent, Nocodazole, on MT dynamics parameters. We also show that TACC3 and XMAP215 can display a synergistic effect and promote axon outgrowth ex vivo. Finally, examination of whole mount *Xenopus* spinal cords shows defects in axon guidance in motor neurons when TACC3 levels are depleted, and manipulation of TACC3 levels impacts the growth cone response to the repellent guidance cue Slit2 in cultured *Xenopus* spinal neurons. Together, these investigations provide new insights into the mechanism by which TACC3 functions either alone or in combination with other + TIPs, such as XMAP215, to regulate MT dynamics during axon outgrowth and guidance.

## Methods

### *Xenopus* embryonic explants

Egg collection and culturing of *Xenopus* embryonic explants (from embryos of either sex) were performed as described [7, 10]. All experiments were approved by the Boston College Institutional Animal Care and Use Committee and were performed according to national regulatory standards.

### Constructs and RNA

Capped mRNA constructs were transcribed and purified as previously described [6, 7] Constructs used were GFP-TACC3 (TACC3 pET30a was gift from the Richter lab, University of Massachusetts Medical School, Worcester, MA), GFP-TACC3-ΔN, GFP-TACC3-ΔΔN, GFP-TACC3-ΔTACC (see Fig. 1e for amino acid residues for full length and each deletion construct, based on GenBank accession number NP-001081964.1) (all TACC3 constructs were subcloned into pSC2+ vector), GFP-MACF 43 (a gift from Hoogenraad Lab) in pCS2+, XMAP215-GFP (a gift from the Hyman lab, Max Planck Institute of Molecular Cell Biology and Genetics, Dresden, Germany; [11]) subcloned into pT7TS. Embryos either at the 2 cell or 4 cell stage received injections 4 times total in 0.1× MMR containing 5% Ficoll with the following total mRNA amount per embryo; 100 pg of GFP-MACF43 as a control for TACC3 or XMAP215 overexpression, 2000 pg of GFP-TACC3

full-length and deletion constructs (deletion constructs are expressed in wildtype embryos), 3000 pg of XMAP215-GFP. For double overexpression studies, 1000 pg of TACC3 and XMAP215 were injected in total.

### Morpholinos

Morpholinos (MOs) were previously described and validated [6, 7]. In knockdown (KD) experiments, TACC3 and control MOs were injected at 80 ng/embryo. For TACC3 and XMAP215 double KD analysis, 20 ng/embryo for TACC3 and control MOs and 2 ng/embryo for XMAP215 MO were injected. In rescue experiments, MO (amounts used as in KD, which is 80 ng/embryo) was injected with mRNA (same amount as in OE which is 2000 pg/embryo for GFP-TACC3 and 3000 pg/embryo for XMAP215-GFP) in the same injection solution. The efficacy of MOs has been previously assessed by Western blot of 35–36 stage embryos, as described [6, 7].

### Whole-mount immunohistochemistry

Two-day-old embryos were fixed, as described [6]. Primary antibody (diluted in blocking buffer made up by 1% DMSO, 1% Triton, 1% BSA, in PBS) to acetylated tubulin (1:1000, monoclonal, clone 6-11B-1, Sigma, St. Louis, MO, USA) and goat anti-mouse Alexa-Fluor 568 conjugate secondary antibody (1:1000, polyclonal, A-1100, Life Technologies) were used. For imaging, the spinal cord was exposed by peeling off skin, and somites were kept intact. Embryos were transferred in a drop of benzoate:benzyl alcohol (BB:BA) to the imaging chamber (made by placing Gene Frame, sticky on both sides, onto a microscope slide). After the tissue was cleared, it was covered with a 1.5× coverslip. Image acquisition and quantitation of fixed and labeled explants were described previously [6]. TACC3 KD-induced change is scored based on the percentage of embryos with disorganized axons in each condition.

### Immunocytochemistry

Embryonic explant cultures were fixed and labelled [12] with primary antibodies (1:1000 diluted in blocking buffer made up by 1% non-fat dry milk in calcium and magnesium free PBS) to tyrosinated tubulin (rat monoclonal, ab6160, Abcam) and de-tyrosinated tubulin (rabbit polyclonal, AB3201, Millipore), and with the secondary antibodies goat anti-rat Alexa Fluor 568 (1:1000, ab175476, Abcam) and goat anti-rabbit Alexa Fluor 488 (1:1000, A-11008, Life Technologies), respectively.

### Growth cone response assay

Recombinant mouse Slit2 protein (R&D Systems) (400 ng/ml) was administered to cultured neural tube explants derived from stage 28 *Xenopus* embryos in 400 µl culture media supplemented with 1% Penicillin/

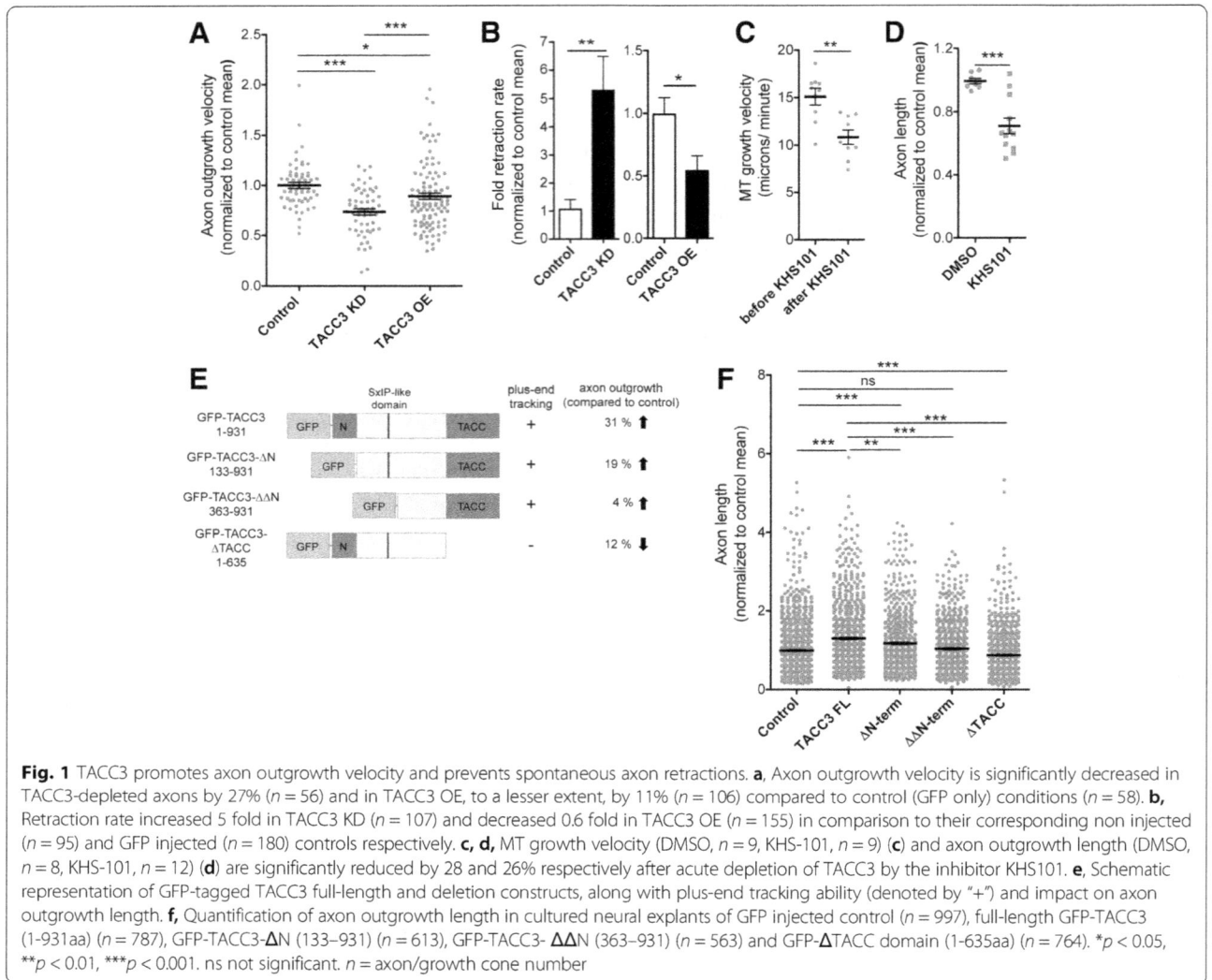

**Fig. 1** TACC3 promotes axon outgrowth velocity and prevents spontaneous axon retractions. **a,** Axon outgrowth velocity is significantly decreased in TACC3-depleted axons by 27% ($n = 56$) and in TACC3 OE, to a lesser extent, by 11% ($n = 106$) compared to control (GFP only) conditions ($n = 58$). **b,** Retraction rate increased 5 fold in TACC3 KD ($n = 107$) and decreased 0.6 fold in TACC3 OE ($n = 155$) in comparison to their corresponding non injected ($n = 95$) and GFP injected ($n = 180$) controls respectively. **c, d,** MT growth velocity (DMSO, $n = 9$, KHS-101, $n = 9$) (**c**) and axon outgrowth length (DMSO, $n = 8$, KHS-101, $n = 12$) (**d**) are significantly reduced by 28 and 26% respectively after acute depletion of TACC3 by the inhibitor KHS101. **e,** Schematic representation of GFP-tagged TACC3 full-length and deletion constructs, along with plus-end tracking ability (denoted by "+") and impact on axon outgrowth length. **f,** Quantification of axon outgrowth length in cultured neural explants of GFP injected control ($n = 997$), full-length GFP-TACC3 (1-931aa) ($n = 787$), GFP-TACC3-$\Delta$N (133–931) ($n = 613$), GFP-TACC3- $\Delta\Delta$N (363–931) ($n = 563$) and GFP-$\Delta$TACC domain (1-635aa) ($n = 764$). *$p < 0.05$, **$p < 0.01$, ***$p < 0.001$. ns not significant. $n$ = axon/growth cone number

Streptomycin and 0.1% BSA. A perfusion chamber was set up to exchange media with Slit2-containing culture media. Time-lapse images of growth cones were acquired for 10 min with 30 s intervals before and immediately after Slit2 addition for 30 min with 30 s intervals, using a Zeiss Axio Observer inverted motorized microscope with a Zeiss 20×/0.8 Plan Apo phase objective. Frame to frame axon growth was tracked manually and retraction or growth cone collapse events were recorded over a movie. Ratio of the number of retracting frames over total frames for each axon was scored. Images given in the figures show the image of growth cone right before adding Slit2 and the image of the growth cone at collapse.

### Nocodazole application

Nocodazole to final concentration of 50 pM was administered in 400 µl culture media. Concentration of Nocodazole was determined after series of titrations and

50 pM was found to be the optimum to keep the MTs intact in order to perform MT dynamics analyses. Time-lapse images of growth cones were acquired for 1 min with 2 s intervals before and 5 min after Nocodazole administration, using a Yokogawa CSU-X1M 5000 spinning disk confocal on a Zeiss inverted motorized microscope with a Zeiss 63× Plan Apo 1.4 NA and a Hamamatsu ORCA R2 CCD camera. MT dynamics were assessed, as described [7].

### PlusTipTracker software analysis

MT dynamics were analyzed from GFP-MACF43 movies using plusTipTracker [10, 13]. Imaging conditions and tracking parameters were previously validated and same parameters were used: maximum gap length is 8 frames; minimum track length is 3 frames; search radius range 5–12 pixels; maximum forward angle, 50°; maximum backward angle, 10°; maximum shrinkage factor, 0.8; fluctuation radius, 2.5 pixels; time interval, 2 s. MT growth lifetime is the measure of persistent outgrowth till MT undergoes catastrophe. MT growth length is the total growth over a movie and MT growth velocity is the average of each MT growth event. MT dynamics parameters were compiled from multiple individual experiments and to avoid day-to-day fluctuations the final complied data were normalized to the mean of the control data for each experiment.

### Image acquisition and analysis

For axon outgrowth imaging, phase contrast images of axons were collected on a Zeiss Axio Observer inverted motorized microscope with a Zeiss 20×/0.5 Plan Apo phase objective and analyzed using ImageJ [7]. Time-lapse images for axon outgrowth velocity was collected for 4 h with 20 min intervals and images were analyzed using plusTipTracker QFSM plugin and velocity was measured as the average of instantaneous velocity per axon as described [6]. Axon retraction events were analyzed from the same data set used to assess axon growth velocity. Frame to frame axon growth was tracked manually and retraction events were recorded over a movie. Ratio of the number of retracting frames over total frames for each axon was scored.

Axon outgrowth and MT dynamics data were normalized to controls, to account for day-to-day fluctuations in room temperature. Image acquisition and quantitation of fluorescence intensity of fixed and labeled explants were described previously [7]. Experiments were performed multiple times to ensure reproducibility. Graphs were made in GraphPad Prism. Statistical differences were determined using unpaired two tailed t-tests when comparing two conditions and one-way analysis of variance with Tukey's *post-hoc* analysis when multiple conditions were compared.

### Results

#### TACC3 promotes persistent axon outgrowth by preventing spontaneous axon retractions

We previously showed that normal axonal outgrowth requires TACC3 [7]. To gain further insight into the mechanism by which TACC3 promotes axon outgrowth, we examined the effect of TACC3 knockdown (KD) and overexpression (OE) on dynamic axon outgrowth parameters. Time-lapse imaging demonstrated that TACC3 KD significantly reduced axon outgrowth velocity by 25% relative to control conditions (TACC3 KD, $0.74 \pm 0.03$, $n = 46$, versus control, $1.04 \pm 0.03$ $n = 57$, ***$p < 0.0001$, Fig. 1a). In addition to the reduced outgrowth velocity, TACC3 reduction dramatically increased axon retraction rates by 5-fold in comparison to control axons (TACC3 KD, $5.27 \pm 1.22$, $n = 107$, versus control, $1.06 \pm 0.35$, $n = 99$, **$p = 0.0015$, Fig. 1b). Conversely, when TACC3 levels were elevated, the frequency of axon

retraction rates was reduced significantly by 45% compared to controls (TACC3 OE, $0.54 \pm 0.12$, $n = 155$, versus control, $0.99 \pm 0.12$, $n = 180$, *$p = 0.01$, Fig. 1b). Although TACC3 OE led to increased axonal length (Fig. 1f), TACC3 OE actually reduced axon outgrowth velocity by 14% ($0.89 \pm 0.32$, $n = 103$, versus control, $1.04 \pm 0.033$, $n = 57$, *$p < 0.0268$, Fig. 1a), suggesting that the increased axonal length may result from reduced axon retraction rather than a change in outgrowth velocity.

To further explore the TACC3 KD phenotype, we examined axon outgrowth of cultured neurons in which TACC3 was acutely inhibited by the TACC3 specific inhibitor, KHS-101 [14]. Consistent with the effect seen in TACC3 KD, KHS-101-induced acute inhibition of TACC3 significantly reduced MT growth velocity by 28% ($15.09 \pm 0.86$ μm/min (before drug treatment); $10.84 \pm 0.75$ μm/min (after drug), **$p < 0.0019$, Fig. 1c). Moreover, acute inhibition led to an immediate retraction of axon length by 26% compared to vehicle treated controls (KHS-101, $0.71 \pm 0.05$, $n = 12$, versus DMSO, $0.96 \pm 0.03$, $n = 9$, ***$p = 0.0007$, Fig. 1d).

In order to determine which domains of TACC3 are involved in axon outgrowth, we tested various truncation mutants of TACC3. We found that, while full-length TACC3 and ΔN (lacking conserved N-terminal domain) significantly increased axon outgrowth by 30% ($1.30 \pm 0.03$, $n = 787$, ***$p < 0.0001$) and 18% ($1.18 \pm 0.31$, $n = 613$, ***$p < 0.0001$) respectively, expression of ΔTACC (lacking the conserved TACC domain, which has been shown to be required for centrosome localization and interaction with the MT polymerase, XMAP215) caused a significant reduction by 12% in axon length ($0.87 \pm 0.021$, $n = 764$, ***$p = 0.0002$) in comparison to wild-type neurons ($0.99 \pm 0.02$, $n = 997$) (Fig. 1f). On the other hand, the larger N-term deletion (lacking both the conserved N-terminus and the putative SxIP-like motif that is known to mediate EB1 interaction for other + TIPs) showed no significant difference ($1.04 \pm 0.028$, $n = 563$, $p = 0.2012$). Additionally, none of the deletion constructs that promoted axon outgrowth were as effective as full-length TACC3 OE (Fig. 1f).

Together, our findings suggest that TACC3 is required for proper axon outgrowth by opposing axonal retracting forces. Additionally, full-length TACC3 is more efficient in promoting axon outgrowth than its truncation mutants, while expression of a version lacking the TACC domain results in a mild dominant negative effect.

#### TACC3 antagonizes nocodazole-induced MT depolymerization but does not affect MT lattice stability

Previously, we determined that TACC3 promotes efficient MT polymerization by enhancing MT growth velocity within growth cones [7]. However, the mechanism by which TACC3 affects MT polymerization remains to be elucidated. Thus, we sought to gain further insight by assessing the impact of low doses of the MT depolymerizing drug, nocodazole, after TACC3 manipulation.

We observed that a low dose of nocodazole led to reduction in several parameters of MT dynamics, and that TACC3 OE could mitigate these effects. While control growth cones exhibited a marked 20% decrease in MT growth speed after treatment with 50 pM nocodazole (before, $1.00 \pm 0.04$, $n = 22$, after treatment, $0.79 \pm 0.03$, $n = 22$, ***$p = 0.0001$), TACC3 OE growth cones showed reduction by only 12% (before, $1.08 \pm 0.04$, $n = 21$, after nocodazole, $0.95 \pm 0.03$, $n = 21$, *$p = 0.0316$, Fig. 2a). Similar trends were observed with MT growth lifetime, in which control growth cones showed a 15% reduction (before, $1.00 \pm 0.03$ s, $n = 22$, after nocodazole, $0.84 \pm 0.03$ s, $n = 22$, ***$p = 0.0008$) versus only a 3% reduction with TACC3 OE (before, $0.91 \pm 0.03$, $n = 21$, after nocodazole, $0.87 \pm 0.03$, $n = 21$, $p = 0.4305$, Fig. 2b), and for MT growth length, there was a 35% reduction in controls (before, $1.00 \pm 0.05$, $n = 22$, after nocodazole, $0.65 \pm 0.03$, $n = 22$, ***$p < 0.0001$) versus 14% in TACC3 OE (before, $1.00 \pm 0.04$, $n = 21$, after nocodazole, $0.85 \pm 0.04$, $n = 21$, *$p = 0.02$, Fig. 2c). These results suggest that TACC3 can mitigate the nocodazole-induced reduction in MT growth dynamics parameters. This mitigation can be more clearly visualized when the nocodazole-induced change is represented as the ratio of after treatment/before treatment. Although the relative reduction in MT growth speed when TACC3 is overexpressed is only slightly less compared to controls and is not quite statistically significant ($0.91 \pm 0.06$ $n = 21$ versus control $0.82 \pm 0.04$ $n = 22$, ns $p = 0.2$, Fig. 2a'), for other MT growth parameters, TACC3 OE significantly dampens the nocodazole-induced reduction in lifetime ($0.99 \pm 0.047$ $n = 21$ versus control $0.86 \pm 0.03$ $n = 22$, *$p = 0.03$, Fig. 2b') and length ($0.91 \pm 0.08$ $n = 21$ versus control $0.68 \pm 0.04$ $n = 22$, *$p = 0.01$, Fig. 2c') compared to controls.

In addition to MT polymerization, MT stabilization is considered to be an important parameter for axon outgrowth and growth cone turning events [12]. Hence, we measured the fluorescence intensities of tyrosinated and de-tyrosinated tubulin in the growth cone and assessed dynamic and stable MT lattice profiles, in TACC3-manipulated growth cones. We found that the ratio of tyrosinated tubulin versus de-tyrosinated tubulin did not statistically differ in TACC3 KD ($0.87 \pm 0.07$, $n = 37$, $p = 0.2394$) nor in TACC3 OE ($1.01 \pm 0.11$, $n = 129$, $p = 0.9673$) growth cones, with respect to control growth cones ($1.00 \pm 0.09$, $n = 143$, Fig. 2d-f). This suggests that TACC3 may not specifically regulate MT lattice stability in growth cones.

## TACC3 and XMAP215 interact to promote axon outgrowth

We previously found that the TACC3 interactor and MT polymerase, XMAP215, also promotes axon outgrowth [6], and that TACC3 and XMAP215 co-localize at the extreme plus-end of MTs in growth cones in a co-dependent manner [7]. However, the consequences of their interaction on axon development have not been elucidated. Therefore, we sought to test whether TACC3 and XMAP215 might cooperate synergistically to promote axon outgrowth by partially elevating or reducing TACC3 and XMAP215 levels alone and in combination with each other. While a very mild TACC3 KD (approximately 20–30% less) led to 10% reduction in axon outgrowth ($204.7 \pm 4.8$ µm, $n = 487$, $p = 0.3528$) and partial XMAP215 KD led to 13% reduction ($185.6 \pm 6.4$ µm, $n = 312$, *$p = 0.0116$), partial knockdown of both reduced axon length significantly by 34% ($140.6 \pm 3.5$ µm, $n = 552$, ***$p < 0.0001$) compared to control axons ($213.6 \pm 9.6$ µm, $n = 219$, Fig. 3a). Conversely, overexpression of both (double OE) increased axon length by 32.7% ($237.7 \pm 5.4$ µm, $n = 654$, ***$p < 0.0001$) while TACC3 OE alone increased by 11% ($198.9 \pm 3.2$, $n = 1585$, ***$p < 0.0001$) and XMAP215 OE increased by 30.9% ($234.5 \pm 4.3$ µm, $n = 1227$, ***$p < 0.0001$) in comparison to controls ($179.1 \pm 3.2$ µm, $n = 1288$, Fig. 3b). Interestingly, while double OE significantly increased axon length in comparison to TACC3 OE alone (***$p < 0.0001$), it did not show a difference when compared to XMAP215 alone ($p = 0.6421$) suggesting that there may be an upper threshold that is reached with XMAP215 OE by itself.

We next asked whether overexpression of one + TIP might rescue the reduced axon length in the absence of the other. We observed that overexpressing XMAP215 in the stronger TACC3 KD background brought axon outgrowth length to control levels (TACC3 KD + XMAP215 OE, $149.4 \pm 5.2$ µm, $n = 313$, **$p = 0.005$, versus control, $148.8 \pm 3.6$ µm, $n = 558$, $p = 0.9331$) by increasing the length 15% in comparison to TACC3 KD ($129.7 \pm 4.477$ µm, $n = 289$, **$p = 0.0015$, Fig. 3c). On the other hand, overexpression of TACC3 in the XMAP215 KD background increased axon outgrowth length by 30% (XMAP215 KD + TACC3 OE, $262.2 \pm 7.8$ µm, $n = 397$, ***$p < 0.0001$) in comparison to XMAP215 KD ($201.3 \pm 7.2$ µm, $n = 299$); however, the rescue was not complete when compared to control axons (Control, $304.9 \pm 8.5$ µm, $n = 463$, ***$p = 0.003$, Fig. 3d). These findings suggest that TACC3 and XMAP215 cooperate during axon outgrowth, with XMAP215 showing more additive effects on TACC3-mediated axon outgrowth.

## TACC3 affects axon guidance in vivo and ex vivo

The direction that the growth cone acquires during outgrowth is a result of local modulation of MT dynamics in response to guidance signals [12, 15–17]. Thus, we

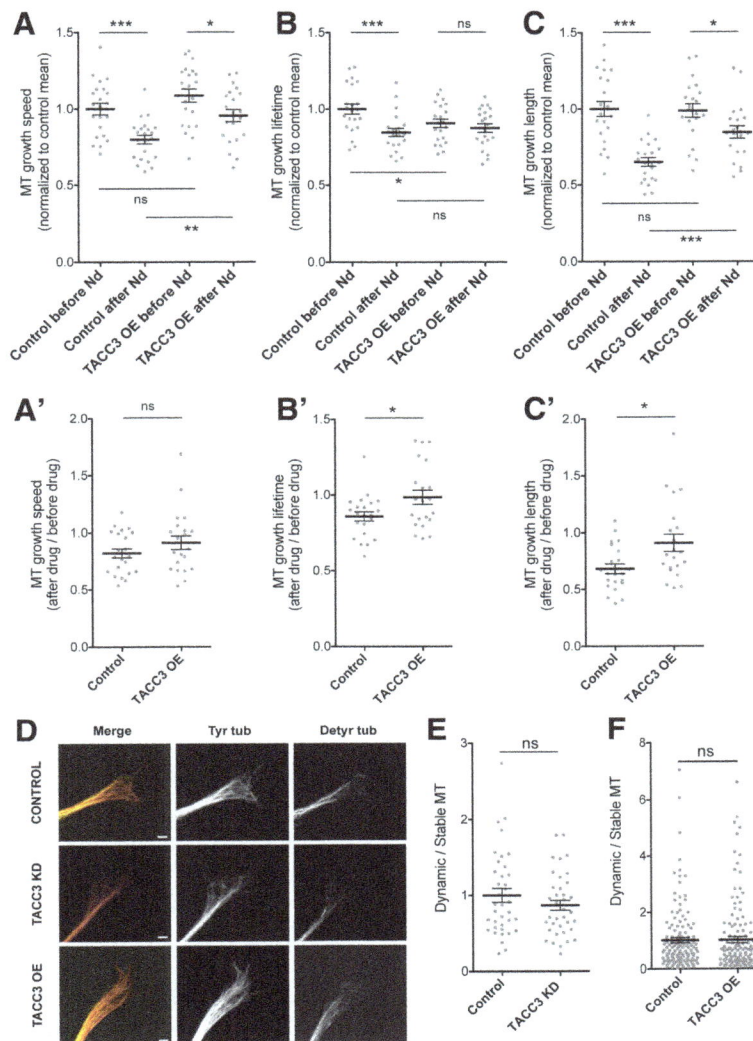

**Fig. 2** TACC3 antagonizes Nocodazole-induced MT depolymerization but does not affect MT stability. **a-c**, Quantification of the MT dynamics shows significant reduction in MT growth speed (**a**), MT lifetime (**b**) and MT growth length (**c**) in control ($n = 22$) and TACC3 OE ($n = 21$) growth cones in response to 50 pM Nocodazole before and 5 min after drug treatment. However, the effect of Nocodazole on TACC3 OE growth cones is dampened compared to controls. **a'-c'**, Although not significant, reduction in MT growth speed (**a'**) is more prominent in control growth cones compared to TACC3 OE growth cones while the reduction in both lifetime (**b'**) and length (**c'**) in control growth cones are significantly higher than the TACC3 OE growth cones (**d**) Representative growth cone images of control, TACC3 KD and TACC3 OE, immunostained for tyrosinated tubulin (*red*) and detyrosinated tubulin (*green*) to label dynamic versus stable MTs, respectively. **e-f**, Quantification of the fluorescence intensity of imaging data in G, with TACC3 KD ($n = 38$) (**e**) and TACC3 OE ($n = 129$) (**f**) growth cones showing no significant changes in dynamic/stable MTs compared to corresponding control growth cones ($n = 37$ and $n = 143$, respectively). *$p < 0.05$, **$p < 0.01$, ***$p < 0.001$. ns not significant. $n$ = growth cone number. Scale bar, 2 μm

wondered whether TACC3 regulation of MT dynamics could play a role during axon guidance. We first examined motor neuron axon outgrowth from the spinal cord in embryos at an early developmental stage (st 28), and we discovered that reduction of TACC3 caused significantly impaired outgrowth and severely disrupted morphology in all embryos examined (Fig. 4a-c). To gain greater insight into whether TACC3 manipulation causes this disorganization under specific guidance signals, we examined growth cone behavior in response to the

guidance molecule, Slit2, applied in culture media. Slit2 is a repellent guidance cue which has been previously studied with other + TIPs, such as CLASP [4], and the response of growth cones of different neuron types isolated from *Xenopus* embryos at different stages has been previously documented [18–20]. We monitored the changes in growth cone behavior for 10 min prior and for 30 min after addition of Slit2. Growth cones that show persistent growth were picked to be analyzed for their behavior after Slit2 addition. Growth cones that

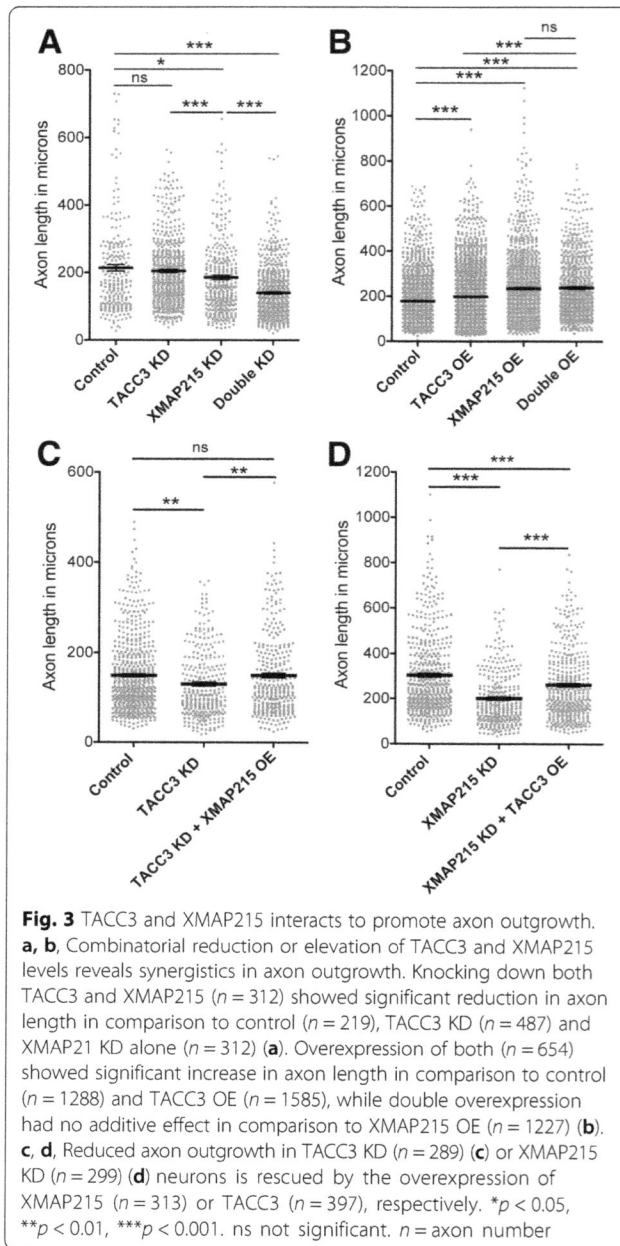

**Fig. 3** TACC3 and XMAP215 interacts to promote axon outgrowth. **a, b**, Combinatorial reduction or elevation of TACC3 and XMAP215 levels reveals synergistics in axon outgrowth. Knocking down both TACC3 and XMAP215 (n = 312) showed significant reduction in axon length in comparison to control (n = 219), TACC3 KD (n = 487) and XMAP21 KD alone (n = 312) (**a**). Overexpression of both (n = 654) showed significant increase in axon length in comparison to control (n = 1288) and TACC3 OE (n = 1585), while double overexpression had no additive effect in comparison to XMAP215 OE (n = 1227) (**b**). **c, d**, Reduced axon outgrowth in TACC3 KD (n = 289) (**c**) or XMAP215 KD (n = 299) (**d**) neurons is rescued by the overexpression of XMAP215 (n = 313) or TACC3 (n = 397), respectively. *p < 0.05, **p < 0.01, ***p < 0.001. ns not significant. n = axon number

during axon outgrowth, guidance decisions and regeneration events [12, 15–17, 21, 22]. Accordingly, MT plus-end tracking proteins (+TIPs) likely play a critical role during axon guidance, as + TIPs dominate the dynamic portion of MTs that reaches the growth cone periphery, where guidance cue receptors reside [2]. However, few + TIPs have been examined within the context of the embryonic growth cone. We previously characterized a MT plus-end tracking function for TACC3 and showed that it can promote MT polymerization and is required for proper axonal development [7]. Here, we sought to uncover new insights into the mechanism underlying axonal regulation by TACC3.

First, we found that the shorter axons that result from reduced levels of TACC3 were due to slower axon outgrowth velocity along with significantly increased retraction rate. Moreover, TACC3 overexpression leads to longer axons, not because of fast axon outgrowth velocity (the outgrowth rate was actually slower than in controls), but because of reduced axon retraction rate. This suggests that TACC3-mediated MT dynamics may be required for opposing the normally-occurring retractive forces within axons. Another possible explanation is that the reduced axon outgrowth velocity and reduced axonal retraction rates after TACC3 OE could be due to stronger anchorage to the underlying substrate and adhesion turnover. While there are some + TIPs that have been implicated to mediate MT − focal adhesion interactions [23], TACC3 has not yet been explored in focal adhesion (or point contacts, in the case of growth cones) regulation. However, since TACC3 has been identified as an interactor of CLASP [24], and given that CLASP is known to function during focal adhesion turnover [25], future studies should examine whether TACC3 also plays a role at focal adhesions/point contacts.

+TIPs modulate MT dynamic instability in various ways; for example, XMAP215 promotes MT growth by catalyzing addition of tubulin dimers [26], while CLASP and APC rescue MT from catastrophe by increasing MT stability [27–29]. Here, we showed that TACC3 OE can dampen nocodazole-induced reduction in MT growth speed, length and lifetime. However, this was not achieved by increased MT lattice stability, as immunofluorescence analysis of dynamic versus stable MTs revealed that TACC3 has no apparent impact on MT stability within the growth cone. It is unclear how TACC3 is able to mitigate the reduction in MT growth speed, length and lifetime as a result of nocodazole application. One possibility could be that TACC3 overexpression, which enhances XMAP215 localization at MT plus ends [7], may simply promote more efficient and processive MT polymerization by XMAP215 to counteract the nocodazole-induced effects.

had reduced lamellipodial area were considered as collapsed. We found that TACC3 OE growth cones had significantly fewer growth cone collapse and axon retraction events (TACC3 OE, 21.28 ± 7.24 n = 76 versus control, 54.72 ± 4.26 n = 44, *p = 0.0164) in response to Slit2, when compared to wild type growth cones (Fig. 4d-e). This suggests that overexpressing TACC3 can counteract Slit2-induced growth cone collapse.

**Discussion**

Dynamic spatial and temporal regulation of MTs within the growth cone is considered to be of key importance

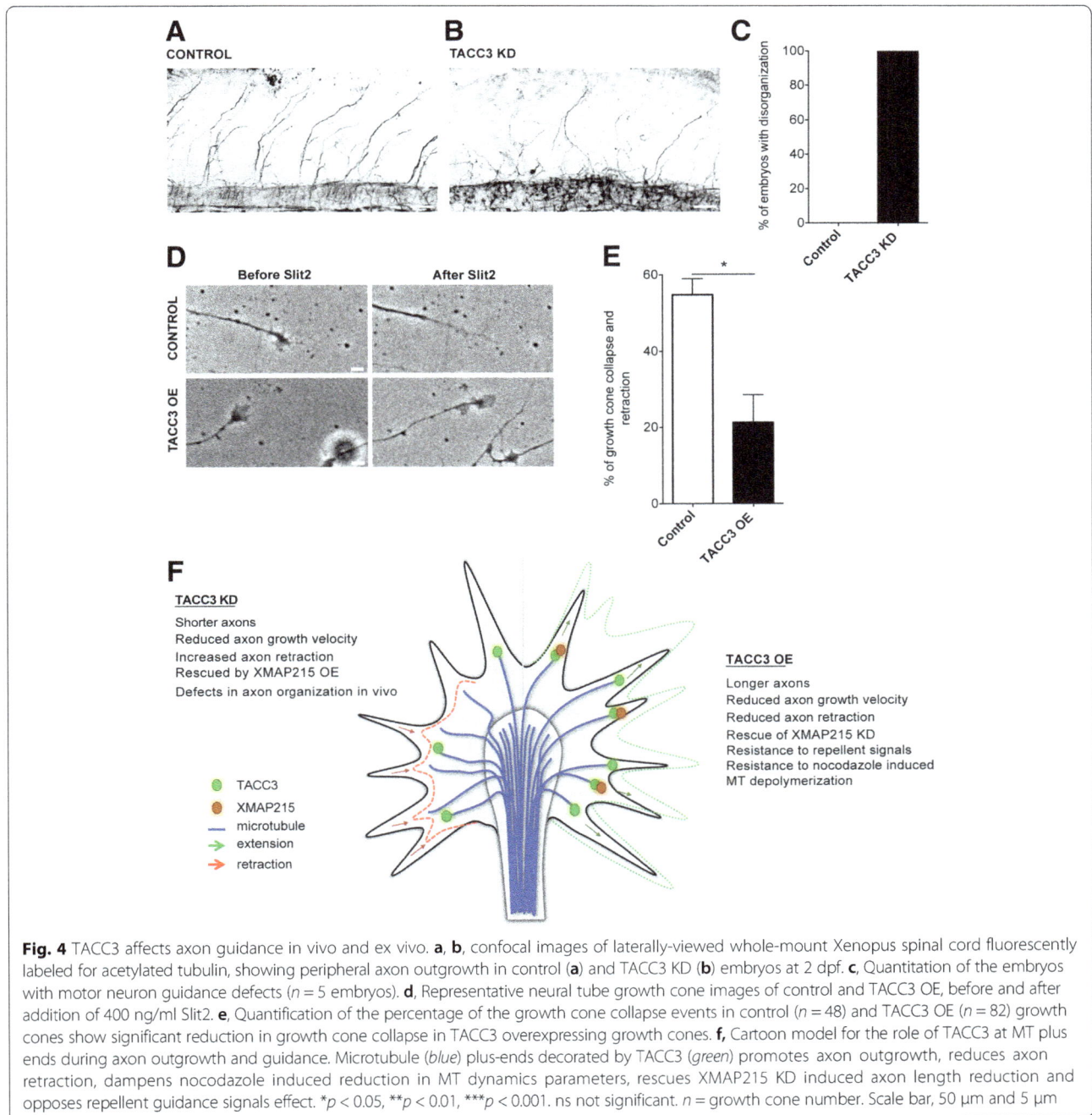

**Fig. 4** TACC3 affects axon guidance in vivo and ex vivo. **a**, **b**, confocal images of laterally-viewed whole-mount Xenopus spinal cord fluorescently labeled for acetylated tubulin, showing peripheral axon outgrowth in control (**a**) and TACC3 KD (**b**) embryos at 2 dpf. **c**, Quantitation of the embryos with motor neuron guidance defects ($n = 5$ embryos). **d**, Representative neural tube growth cone images of control and TACC3 OE, before and after addition of 400 ng/ml Slit2. **e**, Quantification of the percentage of the growth cone collapse events in control ($n = 48$) and TACC3 OE ($n = 82$) growth cones show significant reduction in growth cone collapse in TACC3 overexpressing growth cones. **f**, Cartoon model for the role of TACC3 at MT plus ends during axon outgrowth and guidance. Microtubule (*blue*) plus-ends decorated by TACC3 (*green*) promotes axon outgrowth, reduces axon retraction, dampens nocodazole induced reduction in MT dynamics parameters, rescues XMAP215 KD induced axon length reduction and opposes repellent guidance signals effect. *$p < 0.05$, **$p < 0.01$, ***$p < 0.001$. ns not significant. $n$ = growth cone number. Scale bar, 50 μm and 5 μm

Individual + TIPs comprise a network of proteins at MT plus-ends which can co-localize and function together to modulate MT dynamics. We have previously shown such cooperation between TACC3 and XMAP215 in growth cones, as we demonstrated that TACC3 and XMAP215 co-localize at MT plus-ends in co-dependent manner [7].

Here, we found that TACC3 and XMAP215 interact to promote axon outgrowth (Fig. 3). Partially knocking down both TACC3 and XMAP215 resulted in further reduction in axon outgrowth length, which suggests a synergistic interaction between the two proteins. However, overexpression of both + TIPs did not show further increase in axon length in comparison to XMAP215 OE alone. This might be due to an upper threshold that is reached with overexpression of XMAP215 alone. Conversely, rescue studies show that XMAP215 can fully restore TACC3 KD-mediated reduced axon length to control levels, whereas TACC3 OE fails to show the same impact over XMAP215 KD. As XMAP215 is a processive MT polymerase, reduction in XMAP215 levels may exert more dramatic effect than the reduction in the levels of TACC3, which may play more of an accessory role. Considering that one study suggests that every TACC3 molecule is thought to interact with two molecules of XMAP215 [30], reduced levels of XMAP215 could be a limiting factor. Even though TACC3 OE functions to increase available XMAP215 at MT plus-ends, the reduction in overall XMAP215 levels may result in poor axon outgrowth. While knock down approaches provide supporting evidence regarding the combinatorial role of TACC3 and XMAP215 during axon outgrowth, future studies should utilize mutations that disrupt their interaction [30] in order to understand the dependence of these two proteins on one another during axon outgrowth.

In addition to their role in axon outgrowth, several + TIPs have been implicated in participating in growth cone steering decisions in response to extracellular cues. The first of which is *orbit/MAST*, the fly ortholog of mammalian CLASP, that has been identified to cooperate with Abelson kinase (Abl) downstream of Slit/Robo guidance pathway [4]. In a parallel genetic and proteomic screen in fruit flies, *minispindles* (*msps*), a fly ortholog of Xenopus XMAP215, was identified to function antagonistically against CLASP and Abl during embryonic central nervous system development [5], while another genetic interaction study in flies identified *dtacc* as an antagonist of CLASP [24], reminiscent of the interaction between CLASP and TACC partner, *msps*. Combining these previous works with our findings on the role of TACC3 in axon outgrowth led us to ask whether TACC3 functions during axon guidance. As demonstrated in Fig. 4a, our initial observations revealed that reduction in TACC3 levels impairs the normal organization of axons exiting the spinal cord in embryos at st 28. Stimulation of cultured *Xenopus* retinal neurons at stage 32 or beyond with bath-applied Slit2 has been shown to cause growth cone collapse [19]. Additionally, spinal neurons derived from st 28 *Xenopus* embryos have been previously shown to be repelled by Slit2 [18]. Here, we found that Slit2-induced neural tube growth cone collapse events can be reduced by 60% in TACC3 overexpressing growth cones in comparison to control, suggesting an opposing role for TACC3 in Slit2-induced growth cone collapse. Based on its role in MT polymerization [7], its co-dependent localization at MT plus ends with XMAP215 [7], and their interaction during axon outgrowth (Fig. 3), we propose that TACC3 OE will excessively occupy MT plus-ends, subsequently driving increased recruitment of XMAP215, prompting enhanced MT polymerization in all directions. This global increase in MT polymerization would disturb local MT modulation, which is the underlying mechanism for growth cone steering events and it would result in an aberrant, non-obedient growth cone advance (Fig. 4f).

It remains to be determined whether these effects are specific to Slit2 or if TACC3 could exert similar opposing effects in response to other repellent signals, and/or if TACC3 mediates attractive signals as well. Finally, other TACC members, namely, TACC1 and TACC2, have recently been characterized as + TIPs that can promote MT polymerization in *Xenopus* embryonic cells [31, 32]. Although their expression and MT regulatory function show cell type-specificity, it would be intriguing to study whether other members of the TACC family also play a role in axon outgrowth and guidance decisions.

## Conclusion

This study characterizes the mechanism by which TACC3 regulates MT dynamics within the embryonic neuronal growth cone and promotes axon outgrowth. Using time-lapse imaging of *Xenopus laevis* embryonic axons as they grow in culture, we demonstrated that TACC3 promotes persistent axon outgrowth not by accelerating axon growth velocity but by reducing spontaneous axon retraction events. Moreover, we demonstrate that overexpressing TACC3 can mitigate the reduction in MT dynamics parameters that occur after Nocodazole application, suggesting that TACC3 may be promoting MT dynamics by dampening MT depolymerization. Finally, our data suggests that the + TIP TACC3 mediates axon guidance, as reduction in TACC3 levels results in defects in the normal organization of spinal neuron axons within the spinal cord. Moreover, bath application of the Slit2 repellent guidance molecule into cultured neural tube neurons shows that TACC3 OE reduce the Slit2 induced growth cone collapse events suggesting that TACC3 may involve in generation of response to guidance signals during neuronal development.

**Abbreviations**
+TIPs: Plus-end tracking proteins; ch-TOG: Colonic and hepatic tumor overexpressed gene protein; CLASP: Cytoplasmic linker associated protein; KD: Knockdown; MO: Morpholino; msps: Minispindles; MT: Microtubule; Nd: Nocodazole; OE: Overexpression; TACC3: Transforming acidic coiled-coil; XMAP215: *Xenopus* microtubule associated protein 215

**Acknowledgements**
We thank members of the Lowery Lab for helpful discussions, especially Sangmook Lee, Paula Slater, and Beth Bearce. We also thank Aleks Ostojic, Belinda Nwagbara, Matthew Evans and Jessica Tiber for technical assistance with experiments, and Nancy McGilloway and Todd Gaines for excellent *Xenopus* husbandry.

**Funding**
L.A.L. is funded by NIH R00 MH095768 and R01 MH109651.

## Authors' contributions

BE. and LAL. set up and designed the experiments. BE, GMC, EJL, BCP, AFF and ELR performed the experiments. BE and LAL wrote the manuscript. All authors discussed and edited the manuscript. All authors read and approved the final manuscript.

## Competing interests

The authors declare that they have no competing interests.

## References

1. Lowery LA, Van Vactor D. The trip of the tip: understanding the growth cone machinery. Nat Rev Mol Cell Biol. 2009;10:332–43.
2. Bearce EA, Erdogan B, Lowery LA. TIPsy tour guides: how microtubule plus-end tracking proteins (+TIPs) facilitate axon guidance. Front Cell Neurosci. 2015;9:241.
3. Cammarata GM, Bearce EA, Lowery LA. Cytoskeletal social networking in the growth cone: how + TIPs mediate microtubule-actin cross-linking to drive axon outgrowth and guidance. Cytoskeleton (Hoboken). 2016;73:461–76.
4. Lee H, Engel U, Rusch J, Scherrer S, Sheard K, Van Vactor D. The microtubule plus end tracking protein orbit/MAST/CLASP acts downstream of the tyrosine kinase Abl in mediating axon guidance. Neuron. 2004;42:913–26.
5. Lowery LA, Lee H, Lu C, Murphy R, Obar RA, Zhai B, Schedl M, Van Vactor D, Zhan Y. Parallel genetic and proteomic screens identify Msps as a CLASP-Abl pathway interactor in Drosophila. Genetics. 2010;185:1311–25.
6. Lowery LA, Stout A, Faris AE, Ding L, Baird MA, Davidson MW, Danuser G, Van Vactor D. Growth cone-specific functions of XMAP215 in restricting microtubule dynamics and promoting axonal outgrowth. Neural Dev. 2013;8:22.
7. Nwagbara BU, Faris AE, Bearce EA, Erdogan B, Ebbert PT, Evans MF, Rutherford EL, Enzenbacher TB, Lowery LA. TACC3 is a microtubule plus end-tracking protein that promotes axon elongation and also regulates microtubule plus end dynamics in multiple embryonic cell types. Mol Biol Cell. 2014;25:3350–62.
8. Erdogan B, Ebbert PT, Lowery LA. Using Xenopus laevis retinal and spinal neurons to study mechanisms of axon guidance in vivo and in vitro. Semin Cell Dev Biol. 2016;51:64–72.
9. Slater PG, Hayrapetian L, Lowery LA. Xenopus laevis as a model system to study cytoskeletal dynamics during axon pathfinding. Genesis. 2017;55: e22994.
10. Lowery LA, Faris AE, Stout A, Van Vactor D. Neural Explant Cultures from Xenopus laevis. J Vis Exp. 2012;68:e4232.
11. Widlund PO, Stear JH, Pozniakovsky A, Zanic M, Reber S, Brouhard GJ, Hyman AA, Howard J. XMAP215 polymerase activity is built by combining multiple tubulin-binding TOG domains and a basic lattice-binding region. Proc Natl Acad Sci U S A. 2011;108:2741–6.
12. Challacombe JF, Snow DM, Letourneau PC. Dynamic microtubule ends are required for growth cone turning to avoid an inhibitory guidance cue. J Neurosci. 1997;17:3085–95.
13. Applegate KT, Besson S, Matov A, Bagonis MH, Jaqaman K, Danuser G. plusTipTracker: quantitative image analysis software for the measurement of microtubule dynamics. J Struct Biol. 2011;176:168–84.
14. Wurdak H, Zhu S, Min KH, Aimone L, Lairson LL, Watson J, Chopiuk G, Demas J, Charette B, Halder R, et al. A small molecule accelerates neuronal differentiation in the adult rat. Proc Natl Acad Sci U S A. 2010;107:16542–7.
15. Sabry JH, O'Connor TP, Evans L, Toroian-Raymond A, Kirschner M, Bentley D. Microtubule behavior during guidance of pioneer neuron growth cones in situ. J Cell Biol. 1991;115:381–95.
16. Tanaka E, Kirschner MW. The role of microtubules in growth cone turning at substrate boundaries. J Cell Biol. 1995;128:127–37.
17. Williamson T, GordonWeeks PR, Schachner M, Taylor J. Microtubule reorganization is obligatory for growth cone turning. Proc Natl Acad Sci U S A. 1996;93:15221–6.
18. Stein E, Tessier-Lavigne M. Hierarchical organization of guidance receptors: silencing of netrin attraction by slit through a Robo/DCC receptor complex. Science. 2001;291:1928–38.
19. Piper M, Anderson R, Dwivedy A, Weinl C, van Horck F, Leung KM, Cogill E, Holt C. Signaling mechanisms underlying Slit2-induced collapse of Xenopus retinal growth cones. Neuron. 2006;49:215–28.
20. Myers JP, Robles E, Ducharme-Smith A, Gomez TM. Focal adhesion kinase modulates Cdc42 activity downstream of positive and negative axon guidance cues. J Cell Sci. 2012;125:2918–29.
21. Buck KB, Zheng JQ. Growth cone turning induced by direct local modification of microtubule dynamics. J Neurosci. 2002;22:9358–67.
22. Chen L, Chuang M, Koorman T, Boxem M, Jin Y, Chisholm AD. Axon injury triggers EFA-6 mediated destabilization of axonal microtubules via TACC and doublecortin like kinase. eLife. 2015;4:e08695.
23. Stehbens S, Wittmann T. Targeting and transport: how microtubules control focal adhesion dynamics. J Cell Biol. 2012;198:481–9.
24. Long JB, Bagonis M, Lowery LA, Lee H, Danuser G, Van Vactor D. Multiparametric analysis of CLASP-interacting protein functions during interphase microtubule dynamics. Mol Cell Biol. 2013;33:1528–45.
25. Stehbens SJ, Paszek M, Pemble H, Ettinger A, Gierke S, Wittmann T. CLASPs link focal-adhesion-associated microtubule capture to localized exocytosis and adhesion site turnover. Nat Cell Biol. 2014;16:561–73.
26. Brouhard GJ, Stear JH, Noetzel TL, Al-Bassam J, Kinoshita K, Harrison SC, Howard J, Hyman AA. XMAP215 is a processive microtubule polymerase. Cell. 2008;132:79–88.
27. Mimori-Kiyosue Y, Grigoriev I, Lansbergen G, Sasaki H, Matsui C, Severin F, Galjart N, Grosveld F, Vorobjev I, Tsukita S, Akhmanova A. CLASP1 and CLASP2 bind to EB1 and regulate microtubule plus-end dynamics at the cell cortex. J Cell Biol. 2005;168:141–53.
28. Wen Y, Eng CH, Schmoranzer J, Cabrera-Poch N, Morris EJ, Chen M, Wallar BJ, Alberts AS, Gundersen GG. EB1 and APC bind to mDia to stabilize microtubules downstream of Rho and promote cell migration. Nat Cell Biol. 2004;6:820–30.
29. Zumbrunn J, Kinoshita K, Hyman AA, Näthke IS. Binding of the adenomatous polyposis coli protein to microtubules increases microtubule stability and is regulated by GSK3 beta phosphorylation. Curr Biol. 2001;11:44–9.
30. Mortuza GB, Cavazza T, Garcia-Mayoral MF, Hermida D, Peset I, Pedrero JG, Merino N, Blanco FJ, Lyngso J, Bruix M, et al. XTACC3-XMAP215 association reveals an asymmetric interaction promoting microtubule elongation. Nat Commun. 2014;5:5072.
31. Lucaj CM, Evans MF, Nwagbara BU, Ebbert PT, Baker CC, Volk JG, Francl AF, Ruvolo SP, Lowery LA. Xenopus TACC1 is a microtubule plus-end tracking protein that can regulate microtubule dynamics during embryonic development. Cytoskeleton (Hoboken). 2015;72:225–34.
32. Rutherford EL, Carandang L, Ebbert PT, Mills AN, Bowers JT, Lowery LA. Xenopus TACC2 is a microtubule plus end-tracking protein that can promote microtubule polymerization during embryonic development. Mol Biol Cell. 2016;27:3013–20.

# 5

# Semaphorin-Plexin signaling influences early ventral telencephalic development and thalamocortical axon guidance

Manuela D. Mitsogiannis[1], Graham E. Little[1,2] and Kevin J. Mitchell[1,3,4*]

## Abstract

**Background:** Sensory processing relies on projections from the thalamus to the neocortex being established during development. Information from different sensory modalities reaching the thalamus is segregated into specialized nuclei, whose neurons then send inputs to cognate cortical areas through topographically defined axonal connections. Developing thalamocortical axons (TCAs) normally approach the cortex by extending through the subpallium; here, axonal navigation is aided by distributed guidance cues and discrete cell populations, such as the corridor neurons and the internal capsule (IC) guidepost cells. In mice lacking Semaphorin-6A, axons from the dorsal lateral geniculate nucleus (dLGN) bypass the IC and extend aberrantly in the ventral subpallium. The functions normally mediated by Semaphorin-6A in this system remain unknown, but might depend on interactions with Plexin-A2 and Plexin-A4, which have been implicated in other neurodevelopmental processes.

**Methods:** We performed immunohistochemical and neuroanatomical analyses of thalamocortical wiring and subpallial development in *Sema6a* and *Plxna2*; *Plxna4* null mutant mice and analyzed the expression of these genes in relevant structures.

**Results:** In *Plxna2*; *Plxna4* double mutants we discovered TCA pathfinding defects that mirrored those observed in *Sema6a* mutants, suggesting that Semaphorin-6A – Plexin-A2/Plexin-A4 signaling might mediate dLGN axon guidance at subpallial level.

In order to understand where and when Semaphorin-6A, Plexin-A2 and Plexin-A4 may be required for proper subpallial TCA guidance, we then characterized their spatiotemporal expression dynamics during early TCA development. We observed that the thalamic neurons whose axons are misrouted in these mutants normally express Semaphorin-6A but not Plexin-A2 or Plexin-A4. By contrast, all three proteins are expressed in corridor cells and other structures in the developing basal ganglia.

This finding could be consistent with an hypothetical action of Plexins as guidance signals through Sema6A as a receptor on dLGN axons, and/or with their indirect effect on TCA guidance due to functions in the morphogenesis of subpallial intermediate targets. In support of the latter possibility, we observed that in both *Plxna2*; *Plxna4* and *Sema6a* mutants some IC guidepost cells abnormally localize in correspondence of the ventral path misrouted TCAs elongate into.

**Conclusions:** These findings implicate Semaphorin-6A – Plexin-A2/Plexin-A4 interactions in dLGN axon guidance and in the spatiotemporal organization of guidepost cell populations in the mammalian subpallium.

**Keywords:** Guidepost cells, Plexin-A2, Plexin-A4, Semaphorin-6A, Subpallium, Thalamocortical connectivity

* Correspondence: kevin.mitchell@tcd.ie
[1]Smurfit Institute of Genetics, School of Genetics and Microbiology, Trinity College Dublin, Dublin 2, Ireland
[3]Trinity College Institute of Neuroscience, Trinity College Dublin, Dublin 2, Ireland
Full list of author information is available at the end of the article

# Background

The establishment of specific, finely organized neural circuits comprising often distant central nervous system regions is essential for normal brain functioning. Indeed, many neurological and psychiatric disorders have been characterized as potential neurodevelopmental disconnectivity or abnormal connectivity syndromes [1], including autism spectrum disorders [2–7], schizophrenia [8–16], and attention deficit hyperactivity disorder [17–19].

Growing axonal projections in the brain follow spatially complex, yet remarkably stereotyped pathways en route to their final destinations. Forebrain connections thus develop in a stepwise manner: as axons progressively extend, specific growth instructions are provided by guidance factors located at defined 'decision points' along axonal paths [20]. The correct spatiotemporal distribution of guidance molecules, supported by the development and proper assembly of intermediate targets, is therefore just as essential as their ultimate effects on growth cones for normal brain wiring [21–23]. While a wealth of knowledge has been gained in the past two decades on axon guidance molecules and their roles in steering developing axons, our understanding of the processes underlying intermediate target formation, guidance cue patterning of axonal pathways, and cue presentation to elongating fibers is still relatively limited [22, 24]. One of these process is the migration at intermediate points of "guidepost cells", i.e., discrete, specialized cell populations that finely orient growth cones via short-range cues and direct cell–cell contacts. Interestingly, several lines of evidence have pointed to a role of guidance factors also in guidepost cell migration and positioning, and have shown how these molecules can thus affect axonal pathfinding in an indirect manner (reviewed in Squarzoni, Thion [25]).

In the study of the molecular mechanisms involved in the establishment of topographically arranged neural connections, the thalamocortical system constitutes a unique analytical model. Indeed, in the assembly of neural networks between the cortex and the thalamus, axonal sorting is aided by the presence of guidance molecules patterns, cytoarchitecturally-defined permissive pathways, guidepost cell populations at multiple 'decision points', and axon-axon interactions.

In the mouse, thalamocortical axons (TCAs) from the dorsal thalamus (dTh) first extend ventrally into the prethalamus, then make a sharp turn at the diencephalic-telencephalic boundary (DTB) and proceed in a dorso-lateral direction through the ventral telencephalon (vTel) to reach the pallial-subpallial boundary (PSPB). As TCAs travel within the subpallium, they then diverge along the rostro-caudal axis according to the position of their final cortical targets [21, 26–28]. Navigation of axons in these early stages, taking place

between embryonic day (E) 11–15 [27, 29], has been demonstrated to rely on the presence of intermediate targets and guiding cell populations [21, 27, 30–32], such as the corridor cells and the guidepost cells found in the internal capsule (IC), the axonal bundle containing all reciprocal connections between cortical and subcortical structures.

So far, no specific guidance mechanisms have been identified in axonal pathfinding from each distinct thalamic nucleus. Matching of thalamic axons with appropriate cortical areas appears to emerge from the combinatorial action of several guidance factors and their receptors, expressed in complementary gradients within the dTh and the intermediate targets delineating axonal paths to the neocortex [21, 27]. However, previous studies by our lab have demonstrated a key role of Semaphorin-6A (Sema6A), a member of the semaphorin protein family, in subpallial pathfinding of the visual subset of thalamocortical connections. In *Sema6a* null mice, all dorsal lateral geniculate nucleus (dLGN) axons can be observed to abnormally extend outside the IC and into more ventral areas of the vTel, while projections from other thalamic nuclei develop normally [33–35]. This results in an invasion of the presumptive visual cortex by somatosensory TCAs from the ventrobasal complex (VB) at embryonic stages that persists until early postnatally. A few days after birth, an approximately normal pattern of thalamocortical connectivity is re-established by dLGN axons navigating to the visual cortex via alternative routes, and outcompeting VB-originated axons.

The exact mechanism by which Sema6A influences TCA guidance in such a specific manner has yet to be elucidated. In the central nervous system, two Sema6A binding partners have been so far identified, Plexin-A2 (PlxnA2) and Plexin-A4 (PlxnA4). Sema6A typically acts as a ligand for PlxnA2 and PlxnA4 in the brain, but it is known to be capable of both forward and reverse signaling with the two Plexin protein family members [36, 37]. Moreover, the effects of Sema6A–PlexinAs binding are highly context-dependent, and have been shown to be modulated by association between these proteins *in cis* [38–41]. Experimental evidence indicates that interactions between Sema6A and PlxnA2/PlxnA4 control several fundamental processes in the establishment of neural circuits, such as axon guidance [42, 43], axonal growth [44], laminar connectivity formation [41, 45], neural cell migration [46, 47], and dendritogenesis [48].

Considering all these findings, both Plexin family members might also be hypothesized to mediate Sema6A-induced responses in early visual thalamic axon guidance. Therefore, in this study we investigated the potential role of Sema6A – PlxnA2/PlxnA4 signaling in subpallial TCA pathfinding by analyzing the phenotype of single and double null mutant mouse lines for the two Plexin genes.

In *Plxna2; Plxna4* double mutants we observed a TCA phenotype almost identical to that seen in *Sema6a* mutants. Expression analyses indicate a non-canonical mode of Semaphorin – Plexin interaction-mediated guidance in this case, as both Plexins are not expressed by the misrouted axons, but all proteins are present in the developing subpallium. This suggests either Plexin – Semaphorin reverse signaling taking place, or an indirect effect of Sema6A, PlxnA2 and PlxnA4 on TCA guidance due to earlier functions in ventral forebrain development. A possible indirect guidance role is supported by the finding that a subset of IC guidepost cells is mislocated in both *Sema6a* and *Plxna2; Plxna4* mutants, suggesting that interactions between these molecules are involved in early morphogenesis of subpallial domains delineating TCA pathways.

## Methods
### Animals
All animal procedures were performed in accordance with Irish regulations on the use of animals for scientific purposes (Statutory Instrument No. 566 of 2002 and No. 543 of 2012) and institutional guidelines.

All experiments were performed on embryonic brains taken from C57BL/6 J mice (wild-type) (Jackson Laboratories), a C57BL/6 J strain carrying a null mutation for the *Sema6a* gene, and a *Plxna2; Plxna4* double null mutant C57BL/6 J strain. The *Sema6a* mutation was obtained through the insertion of a gene-trap vector in the 17th intron of *Sema6a*, which results in the production of an intracellularly sequestered N-terminal Sema6A portion–β-galactosidase fusion protein (for further details see Leighton et al. [33] and Mitchell et al. [49]). *Plxna2; Plxna4* knockout mice were generated by crossing single mutant lines obtained using gene-targeting strategies described by Suto and colleagues [41] (*Plxna2*), and Yaron and colleagues [50] (*Plxna4*). The *Plxna4* line was originally generated in a CD1 background and backcrossed to C57BL/6 J for 10 generations. Mice were maintained and bred in a 12:12 h light-dark cycle, in a specific pathogen free animal unit.

Pregnant animals for embryo collection were obtained through timed matings. Embryonic age was calculated considering the day of vaginal plug detection as E0.5. For postnatal mice, the day of birth was designated as P0. Mouse brains were dissected in cold PBS and fixed in 4% paraformaldehyde (PFA)/PBS for 2–4 h at 4 °C. Mouse tail samples (2–5 mm) were also collected for DNA extraction and genotyping.

### Genotyping
Tissue samples were digested overnight at 56 °C in a 1:100 solution of Proteinase K (Roche) in Boston Buffer

(50 mM Tris-HCl pH 8, 2.5 mM EDTA, 50 mM KCl, 0.45% NP-40, and 0.45% Tween 20). The genotype was determined by PCR, using a small aliquot of the digestion solution, a PCR mix (KAPA2G Fast HotStart ReadyMix with dye, KAPA Biosystems) containing dNTPs, a Taq polymerase and a loading dye, and primers for the gene of interest (see Additional file 1: Table S1).

### *In situ* hybridization
Digoxigenin (DIG)-labeled antisense (as) riboprobes for *in situ* hybridization were produced from plasmid templates linearized overnight at 37 °C with appropriate restriction enzymes (see Additional file 1: Table S2). A transcription reaction mix was prepared using 1 µg of linearized plasmid template, 2 µL of 10× RNA transcription buffer, 2 µL of 10× DIG labeling mix (Roche), 0.5 µL of RNase OUT (40 U/µL, Invitrogen), 20 U of T3 RNA polymerase, and brought to 20 µL volume with dH$_2$O. The reaction mix was incubated for 2 h at 37 °C; 1 U of RNase-free DNase I for 15 min at 37 °C were then added to remove the template, followed by 2 µL of 0.2 M EDTA at pH 8.0 to stop this reaction. Synthesized RNA was precipitated by adding 2.5 µL of 4 M LiCl and 75 µL of ethanol and incubating at –20 °C for over an hour, and afterwards pelleted by centrifugation at 4 °C (17,000 g or over, 20 min). RNA pellets were washed with 150 µL of 70% ethanol via centrifugation at 4 °C (17,000 g or over, 2 min), briefly let to air-dry, and resuspended in 1 mM sodium citrate at pH 6.35.

Serial 60 µm thick free-floating brain sections were obtained by slicing brains embedded in 4% w/v RNase free, low melting point agarose/RNase-free phosphate buffered saline (PBS) (obtained by treatment with diethylpyrocarbonate (DEPC)) with a vibratome (VT1000s, Leica), and were collected in DEPC-treated PBS. Sections were washed twice for 5 min in DEPC-treated PBS containing 0.1% Tween-20 (PBT). They were then permeabilized by incubation for 30 min in 0.5% Triton X-100 and 0.2% Tween-20 in DEPC-treated PBS at room temperature (RT), and additionally washed for 5 min in PBT. Next, half of the PBT volume was removed and replaced by pre-hybridization solution (50% deionized formamide, 5× standard saline citrate (SSC), 1% sodium dodecyl sulfate (SDS), 2.5 mg of yeast tRNA, 2.5 mg of heparin in DEPC-treated dH$_2$O) pre-warmed at 65 °C. After a 10 min incubation, sections were further washed with warm pre-hybridization solution for 10 min, and then incubated in fresh pre-warmed pre-hybridization solution for at least 1 h at 65 °C. Warm pre-hybridization solution containing 1 g/mL of the RNA probe of choice was next added to each section series for an overnight incubation at 65 °C in a humidity chamber (pre-equilibrated with 50% formamide/5× SSC in DEPC-treated dH$_2$O).

Following hybridization, three 30 min washes in solution I (50% formamide, 5× SSC, 1% SDS) and three 30 min washes in solution III (50% formamide, 2× SSC, 0.1% Tween-20) were performed at 65 °C. Sections were then washed three times for 5 min in Tris-buffered saline (TBS) containing 1% Tween-20 (TBST) at RT, and incubated in blocking buffer (TBST containing 10% heat-inactivated sheep serum) for at least 1 h. The buffer was subsequently replaced with an alkaline phosphatase (AP) conjugated anti-DIG antibody solution (1:2000 anti-DIG-AP Fab fragment (Roche) in blocking buffer) for an overnight incubation at 4 °C. The next day, sections were washed three times for 5 min in TBST, three times for 2 h in TBST, three times for 10 min in AP buffer (NTMT; 0.1 M Tris-HCl pH 9.5, 0.1 M NaCl, 50 mM $MgCl_2$, 1% Tween-20 in $dH_2O$), and then incubated in the dark in NBT (nitro blue tetrazolium)/BCIP (5-bromo-4-chloro-3-indolyl-phosphate) staining solution (20 μL NBT/BCIP stock solution (Roche) per mL of NTMT) at RT. Once color development was complete, the NBT/BCIP solution was replaced with PBS to stop the staining reaction. Finally, sections were mounted on Superfrost Plus slides (Fisher Scientific) in Aqua-Poly/Mount (Polysciences).

Images were acquired with a camera-equipped Olympus IX51 inverted microscope using Cell^A (Olympus), and further processed with Adobe Photoshop CS6 or ImageJ (U.S. National Institutes of Health).

## Immunohistochemistry

Serial free-floating brain sections were obtained by slicing brains embedded in 4% w/v agarose/PBS with a vibratome (VT1000s, Leica) at 40 μm (E14.5 brains) or 60 μm (E13.5 brains) of thickness, and were collected in PBS. Tissue was permeabilized by washing three times for 10 (40 μm sections) or 15 (60 μm sections) minutes per wash in PBS-Triton X-100 0.2% at RT. Sections were then incubated in blocking buffer (10% solution of normal serum derived from the species in which secondary antibodies were raised in PBS) for at least 1 h at RT, or overnight at 4 °C.

Following blocking, the tissue was incubated with primary antibodies diluted in PBS-NaN$_3$ 0.1% for 24–48 h at 4 °C. Primary antibodies used were mouse anti-neurofilament 2H3 (1:250; Developmental Studies Hybridoma Bank), rabbit anti-Islet1 (1:500; Abcam), mouse anti-Islet1/2 (1:50; Developmental Studies Hybridoma Bank), goat anti-mouse Sema6A (1:100; R&D), Armenian hamster anti-PlexinA4 (Mab-A4F5, 1:500; see Suto et al. [44]), Armenian hamster anti-PlexinA2 (Mab-A2D3, 1:50; see Suto et al. [41]), and mouse anti TAG1 (1:100; Developmental Studies Hybridoma Bank). The monoclonal anti-NF 165 kD (2H3), anti-Islet1/2 homeobox (39.4D5), and anti-TAG1 (4D7)

antibodies, obtained from the Developmental Studies Hybridoma Bank (University of Iowa), were respectively developed by T.M. Jessell and J. Dodd, T.M. Jessell and S. Brenner-Morton, and M. Yamamoto.

Sections were afterwards washed three (40 μm sections) to five (60 μm sections) times for 10′ each in PBS at RT, and incubated for 2 h at RT, or overnight at 4 °C, with species-specific secondary antibodies conjugated with cyanine dyes (Jackson Immunoresearch) or Alexa Fluor® dyes (Invitrogen) in a 1:500 dilution in PBS. They were next washed three to five times in PBS for 10 min each, and post-fixed in 1% PFA/PBS for at least 1 h at RT, or overnight at 4 °C.

After the post-fixation step, sections were counterstained with 4′,6-Diamidino-2-Phenylindole (DAPI) (Invitrogen), and mounted on Superfrost Plus slides in Aqua-Poly/Mount. Slides were examined under an epifluorescence microscope (Axioplan2, Zeiss) connected to a digital CCD camera (DP70, Olympus) or a laser scanning confocal microscope (LSM 700, Zeiss), and pictures acquired using analySISB (Olympus) or ZEN 2009 (Zeiss). Images were further processed and analyzed with Adobe Photoshop CS6 or ImageJ.

## Neuroanatomical tracing experiments

To back-label thalamic neurons projecting abnormally in the ventral telencephalon of *Plxna2*; *Plxna4* double mutant mice, small crystals of 1,1′-dioctadecyl-3,3,3′,3′-tetramethylindocarbocyanine perchlorate (DiI) (Molecular Probes) were inserted with a tungsten dissecting probe (World Precision Instruments) into superficial vTel layers of P0–P2 brain hemispheres. Back-labeling of thalamic neurons from either the primary visual (occipital) or primary somatosensory (parietal) cortex in *Plxna2*; *Plxna4* double mutant/wild-type mice was performed by respectively inserting small crystals of DiI and 4-(4-(dihexadecylamino)styryl)-N-methylpyridinium iodide (DiA) in the superficial cortical layers of P0-P2 brain hemispheres. Following the insertion of dye crystals, brains were kept in 1% PFA/PBS at RT in the dark for 4–6 weeks to allow the complete diffusion of the tracer in the axonal tracts and cell populations of interest.

Similarly, retrograde tracing to label guidepost cells in the vTel of wild-type, *Sema6a* mutant and *Plxna2*; *Plxna4* double mutant mice was carried out by insertion of small DiI crystals in the dTh of E13.5 brains, hemisected with a microsurgical knife (MSP) in order to expose the thalamus. Brains were subsequently kept in 1% PFA/PBS at RT in the dark for two weeks.

At the end of their incubation period, brains were embedded into 4% w/v agarose/PBS, and sectioned with a vibratome at 60 μm of thickness. Sections were counterstained with DAPI, mounted in Aqua-Poly/Mount onto Superfrost Plus slides, and analyzed using an epifluorescence microscope (Zeiss) not more than one day after sectioning, to avoid artifacts due to local dye diffusion at the surface of the sections. For guidepost cells labeling, Z-stacks (4 μm Z-step) of non-saturated DiI signal were acquired with a laser scanning confocal microscope (LSM 700, Zeiss) using the ZEN 2009 (Zeiss) imaging software, and further processed with ImageJ (U.S. National Institutes of Health) to obtain maximum intensity Z-projections of the vTel area.

### Quantification and statistical analyses

Quantification of guidepost cells labeled by DiI in the ventro-caudal area of the vTel was achieved by employing a modified version of the protocol developed by Bielle and colleagues [51]. This approach was preferred over cell counting methods as back-labeled somas can be masked by surrounding neuronal structures in which DiI also diffuses.

Images representative of the caudal DTB and subpallial areas in four consecutive coronal sections (see Fig. 7) were subdivided in dorsal and ventral quadrants. An ImageJ plugin was then employed to integrate the DiI signal intensity within the ventral subpallium quadrant, and across all quadrants. The integrated intensity value measured in the ventral subpallium quadrant was divided by the overall integrated intensity to correct for intra-experimental variations in the amount of DiI diffused along TCAs and guidepost cell projections. Integrated intensity ratios (IIR) were subsequently averaged across the four caudal sections to obtain region-wise values. Welch's ANOVA test was employed to compare mean caudal IIR across genotypes, and a Games-Howell post-hoc test was performed for pair-wise genotype comparisons. All data are reported as mean ± standard deviation. Statistical tests were run using the SPSS software package (IBM); significance was set at $p < 0.05$.

### Results

#### Plxna2; Plxna4 double mutant mice show defects in subpallial TCA guidance

In order to analyze the development of thalamocortical connections in *Plxna2* and *Plxna4* mutant mouse brains, immunohistochemistry for the 165 kDa neurofilament subunit (clone 2H3, Developmental Studies Hybridoma Bank), a pan-axonal marker, was first performed on *Plxna2*$^{-/-}$, *Plxna4*$^{+/+}$, *Plxna2*$^{+/+}$, *Plxna4*$^{-/-}$, *Plxna2*$^{+/-}$; *Plxna4*$^{+/-}$, *Plxna2*$^{+/-}$; *Plxna4*$^{-/-}$, *Plxna2*$^{-/-}$; *Plxna4*$^{+/-}$, and *Plxna2*$^{-/-}$; *Plxna4*$^{-/-}$ early postnatal littermate brains ($n \geq 3$ for all genotypes analyzed) (Fig. 1). No defective TCA phenotype was observed in either single mutants for *Plxna2* and *Plxna4*, nor in *Plxna2*; *Plxna4* double heterozygous mice (Fig. 1a–c). However, *Plxna2*$^{-/-}$; *Plxna4*$^{-/-}$ mice were found to present a

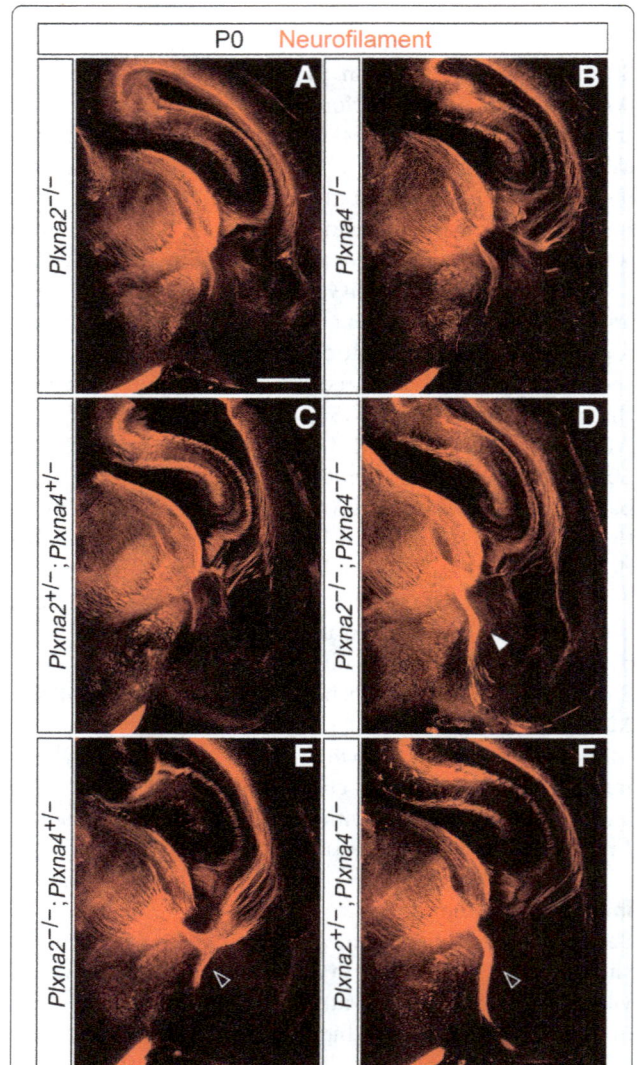

**Fig. 1** Immunohistochemical analysis of TCA development in *Plxna2*; *Plxna4* single and double mutant P0 brains. Immunostaining for neurofilament (*red*) confirms the presence of a *Sema6a*-mutant-like TCA defect in *Plxna2*; *Plxna4* double mutant postnatal brains (**d**; *filled arrowhead*), while no abnormal thalamic projections in the vTel are observed in either *Plxna2* or *Plxna4* single mutants (**a**, **b**). Additionally, misrouted TCAs are not present in *Plxna2*; *Plxna4* double heterozygous brains (**c**). Some TCA guidance defects, similar to those observed in double mutant brains but restricted to only a few thalamic fibers, also characterize *Plxna2*$^{+/-}$; *Plxna4*$^{-/-}$ and *Plxna2*$^{-/-}$; *Plxna4*$^{+/-}$ postnatal brains (**e**, **f**; *empty arrowheads*). Scale: 500 μm

defect in TCA pathfinding at the vTel that is strikingly like that observed in *Sema6a* mutants (Fig. 1d). In all *Plxna2*$^{-/-}$; *Plxna4*$^{-/-}$ specimens analyzed (P0–P2, $n = 5$), caudally-projecting TCAs were found to misproject ventrally in the vTel rather than turning laterally to enter the internal capsule, which these axons completely avoided (Fig. 1d, Additional file 1: Figure S1A, B).

Detailed analysis of the trajectories followed by the misrouted TCAs also highlighted the presence, as in *Sema6a* mutants, of two discrete TCA bundles extending in distinct pathways in the vTel. At a more intermediate level of the rostro-caudal axis, axons were found to travel into the external capsule (Additional file 1: Figure S1C–F), while more caudal TCAs, after their ventral turn, proceeded laterally within superficial vTel layers (Additional file 1: Figure S1G–J). At P2, some of these axons were observed to extend along the pial edge of the vTel and reach the most superficial layers of the neocortex (Additional file 1: Figure S1J), raising the possibility that, in later developmental stages, establishment of normal thalamocortical connections through alternative routes might also occur in *Plxna2*; *Plxna4* double mutants.

A compound effect of *Plxna2* and *Plxna4* loss-of-function mutations on thalamocortical connectivity was further demonstrated by the analysis of $Plxna2^{+/-}$; $Plxna4^{-/-}$ and $Plxna2^{-/-}$; $Plxna4^{+/-}$ mutant P0 brains: immunohistochemistry for neurofilament indeed revealed a few misprojecting caudal thalamic fibers in the vTel of these specimens (Fig. 1e, f).

### Misrouted TCAs in *Plxna2*; *Plxna4* double mutants originate from dorsal lateral dTh nuclei

Retrograde neuroanatomical tracing methods were employed to identify the thalamic origin of the misrouted TCA bundles in the ventral subpallium of $Plxna2^{-/-}$; $Plxna4^{-/-}$ P0 mouse brains ($n = 4$). As in *Sema6a* mutants, placement of DiI crystals at the vTel pial surface labeled thalamic projections that could be back-traced to the dLGN, as well as cell bodies within this nucleus (Fig. 2B, C). In addition, *Plxna2*; *Plxna4* double mutants also showed back-labeling in axons and somas of a small, dorso-lateral portion of the VB (Fig. 2C). Placement of DiI crystals in superficial vTel regions of control (wild-type or $Plxna2^{+/-}$; $Plxna4^{+/-}$ brains, $n = 3$) P0 brains did not result in any dye diffusion in dTh neural populations (Fig. 2A).

### Somatosensory TCAs invade the visual cortex early postnatally in *Plxna2*; *Plxna4* double mutants

To explore the possibility of topographical alterations in the neocortex arising due to defects in subpallial dorso-lateral TCA guidance in $Plxna2^{-/-}$; $Plxna4^{-/-}$ mice, retrograde double tracing experiments were performed from the visual (V1) and somatosensory (S1) cortex of $Plxna2^{-/-}$; $Plxna4^{-/-}$ and wild-type P0 mouse brains ($n = 4$ per genotype) (Fig. 2D–I). In $Plxna2^{-/-}$; $Plxna4^{-/-}$ mice, back-labeling from V1 with DiI resulted in the identification of a subset of misprojecting VB neurons, indicating the invasion by somatosensory TCAs of this cortical region in the absence of dLGN projections (Fig. 2H, I). Connectivity between some $Plxna2^{-/-}$; $Plxna4^{-/-}$ somatosensory TCAs

and their cognate cortical domains appeared to be preserved, as DiA crystals placed in the S1 led to the back-labeling of a ventro-medial VB cell population. Somas of the V1-invading thalamic neurons were observed adjacent ventro-medially to the VB neuronal subset that could be back-labeled from the vTel (Fig. 2I), confirming the extension to somatosensory TCAs of the $Plxna2^{-/-}$; $Plxna4^{-/-}$ miswiring phenotype characterized with vTel tracing experiments.

### Expression patterns of *Sema6a*, *Plxna2* and *Plxna4* during early TCA development

Overall, the phenotypical similarities observed between $Sema6a^{-/-}$ and $Plxna2^{-/-}$; $Plxna4^{-/-}$ mutants provide evidence in support of a role of Sema6A – PlxnA2-PlxnA4 interactions in early dLGN axon guidance. In order to understand where and when these interactions may be required for proper subpallial TCA pathfinding, the spatiotemporal dynamics of *Sema6a*, *Plxna2* and *Plxna4* expression were first analyzed by *in situ* hybridization during TCA extension across the DTB and in the vTel.

Around E14.5, *Sema6a* was found to be expressed in all dorsal thalamic neurons, though more strongly in lateral regions, whereas *Plxna2* and *Plxna4* mRNAs were only detected in medial thalamic nuclei, notably excluding the region that will give rise to the dLGN (Fig. 3a–d). At the same developmental stage, transcription of all three genes was observed in subpallial areas surrounding the IC, both in structures permissive for TCA growth, like the corridor, as well as non-permissive structures, such as the globus pallidus [22]. *Sema6a* mRNA was in addition detected at the vTel pial surface, the region invaded by misrouted TCAs in all of our mutant mice (Fig. 3e–h) ($n = 4$ for each probe).

Overall, these findings suggest that Sema6A, PlxnA2 and PlxnA4 might be present on extending TCAs as they navigate subpallial territories, and furthermore be differentially expressed across axon subsets originating from different thalamic nuclei. Moreover, they indicate that these three guidance molecules are expressed from very early stages (at least as early as E12.5, data not shown) at the level of intermediate 'decision points' delineating TCA pathways in the vTel.

### Sema6A, PlxnA4 and PlxnA2 expression in thalamic neurons, TCAs, and the ventral forebrain in early TCA development

Based on *in situ* hybridization findings, double immunohistochemistry with neurofilament- and either Sema6A-, PlxnA2- or PlxnA4-specific antibodies on wild-type brains at E13.5 and E14.5 (n ≥ 3 per protein investigated) was next performed to analyze the spatiotemporal expression dynamics of these

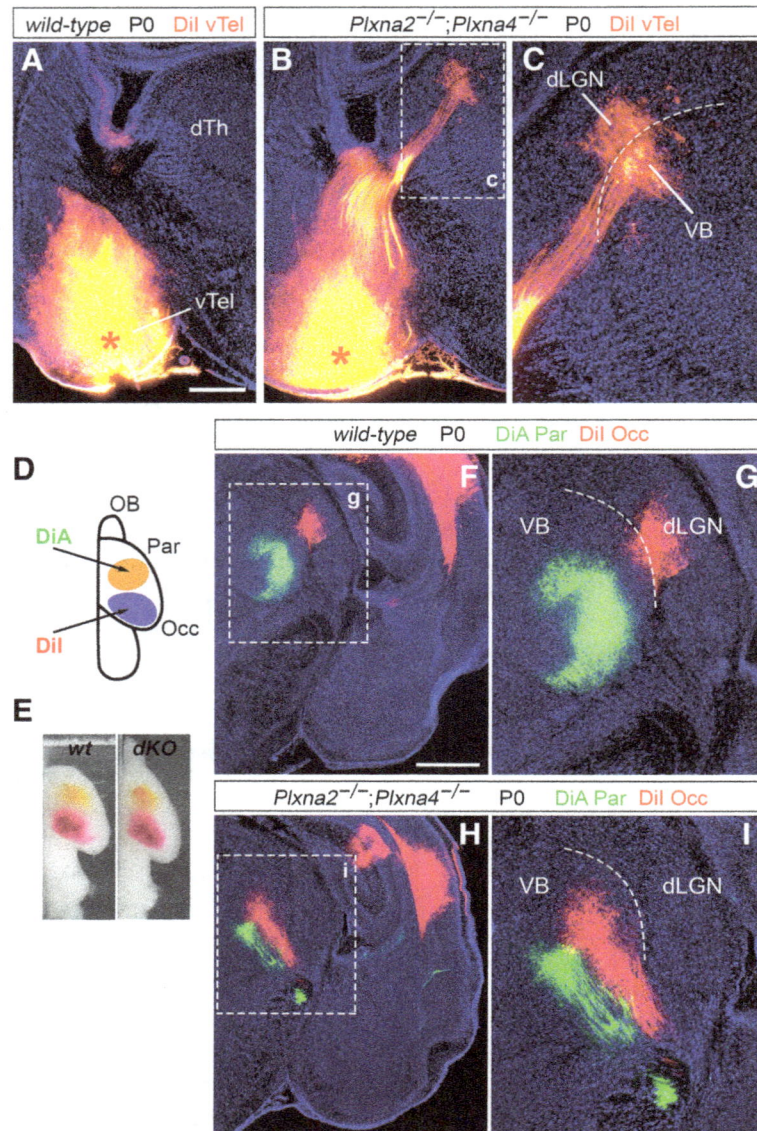

**Fig. 2** Neuroanatomical tracing experiments reveal a *Sema6a* mutant-like TCA phenotype in *Plxna2; Plxna4* double mutant brains. **a–c** Retrograde labeling with carbocyanine dyes from the vTel in wild-type (**a**) versus *Plxna2⁻/⁻; Plxna4⁻/⁻* P0 brains (**b, c**). Insertion of DiI crystals in the vTel (*asterisk*) results in no back-labeling of dTh neurons in wild-type brains; on the other hand, in *Plxna2⁻/⁻; Plxna4⁻/⁻* brains DiI back-labels thalamic axons and cell somas located in the dLGN (**b**), a finding that coincides with data obtained from *Sema6a⁻/⁻* brains. In addition, dye-labeled neurons are also found in the VB, indicating the extension of guidance defects to a subset of thalamic axons normally directed to somatosensory cortical areas. **d–i** Back-labeling of thalamic neurons with two distinct carbocyanine dyes from the visual (occipital) cortex and the somatosensory (parietal) cortex in P0 wild-type (wt) and *Plxna2; Plxna4* double mutant (dKO) brains. **c** Schematic representation of the cortical sites of dye placement in P0 brain hemispheres (OB: olfactory bulb). DiA (*green*) and DiA (*red*) crystals are placed respectively on parietal (Par) and occipital (Occ) regions of the cortex. **e–h** Insertion of DiI crystals in visual cortical areas of *Plxna2⁻/⁻; Plxna4⁻/⁻* brains results in the back-labeling of some thalamic neurons of the dorso-lateral VB (**h**), rather than the dLGN (as instead observed in wild-type brains (**f**)), suggesting a miswiring of somatosensory TCAs to the visual cortex similar to that present in *Sema6a* mutants. Normal connectivity between ventro-medial VB neurons and the somatosensory cortex is preserved, as indicated by back-labeling of these cells by DiA. Scale: **a, b**: 250 μm; **e–h**: 500 μm

guidance molecules in distinct subsets of thalamocortical projections growing in the vTel.

At E13.5, Sema6A was found to be more highly expressed in dorso-lateral thalamic nuclei, while PlxnA4 and PlxnA2 expression appeared to be more restricted to medial thalamic nuclei; all proteins were observed along extending TCAs at moderate levels (Fig. 4A–B', E–F' and Additional file 1: Figure S2, respectively). At E14.5, Sema6A was detected on all thalamic nuclei, but was found to be expressed only on the most caudally-located

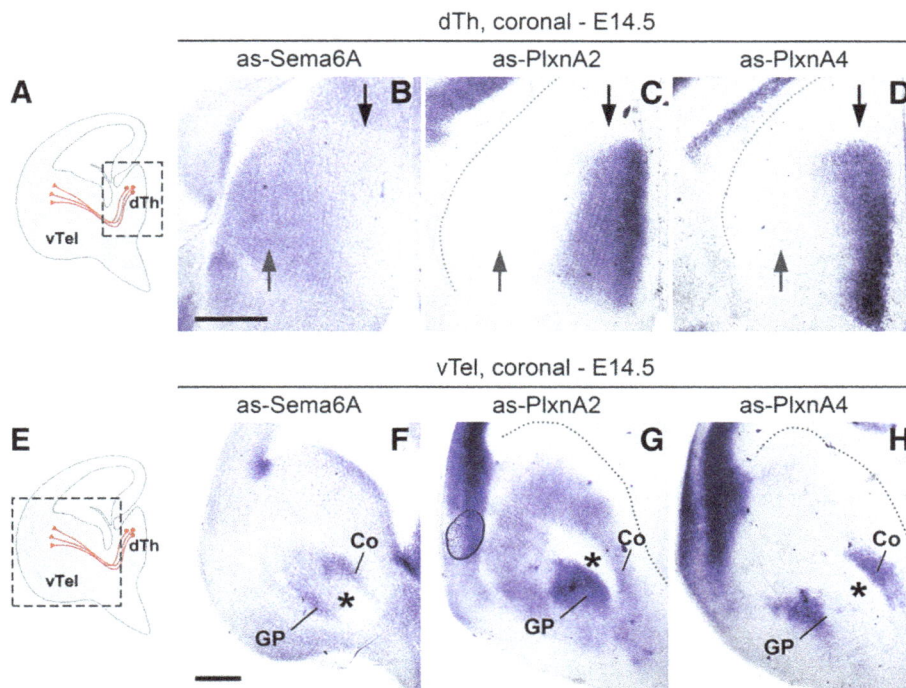

**Fig. 3** Expression of *Sema6a*, *Plxna2* and *Plxna4* mRNA in the E14.5 mouse forebrain. Levels of mRNA expression were detected by *in situ* hybridization with antisense (as) RNA probes. **a–d** mRNA expression in the dTh of E14.5 mouse brains. **a** Schematic representation of a coronal E14.5 section indicating the approximate region of interest (*boxed area*); TCAs are represented in *red*. **b–d** *Sema6a* is strongly expressed in both lateral (*grey arrows*) and medial (*black arrows*) dTh (**b**); in contrast, *Plxna2* and *Plxna4* are highly transcribed only in the medial dTh (**c**, **d**). **e–h** mRNA expression in the subpallium (vTel) of E14.5 mouse brains. **e** Schematic representation of a coronal E14.5 section indicating the approximate region of interest (*boxed area*); TCAs are represented in *red*. (**f–h**) *Sema6a* is highly expressed in areas surrounding the IC (*asterisks*), in the pial surface of the vTel, and the ventricular zone; it is also moderately transcribed in subventricular subpallial regions (**f**). *Plxna2* shows maximum expression in the globus pallidus, ventral to the IC, and strong expression levels in subventricular and mantle layers (**g**), while *Plxna4* is highly transcribed in two discrete bands located dorsal and ventral to the IC (**h**). Scale: **a–d**, 500 μm; **e–h**, 500 μm. Coronal section schemes adapted from López-Bendito et al. [22]

TCAs (which originate dorso-laterally in the thalamus) (Fig. 4C–D'); PlxnA4 expression was observed only in medial thalamic nuclei and the rostrally-projecting TCAs originating from them, but some protein expression was surprisingly found on more caudally-located axons as well (Fig. 4G–H'). However, at this caudal level the high degree of TCA fasciculation might not allow to completely distinguish projections directed to the somatosensory cortex from those directed to the visual cortex. Hence, PlxnA4 expression was also analyzed in *Sema6a* mutants at E15.5, a time-point at which misrouted thalamic fibers from the dLGN start to be clearly detectable as a bundle extending within the subpallial pial surface, completely detached from the IC. Immunostaining of tissue at caudal vTel levels revealed that, while PlxnA4 is present on TCAs elongating within the IC and presumably originating from the VB, this protein is not expressed by misprojecting dLGN axons (Fig. 4I, J; *n* = 3). Taken comprehensively, these findings confirm *in situ* hybridization results at E14.5 showing differential expression in distinct thalamic nuclei.

In addition, immunohistochemistry data highlighted areas of Sema6A, PlxnA2 and PlxnA4 expression in

developing vTel domains surrounding the extending TCA bundle. For Sema6A, immunostaining could be detected in a restricted band dorsal to the IC, and in ventral domains extending to mantle and pial surface areas (particularly at intermediate/caudal levels) at E13.5; high expression appeared to additionally occur at the level of the lateral olfactory tract (Fig. 4A). At E14.5, Sema6A could be moderately observed in areas possibly corresponding to corridor cell populations and in presumptive amygdalar territories; intense expression of the protein could be furthermore found at the level of the globus pallidus (Fig. 4C, D).

For PlxnA4, immunostaining at E13.5 revealed the presence of this protein at intermediate vTel levels, in discrete domains surrounding dorso-medially and ventro-laterally the IC bundle, and a sparse expression in mantle/pial surface regions of the caudal vTel (Fig. 4E, F). Staining could be observed also at E14.5 in a very small domain dorsal to the IC, but not in contact with the axons (Fig. 4G).

For PlxnA2, immunostaining could be observed in a region likely overlapping the corridor at more intermediate levels of the E13.5 vTel; the protein was also found in

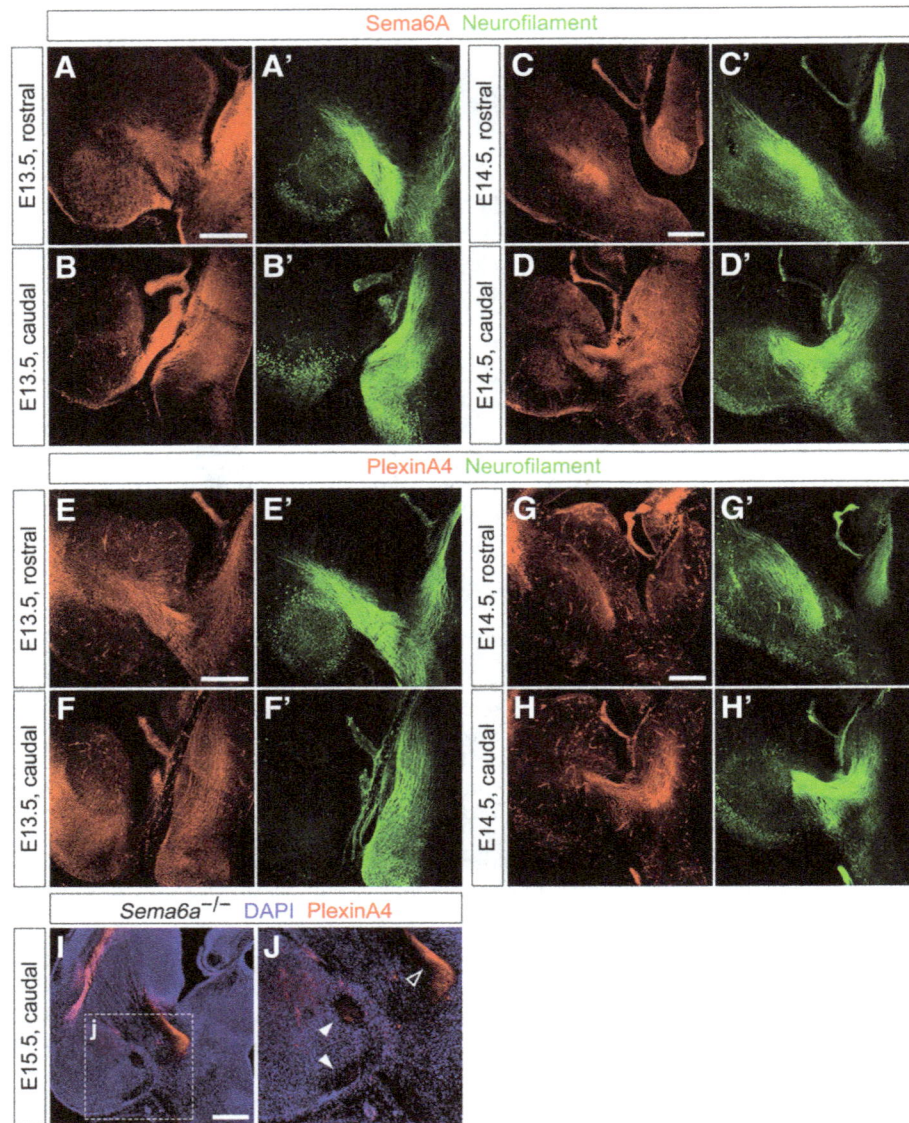

**Fig. 4** Expression of Sema6A and PlxnA4 on thalamic neurons and TCAs during axonal growth into the subpallium. **a–b′** Double immunohistochemistry for Sema6A (*red*) and neurofilament (*green*) on wild-type E13.5 coronal brain sections indicates expression of Sema6A in thalamic neurons, in particularly in dorso-lateral populations (**b, b′**), as well as on extending TCAs; the protein can also be found in vTel areas ventral to the IC (**a, a′**). **c–d′** Double immunohistochemistry for Sema6A (*red*) and neurofilament (*green*) on coronal sections of wild-type E14.5 brains shows expression of Sema6A extending to all thalamic nuclei (**d, d′**); the protein is furthermore expressed along TCAs positioned more caudally along the rostro-caudal axis (**d, d′**), while it is not found on TCAs projecting more rostrally (**c, c′**). **e–f′** Double immunohistochemistry for PlxnA4 (*red*) and neurofilament (*green*) in wild-type E13.5 coronal brain sections reveals that expression of PlxnA4 is mostly concentrated in medial thalamic neural populations, and is present on TCAs. Immunostaining can also be observed on some fibers in the IC contacting the axon bundle dorso-medially and ventro-laterally, and in mantle and pial surface areas of the caudal vTel (**e, e′**). **g–h′** Double immunohistochemistry for PlxnA4 (*red*) and neurofilament (*green*) on coronal sections of wild-type E14.5 brains demonstrates localization of PlxnA4 in medial thalamic neural populations (**h, h′**), as well as along TCAs projecting rostrally (**g, g′**). PlexinA4 seems to be further localized in some caudally-located TCAs (**h, h′**). **i–j** Immunohistochemistry for PlxnA4 (*red*) on coronal sections of *Sema6a*−/− E15.5 brains shows the presence of PlxnA4 on caudally-located TCAs extending within the IC (*empty arrowhead*), which presumably correspond to VB-originated axons. On the other hand, no immunostaining can be detected on misrouted projections corresponding to dLGN-originated fibers (*filled arrowheads*). Scale: **a–b′**, 300 μm; **c–d′**, 300 μm; **e–f′**, 300 μm; **g–h′**, 300 μm; **i–j**, 300 μm

medial-ventral areas of the caudal vTel (Additional file 1: Figure S2A, B).

## Sema6A, PlxnA4, and PlxnA2 expression in vTel intermediate targets and guidepost neural populations

*In situ* hybridization and double immunohistochemistry experiments highlighted the expression of all our genes of interest in subpallial domains delineating TCA pathways in the vTel, and likely corresponding to structures crucial for proper guidance in these regions (e.g., the corridor). To better investigate spatiotemporal expression dynamics within intermediate TCA guidance targets, double immunohistochemistry for either Sema6A, PlxnA2 or PlxnA4 and Islet1, a marker for corridor cells and LGE-derived striatal neurons (Fig. 5A), was performed on E13.5 (Fig. 5B–H) and E14.5 (Additional file 1: Figure S3, S4) wild-type brains ($n \geq 3$ per experimental condition).

These experiments confirmed that Sema6A is consistently expressed during these developmental stages by corridor neurons and cells within the MGE-derived globus pallidus (Fig. 5B–C). Furthermore, data indicated that Sema6A is present on most caudally-projecting TCAs, but also on other axonal tracts contained within the IC bundle: in particular, Sema6A appears to be expressed on nigrostriatal axons, that travel within the IC ventrally to and in close contact with TCAs, and are also labeled by neurofilament immunostaining [52] (Additional file 1: Figure S3).

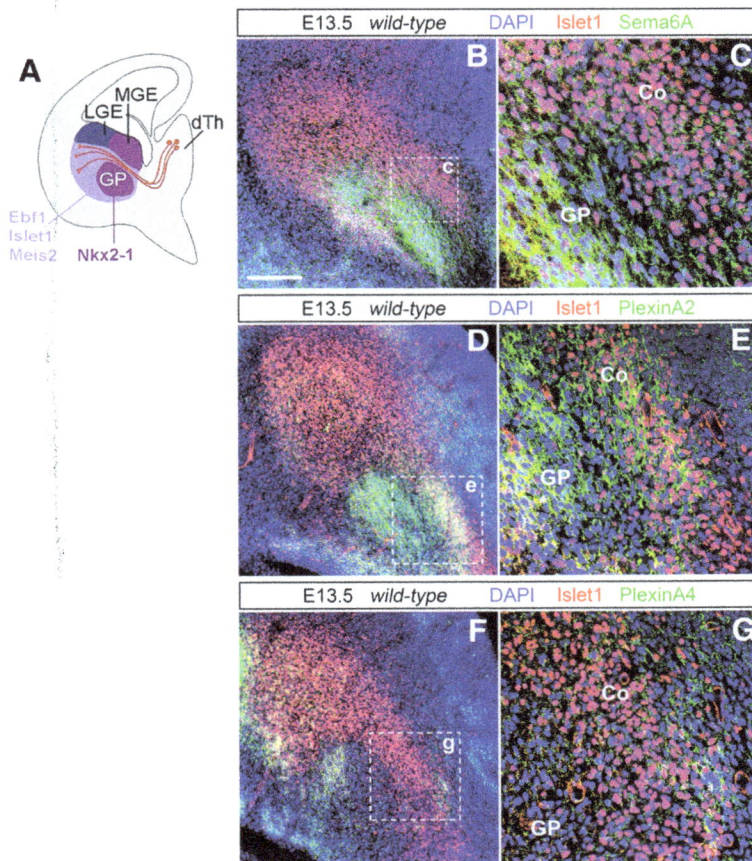

**Fig. 5** Expression of Sema6A, PlxnA2 and PlxnA4 in corridor cells and other subpallial structures at E13.5. **a** Diagram illustrating the spatial expression patterns of LGE- and MGE-derived neural population markers. The transcription factors Ebf1, Islet1, and Meis2 are detected in striatal and corridor regions of the vTel (*light purple*), both derivatives of the LGE, but not in the GP and the ventricular/subventricular zone of the MGE (*dark purple*). These territories in turn express a transcription factor, Nkx2-1, not present in LGE-derived territories. (Adapted from López-Bendito et al. [22].). **b, c** Double immunohistochemistry for the corridor cell marker Islet1 (*red*) and Sema6A (*green*) on coronal wild-type brain sections demonstrates the expression of Sema6A on corridor cells (Co) during the growth of TCAs into subpallial populations. Sema6A is also highly expressed in globus pallidus (GP) cells (**c**). **d–g** Double immunohistochemistry for PlxnA2 (*green*) and Islet1 (*red*) (**d, e**), or PlxnA4 (*green*) and Islet1 (*red*) (**f, g**) on coronal wild-type brain sections indicates a strong presence of PlxnA2 within the corridor and in the globus pallidus (**e**); PlxnA4 is also moderately present on most dorso-medial corridor domains (**g**), and in the lateral half of the globus pallidus area (**f**). Both molecules are additionally lightly expressed in the vTel subventricular zone and pial surface, in an area close to the IC, and in a discrete band at the ventral edge of the striatum (PlxnA4 is particularly present here) (**d, f**). Scale: 150 µm

Likewise, immunohistochemistry results for PlxnA2 confirmed the presence of this protein in corridor cells, and within the globus pallidus. PlxnA2 expression seems to extend, similarly to Sema6A, to multiple axonal projections extending within the IC more ventrally in respect to TCAs (Fig. 5D–E). Concerning PlxnA4, immunohistochemistry data showed moderate expression of the protein in the corridor and in the globus pallidus at both E13.5 and E14.5 (Fig. 5F–G, Additional file 1: Figure S4). Compared to Sema6A and PlxnA2, PlxnA4 expression at E13.5 was observed in more limited domains overlapping with dorsal regions of the corridor, and lateral regions of the globus pallidus (Fig. 5F). Interestingly, at E14.5 PlxnA4 was still found not only in the corridor, but also in discrete areas, particularly evident at caudal vTel positions, surrounding Islet-positive territories both dorso-medially and ventro-laterally (Additional file 1: Figure S4).

Taken together, these results support a potential function of Sema6A, PlxnA2 and PlxnA4 not solely in the control of TCA guidance within subpallial territories, but also in corridor morphogenesis.

### Preserved corridor formation in *Sema6a* and *Plxna2; Plxna4* mutants

In order to investigate whether Sema6A, PlxnA2 and PlxnA4 might play a role in shaping the corridor domain, expression patterns for the corridor marker Islet1 in the vTel of wild-type, *Sema6a*$^{-/-}$, *Plxna2*$^{+/-}$; *Plxna4*$^{+/-}$ and *Plxna2*$^{-/-}$; *Plxna4*$^{-/-}$ mice were examined at E13.5 and E14.5, at a time when LGE-derived neurons have terminated their migration while TCAs are extending into the IC, after crossing the DTB. Double immunohistochemistry for Islet1 and neurofilament on coronal brain sections revealed comparable patterns of the corridor cell marker's expression in both striatal and IC regions between wild-type and mutant brains at E13.5 (Fig. 6) and E14.5 (Additional file 1: Figure S5) ($n \geq 3$ for all genotypes in each experiment). At IC level, Islet1 was detected in a narrow band of cells lining a pathway for TCAs between the globus pallidus and the subventricular MGE zone, corresponding to the normal location of corridor neurons at these developmental stages. Additionally, immunostaining could be observed as normally expected in LGE-derived striatal territories, where TCA begin to rostro-caudally segregate in a fan-like shape. The local spatial distribution and density of corridor cells at E14.5 appeared to be fully preserved in all mutants (Additional file 1: Figure S5, S6).

At these early subpallial navigation stages, neurofilament immunostaining could not consistently reveal misrouted TCAs at the pial surface of the vTel in any of the mutants analyzed. This finding is suggestive of a brief stall of TCAs at the DTB in the absence of Sema6A, PlxnA2 and PlxnA4 activity. As the IC bundle

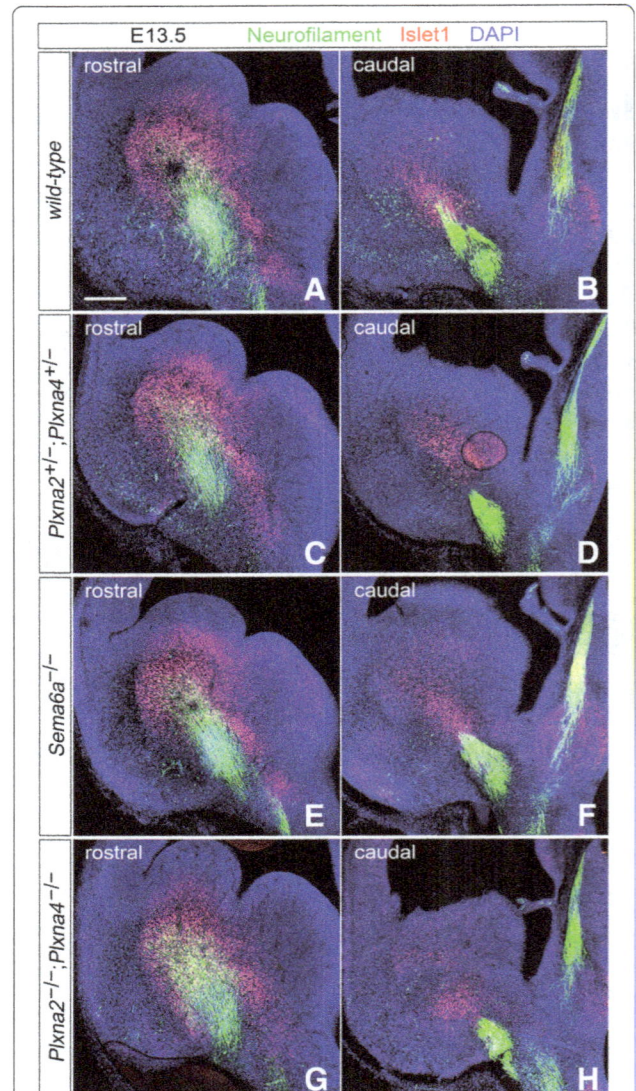

**Fig. 6** Normal overall expression of Islet1 in the vTel of *Sema6a* mutants and *Plxna2; Plxna4* double mutants at E13.5. Double immunohistochemistry for neurofilament (*green*) and Islet1 (*red*) on E13.5 coronal brain sections indicates the preserved organization, at this stage, of Islet1-positive cell domains in the developing subpallium of *Sema6a*$^{-/-}$ (**e, f**), *Plxna2*$^{+/-}$; *Plxna4*$^{+/-}$ (**c, d**), *Plxna2*$^{-/-}$; *Plxna4*$^{-/-}$ (**g, h**) mouse brains, as compared to wild-type (**a, b**). Islet1-positive neurons are present in a narrow band situated immediately dorsal to extending TCAs, between the vTel subventricular zone and the globus pallidus (characterized by the absence of Islet1 immunostaining), and throughout the striatum, where neurofilament-expressing thalamocortical fibers can be observed to segregate (**a, c, e, g**). Caudally, a slight reduction and disorganization of the most posteriorly-located subset of Islet1-positive cells can be observed in the *Plxna2*$^{-/-}$; *Plxna4*$^{-/-}$ mouse vTel (**h**). Scale: 200 μm

comprises several highly fasciculated axonal tracts (thalamocortical, corticothalamic, striatonigral, nigrostriatal, corticospinal, etc.), the stall could be explained in terms of TCAs encountering multiple physical obstacles in their growth outside the IC and into the vTel. It should also be noted that neurofilament is a broad-spectrum, high-density-labeling axonal marker characterizing IC tracts, such as the striatonigral/nigrostriatal pathways or cerebral peduncle fibers, that closely traverse the DTB ventral or adjacent to thalamocortical/corticothalamic bundles [52, 53]. At early developmental stages, therefore, other neurofilament-positive axonal projections might obscure the abnormal trajectories taken by caudal TCAs that have just started to cross the DTB.

Since dLGN axons are the first projections that cross the DTB during thalamocortical connectivity development, failure of pioneer caudally-directed axons to elongate with other thalamic fibers in the IC in Sema6a- and Plxna2; Plxna4-deficient mice could be due, for instance, to a delay in corridor cell migration. Thus, immunohistochemistry for Islet1 was performed on coronal brain sections of wild-type, Sema6A$^{-/-}$ and Plxna2$^{-/-}$; Plxna4$^{-/-}$ E12.5 brains (when corridor formation is in its latest stages, and the first TCAs start crossing the DTB) to investigate the migration process of LGE-derived neurons to MGE-derived territories ($n \geq 3$ for all genotypes). Comparison of Islet1 vTel expression pattern between wild type and mutant brain sections demonstrated the absence of any evident delay or corridor malformations: in all cases, Islet1-positive cells could be distinguished in the mantle zone of the MGE-derived subpallial region (Additional file 1: Figure S7).

Taken comprehensively, these findings suggest that loss of function of Sema6A, PlxnA2 and PlxnA4 does not impact on the overall development and spatiotemporal organization of the LGE-derived corridor and striatal populations in the mouse vTel.

## Misplacement of a subset of guidepost cells in Sema6a and Plxna2; Plxna4 mutants

Guidance of TCAs across the subpallium has been suggested to rely not only on corridor cells, but also on IC-localized guidepost cells which form projections to the dTh just as TCAs start extending in the vTel (around E12.5). As there are no known molecular markers for these cells, they have been so far identified and studied by retrograde dye tracings experiments from the dTh [27]. Thalamic tracings with the carbocyanine dye DiI (Fig. 7a–c) were therefore performed in Plxna2$^{+/-}$; Plxna4$^{+/-}$ and Plxna2$^{-/-}$; Plxna4$^{-/-}$ E13.5 brains from littermates to investigate whether loss of function of these guidance factors is associated with guidepost cell defects that might explain the TCA misrouting phenotype observed in Plxna2; Plxna4 double mutants. E13.5 was selected as an optimal time-point as it lead to a more consistent back-labeling of cells in the IC area compared to E12.5, while allowing the identification of subpallial cell bodies due to the still limited axonal

growth of TCAs, in particular those misrouted in Plxna2$^{-/-}$; Plxna4$^{-/-}$ mutants, in the developing vTel.

In Plxna2$^{+/-}$; Plxna4$^{+/-}$ brains, as expected, dye tracings from the dTh resulted in the back-labeling of cell bodies in the IC, in the proximity of anterograde-labeled TCAs and along the dorso-lateral pathway followed normally by TCAs during navigation into the subpallium ($n = 7/7$) (Fig. 7h–k). In Plxna2$^{-/-}$; Plxna4$^{-/-}$ brains, however, some back-labeled cell bodies were additionally found at a more superficial level of the vTel, in the presumptive amygdala; this group of cells was also observed more caudally in respect to the IC ($n = 6/6$) (Fig. 7l–o).

Similar dye tracing experiments were next performed on Sema6a$^{-/-}$ E13.5 brains to examine the spatial distribution of IC guidepost cells in these mutants (Fig. 7p–s) (late E13.5 wild-type brains ($n = 10$) were used as an extra control group (Fig. 7d–g)). Like in Plxna2$^{-/-}$; Plxna4$^{-/-}$ brains, along with somas normally localized in the IC region, some cell bodies were identified via back-labeling in posterior vTel surface areas of Sema6a-deficient specimens (these cells were not detected by retrograde tracing in wild-type brains) ($n = 11/11$). Quantification of the DiI signal in the caudal region of the ventral subpallium confirmed a significant presence of back-labeled subpallial neurons in the most caudo-ventral portions of the vTel in Plxna2$^{-/-}$; Plxna4$^{-/-}$ and Sema6a$^{-/-}$ brains, compared to wild-type and Plxna2$^{+/-}$; Plxna4$^{+/-}$ brains (Fig. 7t). In general, the positioning of these retrograde-labeled cells appeared to be less severely affected in Sema6a$^{-/-}$ brains, although statistical analysis did not detect a significant difference between average DiI signal intensities measured in the caudal vTel of Plxna2$^{-/-}$; Plxna4$^{-/-}$ and Sema6a$^{-/-}$ specimens. In some cases, only a very small number of cell bodies ($n < 10$) could be observed in aberrant sites throughout the vTel of these mutants.

Overall, these finding suggests that loss of Sema6A, PlxnA2 and PlxnA4 function in subpallial areas leads to the caudo-ventral misplacement of a subset of IC guidepost cells, which could explain the abnormal extension into the amygdala of more caudally-projecting TCAs.

## Caudally-projecting TCAs fasciculate and elongate normally in the dorsal thalamus and prethalamus of Plxna2; Plxna4 double mutants

In the developing dorsal thalamus Sema6A and PlxnA2/PlxnA4 are distinctly expressed across TCA subsets that navigate diencephalic and telencephalic territories in close contact with each other. The formation or the disaggregation of neurite bundles represent critical events in axon guidance, and Semaphorins are known to play diverse roles in axonal fasciculation [54]. Motor axon fasciculation in Drosophila, for instance, has been shown to be mediated by transmembrane reverse

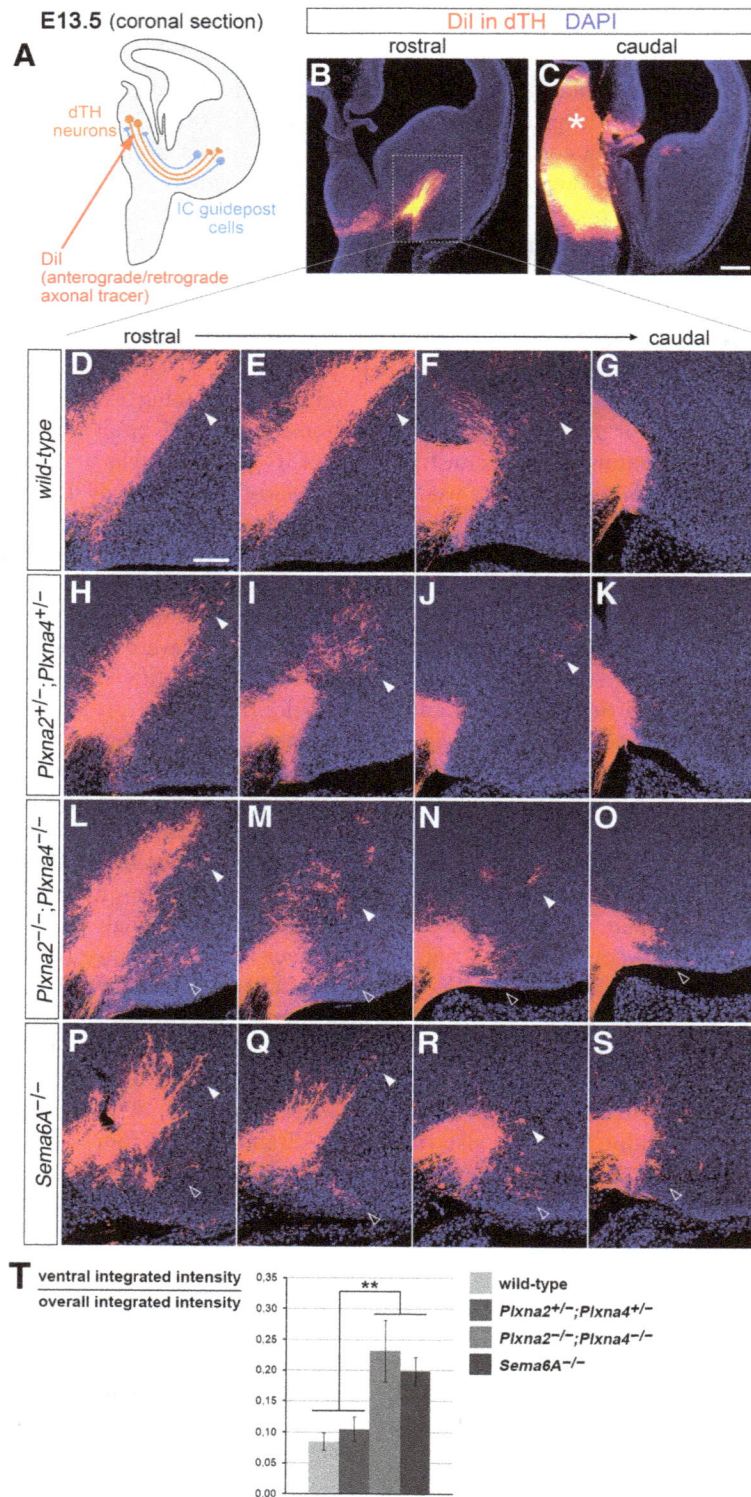

**Fig. 7** (See legend on next page.)

(See figure on previous page.)
**Fig. 7** A subset of IC guidepost cells is misplaced in *Sema6a* mutant and *Plxna2; Plxna4* double mutant E13.5 brains. **a** Schematic representation of the dye tracing experiments performed. DiI crystals were inserted into the dTh of E13.5 $Plxna2^{+/-}$; $Plxna4^{+/-}$ and $Plxna2^{-/-}$; $Plxna4^{-/-}$ mouse brains; from this position, the dye diffuses along TCAs in an anterograde fashion, and on guidepost cell projections reaching the dTh. (Adapted from Garel and López-Bendito [21].). **b, c** Coronal sections of E13.5 brains illustrating the labeled IC (**b**) and the exact location of dye placement in the dTh (*asterisk* in **c**). **d–s** DiI labels growing TCAs as well as guidepost cell bodies in the IC area, along the dorso-lateral path which TCAs will follow to proceed further into the subpallium (*solid arrowheads*), in late E13.5 wild-type (**d–g**), E13.5 $Plxna2^{+/-}$; $Plxna4^{+/-}$ (**h–k**), E13.5 $Plxna2^{-/-}$; $Plxna4^{-/-}$ (**l–o**), and E13.5 $Sema6a^{-/-}$ (**p–s**) mouse brains. In $Plxna2^{-/-}$; $Plxna4^{-/-}$ and $Sema6a^{-/-}$ sections, however, back-labeling identifies a group of cells projecting to the dTh in an abnormal caudo-ventral position in the vTel, close to the pial surface, corresponding to presumptive amygdala territories (**l–s**, *empty arrowheads*). No dye can be detected in this domain in either wild-type or $Plxna2^{+/-}$; $Plxna4^{+/-}$ brains. Scale: **b, c**: 250 μm; **d–s**: 100 μm. **t** Quantification and comparison of DiI signal intensities in the caudo-ventral subpallium, expressed as ventral vTel/overall (DTB and vTel) integrated intensity ratios (IRRs), between wild-type, $Plxna2^{+/-}$; $Plxna4^{+/-}$, $Plxna2^{-/-}$; $Plxna4^{-/-}$, and $Sema6a^{-/-}$ E13.5 brains. A significantly higher DiI signal intensity compared to both wild-type ($n = 10$) and $Plxna2^{+/-}$; $Plxna4^{+/-}$ ($n = 7$) measurements was detected in case of $Plxna2^{-/-}$; $Plxna4^{-/-}$ ($n = 6$) as well as $Sema6a^{-/-}$ ($n = 11$) specimens. $IRR_{wild-type} = 0.09 \pm 0.01$; $IRR_{Plxna2+/-; Plxna4+/-} = 0.10 \pm 0.02$; $IRR_{Plxna2-/-; Plxna4-/-} = 0.23 \pm 0.06$; $IRR_{Sema6a-/-} = 0.20 \pm 0.02$; $p < 0.01$

signaling via Sema-1a, the invertebrate semaphorin most closely related to the Sema6 class [55, 56]. Considering this evidence, the spatial navigation and the responsiveness to environmental cues of Sema6A-expressing thalamic projections might depend, in some part, to axon-axon interactions between subsets differentially expressing PlxnA2/PlxnA4. This being the case, subtle TCA fasciculation and guidance defects would be expected to be present at diencephalic level during early TCA growth as a result of disrupted Sema6A–PlxnA2/PlxnA4 reverse signaling. Therefore, Sema6A expression was investigated in the developing $Plxna2^{-/-}$; $Plxna4^{-/-}$ mouse forebrain in order to elucidate whether Sema6A-positive, caudally-projecting TCAs properly navigate the dorsal thalamus and prethalamus areas in the absence of PlxnA2/PlxnA4s on rostrally-projecting TCAs.

At E13.5, the comparison between immunohistochemistry results from $Plxna^{+/-}$; $Plxna4^{+/-}$ and $Plxna2^{-/-}$; $Plxna4^{-/-}$ mouse brain sections (Fig. 8A–F; $n = 3$ per genotype) revealed unchanged fasciculation levels and a normal diencephalic pathfinding for Sema6A-expressing TCAs in animals lacking PlxnA2/PlxnA4. Hence, findings tend to exclude the involvement of axon-axon Sema6A–PlxnA2/PlxnA4 interactions in the guidance of caudally-directed TCA subsets.

## Additional ventral subpallium guidance and cytoarchitectural defects in *Sema6A* and *PlxnA2; PlxnA4* mutants

In light of the observed misplacement of IC guidepost cells in PlxnA2; PlxnA4-deficient mice, and considering that Sema6A, PlxnA2 and PlxnA4 are expressed in many populations surrounding the IC, it might be for instance hypothesized that, in absence of PlxnA2/PlxnA4 activity in the caudal vTel (where PlxnA4 is present in corridor cells and in IC-proximal domains), some Sema6A-positive guidepost cells might fail to properly locate at the IC level. Therefore, further immunohistochemical analyses of Sema6A vTel expression were performed in

E13.5 wild-type and *PlxnA2; PlxnA4* mutant mouse brains to investigate this possibility (Fig. 8G–J').

In $PlxnA2^{-/-}$; $PlxnA4^{-/-}$ ($n = 3$) or $PlxnA2^{+/-}$; $PlxnA4^{-/-}$ ($n = 2$) specimens no changes were observed in Sema6A immunoreactivity in the areas of the corridor, the globus pallidus, and the region immediately ventral to this latter structure as compared to $PlxnA2^{+/-}$; $PlxnA4^{+/-}$ ($n = 3$) or wild-type ($n = 2$) brains. However, a Sema6A-expressing complex of fibers morphologically correspondent to the lateral olfactory tract (LOT) was found to deviate dorsally from its normal superficial trajectory across the vTel and invade the subpallium, reaching the mantle zone (Fig. 8H, J). Double immunohistochemistry with TAG1, a molecular marker for specific subsets of LOT fibers [57], in wild-type and $PlxnA2^{+/-}$; $PlxnA4^{-/-}$ E13.5 mouse brains confirmed the anatomically-inferred identity of these projections (Fig. 8I–J').

Taken together with evidence of LOT defects being present in *Sema6A* null mutants [35], these findings implicate Sema6A–PlxnA2/PlxnA4 signaling in the subpallial guidance of an additional axonal tract. Furthermore, they raise the possibility that a subtle, but widespread cytoarchitectural disruption of the most superficial vTel area in Sema6A- or PlxnA2; PlxnA4-deficient mice might impact on subsequent patterning and pathfinding processes in the vTel.

## Discussion

### Sema6A, PlxnA2 and PlxnA4 act together in caudally-directed TCA navigation through the subpallium

Our investigation revealed that PlxnA2 and PlxnA4 act together in the guidance of the same thalamic fiber subset miswired in *Sema6a* null mutants, at the level of the same subpallial structures. As *Plxna2* and *Plxna4* single mutants do not show any defect in TCA guidance, the two proteins appear to have an at least partially redundant role in dLGN axon pathfinding. These results add to the body of evidence showing functional redundancy between

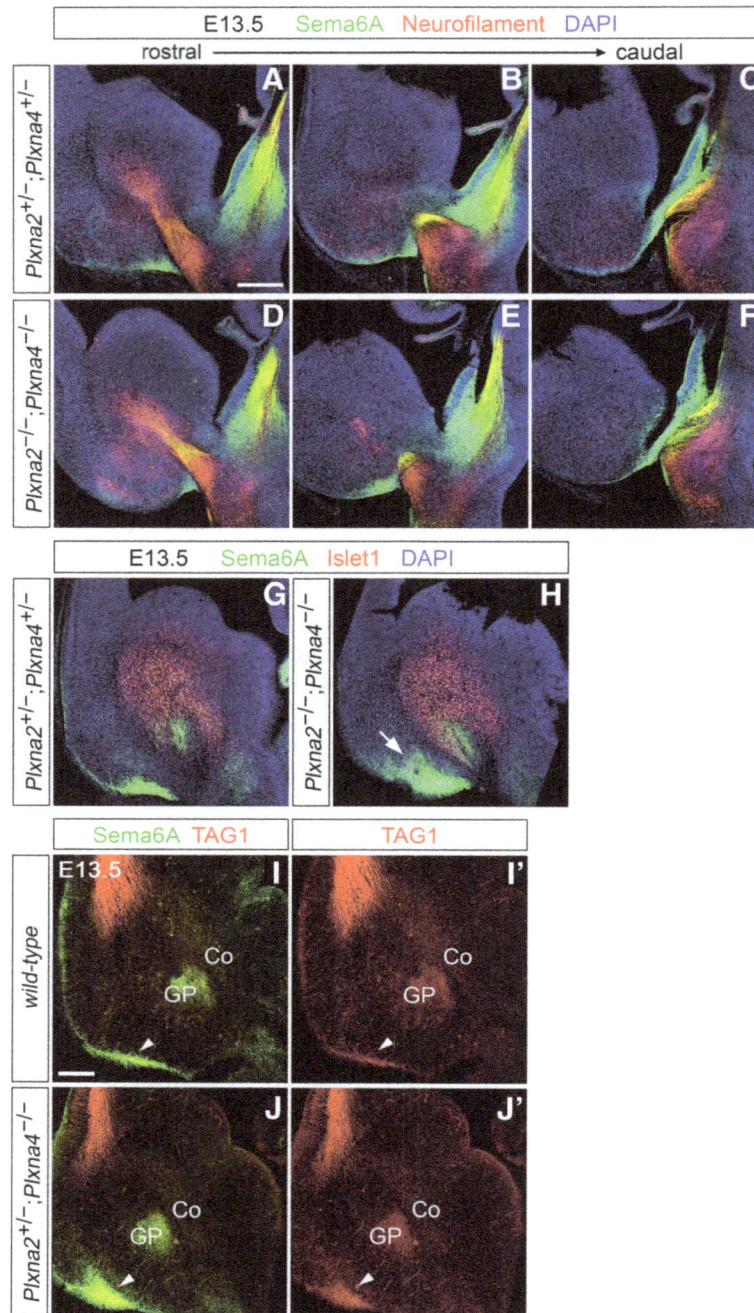

**Fig. 8** Sema6A expression in the dorsal thalamus, prethalamus, developing basal ganglia and lateral olfactory tract in *Plxna2; Plxna4* double mutant E13.5 brains. **a–f** Double immunohistochemistry for neurofilament (*red*) and Sema6A (*green*) on E13.5 coronal brain sections reveals the normal fasciculation and spatial navigation of Sema6A-positive caudally-projecting TCAs at dorsal thalamic and prethalamic level in *Plxna2*$^{-/-}$; *Plxna4*$^{-/-}$ (**a–c**) mouse brains, as compared to *Plxna2*$^{+/-}$; *Plxna4*$^{+/-}$ specimens (**d–f**). **g, h** Double immunohistochemistry for Islet1 (*red*) and Sema6A (*green*) on E13.5 coronal *Plxna2*$^{+/-}$; *Plxna4*$^{+/-}$ and *Plxna2*$^{-/-}$; *Plxna4*$^{-/-}$ brain sections demonstrates the preserved corridor region co-expression of the two proteins in the absence of PlxnA2/PlnxA4 function, as well as the normal presence of Sema6A in the globus pallidus and other subpallial areas. However, a Sema6A-positive axonal bundle, which normally elongates within the ventral vTel surface, can be observed to invade the subpallium in a ventro-dorsal direction in *Plxna2*$^{-/-}$; *Plxna4*$^{-/-}$ brains (*arrow* in **h**). **i–j'** Double immunohistochemistry for TAG1 (*red*) and Sema6A (*green*) on E13.5 coronal wild-type and *Plxna2*$^{+/-}$; *Plxna4*$^{-/-}$ brain sections indicates that the Sema6A-positive axonal bundle invading the subpallium in mice lacking PlxnA2/PlxnA4 (*arrowheads*) co-expresses TAG1, and thus corresponds to the lateral olfactory tract. Moreover, immunohistochemical data confirms the normal expression of Sema6A in developing basal ganglia structures in *Plxna2; Plxna4* null mutants. Co: corridor cells; GP: globus pallidus. Scale: **a–g**: 250 µm; **i–j'**: 200 µm

Plexins, including PlxnA2/PlxnA4, in diverse neurodevelopmental contexts [37, 50, 58].

Furthermore, our findings highlighted an almost exact correspondence in several defects involving thalamocortical connections emerging as a result of either *Sema6A* or *Plxna2*; *Plxna4* ablation. Like in *Sema6a* null mutants, in *Plxna2*$^{-/-}$; *Plxna4*$^{-/-}$ dLGN fibers turn ventrally once having crossed the DTB, instead of entering the IC, then proceed rostrally along the external capsule (eventually rejoining the IC axon bundle at the PSPB), or caudally within the pial surface of the vTel. Moreover, at P2 these latter misrouted axons can be observed to elongate dorsally in caudal pallial areas, at the level of the outermost neocortical layers. This finding might be indicative of an early postnatal recovery of visual thalamic nuclei–visual cortical areas connections via alternative axonal routes in superficial vTel and cortical territories, which is also characteristic of *Sema6a* mutants [34].

Another aspect of the *Plxna2*$^{-/-}$; *Plxna4*$^{-/-}$ TCA pathfinding phenotype that mirrors that of *Sema6a*$^{-/-}$ mice is the invasion of visual cortical domains by somatosensory thalamic fibers originating from dorso-lateral VB regions. In *Sema6a*-deficient mouse brains, this caudal shift in TCA targeting is clearly observable around birth, but does not persist beyond P4, possibly due to somatosensory axons being out-competed by recovering visual projections in the innervation of the presumptive V1 [34]. Accordingly, the same shift in thalamocortical topography can be seen in P0 *Plxna2*$^{-/-}$; *Plxna4*$^{-/-}$ mouse brains.

Interestingly, data here presented show that defects in TCA guidance in *Plxna2*$^{-/-}$; *Plxna4*$^{-/-}$ mice extend to a small population of VB neurons located at the interface between visual and somatosensory thalamic nuclei. This observation suggests that additional cues might participate in PlxnA2/PlxnA4-dependent TCA guidance mechanisms, and indeed both Plexins have been shown to mediate signaling of other Semaphorin family members. The association of PlxnA2 with Semaphorin-6B and Semaphorin-5A plays an essential role during commissural and hippocampal axon guidance [44, 59, 60], and in the regulation of dentate gyrus granule cell synaptogenesis [61], respectively. As for PlxnA4, this guidance protein has been demonstrated to mediate axon-repulsive responses by binding to Semaphorin-6B [44], and to cooperate with other Semaphorin/Plexin cues in sensory and sympathetic axon pathfinding by interacting with Semaphorin-3A [44, 50]. PlxnA2 and PlxnA4 might therefore participate with additional Plexins and other Semaphorin receptor components in the subpallial guidance of specific VB axon subsets.

Together with other findings generated by studies of mutant mouse lines presenting defects in TCA pathfinding within the basal forebrain, our results also support the notion that the switch from an external to an internal axonal path in the mammalian subpallium, due to changes in guidance cue patterning, is an evolutionarily recent trait connected with neocortical development in mammals [51]. Our mutant mouse lines specifically show that, in the event of a cytoarchitectural and/or functional disruption of structures delineating this internal path, thalamocortical connectivity can be eventually re-established following ancestral trajectories; however, this might occur at the expense of the proper functionality of the mature thalamocortical system [34, 62, 63].

## Complementary and overlapping *Sema6a*, *Plxna2* and *Plxna4* expression patterns in thalamic fibers and vTel guidepost cells during early TCA development

In this study, we expanded upon previous knowledge specific to late stages of TCA subpallial development by examining expression profiles of all our genes of interest throughout critical steps of TCA subcortical navigation. Our results confirmed previous findings obtained by *in situ* hybridization studies of Sema6A, PlxnA2 and PlxnA4 mRNA expression [34, 64, 65].

At E13.5 and E14.5, Sema6A, PlxnA2 and PlxnA4 present subpopulation-specific expression profiles in thalamic neurons and their projections, as well as the vTel. In the dTh, Sema6A is expressed broadly, in a high-dorsal to low-medial gradient, while PlxnA2 and PlxnA4 are observed restrictedly in medial thalamic nuclei. Notably, this region excludes the developing dLGN. These proteins are also present on TCAs; at E14.5 Sema6A is present on caudally-located axons, but absent in rostrally-projecting fibers, while PlexinA4 was observed to principally localize on these latter projections. Consistent with the *in situ* hybridization patterns, PlxnA4 immunoreactivity was absent from misrouted dLGN axons in *Sema6a* mutants. These data indicate that the effects on dLGN axon projections seen in *Plxna2*; *Plxna4* double mutants must be cell-non-autonomous.

During TCA elongation in the subpallium, Sema6A, PlxnA2 and PlxnA4 are also present in several regions of the vTel, including structures, such as the corridor and the globus pallidus, suggested to play a role in directing TCA guidance during the first steps of subpallial axonal growth [21, 22, 27, 52, 66]. Combining these observations with recent evidence indicating that PlxnA2/PlxnA4 – Sema6A reverse signaling occurs in vitro [36] and regulates axon guidance and targeting during murine optic system development [37], it can be hypothesized that PlxnA2 and PlxnA4 may act as a guidance cue for dLGN axons in the vTel, at the level of the IC. In this scenario, PlxnA2/PlxnA4 could provide, for instance, a repellent signal constraining axonal growth within the IC and acting specifically on Sema6A-positive dLGN projections. At the same time, PlxnA2/PlxnA4-positive axons originating from other thalamic nuclei might be unresponsive to subpallial Sema6A due to *cis* PlxnA2/A4–Sema6A interactions in those thalamic axon populations [36, 38].

On the other hand, the expression of all three proteins in the developing basal ganglia suggests that Sema6A – PlxnA2-PlxnA4 interactions might intervene in the correct patterning of these important ventral forebrain regions. Since all proteins are present in partially overlapping patterns in several subpallial domains, both forward and reverse signaling mechanisms might be here involved, and could be modulated by *cis* as well as *trans* binding events.

### Sema6A, PlxnA2 and PlxnA4 cooperate in morphogenetic processes involving caudal guidepost cell populations

Our analysis of vTel development in *Plxna2*$^{-/-}$; *Plxna4*$^{-/-}$ and *Sema6a*$^{-/-}$ mice focused on two specific cell populations suggested by several studies to play a role in subpallial TCA guidance, the corridor cells and the IC guidepost cells.

In case of the LGE-derived corridor neurons, we observed an overall preserved spatial and temporal organization of these cells within basal forebrain territories of both *Sema6a*- and *Plxna2*; *Plxna4*-deficient mouse brains. Specifically, findings demonstrated that corridor cell migration proceeds normally in all null mutant brains, indicating that a cooperative action of Sema6A, PlxnA2 and PlxnA4 is not required during these early patterning events of the vTel. Moreover, the corridor domain's cytoarchitectural features were found to be, for the most part, comparable between wild-type and mutant mouse brains at later developmental stages, when TCAs are elongating into presumptive basal ganglia regions of the vTel.

Considering IC guidepost cells, evident abnormalities in the spatiotemporal organization of this neural population were observed in both *Sema6a* and *Plxna2*; *Plxna4*-deficient mouse brains. At E13.5, when TCAs have begun their extension into the subpallium, guidepost cells could be back-labeled via retrograde dye tracing from the dTh in normal, IC-proximal positions in both *Sema6a*$^{-/-}$ and *Plxna2*$^{-/-}$; *Plxna4*$^{-/-}$ mutant brains. However, in the posterior part of the vTel, a small population of retrograde-labeled cell bodies was observed in a more ventro-caudal site with respect to the IC, which corresponds to a presumptive amygdala area invaded by misprojecting TCAs in the examined mutants. This clearly suggests that Sema6A, PlxnA2 and PlxnA4 together play a role in specifying the proper localization of a caudal subset of dTh-projecting guidepost cells.

Taken comprehensively, results from our investigation suggest that Sema6A–Plxna2-PlxnA4 interactions may participate, by acting on the formation of intermediate guidance structures, in indirect mechanisms of TCA axon guidance at the level of the subpallium. As a consequence, the more severe subpallial TCA miswiring observed in *PlxnA2*; *PlxnA4*-deficient mice compared to *Sema6A*$^{-/-}$ mutants might be deemed to result from a relatively worse defect in the final positioning of IC guidepost cells (which, in turn, could be due to previously discussed additional interactions of PlxnA2/PlxnA4 with other Semaphorins).

This possibility does not completely exclude, however, a hypothetical role of Sema6A reverse signaling in directing axonal growth in PlxnA2/PlxnA4-expressing intermediate subpallial targets. The striking specificity of TCA defects resulting from *Sema6A* ablation seems to indicate instead that multiple modes of interactions among the guidance factors here examined might, together, control caudal TCA guidance. Moreover, our experiments cannot definitively rule out that the response of these projections to environmental cues might depend, in some part, to axon-axon interactions between subsets differentially expressing PlxnA2-PlxnA4. This said, analysis of Sema6A expression in *PlxnA2*; *PlxnA4* double mutant brains, which indicates that caudally-projecting TCAs fasciculate with other axons lacking PlxnA2/PlxnA4 and navigate the dorsal thalamus and prethalamus normally, seems to suggests that Sema6A–PlxnA2/PlxnA4-dependent axon-axon interactions are generally dispensable for caudally-directed thalamic fiber guidance.

Considering that in *PlxnA2*$^{-/-}$; *PlxnA4*$^{-/-}$ brains Sema6A expression patterns in the corridor, the globus pallidus and the most ventral subpallial territories appear similar to those observed in wild-type and *PlxnA2*$^{+/-}$; *PlxnA4*$^{+/-}$ brains, the guidepost population phenotypes characterizing *Sema6a*- and *PlxnA2*; *PlxnA4*-deficient mice are unlikely to be induced by a defective migration of Sema6A-expressing (corridor or IC) guidepost cells in absence of directive signals provided by PlxnA2/PlxnA4 caudally. Whether PlxnA2/PlxnA4-expressing cells found in the corridor and the globus pallidus might, conversely, fail to position properly in the presumptive IC region due to ablation of Sema6A in the vTel, or lack of responsiveness to Sema6A, in the mutants here analyzed remains to be explored.

In relation to a potential cell-non-autonomous mechanism of Sema6A action in visual axon guidance, it is worth to examine findings from previous studies on *Ebf1*, *Inpp5e* and *Lhx2* null mutant mice, which all show disruption of Sema6A subpallial expression profiles in concomitance with TCA pathfinding errors. The loss of *Sema6a* mRNA expression domains in the developing vTel of *Ebf1*- and *Inpp5e*-deficient mice is correlated to a disorganization of cell populations in the developing basal ganglia (which in these cases includes corridor cells), and the ectopic growth of caudally-projecting TCAs in the presumptive amygdala [64, 65]. On the other hand, in *Lhx2* knockout mutants, *Sema6a* is over-expressed in the caudal vTel, guidepost cells cannot be back-labeled from the dTh in the IC region, and TCAs fail to extend in the vTel [67]. Our results are thus in line with evidence supporting a direct function of Sema6A in the morphogenesis of the IC, and provide new mechanistic insights on its role in the positioning of IC guidepost cells.

The fact that no Islet1-positive cells were observed in the vTel pial surface of our mutants, where some IC guidepost cells are found to mislocalize, supports the idea that at least part of this latter population may be unrelated to Islet1-positive corridor neurons [52, 66, 68, 69]. Indeed, it has been recently shown that some Dlx5/6-positive, Islet1-negative cells participate in forming the axonal bridge that allows TCAs to cross the DTB [68].

Our data is also in accordance with evidence showing that abnormalities, such as cell loss or misplacement, at the level of the most caudal parts of the corridor domain or the globus pallidus are associated with severe defects in TCA subpallial pathfinding (involving, in some cases, almost all fibers) [52, 63, 66, 70, 71]. Furthermore, these findings support the scaffolding model of axon guidance that has been proposed for IC guidepost cells [27, 68]. This said, it must be noted that a somewhat similarly compromised IC guidepost cells localization in concomitance to partial TCA guidance miswiring in the ventral subpallium has been described, so far, only in mice lacking the transcription factor Emx2 [72]. However, IC guidepost cells have yet to be exhaustively investigated in several mutant lines presenting an abnormal growth of caudal TCAs towards the presumptive amygdala.

## Conclusions

Overall, our investigation of vTel development in mouse brains lacking Sema6A or PlxnA2/PlxnA4 suggests that Sema6A–PlxnA2-PlxnA4 interactions may participate, by acting on the formation of intermediate guidance structures, in indirect mechanisms of TCA axon guidance at the level of the subpallium. Our findings do not exclude, however, a potential additional role of Sema6A reverse signaling in directing axonal growth with respect to PlxnA2/PlxnA4-expressing intermediate subpallial targets. On the other hand, our analyses indicate that the proper growth of these axons, or their responsiveness to guidance cues along their trajectories, is unlikely to be influenced by axon-axon interactions between TCA subsets differentially expressing Sema6A, PlxnA2 and PlxnA4.

More generally, this study illustrates how even subtle defects in early neurodevelopmental events can have substantial effects on contingent processes, such as guidance of major axonal tracts.

## Abbreviations

DAPI: 4',6-Diamidino-2-Phenylindole; DiA: 4-(4-(dihexadecylamino)styryl)-N-methylpyridinium iodide; DiI: 1,1'-dioctadecyl-3,3,3',3'-tetramethylindocarbocyanine perchlorate; dLGN: Dorsal lateral geniculate nucleus; DTB: Diencephalic–telencephalic boundary; dTh: Dorsal thalamus; GP: Globus pallidus; IC: Internal capsule; LGE: Lateral ganglionic eminence; LOT: Lateral olfactory tract; MGE: Medial ganglionic eminence; PlxnA2: Plexin-A2; PlxnA4: Plexin-A4; PSPB: Pallial–subpallial boundary; RT: Room temperature; S1: Primary somatosensory cortex; Sema6A: Semaphorin-6A; TCA: Thalamocortical axon; V1: Primary visual cortex; VB: Ventrobasal complex; vTel: Ventral telencephalon

## Acknowledgements

We would like to thank Hajime Fujisawa's group at Nagoya University, Japan, for providing the Plexin-A2- and Plexin-A4-specific antibodies that were employed throughout this study. We are additionally grateful to Jackie Dolan, Olivia Bibollet-Bahena, Daniel Shanley, Ash Watson, and Trinity College Dublin's Bioresources staff for their precious technical assistance and useful comments.

## Funding

This work was supported by grant 09/IN.1/B2614 from Science Foundation Ireland to KJM. MDM has been supported by a Trinity College Postgraduate Research Studentship. GEL has been supported by a Government of Ireland Scholarship, awarded by the Irish Research Council of Science, Engineering and Technology. The funders had no role in study design, data collection and analysis, decision to publish, or preparation of the manuscript.

## Authors' contributions

MDM and KJM conceived and designed the study. MDM performed all immunohistological and neuroanatomical tracing experiments. GEL and MDM performed *in situ* hybridization experiments. MDM and KJM analyzed and interpreted all data, and wrote the manuscript. All authors read and approved the final manuscript.

## Competing interests

The authors declare that they have no competing interests.

## Author details

[1]Smurfit Institute of Genetics, School of Genetics and Microbiology, Trinity College Dublin, Dublin 2, Ireland. [2]MRC Clinical Sciences Centre, Imperial College London, Hammersmith Hospital Campus, Du Cane Road, London W12 0NN, United Kingdom. [3]Trinity College Institute of Neuroscience, Trinity College Dublin, Dublin 2, Ireland. [4]Developmental Neurogenetics, Smurfit Institute of Genetics, Trinity College Dublin, Dublin 2, Ireland.

## References

1. Van Battum EY, Brignani S, Pasterkamp RJ. Axon guidance proteins in neurological disorders. Lancet Neurol. 2015;14(5):532–46.
2. Amaral DG, Schumann CM, Nordahl CW. Neuroanatomy of autism. Trends Neurosci. 2008;31(3):137–45.
3. Ameis SH, Catani M. Altered white matter connectivity as a neural substrate for social impairment in Autism Spectrum Disorder. Cortex. 2015;62:158–81.
4. Belmonte MK, et al. Autism and abnormal development of brain connectivity. J Neurosci. 2004;24(42):9228–31.
5. Geschwind DH, Levitt P. Autism spectrum disorders: developmental disconnection syndromes. Curr Opin Neurobiol. 2007;17(1):103–11.
6. McFadden K, Minshew NJ. Evidence for dysregulation of axonal growth and guidance in the etiology of ASD. Front Hum Neurosci. 2013;7:671.
7. Wass S. Distortions and disconnections: disrupted brain connectivity in autism. Brain Cogn. 2011;75(1):18–28.
8. Barch DM. Cerebellar-thalamic connectivity in schizophrenia. Schizophr Bull. 2014;40(6):1200–3.
9. Canu E, Agosta F, Filippi M. A selective review of structural connectivity abnormalities of schizophrenic patients at different stages of the disease. Schizophr Res. 2015;161(1):19–28.
10. Fornito A, Bullmore ET. Reconciling abnormalities of brain network structure and function in schizophrenia. Curr Opin Neurobiol. 2015;30:44–50.
11. Friston KJ, Frith CD. Schizophrenia: a disconnection syndrome. Clin Neurosci. 1995;3(2):89–97.
12. Innocenti GM, Ansermet F, Parnas J. Schizophrenia, neurodevelopment and corpus callosum. Mol Psychiatry. 2003;8(3):261–74.
13. Karlsgodt KH, et al. Developmental disruptions in neural connectivity in the pathophysiology of schizophrenia. Dev Psychopathol. 2008;20:1297–327.
14. Pantelis C, et al. Early and late neurodevelopmental disturbances in schizophrenia and their functional consequences. Aust N Z J Psychiatry. 2003;37(4):399–406.
15. Pantelis C, et al. Structural brain imaging evidence for multiple pathological processes at different stages of brain development in schizophrenia. Schizophr Bull. 2005;31(3):672–96.
16. Woodward ND, Karbasforoushan H, Heckers S. Thalamocortical dysconnectivity in schizophrenia. Am J Psychiatr. 2012;169(10):1092–9.
17. Cao M, et al. Imaging functional and structural brain connectomics in attention-deficit/hyperactivity disorder. Mol Neurobiol. 2014;50(3):1111–23.
18. Konrad K, Eickhoff SB. Is the ADHD brain wired differently? A review on structural and functional connectivity in attention deficit hyperactivity disorder. Hum Brain Mapp. 2010;31(6):904–16.
19. Qiu M-G, et al. Changes of brain structure and function in ADHD children. Brain Topogr. 2011;24(3–4):243–52.
20. Braisted JE, Tuttle R, O'Leary DDM. Thalamocortical axons are influenced by chemorepellent and chemoattractant activities localized to decision points along their path. Dev Biol. 1999;208(2):430–40.
21. Garel S, López-Bendito G. Inputs from the thalamocortical system on axon pathfinding mechanisms. Curr Opin Neurobiol. 2014;27:143–50.
22. López-Bendito G, et al. Tangential neuronal migration controls axon guidance: a role for Neuregulin-1 in thalamocortical axon navigation. Cell. 2006;125(1):127–42.
23. Marín O, et al. Guiding neuronal cell migrations. Cold Spring Harb Perspect Biol. 2010;2(2):a001834.
24. Raper J, Mason C. Cellular strategies of axonal pathfinding. Cold Spring Harb Perspect Biol. 2010;2(9):a001933.
25. Squarzoni P, Thion MS, Garel S. Neuronal and microglial regulators of cortical wiring: usual and novel guideposts. Front Neurosci. 2015;9:248.
26. López-Bendito G, Molnár Z. Thalamocortical development: how are we going to get there? Nat Rev Neurosci. 2003;4(4):276–89.
27. Molnár Z, et al. Mechanisms controlling the guidance of thalamocortical axons through the embryonic forebrain. Eur J Neurosci. 2012;35(10):1573–85.
28. Price DJ, et al. The development of cortical connections. Eur J Neurosci. 2006;23(4):910–20.
29. Auladell C, et al. The early development of thalamocortical and corticothalamic projections in the mouse. Anat Embryol. 2000;201(3):169–79.
30. Garel S, Rubenstein JLR. Intermediate targets in formation of topographic projections: inputs from the thalamocortical system. Trends Neurosci. 2004;27(9):533 9.
31. Leyva-Díaz E, López-Bendito G. In and out from the cortex: development of major forebrain connections. Neuroscience. 2013;254:26–44.
32. Vanderhaeghen P, Polleux F. Developmental mechanisms patterning thalamocortical projections: intrinsic, extrinsic and in between. Trends Neurosci. 2004;27(7):384–91.
33. Leighton PA, et al. Defining brain wiring patterns and mechanisms through gene trapping in mice. Nature. 2001;410(6825):174–9.
34. Little GE, et al. Specificity and plasticity of thalamocortical connections in Sema6A mutant mice. PLoS Biol. 2009;7(4):e1000098.
35. Rünker AE, et al. Mutation of Semaphorin-6A disrupts limbic and cortical connectivity and models neurodevelopmental psychopathology. PLoS ONE. 2011;6(11):e26488.
36. Perez-Branguli F, et al. Reverse signaling by Semaphorin-6A regulates cellular aggregation and neuronal morphology. PLoS ONE. 2016;11(7): e0158686.
37. Sun LO, et al. Functional assembly of accessory optic system circuitry critical for compensatory eye movements. Neuron. 2015;86(4):971–84.
38. Haklai-Topper L, et al. Cis interaction between Semaphorin6A and Plexin-A4 modulates the repulsive response to Sema6A. EMBO J. 2010;29(15):2635–45.
39. Jongbloets BC, Pasterkamp RJ. Semaphorin signalling during development. Development. 2014;141(17):3292–7.
40. Sun LO, et al. On and off retinal circuit assembly by divergent molecular mechanisms. Science. 2013;342(6158):1241974.
41. Suto F, et al. Interactions between plexin-A2, plexin-A4, and semaphorin 6A control lamina-restricted projection of hippocampal mossy fibers. Neuron. 2007;53(4):535–47.
42. Faulkner RL, et al. Dorsal turning of motor corticospinal axons at the pyramidal decussation requires plexin signaling. Neural Dev. 2008;3:21.
43. Rünker AE, et al. Semaphorin-6A controls guidance of corticospinal tract axons at multiple choice points. Neural Dev. 2008;3(1):1–19.
44. Suto F, et al. Plexin-a4 mediates axon-repulsive activities of both secreted and transmembrane semaphorins and plays roles in nerve fiber guidance. J Neurosci. 2005;25(14):3628–37.
45. Matsuoka RL, et al. Transmembrane semaphorin signalling controls laminar stratification in the mammalian retina. Nature. 2011;470(7333):259–63.
46. Bron R, et al. Boundary cap cells constrain spinal motor neuron somal migration at motor exit points by a semaphorin-plexin mechanism. Neural Dev. 2007;2:21.
47. Renaud J, et al. Plexin-A2 and its ligand, Sema6A, control nucleus-centrosome coupling in migrating granule cells. Nat Neurosci. 2008;11(4):440–9.
48. Zhuang BQ, Su YRS, Sockanathan S. FARP1 promotes the dendritic growth of spinal motor neuron subtypes through transmembrane Semaphorin6A and PlexinA4 signaling. Neuron. 2009;61(3):359–72.
49. Mitchell KJ, et al. Functional analysis of secreted and transmembrane proteins critical to mouse development. Nat Genet. 2001;28(3):241–9.
50. Yaron A, et al. Differential requirement for Plexin-A3 and -A4 in mediating responses of sensory and sympathetic neurons to distinct class 3 Semaphorins. Neuron. 2005;45(4):513–23.
51. Bielle F, et al. Slit2 activity in the migration of guidepost neurons shapes thalamic projections during development and evolution. Neuron. 2011;69(6): 1085–98.
52. Uemura M, et al. OL-Protocadherin is essential for growth of striatal axons and thalamocortical projections. Nat Neurosci. 2007;10(9):1151–9.
53. Wang Y, et al. Axonal growth and guidance defects in Frizzled3 knock-out mice: a comparison of diffusion tensor magnetic resonance imaging, neurofilament staining, and genetically directed cell labeling. J Neurosci. 2006;26(2):355–64.
54. Yoshida Y. Semaphorin signaling in vertebrate neural circuit assembly. Front Mol Neurosci. 2012;5:71.
55. Hsieh H-H, et al. Control of axon–axon attraction by Semaphorin reverse signaling. Proc Natl Acad Sci U S A. 2014;111(31):11383–8.
56. Jeong S, Juhaszova K, Kolodkin AL. The control of Semaphorin-1a-mediated reverse signaling by opposing pebble and RhoGAPp190 functions in Drosophila. Neuron. 2012;76(4):721–34.
57. Inaki K, et al. Laminar organization of the developing lateral olfactory tract revealed by differential expression of cell recognition molecules. J Comp Neurol. 2004;479(3):243–56.
58. Schwarz Q, et al. Plexin A3 and plexin A4 convey semaphorin signals during facial nerve development. Dev Biol. 2008;324(1):1–9.

59. Andermatt I, et al. Semaphorin 6B acts as a receptor in post-crossing commissural axon guidance. Development. 2014;141(19):3709–20.

60. Tawarayama H, et al. Roles of semaphorin-6B and plexin-A2 in lamina-restricted projection of hippocampal mossy fibers. J Neurosci. 2010;30(20):7049–60.

61. Duan Y, et al. Semaphorin 5A inhibits synaptogenesis in early postnatal- and adult-born hippocampal dentate granule cells. eLife. 2014;3:e04390.

62. Gezelius, H., et al. Genetic labeling of nuclei-specific thalamocortical neurons reveals putative sensory-modality specific genes. Cereb Cortex. 2016;1:16.

63. Lokmane L, et al. Sensory map transfer to the neocortex relies on pretarget ordering of thalamic axons. Curr Biol. 2013;23(9):810–6.

64. Garel S, et al. The early topography of thalamocortical projections is shifted in Ebf1 and Dlx1/2 mutant mice. Development. 2002;129(24):5621–34.

65. Magnani D, et al. The ciliogenic transcription factor Rfx3 is required for the formation of the thalamocortical tract by regulating the patterning of prethalamus and ventral telencephalon. Hum Mol Genet. 2015;24(9):2578–93.

66. Jia Z, et al. Regulation of the protocadherin Celsr3 gene and its role in globus pallidus development and connectivity. Mol Cell Biol. 2014;34(20): 3895–910.

67. Lakhina V, et al. Early thalamocortical tract guidance and topographic sorting of thalamic projections requires LIM-homeodomain gene Lhx2. Dev Biol. 2007;306(2):703–13.

68. Feng J, et al. Celsr3 and Fzd3 organize a pioneer neuron scaffold to steer growing thalamocortical axons. Cereb. Cortex. 2016;26(7):3323–34.

69. Tuttle R, et al. Defects in thalamocortical axon pathfinding correlate with altered cell domains in Mash-1-deficient mice. Development. 1999;126(9): 1903–16.

70. Mandai K, et al. LIG family receptor tyrosine kinase-associated proteins modulate growth factor signals during neural development. Neuron. 2009; 63(5):614–27.

71. Morello F, et al. Frizzled3 controls axonal polarity and intermediate target entry during striatal pathway development. J Neurosci. 2015;35(42):14205–19.

72. López-Bendito G, et al. Role of Emx2 in the development of the reciprocal connectivity between cortex and thalamus. J Comp Neurol. 2002;451(2):153–69.

# 6

# Expression and functional analysis of the Wnt/beta-catenin induced *mir-135a-2* locus in embryonic forebrain development

Giuliana Caronia-Brown[*], Angela Anderegg and Rajeshwar Awatramani

## Abstract

**Background:** Brain size and patterning are dependent on dosage-sensitive morphogen signaling pathways – yet how these pathways are calibrated remains enigmatic. Recent studies point to a new role for microRNAs in tempering the spatio-temporal range of morphogen functions during development. Here, we investigated the role of *miR-135a*, derived from the *mir-135a-2* locus, in embryonic forebrain development.

**Method:** 1. We characterized the expression of *miR-135a*, and its host gene *Rmst*, by in situ hybridization (*ish*). 2. We conditionally ablated, or activated, beta-catenin in the dorsal forebrain to determine if this pathway was necessary and/or sufficient for *Rmst/miR-135a* expression. 3. We performed bioinformatics analysis to unveil the most predicted pathways targeted by *miR-135a*. 4. We performed gain and loss of function experiments on *mir-135a-2* and analyzed by *ish* the expression of key markers of cortical hem, choroid plexus, neocortex and hippocampus.

**Results:** 1. *miR-135a*, embedded in the host long non-coding transcript *Rmst*, is robustly expressed, and functional, in the medial wall of the embryonic dorsal forebrain, a Wnt and TGFβ/BMP-rich domain. 2. Canonical Wnt/beta-catenin signaling is critical for the expression of *Rmst* and *miR-135a*, and the cortical hem determinant *Lmx1a*. 3. Bioinformatics analyses reveal that the Wnt and TGFβ/BMP cascades are among the top predicted pathways targeted by *miR-135a*. 4. Analysis of *mir-135a-2* null embryos showed that dorsal forebrain development appeared normal. In contrast, modest *mir-135a-2* overexpression, in the early dorsal forebrain, resulted in a phenotype resembling that of mutants with Wnt and TGFβ/BMP deficits - a smaller cortical hem and hippocampus primordium associated with a shorter neocortex as well as a less convoluted choroid plexus. Interestingly, late overexpression of *mir-135a-2* revealed no change.

**Conclusions:** All together, our data suggests the existence of a *Wnt/miR-135a* auto-regulatory loop, which could serve to limit the extent, the duration and/or intensity of the Wnt and, possibly, the TGFβ/BMP pathways.

**Keywords:** *Wnts, Rmst, miR-135a, Forebrain, Lmx1a, beta-catenin*

## Background

MicroRNAs are micro-modulators of gene expression, eliciting small changes in the expression of a wide array of targets [1]. In the last ten years, their role in almost every facet of nervous system development and function has been considered including neuronal and glial differentiation, synaptogenesis, and neuro-degeneration [2–10]. Yet only recently, some studies have focused on their role in modulating the dosage or duration of the most fundamental developmental molecules – morphogens [11, 12]. Given the exquisite dosage sensitivity of morphogens, an argument has been proposed that these pathways are prime substrates for microRNA micro-management [12].

Wnt and TGFβ/BMP morphogens expressed by the roof plate, or adjacent neuroepithelium, act through signaling cascades implicated in various facets of dorsal neural tube development [13]. Throughout the Central Nervous System (CNS), various studies have revealed a role for Wnt signaling in the expansion of the brain via increases in cell proliferation and survival [14–18].

* Correspondence: giuliana.caronia-brown@northwestern.edu
Department of Neurology and Center for Genetic Medicine, Northwestern University Feinberg School of Medicine, 7-113 Lurie Bldg., 303 E. Superior Street, Chicago, IL 60611, USA

Other studies have revealed roles in specification of key neuronal progenitor types, as well as in the timing of neurogenesis [16, 19–22]. Additionally, several studies have suggested that the dosage of the Wnt pathway is critical for normal specification, neurogenesis and differentiation [15, 19, 23, 24]. TGFβ/BMP signaling has also been implicated in proliferation, specification, neurogenesis and gliogenesis [25–31]. Akin to the Wnt pathway, several studies have suggested that the TGFβ/BMP pathway is exquisitely dosage sensitive [32, 33]. Despite an emerging literature on the cross talk between these two key pathways [31, 34], the potential nodes of intersection and their net molecular outputs remain to be fully elucidated. It is likely that the molecular synchronization of these pathways is required for dorsal neural tube development.

The cortical hem, positioned adjacent to the hippocampus, between the choroid plexus on the medial side and the cortical neuroepithelium on the lateral side, is a Wnts and TGFβ/BMPs-rich embryonic structure [29, 35, 36]. The hem has been demonstrated to specify the hippocampus primordium [37–42], to serve as a source of Cajal-Retzius cells [43], to be required for choroid plexus formation [16, 29, 36] and to play a role in regulating the size and patterning of the neocortex [44].

Previously, we identified a microRNA, miR-135a, whose expression was correlated to the long non-coding transcript Rhabdomyosarcoma 2 associated transcript (Rmst). We deduced that miR-135a was derived from mir-135a-2 locus embedded in Rmst and we demonstrated that Rmst and miR-135a are co-expressed in the ventral midbrain, isthmus, as well as dorsal regions of the neural tube [11]. At least in the midbrain, modest and early overexpression of this microRNA yields phenotypes consistent with a reduction of Wnt signaling [11]. Given the potential importance of this microRNA, we have explored its expression, activity and induction in the dorsal forebrain as well as generated mir-135a-2 knockout and overexpressor mice. We reveal that miR-135a is strongly expressed, and is functional, in the medial wall of the telencephalon including the cortical hem and hippocampus primordium, but more weakly expressed in the choroid plexus and in the neocortex. We show that canonical Wnt/beta-catenin signaling is critical for Rmst and miR-135a expression, and also for Lmx1a expression, a key cortical hem determinant. While mir-135a-2 loss of function did not result in appreciable changes in the cortical hem and neocortex sizes or in choroid plexus complexity, its modest over-expression resulted in smaller cortical hem and neocortical domains and also in a less convoluted choroid plexus. All together, our data lead us to conclude that this Wnt induced microRNA is a potential modulator of the Wnt and TGFβ/BMP signaling pathways during dorsal forebrain development.

## Methods

### Nomenclature

miRbase uses a 3 or 4 letter prefix to designate the microRNA species, such that 'mmu' refers to the mouse. The un-capitalized 'mir' refers to the pre-microRNA (mmu-mir-135). In this manuscript, we have only investigated the murine mir-135 therefore we have omitted the prefix. Distinct genomic loci that belong to the same family (mir-135) are typically indicated with an additional letter and number such as mir-135a-1, mir-135a-2 and mir-135b. The capitalized 'miR' refers to the mature form (miR-135). mir-135a-1 and mir-135a-2 give rise to only one mature form called mmu-miR-135a-5p. For simplicity, we will refer to the mature form as miR-135a. However, our experiments on mir-135a-2 knockout mice imply that the predominant mature form of miR-135a in the dorsal forebrain is produced from the mir-135a-2 locus.

### Mouse lines

Animals were maintained in compliance with National Institutes of Health guidelines. The Northwestern University IACUC approved the protocols for this study. E0.5 designates the morning of the day when a vaginal plug was detected. For beta-catenin gain and loss of function experiments, Ctnnb1$^{lox(ex3)}$ [45] or beta-catenin floxed mice (Ctnnb1$^{flox/flox}$) [46], were crossed with Emx1::IRES-Cre [47] and embryos were used for in situ hybridization (ish) or RT-qPCR experiments. The miR-135a "sensor" construct was previously described [11]. To evaluate miR-135b expression, we used mir-135b$^{flox/flox}$ mice (Jackson lab) [48], which harbor a LacZ cassette and crossed them to wild type females. E12.5 embryos of the mir-135b$^{flox/+}$ genotype were stained for Xgal as previously described [49]. To generate the mir-135a-2 knockout mice, we utilized ZFN technology (Sigma). One advantage of this approach is that no selection cassette or residual FRT, or loxP sites, will remain in the intron, and the resultant deletion will be clean. Sixteen different ZFNs were custom designed to bind and cleave the mir-135a-2 locus, within 100 bp upstream or downstream of the stem-loop precursor. The ZFN (GCCATCAGGATAGC nAACTATAGCCTGTGGAC) that demonstrated the highest activity, in an in vitro Mouse Neuro2a cell screen, was chosen for large-scale production and microinjection in mice. The ZFN mRNA was diluted to 2.5 ng/μl in injection buffer and microinjected into early stage FVB embryos. 152 mice were screened with ZFN-F: GGTC CTCGTAGCGAAGAATG and ZFN-R: AATCGGTGGT CAGGAAGATG PCR primers. Five heterozygous mice were identified with one wild type allele and one allele containing a deletion near the mir-135a-2 locus. After sequence analysis, we found that each deletion was unique and ranged from 2 bp to 294 bp. Line #4 had the largest deletion, which removed the entire *mir-135a-2* precursor, and was used for the experiments here described. RT-qPCR with TaqMan primers was used to confirm drastic reduction of the mature form *miR-135a*.

Sensor transgenic embryos (*n* = 4), and *mir-135a-2* knockout (*mir-135a-2KO*) mice were generated at the Northwestern Transgenic and Targeted Mutagenesis Laboratory.

Generation and genotyping of *mir-135a-2* overexpressor transgenic mouse line have been previously described in [11]. To generate conditional *mir-135a-2OE* embryos, *mir-135a-2OE* mouse line was crossed with *Emx1::IRES-Cre* (henceforth *Emx1::Cre*) [47] or *Nestin::Cre* (henceforth *Nes::Cre*) [50]. As controls for these experiments, we used littermates negative for *Cre*. To generate *Emx1::Cre;mir-135a-2OE;mir-135a-2^{+/-}* embryos, *Emx1::Cre;mir-135a-2OE* adult mice were crossed with *mir-135a-2* knockout mice.

### Tissue processing

Brains were fixed with 4 % PFA and either embedded in 30 % sucrose-10 % gelatin-PBS and sectioned with a Leica SM2010R sliding microtome, or in OCT and sectioned with a Leica cryostat. Sections (20–40 μm) were processed for *ish* with Digoxigenin (Dig)-labeled riboprobes [43]. Bound Dig was detected with anti-Dig antibody (1:5000, Roche). To detect *Rmst*, we used two probes as described in [11]. To detect *miR-135a*, we performed locked-nucleic acid (LNA) *ish* with Exiqon probe # 39037-01 and followed recommended protocol for non-radioactive hybridization by Dr. Wigard Kloosterman, the Plasterk Group, Hubrecht Laboratory, Utrecht, The Netherlands, with the following modifications: no de-paraffinization step; PK treatment 5'–10' at 37C (20-40 μm sections); T hyb 53C; probe [25nM]; blocking solution 10 % lamb serum-TBST; anti-Dig-AP was diluted 1:5000 in 1 % lamb serum-TBST. eGFP expression, in double transgenic embryos, was detected by immunofluorescence with anti-GFP rabbit polyclonal (1:1500, Invitrogen) without antigen retrieval on 20 μm cryostat sections. Secondary antibody was donkey anti-rabbit 488 (Invitrogen). No immunostaining was necessary to detect tdTomato expression. For Xgal staining, brains were lightly fixed in 2 % PFA-PIPES solution, washed in PBS and Xgal stained from few hours to overnight at 37C. To generate coronal sections, after Xgal staining, brains were fixed in 4 % PFA overnight and processed for cryostat sectioning (50 μm). For immunohistochemistry (IHC) assay, brains were also fixed in 4 % PFA overnight and sectioned at 20 μm with a Leica cryostat. After citrate antigen retrieval, sections were incubated with anti-phospho-Smad 1/5/8 rabbit polyclonal (1:50, Cell signaling). Secondary antibody was biotinylated anti-rabbit polyclonal from ABC KIT (1:200, Vectastain). In this study, gene expression comparisons between control and mutant mice were based on at least 3 brains per group per age for each gene.

### Quantification of cortical tissue and cortical hem area

At E12.5, the length of the neocortex was measured from the pallium-subpallium boundary (PSB), chosen as a landmark, to the cortical hem. Quantification was performed at three levels of the brain, 80 μm apart, along the rostrocaudal axis. At the same stage, we additionally quantified the cortical hem area (*Lmx1a+*). For all of the measurements, we used ImageJ software (series 1.4, NIH, public domain). Data are expressed as a mean ± the standard error (SEM) (*n* = 3).

### RT-qPCR

For RT-qPCR experiments, dorsal or ventral forebrain tissue was dissected from controls (wild types) and mutants (*Emx1::Cre;Ctnnb1^{lox(ex3)}*, *Emx1::Cre;Ctnnb1* cKO, *mir-135a-2* knockout and overexpressor) (*n* = 3). Briefly, E12.5 embryos were collected in ice cold PBS, the forebrain was exposed, and a piece of the dorsal, or ventral, forebrain tissue was snipped with forceps and processed for RNA extraction. Total RNA, including small RNAs, was extracted using the *mir*Vana kit (Ambion). To quantify *miR-135a* and *miR-135b* expression levels, we used the TaqMan PCR Assay (ID 000460 and ID 002261, Applied Biosystems) and normalized our data to microRNA *sno202* (ID 001232, Applied Biosystems).

### Statistical analysis

To determine statistical significance of our quantification experiments, we first determined if data followed the normal distribution by the Anderson-Darling Test for Normality. All of our data sets had a p value > 0.05, indicating normality. To assess the statistical significance of changes in the cortical hem area and neocortical domain length, the two experimental groups (control and mutant mice) were compared with two samples equal variance, two tailed, Student's *t*-test. To calculate the relative fold changes in *miR-135a* and *miR-135b* expression by RT-qPCR experiments, we applied the comparative C(T) method also referred to as the 2 (-DeltaDeltaC(T)) method [51] and normalized our data to microRNA *sno202*. Unpaired Student's *t* test was applied to determine statistical significance.

### Bioinformatics analysis

To determine *miR-135a* most predicted targeted pathways, we used the Diana-miRPath, a microRNA pathway analysis web server that combines predicted and validated microRNA targets in CDS or 3'-UTR regions with sophisticated merging and meta-analysis algorithms [52].

## Results

### Rmst and miR-135a expression and activity in the embryonic forebrain

Previously, we identified *miR-135a* through a screen for microRNAs that were robustly expressed in the Wnt-rich ventral midbrain region of the embryonic Central Nervous System (CNS) [11]. We provided evidence that *miR-135a* expression was correlated with *Rmst*, and deduced that *miR-135a* was derived from *mir-135a-2* locus located in the final detected intron of *Rmst* [11, 53]. Since the embryonic dorsal forebrain is known to be a Wnt-rich region and dependent on Wnt signaling [36, 54, 55], we determined if *Rmst* and *miR-135a* were also co-expressed in this region of the CNS. We therefore first characterized *Rmst* expression at embryonic and adult stages (Fig. 1 and Additional file 1: Figure S1). In embryonic forebrain sections *Rmst* is robustly detected in the medial wall of the telencephalon, encompassing a Wnt and TGFβ/BMP-rich signaling center, the cortical hem [35, 56]. At E12.5, *Rmst* was strongly expressed in the dorsal telencephalon in a medial$^{High}$ to dorso-lateral$^{Low}$ gradient (Fig. 1a). Expression was robust in the cortical hem and the adjacent hippocampus primordium. A very weak hybridization signal was detected in the choroid plexus and along the neocortical domain. *Rmst* was also strongly expressed in the septum, diencephalon, and eminentia thalami. At later stages, *Rmst* expression was localized to various forebrain nuclei, and the fimbria (Additional file 1: Figure S1). We next performed Locked Nucleic Acid (LNA) *ish*

experiments to detect mature *miR-135a*, focusing on the embryonic forebrain. We found that this microRNA species, like *Rmst*, was expressed in the medial wall of the telencephalon in a medial$^{High}$ to dorso-lateral$^{Low}$ gradient (Fig. 1b). Expression was robust in the cortical hem and the adjacent hippocampus primordium. A very weak hybridization signal was detected in the choroid plexus and along the neocortical domain. Some signal was also detected in the LGE, however, since *Rmst* is not expressed in this region, this signal could represent cross hybridization with a closely related microRNA. Alternatively, in this region *miR-135a* and *Rmst* expression could be uncoupled.

To demonstrate that *miR-135a* is functional in these domains, we generated double transgenic embryos harboring a "sensor" and a control transgene. A "sensor" construct contains a constitutively expressed reporter gene (eGFP), under control of a CAG promoter, and multiple binding sites for *miR-135a* in the 3' UTR region (Fig. 1c, cartoon, yellow bars). In cells expressing *miR-135a*, its perfect complementarity to sequences in the 3' UTR should result in suppression of the eGFP reporter. A control transgene construct contains a tdTomato reporter, but lacks the *miR-135a* binding sites and, therefore, should be

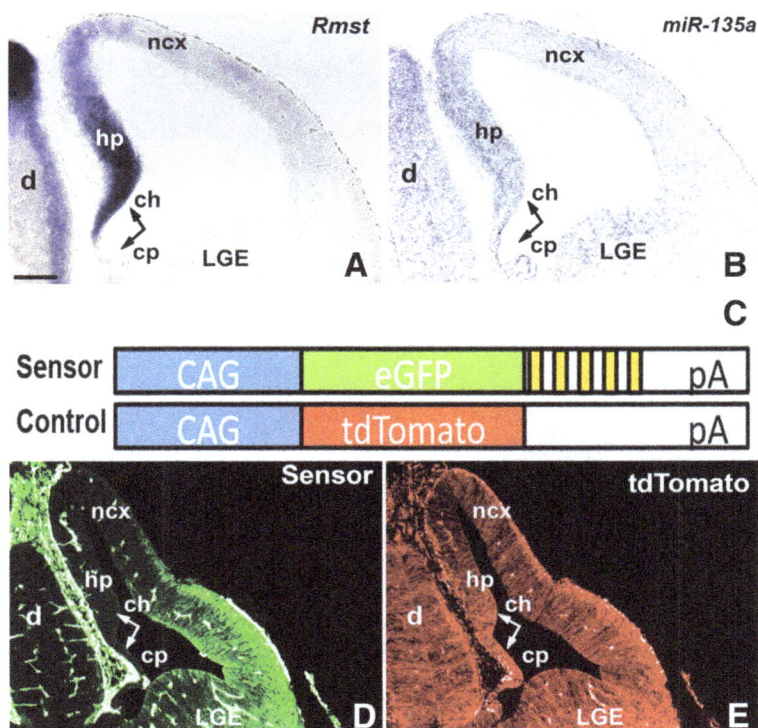

**Fig. 1** *Rmst and miR-135a* expression and activity in the embryonic dorsal forebrain. (**a-b** and **d-e**). Forebrain coronal sections of E12.5 wild type (**a**, **b**) and double transgenic mice (**d**, **e**). **a** *ish* for *Rmst*. **b** LNA *ish* for mature *miR-135a*. **d**, **e** Double transgenic embryos harboring eGFP "sensor" and tdTomato control constructs represented in **c** (cartoon; yellow bars indicate *miR-135a* binding sites). **d** eGFP immunolabeling **e** tdTomato fluorescence. ch, cortical hem; hp, hippocampus primordium; cp, choroid plexus; LGE, lateral ganglionic eminences; ncx, neocortex; d, diencephalon. Scale bar 100 μm

constitutively active. In E12.5 double transgenic embryos, we found that the eGFP reporter (Fig. 1d), but not tdTomato (Fig. 1e), was selectively reduced in the medial wall of the telencephalon where *miR-135a* is strongly expressed, as well as in the choroid plexus and in the dorsal neocortical domain, where *Rmst* and *miR-135a* are more weakly expressed. eGFP was also not detected in the diencephalon (Fig. 1d). Thus, *miR-135a* is expressed, and displays activity, in the embryonic dorsal forebrain.

### beta-catenin signaling induces Rmst and miR-135a expression

Previously, we reported that in the embryonic midbrain, the transcription factor *Lmx1b* induces Wnt1/Wnt signaling as well as *Rmst* and *mir-135a-2* locus [11]. Since *Lmx1b* and *Lmx1a* are partially redundant, we postulated that *Lmx1a* might also be a regulator of *Rmst* and *mir-135a-2*. However, since, in the dorsal forebrain, *Rmst* and *miR-135a* expressions exceed the *Lmx1a* domain, one possibility is that in addition to *Lmx* genes, Wnt signaling abets the induction of the *Rmst* and *mir-135a-2* locus. To address this question, we performed gain and loss of function experiments of beta-catenin, a key effector of Wnt signaling pathway [57]. *Emx1::Cre* mouse line was used to drive recombination throughout the dorsal, but not ventral, forebrain [47]. For gain of function experiments, by conditionally deleting beta-catenin exon 3 (*Ctnnb1$^{lox(ex3)}$*), which encompasses GSK3β phosphorylation sites, we effectively elevated Wnt signaling [23, 45]. In mutants (*Emx1::Cre;Ctnnb1$^{lox(ex3)}$*) (Fig. 2b), but not in controls (Fig. 2a), *Rmst* was detected throughout the dorsal forebrain. Conversely, for loss of function experiments, we conditionally removed exons 2-6 of beta-catenin to prevent formation of a functional beta-catenin protein thus impairing Wnt signaling [46]. In mutants (*Emx1::Cre;Ctnnb1* cKO) (Fig. 2c), but not in

controls (Fig. 2a), we observed drastic loss of *Rmst* expression throughout the dorsal forebrain and in the remaining cortical hem tissue (Fig. 2c, asterisk). *miR-135a* expression levels, quantified by RT-qPCR on E12.5 dissected dorsal telencephalon, were strongly induced in *Emx1::Cre;Ctnnb1$^{lox(ex3)}$* mutants, and reduced in *Emx1::Cre;Ctnnb1* cKOs (Fig. 2d). Overall, these data demonstrate that beta-catenin signaling is necessary and sufficient for *Rmst* and *miR-135a* expression in the dorsal forebrain.

### beta-catenin signaling is necessary for Lmx1a expression

We also determined if *Lmx1a*, a key cortical hem determinant [58], is a target of Wnt/beta-catenin signaling in the forebrain, as in other brain regions [11, 22, 23]. While in *Emx1::Cre;Ctnnb1$^{lox(ex3)}$* embryos (Fig. 2f), we did not observe a drastic change in the cortical hem size (*Lmx1a+*, Fig. 2f and *Wnt3a+*, Additional file 2: Figure S2) or in *Lmx1a* expression (Fig. 2f) with respect to controls (Fig. 2e), in *Emx1::Cre;Ctnnb1* cKOs, we observed a drastic reduction of *Lmx1a* signal in the remaining cortical hem tissue (Fig. 2g, asterisk). *Lmx1a* was detected in the choroid plexus of both mutants (Fig. 2f and g). These results suggest that Wnt/beta-catenin signaling is necessary, but not sufficient, for *Lmx1a* expression in the dorsal forebrain. Given that *Lmx1a* in part functions to repress *Lhx2* [58], a negative regulator of the hem [39], Wnt/beta-catenin induction of *Lmx1a* is likely to be an important event in the cortical hem establishment and/or maintenance.

### miR-135a is predicted to target the Wnt and TGFβ/BMP pathways, but loss of function does not affect dorsal forebrain development

To begin to elucidate *miR-135a* functions, we performed bioinformatics analysis to determine the most common pathways targeted by *miR-135a*. To do that, we took advantage of the Diana–miRPath software [52], which

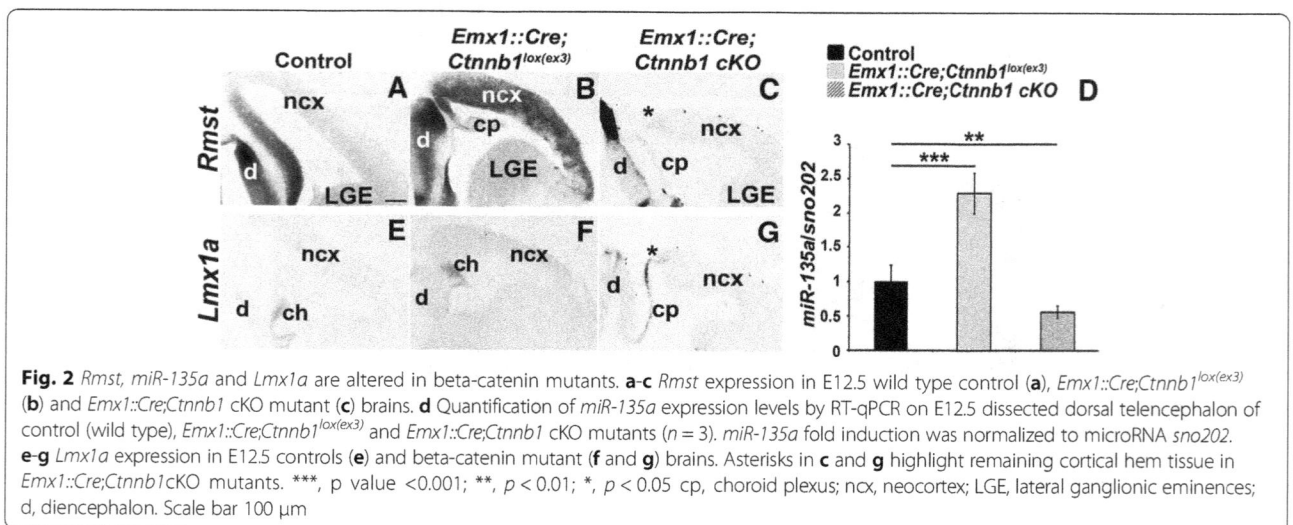

**Fig. 2** *Rmst, miR-135a* and *Lmx1a* are altered in beta-catenin mutants. **a–c** *Rmst* expression in E12.5 wild type control (**a**), *Emx1::Cre;Ctnnb1$^{lox(ex3)}$* (**b**) and *Emx1::Cre;Ctnnb1* cKO mutant (**c**) brains. **d** Quantification of *miR-135a* expression levels by RT-qPCR on E12.5 dissected dorsal telencephalon of control (wild type), *Emx1::Cre;Ctnnb1$^{lox(ex3)}$* and *Emx1::Cre;Ctnnb1* cKO mutants (n = 3). *miR-135a* fold induction was normalized to microRNA *sno202*. **e–g** *Lmx1a* expression in E12.5 controls (**e**) and beta-catenin mutant (**f** and **g**) brains. Asterisks in **c** and **g** highlight remaining cortical hem tissue in *Emx1::Cre;Ctnnb1*cKO mutants. ***, p value <0.001; **, p < 0.01; *, p < 0.05 cp, choroid plexus; ncx, neocortex; LGE, lateral ganglionic eminences; d, diencephalon. Scale bar 100 μm

utilizes predicted, and validated, microRNA targets to perform a hierarchical clustering of microRNA and pathways based on their interactions. We found that Wnt and TGFβ/BMP signaling pathways are among the top pathways targeted by *miR-135a* with an extremely high statistical significance (p value of approximately 2.9E-07 and 3.6E-10, respectively) (Additional file 3: Figure S3A). It is worth noticing that the genes targeted by *miR-135a* in the TGFβ/BMP (Additional file 3: Figure S3B) and Wnt pathways (Additional file 4: Figure S4) include ligands, receptors and downstream transcriptional regulators suggesting that this microRNA likely acts through multiple levels of the Wnt and TGFβ/BMP cascades to modulate the outcome of their signaling.

To determine the role of *miR-135a* in embryonic dorsal forebrain development, we generated a mouse line in which *mir-135a-2* was deleted by pronuclear injection of a specific Zn finger nuclease (Fig. 3a and b), designed to cleave <100 bp from the mature sequence. Of ~60 pups examined, 1 harbored a ~294 bp deletion (Fig. 3c and d) and was used to generate a line for the experiments here described. RT-qPCR on dissected E12.5 dorsal forebrain tissue confirmed a drastic reduction in *miR-135a* expression levels (Fig. 3e). We thus deduced that, in the dorsal forebrain akin to the ventral midbrain, *miR-135a* is predominantly produced from *mir-135a-2* locus.

Because a growing literature has described interactions between microRNAs and long non-coding RNAs (lncRNAs) as a novel mechanism to regulate gene expression as well as microRNA function [59–61], we investigated the possibility of an interaction between *Rmst* and *miR-135a*. A search on miRcode web site, which represents a comprehensive map of putative microRNA target sites across the GENCODE long non-coding transcriptome [62], indicated lack of *miR-135a* responsive elements in *Rmst*. To confirm the bioinformatics prediction, we performed *ish* for *Rmst* on E12.5 coronal sections of *mir-135a-2* knockout mice and we did not observe any change in its expression (Fig. 4a and b). These data seem to therefore exclude the possibility of *Rmst* being a potential target of *miR-135a*. Next, we performed in situ hybridization with *Lmx1a* (Fig. 4c and d), a marker for the cortical hem and the choroid plexus to investigate any possible change in proper development of these Wnt and TGFβ/BMP responsive domains. We did not, however, observe any apparent change in the cortical hem size (Fig. 4d) as was also confirmed by quantification analysis at three levels of the forebrain, equally spaced along the rostro-caudal axis (referred to as Rostral, Mid and Caudal) (Fig. 4e). No difference was detected in the extent of the cortical domain (Fig. 4d), which was again measured at three levels of the forebrain, equally spaced along the rostro-caudal axis (Rostral, Mid and Caudal) from the inflection that marks the pallium-subpallium boundary (PSB), chosen as a

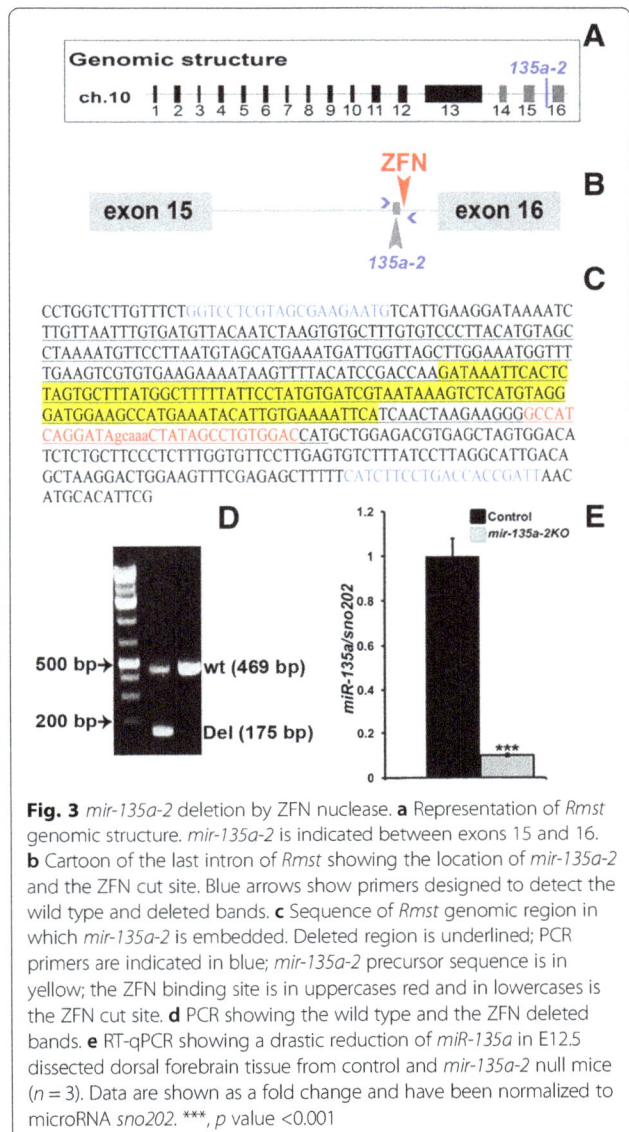

**Fig. 3** *mir-135a-2* deletion by ZFN nuclease. **a** Representation of *Rmst* genomic structure. *mir-135a-2* is indicated between exons 15 and 16. **b** Cartoon of the last intron of *Rmst* showing the location of *mir-135a-2* and the ZFN cut site. Blue arrows show primers designed to detect the wild type and deleted bands. **c** Sequence of *Rmst* genomic region in which *mir-135a-2* is embedded. Deleted region is underlined; PCR primers are indicated in blue; *mir-135a-2* precursor sequence is in yellow; the ZFN binding site is in uppercases red and in lowercases is the ZFN cut site. **d** PCR showing the wild type and the ZFN deleted bands. **e** RT-qPCR showing a drastic reduction of *miR-135a* in E12.5 dissected dorsal forebrain tissue from control and *mir-135a-2* null mice (n = 3). Data are shown as a fold change and have been normalized to microRNA *sno202*. ***, p value <0.001

landmark, to the cortical hem (Fig. 4f). No change in the choroid plexus complexity was observed (Fig. 4d).

The cortical hem is a signaling center known to induce and pattern the adjacent hippocampus [38, 41]. We therefore performed in situ hybridization with neuronal marker *NeuroD2* to assess any morphological changes in the hippocampal complex at post-natal and adult stages of *mir-135a-2* knockouts. No changes were observed (Fig. 4g-j). These findings clearly demonstrate that, at least by these criteria, *mir-135a-2* loss of function does not alter forebrain development.

microRNAs often display redundancy with family members [63, 64]. To determine whether *miR-135b*, a closely related microRNA was expressed in a similar domain, we obtained mice in which LacZ had been inserted into the *mir-135b* locus. In E12.5 whole mount

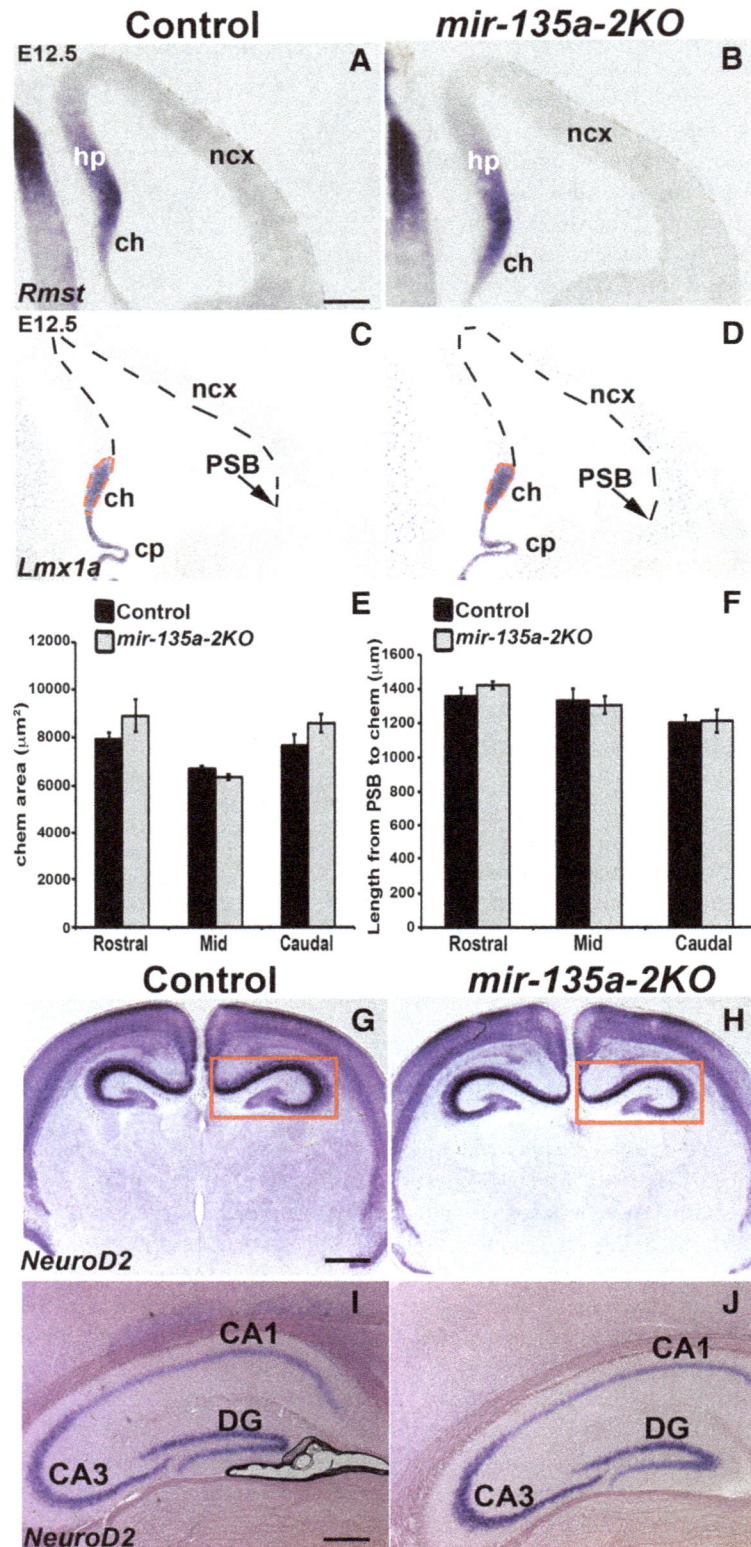

**Fig. 4** (See legend on next page.)

(See figure on previous page.)
**Fig. 4** *mir-135a-2* loss of function characterization. **a-b** E12.5 coronal sections of control (*mir-135a-2*^+/^) and *mir-135a-2*KO brains (*mir-135a-2*^-/-^) processed for *ish* for *Rmst* showing no change in its expression. **c-d** *ish* for *Lmx1a* in control (**c**) and *mir-135a-2*KO (**d**) brains. Dashed lines highlight the cortical hem area and the neocortical domain size. **e** Quantification of the cortical hem area (μm² ± SEM) along the rostro-caudal axis (*n* = 3). **f** Quantification of the neocortex length (μm ± SEM) from the PSB to the hem at the same levels (*n* = 3). **g-j** *ish* for *NeuroD2* on coronal sections of post-natal P1 (**g-h**) and adult (**i-j**) control and mutant brains showing no change in hippocampus morphology (boxed in **g** and **h**). ch, cortical hem; cp, choroid plexus; hp, hippocampus; PSB, pallium-subpallium boundary; ncx, neocortex; CA1, CA3, hippocampus fields; DG, dentate gyrus. Scale bar 100 μm in panels **a-d**, 400 μm in panels **g** and **h**; 200 μm in panels **i** and **j**

(Fig. 5a) and forebrain sections (Fig. 5b and c), we did not observe any LacZ staining in the dorsal forebrain (Fig. 5a and b) whereas we found LacZ expression in cells emanating from the ganglionic eminences in the ventral forebrain (Fig. 5c). Consistent with this, RT-qPCR experiments for *miR-135b* on wild type dorsal and ventral forebrain dissected tissues, revealed a ventral enrichment of this microRNA (Fig. 5d). These data suggest that *miR-135b* does not serve a redundant function in the dorsal forebrain.

### Early mir-135a-2 overexpression affects dorsal forebrain development

To complement our loss of function results, we took advantage of previously generated transgenic mice to conditionally express *mir-135a-2* for gain of function experiments. This time, we reasoned that if the *Wnt/miR-135a* circuitry identified in the midbrain [11] is functionally conserved in the forebrain, *mir-135a-2* overexpression might result in Wnts related phenotypes. To test this hypothesis, mice in which *mir-135a-2* precursor expression is under control of a CAG promoter [11] (henceforth *mir-135a-2OE*), were crossed with *Emx1::Cre* line [47] to overexpress *mir-135a-2* throughout the *Emx1* domain of the dorsal, but not ventral, forebrain as early as E9.5 [43]. RT-qPCR on dissected E12.5 dorsal forebrain tissue confirmed that *miR-135a* expression levels, in *Emx1::Cre;mir-135a-2OE* mutants, were 1.5 fold more than in controls (Additional file 5: Figure S5). In such mutants we observed a clear reduction in the size of the cortical hem (*Wnt3a+*, *Wnt8b+*) and the hippocampus primordium (*Wnt8b+*) (Fig. 6a-d). Additionally, we observed a reduction in size of the neocortical domain (Fig. 6a-b, dashed lines), a phenotype previously shown in mice with genetic ablation of the cortical hem [44, 65], but not reported in *BmpRIA/IB* cKOs which display a smaller cortical hem [42]. The choroid plexus, normally specified by TGFβ/BMPs [29, 42] and demarcated by *rTtr1*, was overall less

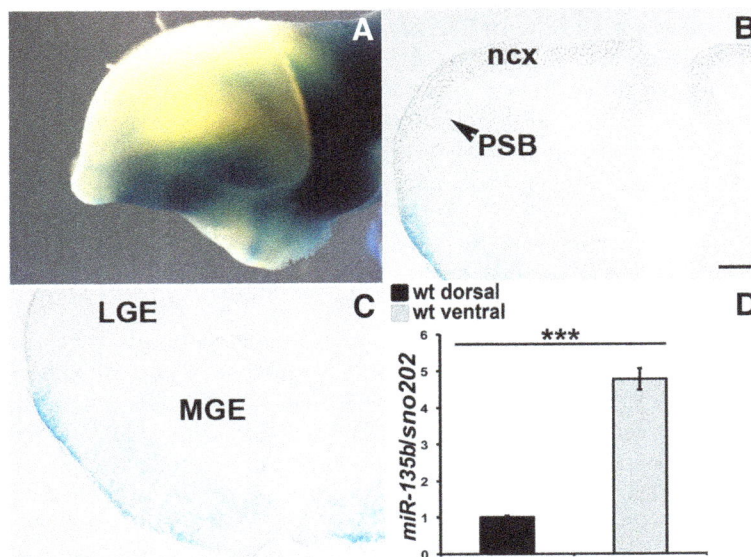

**Fig. 5** *miR-135b* expression in the embryonic forebrain. **a-c** Xgal staining of E12.5 whole mount (lateral view) (**a**) and E12.5 coronal sections (**b-c**), showing expression of *lacZ* exclusively in the ventral forebrain of *mir-135b*^flox/+^ mice harboring a LacZ reporter gene in the *mir-135b* locus. **d** RT-qPCR on wild type dorsal and ventral forebrain tissue samples (*n* = 3). *miR-135b* fold induction was normalized to microRNA *sno202*. ***, *p* value <0.001. LGE, lateral ganglionic eminences; MGE, medial ganglionic eminences; PSB, pallium-subpallium boundary; ncx, neocortex. Scale 200 μm in panels **b** and **c**

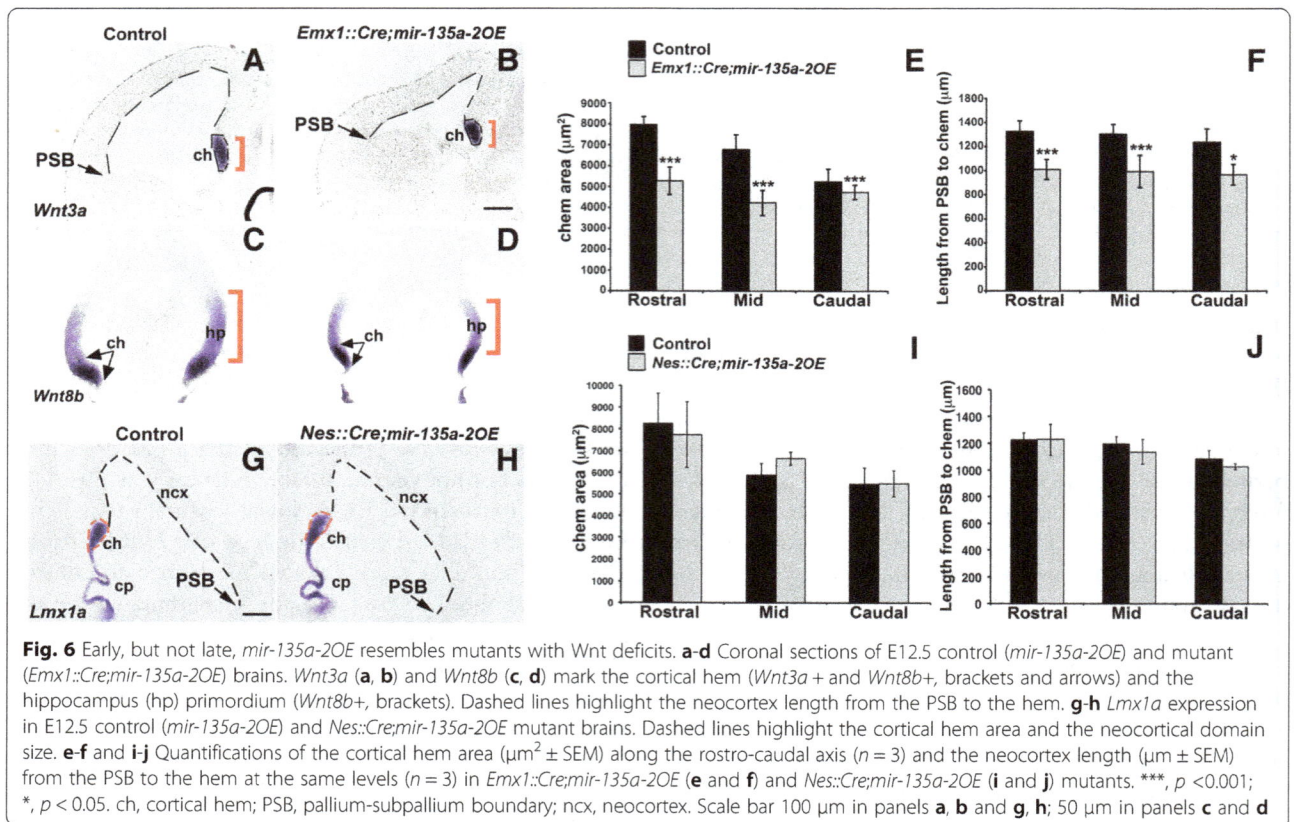

**Fig. 6** Early, but not late, *mir-135a-2OE* resembles mutants with Wnt deficits. **a-d** Coronal sections of E12.5 control (*mir-135a-2OE*) and mutant (*Emx1::Cre;mir-135a-2OE*) brains. *Wnt3a* (**a**, **b**) and *Wnt8b* (**c**, **d**) mark the cortical hem (*Wnt3a* + and *Wnt8b+*, brackets and arrows) and the hippocampus (hp) primordium (*Wnt8b+*, brackets). Dashed lines highlight the neocortex length from the PSB to the hem. **g-h** *Lmx1a* expression in E12.5 control (*mir-135a-2OE*) and *Nes::Cre;mir-135a-2OE* mutant brains. Dashed lines highlight the cortical hem area and the neocortical domain size. **e-f** and **i-j** Quantifications of the cortical hem area ($\mu m^2 \pm$ SEM) along the rostro-caudal axis ($n = 3$) and the neocortex length ($\mu m \pm$ SEM) from the PSB to the hem at the same levels ($n = 3$) in *Emx1::Cre;mir-135a-2OE* (**e** and **f**) and *Nes::Cre;mir-135a-2OE* (**i** and **j**) mutants. ***, $p < 0.001$; *, $p < 0.05$. ch, cortical hem; PSB, pallium-subpallium boundary; ncx, neocortex. Scale bar 100 $\mu m$ in panels **a**, **b** and **g**, **h**; 50 $\mu m$ in panels **c** and **d**

convoluted (Additional file 6: Figure S6). Altogether, *Emx1::Cre;mir-135a-2OE* mutants show characteristics previously described in mice deficient for Wnt or TGFβ/BMP activity, or in which the cortical hem has been genetically ablated [16, 29, 42, 44, 65, 66], although they display a milder phenotype.

Next, we quantified the cortical hem area along the rostro-caudal axis. We estimated a reduction in its size of ~34 % at rostral level, ~38 % at mid level and ~18 % at caudal level (Fig. 6e) in mutants compared to controls. Finally, we quantified the extent of the neocortical domain and found a significant reduction in size of the mutant neocortices in comparison to controls (Fig. 6f). Since the cortical hem and the hippocampus primordium are reduced in *Emx1*::Cre;*mir-135a-2OE* embryos, these mutants showed a significant reduction of all hippocampal structures (CA fields and dentate gyrus) from postnatal stage P1 (Additional file 7: Figure S7, A-B and E) to adulthood (Additional file 7: Figure S7C and D) when compared to controls.

Finally, we examined the expression of several bioinformatically predicted *miR-135a* targets. Of these, only phospho-Smad (1/5/8) and *Msx2* revealed consistent changes, showing apparent reduction in their level and expression domain extent (Additional file 8: Figure S8). Their reduction might be due to direct repression, overall net down regulation of these pathways, or both.

### Late mir-135a-2 overexpression does not affect dorsal forebrain development

Conditional transgenes in neural progenitor cells have been associated with non-specific phenotypes [67]. To rule out non-specific effects of *mir-135a-2* overexpression, we also overexpressed *mir-135a-2* by using *Nes::Cre* driver [50], which like *Emx1::Cre*, is active in the hippocampus primordium, along the neocortical domain, and reported to mediate Cre recombination in the hem at ~ E12.5 [10, 68–71]. *Nes::Cre* driven overexpression of *mir-135a-2* was additionally useful to determine whether the phenotype resulting from *mir-135a-2* overexpression in *Emx1::-Cre;mir-135a-2OE* mice, was time sensitive. In E12.5 (Fig. 6g and h) and E13.5 (Additional file 9: Figure S9) *Nes::Cre;mir-135a-2OE* mutants, we did not observed microcephaly. Both the cortical hem and neocortical sizes were not affected (Fig. 6i and j). Also, no change was observed in the choroid plexus (Fig. 6g and h). These data suggest that late overexpression of this microRNA in neural progenitors, does not affect forebrain development, and that the transgene does not appear to display significant toxicity in neuronal progenitors.

## mir-135a-2 overexpression in mir-135a-2$^{+/-}$ mice does not result in forebrain abnormalities

To further demonstrate the specificity of our results, we removed one copy of endogenous *mir-135a-2* from embryos conditionally overexpressing *mir-135a-2*. We reasoned that if the phenotype observed in *Emx1::Cre;-mir-135a-2OE* mutants is due to *mir-135a-2* overexpression, then, removal of one copy of the endogenous *mir-135a-2* should alleviate this phenotype. E12.5 embryos of *Emx1::Cre;mir-135a-2OE;mir-135a-2$^{+/-}$* (mutants) and *Emx1::Cre;mir-135a-2$^{+/-}$* (controls) genotypes were analyzed for the expression of *Lmx1a* (Fig. 7a and b) and *Wnt3a* (Additional file 10: Figure S10). The cortical hem area and the extent of the cortical domain were quantified as previously described (Fig. 7c and d). No alterations in these domains and in the choroid plexus were observed,

suggesting that normal *miR-135a* levels are important for embryonic forebrain development.

## Discussion

From the present study we deduced six prominent conclusions. First, *miR-135a*, and *Rmst*, are expressed and functional in the embryonic dorsal forebrain. Second, in the dorsal forebrain, mature *miR-135a* is predominantly derived from the *mir-135a-2* locus. Third, *miR-135a* is dispensable for forebrain development. Fourth, modest *mir-135a-2* overexpression, within an early but not late time window, results in a phenotype consistent with Wnt and TGFβ/BMP signaling deficits – a reduced cortical hem, hippocampus primordium and neocortex, and a less convoluted choroid plexus. Fifth, Wnt/beta-catenin pathway is necessary and sufficient to induce *Rmst* and *miR-135a* expression pointing to the existence of a *Wnt/miR-135a* auto-regulatory loop, which could serve to limit the extent, the duration and/or intensity of the Wnt pathway. Finally, Wnt/beta-catenin pathway is also necessary

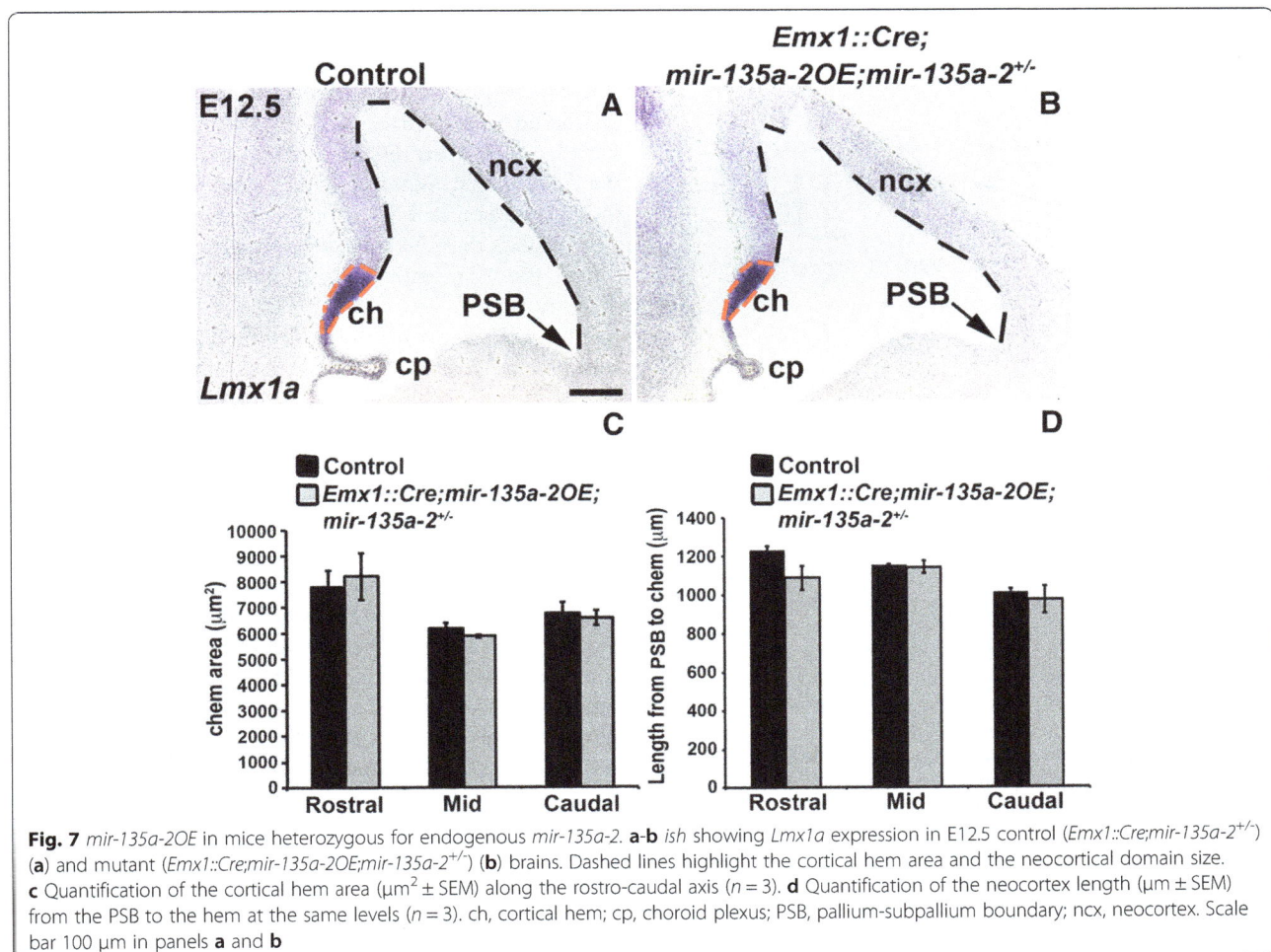

**Fig. 7** *mir-135a-2OE* in mice heterozygous for endogenous *mir-135a-2*. **a-b** *ish* showing *Lmx1a* expression in E12.5 control (*Emx1::Cre;mir-135a-2$^{+/-}$*) (**a**) and mutant (*Emx1::Cre;mir-135a-2OE;mir-135a-2$^{+/-}$*) (**b**) brains. Dashed lines highlight the cortical hem area and the neocortical domain size. **c** Quantification of the cortical hem area (μm$^2$ ± SEM) along the rostro-caudal axis (*n* = 3). **d** Quantification of the neocortex length (μm ± SEM) from the PSB to the hem at the same levels (*n* = 3). ch, cortical hem; cp, choroid plexus; PSB, pallium-subpallium boundary; ncx, neocortex. Scale bar 100 μm in panels **a** and **b**

for *Lmx1a* expression, a key cortical hem determinant. A model of these interactions is depicted in Fig. 8.

Wnt and TGFβ/BMP morphogens act through gradients of signaling cascades and have been implicated in various facets of dorsal neural tube development [16, 19–22].

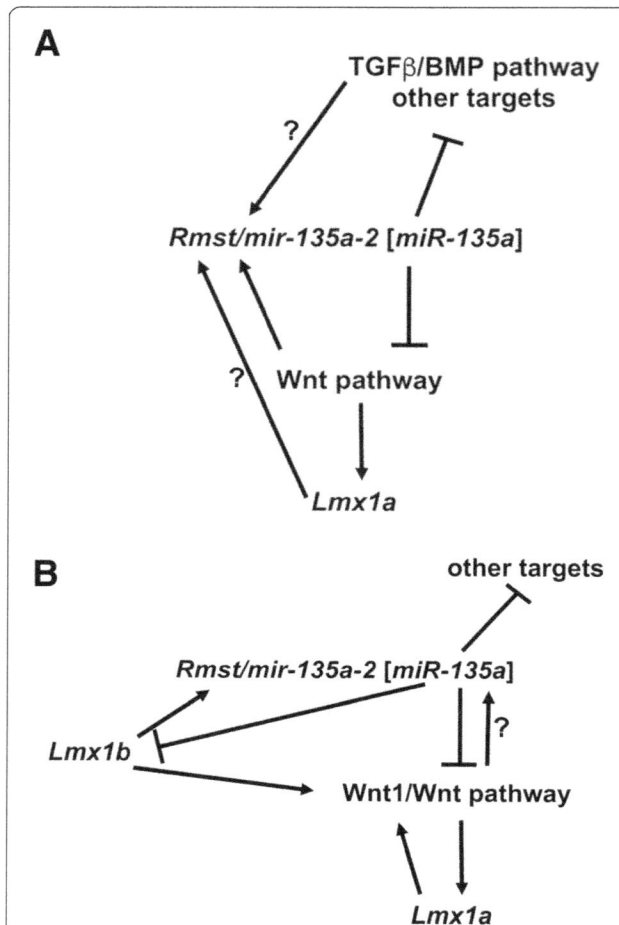

**Fig. 8** Schematic representation of interactions between *Lmx1* genes, the Wnt pathway and *Rmst/mir-135a-2 [miR-135a]*. **a** In the embryonic forebrain, canonical Wnt/beta-catenin pathway induces *Rmst/mir-135a-2 [miR-135a]*, as well as the cortical hem determinant *Lmx1a*. *miR-135a*, in turn, negatively targets Wnt pathway mRNAs establishing an auto-regulatory loop. *miR-135a* is also predicted to target TGFβ/BMP pathway mRNAs as well as other targets. It is possible that the TGFβ/BMP pathway is also able to induce *Rmst/mir-135a-2 [miR-135a]* and establish a *miR-135a*/TGFβ/BMP auto-regulatory loop. It is also possible that *Lmx1a* contributes to *Rmst/mir-135a-2 [miR-135a]* expression. However, these interactions remain to be demonstrated. Ultimately, this complex network of positive and negative interactions plays a role in determining proper dorsal forebrain size (cortical hem, hippocampus primordium, choroid plexus and neocortex). **b** A similar scenario was previously identified in the embryonic midbrain [11] where *Lmx1b* drives the expression of Wnt1/Wnt pathway and of *Rmst/mir-135a-2 [miR-135a]*, which in turn negatively modulates the levels of *Lmx1b*, Wnt1/Wnt pathway and other targets. Additionally, Wnt1/Wnt pathway and *Lmx1a* interactions have been demonstrated. All together these interactions are critical for midbrain dopamine progenitor pool patterning and expansion

Several studies have suggested that the dosage of the Wnt and TGFβ/BMP pathways is critical and has to be tightly controlled through intricate networks of positive and negative feedback loops [15, 19, 23, 32, 33]. It is therefore challenging to understand how these pathways are modulated in time and space during embryonic development, how cells receive and integrate multiple signals and whether potential nodes of intersection exist. Recently, it has been demonstrated that microRNAs contribute to gene networks that transform the graded activity of a morphogen in robust cell fate decisions by establishing context-dependency, threshold responses and sharpening temporal and spatial expression patterns [4, 12, 72]. *miR-135a* and its host long non-coding transcript, *Rmst*, were shown to be expressed and functional in the embryonic Wnt-rich domain of the midbrain [11]. Here, we have shown that *miR-135a* and *Rmst* are also co-expressed in the Wnt and TGFβ/BMP-rich domains of the embryonic dorsal forebrain suggesting a correlation between this microRNA, the Wnts and TGFβ/BMPs-rich domains across the embryonic CNS. Interestingly, akin to several Wnts and TGFβ/BMPs, strong expression of *Rmst* in the embryonic hippocampal primordium declines over time and, at post-natal stages, become restricted to the fimbria and virtually undetectable in the adult hippocampus. *Rmst* expression has also been detected in human fetal cortical radial glia, suggesting a conserved role for this locus [73]. Taking together, the *Rmst*/*miR-135a* expression pattern in mice and humans, the finding that Wnt signaling is indeed able to induce their expression and the strong bioinformatics predictions, we postulate that this microRNA might play a role in fine-tuning the Wnt pathway and, possibly, the TGFβ/BMP pathway.

Embryos lacking *Wnt3a* [16], functional LEF1 [66], or with genetic ablation of the cortical hem [44, 65], display loss of the hippocampus and shrinkage of the neocortex [44, 65], while mice with disrupted TGFβ/BMP signaling fail to develop or properly differentiate the choroid plexus [29]. Modest *mir-135a-2* overexpression appears to recapitulate these phenotypes, albeit in a milder fashion. Coupled with the findings that this microRNA is bioinformatically predicted to target both positive and negative regulators in the Wnt and TGFβ/BMP pathways, the Wnt related phenotypes observed in the midbrain [11], and proven interactions between *miR-135a* and targets like *GSK*, *Tcf7l2*, *Ccnd1* and *APC* in heterologous systems or cancer cell lines [11, 74–78], we posit that *miR-135a* modulates the Wnt and TGFβ/BMP signaling cascade in the developing forebrain.

*mir-135a-2* loss of function embryos did not display overt forebrain phenotypes, at least by the criteria that we assayed. One plausible explanation comes from the observation that members of a microRNA family are often predicted to target the same or overlapping sets of genes and therefore to act in a functionally redundant manner [63]. Supporting this idea, single microRNA loss of function or single microRNA silencing, through antisense oligonucleotides and sponge techniques, typically results in subtle or no phenotypes [64, 79–81]. Because *mir-135b* was expressed in the embryonic ventral forebrain, we ruled out any compensatory effect due to this microRNA. We considered the possibility that the other member of this family, *mir-135a-1* might be expressed in a similar and overlapping pattern. Because *mir-135a-1* and *mir-135a-2* produce an identical mature form, it is not possible to analyze their differential expression by standard techniques. However, RT-qPCR experiments for mature *miR-135a* on dorsal forebrain tissue of *mir-135a-2* null embryos revealed greatly reduced expression levels. Therefore, we concluded that the main *miR-135a* mature form in the dorsal forebrain could be attributed to *mir-135a-2* precursor. Redundancy, on the other hand, can either be attributed to very low levels of *miR-135a* produced by the *mir-135a-1* precursor or to some other microRNA having a similar seed sequence. This latter, more likely, possibility has been raised in the recent literature [82].

Identifying regulators of the Wnt pathway has been highlighted as an important goal [83]. *miR-135a* is up regulated in several tumor types characterized by high levels of Wnt/beta-catenin signaling, including colorectal tumors as well as certain subtypes of medulloblastomas [74, 76]. It is possible that, in these tumors, Wnt signaling, in accordance with our data in the forebrain, induces *miR-135a*. If so, *miR-135a* would serve as a useful marker for aberrant Wnt signaling in these tumors, and possibly others, and in therapeutic protocols designed to circumscribe unrestrained Wnt signaling. In colorectal cancers, *miR-135a* has been proposed to act as a positive regulator of Wnt signaling by targeting APC, a key molecule of the beta-catenin destruction complex [74]. Thus, while it is emerging that this microRNA is intimately correlated with Wnt signaling in the embryonic CNS ([11]and this work), in tumors [74–76] and in other cell types with high Wnt signaling [77, 78], it is possible that the net effect of *miR-135a* depends on the physiological milieu. Elucidating the targets may reveal how a single microRNA, predicted to target both positive and negative regulators of a signaling pathway, may have distinct outcomes depending on the context. Ultimately, an array of biochemical and genetic approaches will be required to accurately define direct *miR-135a* targets and the molecular underpinnings of *mir-135a-2* mutant phenotypes.

Finally, our study has highlighted a role for Wnt/beta-catenin signaling in the expression of cortical hem determinant *Lmx1a*, a LIM-homeodomain transcription factor.

Wnt1/Wnt signaling has been shown to form an autoregulatory loop with *Lmx1a* to control dopaminergic neurons differentiation in the embryonic ventral midbrain [22, 23, 84, 85]. In the dorsal embryonic forebrain, *Lmx1a* is expressed in the cortical hem, a Wnt-rich region. While *Lmx1a* is not required for cortical hem induction, it is critical for proper regulation of cell fate decisions [58]. In the absence of *Lmx1a*, the hippocampal selector gene *Lhx2* is ectopically expressed in the cortical hem leading to excessive production of hippocampal cells and decreased production of Cajal-Retzius cells [58]. Here, through gain and loss of function experiments of beta-catenin, we show that, in the dorsal forebrain akin to the ventral midbrain [22, 24], Wnt/beta-catenin signaling is necessary, but not sufficient, for *Lmx1a* expression. Wnt/beta-catenin induction of *Lmx1a* is likely to be a key event in the proper cortical hem cell fate establishment and/or maintenance.

## Additional files

**Additional file 1: Figure S1.** *Rmst* expression during forebrain development. (A-F) *Rmst ish* on coronal sections of wild type brains from E11.5 to adult stage. (A) At E11.5, *Rmst* is expressed in the epithalamus, medial wall of the dorsal telencephalon, the eminentia thalami, and the septum. (B) At E12.5 (as in Fig. 1), *Rmst* was detected in the medial wall of the telencephalon and in the diandephalon. (C) At E14.5, *Rmst* is still highly expressed in the cortical hem and hippocampus primordium, thalamus and hypothalamus. (D) At E16.5, *Rmst* expression is high in the hippocampus and fimbria but low in scattered cells of the migratory stream. Expression in the thalamus is maintained. (E) At post-natal stages P1, *Rmst* is restricted to the fimbria, yet expressed outside of the hippocampal formation to become virtually undetectable in the hippocampus of adult mice (F) (hippocampal staining is not considered specific to the *Rmst* probe). dm, dorso-medial wall of telencephalon; emT, eminentia thalami; Et, epithalamus; tel, telencephalon; v3, third ventricle; lv, lateral ventricle; Sp, septum; d, diencephalon; hp, hippocampus; ch, cortical hem; cp, choroid plexus; ncx, neocortex; LGE, lateral ganglionic eminences; th, thalamus, hy, hypothalamus; fm, fimbria; ms, migratory stream; CA1 and CA3, hippocampal fieds; DG, dentate gyrus. Scale bar 400 μm in panels A, C and D; 100 μm in panel B; 200 μm in panels E and F. (TIF 1931 kb)

**Additional file 2: Figure S2.** *Wnt3a* expression in mice with elevated beta-catenin. (A-B) *Wnt3a in situ* hybridization on control (A) and mutant (*Emx1::Cre;Ctnnb1lox(ex3)*) E12.5 coronal sections. Brackets highlight the cortical hem. ch, cortical hem; cp, choroid plexus. Scale bar 100 μm. (TIF 2822 kb)

**Additional file 3: Figure S3.** *miR-135a* bioinformatics analysis. A) Top pathways targeted by *miR-135a*. TGFβ/BMP and Wnt signaling pathways rank at position number 2 and 3 with high statistical significance. P values and number of genes targeted in each pathway are indicated. B) Overview of TGFβ/BMP cascade with highlighted, and listed, 16 genes targeted by *miR-135a*. It is worth noticing that the number of listed genes reflects only the data available on the Diana web site and the algorithm used for the search, as a higher number of putative *miR-135a* targets have already been reported using multiple search engines [11]. (TIF 1865 kb)

**Additional file 4: Figure S4.** *miR-135a* targets several mRNAs in the Wnt pathway. Schematic representation of *miR-135a* predicted targets in the Wnt signaling pathway, as generated by the Diana-miRPath software [52]. The 22 genes predicted to be *miR-135a* targets are highlighted and listed. As for the TGFβ/BMP pathway, the number of genes here listed reflects the data available on the Diana web site and the algorithm used for the search. (TIF 1741 kb)

**Additional file 5: Figure S5.** Quantification of *miR-135a* expression in *Emx1::Cre;mir-135a-2OE* mice. RT-qPCR showing a 1.5 fold change in *miR-135a* expression level in E12.5 dissected dorsal forebrain tissue from mutant mice compared to controls (*n* = 3). Data are shown as a fold change and have been normalized to microRNA *sno202*. ***, *p* value <0.001. (TIF 145 kb)

**Additional file 6: Figure S6.** Early *mir-135a-2* overexpression affects choroid plexus development. (A-B) Coronal sections of E12.5 control (*mir-135a2-OE*) and mutant brains (*Emx1::Cre;mir-135a-2OE*) showing expression of choroid plexus specific marker *rTtr1*. The dashed red line is used to highlight the change in choroid plexus complexity. cp, choroid plexus. Scale bar 100 μm. (TIF 2429 kb)

**Additional file 7: Figure S7.** Early *mir-135a-2* overexpression affects hippocampus development. (A-D) Coronal sections of post-natal stage P1 and adult brains processed for *ish* for *NeuroD2*. Panels A, B show overall morphology and size of the hippocampus. Asterisks point towards the pallium-subpallium boundary. Insets show the extent of the hippocampus from the CA1 field to the tip of the dentate gyrus, quantification of which, at mid and caudal level of the brain, is reported in panel E. Length is expressed in μm ± SEM (*n* = 4). Consistent with a reduced cortical hem size at embryonic stages, the hippocampus was significantly reduced in its extent in mutant brains with respect to controls. ***, *p* <0.001. Abbreviations: pSub, para subiculum; Sub, subiculum; DG, dentate gyrus; Cng, cingulate cortex. Scale bar 400 μm in panels A and B; 200 μm in panels C and D. (TIF 2162 kb)

**Additional file 8: Figure S8.** Expression of bioinformatically predicted *miR-135a* targets. (A-D) Coronal sections of E12.5 controls (*mir-135a-2OE*) and mutant (*Emx1::Cre;mir-135a2-OE*) brains, processed for immunohistochemistry (IHC) (A-B) or in situ hybridization (C, D). phospho-Smad (1/5/8) IHC on control (A) and mutant (B) brain coronal sections shows reduced signal in the cortical hem and the choroid plexus domains of mutants (arrowheads). Panels C and D show a reduced *Msx2* expression domain. ch, cortical hem; cp, choroid plexus. Scale bar 25 μm in panels A and B; 50 μm in panels C and D. (TIF 5061 kb)

**Additional file 9: Figure S9.** Late *mir-135a-2* overexpression does not overtly affect forebrain development. Coronal sections of E13.5 control (*mir-135a-2OE*) and mutant brains (*Nes::Cre;mir-135a-2OE*) processed for *in situ* hybridization for *Lmx1a*. Little to no change was observed in the cortical hem and neocortical domain (dashed lines) or in the choroid plexus. ch, cortical hem; cp, choroid plexus; ncx, neocortex. Scale bar 400 μm. (TIF 2507 kb)

**Additional file 10: Figure S10.** Little to no change in cortical hem of *Emx1::Cre;mir-135a-2OE;mir-135a-2+/-* mutant mice. (A-B) *ish* showing cortical hem marker *Wnt3a* in E12.5 control (*Emx1::Cre;mir-135a-2+/-*) (A) and mutant (*Emx1::Cre;mir-135a-2OE;mir-135a-2+/-*) (B) brains. ch, cortical hem. Scale bar 100 μm. (TIF 542 kb)

**Competing interests**
The authors declare that they have no competing interests.

**Authors' contributions**
GCB and RA conceived the experiments and wrote the manuscript; GCB performed the experiments and analyzed the data; AA generated *mir-135a-2* knockout, *mir-135a-2* overexpressor mice lines and the "sensor" construct to determine *miR-135a* activity. All authors read and approved the final manuscript.

**Acknowledgements**
We thank Makoto Taketo for *Ctnnb1^lox(ex3)* mouse line. Northwestern Transgenic and Targeted Mutagenesis Laboratory for pronuclear injections. We thank Profs. Elizabeth Grove and Shubha Tole for their feedback on the manuscript.

**Funding**
This work was supported by the Brain Research Foundation, the National Institute of Health (grant number 1R01NS071081-01) and National Institute of Neurological Disorder (grant number 1F31NS065670-01A2). The funders had no role in study design, data collection and analysis, decision to publish or preparation of the manuscript.

**References**
1. Lewis BP, Burge CB, Bartel DP. Conserved seed pairing, often flanked by adenosines, indicates that thousands of human genes are microRNA targets. Cell. 2005;120(1):15–20. doi:10.1016/j.cell.2004.12.035.
2. Fineberg SK, Kosik KS, Davidson BL. MicroRNAs potentiate neural development. Neuron. 2009;64(3):303–9. doi:10.1016/j.neuron.2009.10.020.
3. Yun B, Anderegg A, Menichella D, Wrabetz L, Feltri ML, Awatramani R. MicroRNA-deficient Schwann cells display congenital hypomyelination. J Neurosci. 2010;30(22):7722–8. doi:10.1523/JNEUROSCI.0876-10.2010. PubMed PMID: 20519547, PubMed Central PMCID: PMC2906453.
4. Chen JA, Huang YP, Mazzoni EO, Tan GC, Zavadil J, Wichterle H. Mir-17-3p controls spinal neural progenitor patterning by regulating Olig2/Irx3 cross-repressive loop. Neuron. 2011;69(4):721–35. doi:10.1016/j.neuron.2011.01.014. PubMed PMID: 21338882, PubMed Central PMCID: PMC3062262.
5. Haramati S, Chapnik E, Sztainberg Y, Eilam R, Zwang R, Gershoni N, et al. miRNA malfunction causes spinal motor neuron disease. Proc Natl Acad Sci U S A. 2010;107(29):13111–6. doi:10.1073/pnas.1006151107. PubMed PMID: 20616011, PubMed Central PMCID: PMC2919953.
6. Li X, Carthew RW. A microRNA mediates EGF receptor signaling and promotes photoreceptor differentiation in the Drosophila eye. Cell. 2005;123(7):1267–77. doi:10.1016/j.cell.2005.10.040.
7. Lin HP, Oksuz I, Hurley E, Wrabetz L, Awatramani R. Microprocessor complex subunit DiGeorge syndrome critical region gene 8 (Dgcr8) is required for schwann cell myelination and myelin maintenance. J Biol Chem. 2015; 290(40):24294–307. doi:10.1074/jbc.M115.636407. PubMed PMID: 26272614; PubMed Central PMCID: PMC4591815.
8. Nowakowski TJ, Mysiak KS, Pratt T, Price DJ. Functional dicer is necessary for appropriate specification of radial glia during early development of mouse telencephalon. PLoS One. 2011;6(8):e23013. doi:10.1371/journal.pone. 0023013. PubMed PMID: 21826226, PubMed Central PMCID: PMC3149632.
9. Kawase-Koga Y, Otaegi G, Sun T. Different timings of Dicer deletion affect neurogenesis and gliogenesis in the developing mouse central nervous system. Dev Dyn. 2009;238(11):2800–12. doi:10.1002/dvdy.22109. PubMed PMID: 19806666, PubMed Central PMCID: PMC2831750.
10. Davis TH, Cuellar TL, Koch SM, Barker AJ, Harfe BD, McManus MT, et al. Conditional loss of Dicer disrupts cellular and tissue morphogenesis in the cortex and hippocampus. J Neurosci. 2008;28(17):4322–30. doi:10.1523/JNEUROSCI.4815-07.2008.
11. Anderegg A, Lin HP, Chen JA, Caronia-Brown G, Cherepanova N, Yun B, et al. An Lmx1b-miR135a2 Regulatory Circuit Modulates Wnt1/Wnt Signaling and Determines the Size of the Midbrain Dopaminergic Progenitor Pool. PLoS Genet. 2013;9(12):e1003973. doi:10.1371/journal.pgen 1003973. PubMed PMID: 24348261, PubMed Central PMCID: PMC3861205.
12. Inui M, Montagner M, Piccolo S. miRNAs and morphogen gradients. Curr Opin Cell Biol. 2012;24(2):194–201. doi:10.1016/j.ceb.2011.11.013.
13. Inestrosa NC, Arenas E. Emerging roles of Wnts in the adult nervous system. Nat Rev Neurosci. 2010;11(2):77–86. doi:10.1038/nrn2755.
14. Chenn A, Walsh CA. Regulation of cerebral cortical size by control of cell cycle exit in neural precursors. Science. 2002;297(5580):365–9. doi:10.1126/science.1074192.
15. Megason SG, McMahon AP. A mitogen gradient of dorsal midline Wnts organizes growth in the CNS. Development. 2002;129(9):2087–98.
16. Lee SM, Tole S, Grove E, McMahon AP. A local Wnt-3a signal is required for development of the mammalian hippocampus. Development. 2000;127(3):457–67. Epub 2000/01/13.
17. McMahon AP, Joyner AL, Bradley A, McMahon JA. The midbrain-hindbrain phenotype of Wnt-1-/Wnt-1- mice results from stepwise deletion of engrailed-expressing cells by 9.5 days postcoitum. Cell. 1992;69(4):581–95.
18. Machon O, Backman M, Machonova O, Kozmik Z, Vacik T, Andersen L, et al. A dynamic gradient of Wnt signaling controls initiation of neurogenesis in the mammalian cortex and cellular specification in the hippocampus. Dev Biol. 2007;311(1):223–37. doi:10.1016/j.ydbio.2007.08.038.
19. Tang M, Villaescusa JC, Luo SX, Guitarte C, Lei S, Miyamoto Y, et al. Interactions of Wnt/beta-catenin signaling and sonic hedgehog regulate the neurogenesis of ventral midbrain dopamine neurons. J Neurosci. 2010;30(27):9280–91. doi:10.1523/JNEUROSCI.0860-10.2010. PubMed PMID: 20610763, PubMed Central PMCID: PMC3578394.

20. Galceran J, Farinas I, Depew MJ, Clevers H, Grosschedl R. Wnt3a-/–like phenotype and limb deficiency in Lef1(-/-)Tcf1(-/-) mice. Genes Dev. 1999;13(6):709–17. PubMed PMID: 10090727, PubMed Central PMCID: PMC316557, Epub 1999/03/25.

21. Woodhead GJ, Mutch CA, Olson EC, Chenn A. Cell-autonomous beta-catenin signaling regulates cortical precursor proliferation. J Neurosci. 2006;26(48): 12620–30. doi:10.1523/JNEUROSCI.3180-06.2006. PubMed PMID: 17135424, PubMed Central PMCID: PMC2867669.

22. Joksimovic M, Yun BA, Kittappa R, Anderegg AM, Chang WW, Taketo MM, et al. Wnt antagonism of Shh facilitates midbrain floor plate neurogenesis. Nat Neurosci. 2009;12(2):125–31. doi:10.1038/nn.2243. Epub 2009/01/06.

23. Joksimovic M, Awatramani R. Wnt/beta-catenin signaling in midbrain dopaminergic neuron specification and neurogenesis. J Mol Cell Biol. 2014. doi:10.1093/jmcb/mjt043.

24. Nouri N, Patel MJ, Joksimovic M, Poulin JF, Anderegg A, Taketo MM, et al. Excessive Wnt/beta-catenin signaling promotes midbrain floor plate neurogenesis, but results in vacillating dopamine progenitors. Mol Cell Neurosci. 2015;68:131–42. doi:10.1016/j.mcn.2015.07.002. PubMed PMID: 26164566; PubMed Central PMCID: PMCPMC4633300.

25. Furuta Y, Piston DW, Hogan BL. Bone morphogenetic proteins (BMPs) as regulators of dorsal forebrain development. Development. 1997;124(11):2203–12.

26. Liem Jr KF, Tremml G, Jessell TM. A role for the roof plate and its resident TGFbeta-related proteins in neuronal patterning in the dorsal spinal cord. Cell. 1997;91(1):127–38. Epub 1997/10/23 22:32.

27. Augsburger A, Schuchardt A, Hoskins S, Dodd J, Butler S. BMPs as mediators of roof plate repulsion of commissural neurons. Neuron. 1999;24(1):127–41. Epub 2000/02/17.

28. Samanta J, Burke GM, McGuire T, Pisarek AJ, Mukhopadhyay A, Mishina Y, et al. BMPR1a signaling determines numbers of oligodendrocytes and calbindin-expressing interneurons in the cortex. J Neurosci. 2007;27(28):7397–407.

29. Hebert JM, Mishina Y, McConnell SK. BMP signaling is required locally to pattern the dorsal telencephalic midline. Neuron. 2002;35(6):1029–41. Epub 2002/10/02.

30. See J, Mamontov P, Ahn K, Wine-Lee L, Crenshaw 3rd EB, Grinspan JB. BMP signaling mutant mice exhibit glial cell maturation defects. Mol Cell Neurosci. 2007;35(1):171–82.

31. Choe Y, Kozlova A, Graf D, Pleasure SJ. Bone morphogenic protein signaling is a major determinant of dentate development. J Neurosci. 2013;33(16):6766–75. doi:10.1523/JNEUROSCI.0128-13.2013. PubMed PMID: 23595735, PubMed Central PMCID: PMC3684166.

32. Doan LT, Javier AL, Furr NM, Nguyen KL, Cho KW, Monuki ES. A Bmp reporter with ultrasensitive characteristics reveals that high Bmp signaling is not required for cortical hem fate. PLoS One. 2012;7(9):e44009. doi:10.1371/journal.pone.0044009. PubMed PMID: 22984456, PubMed Central PMCID: PMC3439469.

33. Hu JS, Doan LT, Currle DS, Paff M, Rheem JY, Schreyer R, et al. Border formation in a Bmp gradient reduced to single dissociated cells. Proc Natl Acad Sci U S A. 2008;105(9):3398–403. doi:10.1073/pnas.0709100105. PubMed PMID: 18292231, PubMed Central PMCID: PMC2265170.

34. Itasaki N, Hoppler S. Crosstalk between Wnt and bone morphogenic protein signaling: a turbulent relationship. Dev Dyn. 2010;239(1):16–33. doi:10.1002/dvdy.22009.

35. Subramanian L, Remedios R, Shetty A, Tole S. Signals from the edges: the cortical hem and antihem in telencephalic development. Semin Cell Dev Biol. 2009;20(6):712–8. doi:10.1016/j.semcdb.2009.04.001. Epub 2009/05/19. PubMed PMID: 19446478; PubMed Central PMCID: PMC2791850.

36. Grove EA, Tole S, Limon J, Yip L, Ragsdale CW. The hem of the embryonic cerebral cortex is defined by the expression of multiple Wnt genes and is compromised in Gli3-deficient mice. Development. 1998;125(12):2315–25.

37. Monuki ES, Porter FD, Walsh CA. Patterning of the dorsal telencephalon and cerebral cortex by a roof plate-Lhx2 pathway. Neuron. 2001;32(4):591–604. Epub 2001/11/24 doi: S0896-6273(01)00504-9 [pii].

38. Tole S, Grove EA. Detailed field pattern is intrinsic to the embryonic mouse hippocampus early in neurogenesis. J Neurosci. 2001;21(5):1580–9. Epub 2001/02/27.

39. Mangale VS, Hirokawa KE, Satyaki PR, Gokulchandran N, Chikbire S, Subramanian L, et al. Lhx2 selector activity specifies cortical identity and suppresses hippocampal organizer fate. Science. 2008;319(5861):304–9. doi:10.1126/science.1151695. PubMed PMID: 18202285, PubMed Central PMCID: PMC2494603.

40. Zhou CJ, Zhao C, Pleasure SJ. Wnt signaling mutants have decreased dentate granule cell production and radial glial scaffolding abnormalities.

41. J Neurosci. 2004;24(1):121–6. doi:10.1523/JNEUROSCI.4071-03.2004. Epub 2004/01/13. PubMed PMID: 14715945.

41. Grove EA, Tole S. Patterning events and specification signals in the developing hippocampus. Cereb Cortex. 1999;9(6):551–61. Epub 1999/09/25.

42. Caronia G, Wilcoxon J, Feldman P, Grove EA. Bone morphogenetic protein signaling in the developing telencephalon controls formation of the hippocampal dentate gyrus and modifies fear-related behavior. J Neurosci. 2010;30(18):6291–301. doi:10.1523/JNEUROSCI.0550-10.2010. Epub 2010/05/07.

43. Yoshida M, Assimacopoulos S, Jones KR, Grove EA. Massive loss of Cajal-Retzius cells does not disrupt neocortical layer order. Development. 2006;133(3):537–45. doi:10.1242/dev.02209.

44. Caronia-Brown G, Yoshida M, Gulden F, Assimacopoulos S, Grove EA. The cortical hem regulates the size and patterning of neocortex. Development. 2014;141(14):2855–65. doi:10.1242/dev.106914.

45. Harada N, Tamai Y, Ishikawa T, Sauer B, Takaku K, Oshima M, et al. Intestinal polyposis in mice with a dominant stable mutation of the beta-catenin gene. EMBO J. 1999;18(21):5931–42. doi:10.1093/emboj/18.21.5931. PubMed PMID: 10545105, PubMed Central PMCID: PMC1171659.

46. Brault V, Moore R, Kutsch S, Ishibashi M, Rowitch DH, McMahon AP, et al. Inactivation of the beta-catenin gene by Wnt1-Cre-mediated deletion results in dramatic brain malformation and failure of craniofacial development. Development. 2001;128(8):1253–64.

47. Gorski JA, Talley T, Qiu M, Puelles L, Rubenstein JL, Jones KR. Cortical excitatory neurons and glia, but not GABAergic neurons, are produced in the Emx1-expressing lineage. J Neurosci. 2002;22(15):6309–14. doi: 20026564.

48. Park CY, Jeker LT, Carver-Moore K, Oh A, Liu HJ, Cameron R, et al. A resource for the conditional ablation of microRNAs in the mouse. Cell Reports. 2012;1(4):385–91. doi:10.1016/j.celrep.2012.02.008. PubMed PMID: 22570807, PubMed Central PMCID: PMC3345170.

49. Awatramani R, Soriano P, Rodriguez C, Mai JJ, Dymecki SM. Cryptic boundaries in roof plate and choroid plexus identified by intersectional gene activation. Nat Genet. 2003;35(1):70–5. doi:10.1038/ng1228.

50. Tronche F, Kellendonk C, Kretz O, Gass P, Anlag K, Orban PC, et al. Disruption of the glucocorticoid receptor gene in the nervous system results in reduced anxiety. Nat Genet. 1999;23(1):99–103. doi:10.1038/12703.

51. Schmittgen TD, Livak KJ. Analyzing real-time PCR data by the comparative C(T) method. Nat Protoc. 2008;3(6):1101–8.

52. Vlachos IS, Kostoulas N, Vergoulis T, Georgakilas G, Reczko M, Maragkakis M, et al. DIANA miRPath v.2.0: investigating the combinatorial effect of microRNAs in pathways. Nucleic Acids Res. 2012;40(Web Server issue): W498–504. doi:10.1093/nar/gks494. PubMed PMID: 22649059; PubMed Central PMCID: PMC3394305.

53. Uhde CW, Vives J, Jaeger I, Li M. Rmst is a novel marker for the mouse ventral mesencephalic floor plate and the anterior dorsal midline cells. PLoS One. 2010;5(1):e8641. doi:10.1371/journal.pone.0008641. PubMed PMID: 20062813, PubMed Central PMCID: PMC2799666.

54. Backman M, Machon O, Mygland L, van den Bout CJ, Zhong W, Taketo MM, et al. Effects of canonical Wnt signaling on dorso-ventral specification of the mouse telencephalon. Dev Biol. 2005;279(1):155–68. doi:10.1016/j.ydbio.2004.12.010. Epub 2005/02/15.

55. Kim AS, Lowenstein DH, Pleasure SJ. Wnt receptors and Wnt inhibitors are expressed in gradients in the developing telencephalon. Mech Dev. 2001;103(1-2):167–72. Epub 2001/05/04.

56. Bulchand S, Grove EA, Porter FD, Tole S. LIM-homeodomain gene Lhx2 regulates the formation of the cortical hem. Mech Dev. 2001;100(2):165–75.

57. Willert J, Epping M, Pollack JR, Brown PO, Nusse R. A transcriptional response to Wnt protein in human embryonic carcinoma cells. BMC Dev Biol. 2002;2:8. PubMed PMID: 12095419, PubMed Central PMCID: PMC117803.

58. Chizhikov VV, Lindgren AG, Mishima Y, Roberts RW, Aldinger KA, Miesegaes GR, et al. Lmx1a regulates fates and location of cells originating from the cerebellar rhombic lip and telencephalic cortical hem. Proc Natl Acad Sci U S A. 2010;107(23):10725–30. doi:10.1073/pnas.0910786107. Epub 2010/05/26. PubMed PMID: 20498066; PubMed Central PMCID: PMC2890798.

59. Quan M, Chen J, Zhang D. Exploring the secrets of long noncoding RNAs. Int J Mol Sci. 2015;16(3):5467–96. doi:10.3390/ijms16035467. PubMed PMID: 25764159; PubMed Central PMCID: PMCPMC4394487.

60. Tan JY, Sirey T, Honti F, Graham B, Piovesan A, Merkenschlager M, et al. Corrigendum: Extensive microRNA-mediated crosstalk between lncRNAs and mRNAs in mouse embryonic stem cells. Genome Res. 2015;25(9):1410.1. PubMed PMID: 26330573; PubMed Central PMCID: PMCPMC4561499.

61. Jalali S, Bhartiya D, Lalwani MK, Sivasubbu S, Scaria V. Systematic transcriptome wide analysis of lncRNA-miRNA interactions. PLoS One. 2013;8(2):e53823. doi:10.1371/journal.pone.0053823. PubMed PMID: 23405074; PubMed Central PMCID: PMCPMC3566149.

62. Jeggari A, Marks DS, Larsson E. miRcode: a map of putative microRNA target sites in the long non-coding transcriptome. Bioinformatics. 2012;28(15):2062–3. doi:10.1093/bioinformatics/bts344. PubMed PMID: 22718787; PubMed Central PMCID: PMCPMC3400968.

63. Fischer S, Handrick R, Aschrafi A, Otte K. Unveiling the principle of microRNA-mediated redundancy in cellular pathway regulation. RNA Biol. 2015;12(3):238–47. doi:10.1080/15476286.2015.1017238.

64. Mendell JT, Olson EN. MicroRNAs in stress signaling and human disease. Cell. 2012;148(6):1172–87. doi:10.1016/j.cell.2012.02.005. PubMed PMID: 22424228, PubMed Central PMCID: PMC3308137.

65. Caronia-Brown G, Grove EA. Timing of Cortical Interneuron Migration Is Influenced by the Cortical Hem. Cereb Cortex. 2010. doi:10.1093/cercor/bhq142. Epub 2010/08/18.

66. Galceran J, Miyashita-Lin EM, Devaney E, Rubenstein JL, Grosschedl R. Hippocampus development and generation of dentate gyrus granule cells is regulated by LEF1. Development. 2000;127(3):469–82. Epub 2000/01/13.

67. Qiu L, Rivera-Perez JA, Xu Z. A non-specific effect associated with conditional transgene expression based on Cre-loxP strategy in mice. PLoS One. 2011;6(5):e18778. doi:10.1371/journal.pone.0018778. PubMed PMID: 21572998, PubMed Central PMCID: PMC3091857.

68. Hodge RD, Garcia III AJ, Elsen GE, Nelson BR, Mussar KE, Reiner SL, et al. Tbr2 expression in Cajal-Retzius cells and intermediate neuronal progenitors is required for morphogenesis of the dentate gyrus. J Neurosci. 2013;33(9): 4165–80. doi:10.1523/JNEUROSCI.4185-12.2013. PubMed PMID: 23447624; PubMed Central PMCID: PMCPMC3623668.

69. Konno D, Iwashita M, Satoh Y, Momiyama A, Abe T, Kiyonari H, et al. The mammalian DM domain transcription factor Dmrta2 is required for early embryonic development of the cerebral cortex. PLoS One. 2012;7(10):e46577. doi:10.1371/journal.pone.0046577. PubMed PMID: 23056351; PubMed Central PMCID: PMCPMC3462758.

70. Li Q, Bian S, Hong J, Kawase-Koga Y, Zhu E, Zheng Y, et al. Timing specific requirement of microRNA function is essential for embryonic and postnatal hippocampal development. PLoS One. 2011;6(10):e26000. doi:10.1371/journal.pone.0026000. PubMed PMID: 21991391; PubMed Central PMCID: PMCPMC3186801.

71. Lavado A, He Y, Pare J, Neale G, Olson EN, Giovannini M, et al. Tumor suppressor Nf2 limits expansion of the neural progenitor pool by inhibiting Yap/Taz transcriptional coactivators. Development. 2013;140(16):3323–34. doi:10.1242/dev.096537. PubMed PMID: 23863479; PubMed Central PMCID: PMCPMC3737715.

72. Shi Y, Zhao X, Hsieh J, Wichterle H, Impey S, Banerjee S, et al. MicroRNA regulation of neural stem cells and neurogenesis. J Neurosci. 2010;30(45):14931–6. doi:10.1523/JNEUROSCI.4280-10.2010. PubMed PMID: 21068294, PubMed Central PMCID: PMC3071711.

73. Johnson MB, Wang PP, Atabay KD, Murphy EA, Doan RN, Hecht JL, et al. Single-cell analysis reveals transcriptional heterogeneity of neural progenitors in human cortex. Nat Neurosci. 2015;18(5):637–46. doi:10.1038/nn.3980.

74. Nagel R, le Sage C, Diosdado B, van der Waal M, Oude Vrielink JA, Bolijn A, et al. Regulation of the adenomatous polyposis coli gene by the miR-135 family in colorectal cancer. Cancer Res. 2008;68(14):5795–802. doi:10.1158/0008-5472.CAN-08-0951.

75. Leung CO, Deng W, Ye TM, Ngan HY, Tsao SW, Cheung AN, et al. miR-135a leads to cervical cancer cell transformation through regulation of beta-catenin via a SIAH1-dependent ubiquitin proteosomal pathway. Carcinogenesis. 2014;35(9):1931–40. doi:10.1093/carcin/bgu032.

76. Gokhale A, Kunder R, Goel A, Sarin R, Moiyadi A, Shenoy A, et al. Distinctive microRNA signature of medulloblastomas associated with the WNT signaling pathway. J Cancer Res Ther. 2010;6(4):521–9. doi:10.4103/0973-1482.77072.

77. Chen C, Peng Y, Peng Y, Peng J, Jiang S. miR-135a-5p inhibits 3T3-L1 adipogenesis through activation of canonical Wnt/beta-catenin signaling. J Mol Endocrinol. 2014;52(3):311–20. doi:10.1530/JME-14-0013.

78. Yang X, Wang X, Nie F, Liu T, Yu X, Wang H, et al. miR-135 family members mediate podocyte injury through the activation of Wnt/beta-catenin signaling. Int J Mol Med. 2015;36(3):669–77. doi:10.3892/ijmm.2015.2259. PubMed PMID: 26134897; PubMed Central PMCID: PMCPMC4533775.

79. Krutzfeldt J, Rajewsky N, Braich R, Rajeev KG, Tuschl T, Manoharan M, et al. Silencing of microRNAs in vivo with 'antagomirs'. Nature. 2005;438(7068):685–9. doi:10.1038/nature04303.

80. Ebert MS, Sharp PA. MicroRNA sponges: progress and possibilities. RNA. 2010;16(11):2043–50. doi:10.1261/rna.2414110. PubMed PMID: 20855538, PubMed Central PMCID: PMC2957044.

81. Park CY, Choi YS, McManus MT. Analysis of microRNA knockouts in mice. Hum Mol Genet. 2010;19(R2):R169–75. doi:10.1093/hmg/ddq367. PubMed PMID: 20805106, PubMed Central PMCID: PMC2981466.

82. Bertero T, Grosso S, Robbe-Sermesant K, Lebrigand K, Henaoui IS, Puissegur MP, et al. "Seed-Milarity" confers to hsa-miR-210 and hsa-miR-147b similar functional activity. PLoS One. 2012;7(9):e44919. doi:10.1371/journal.pone.0044919. PubMed PMID: 23028679; PubMed Central PMCID: PMC3441733.

83. Clevers H, Nusse R. Wnt/beta-catenin signaling and disease. Cell. 2012; 149(6):1192–205. doi:10.1016/j.cell.2012.05.012.

84. Chung S, Leung A, Han BS, Chang MY, Moon JI, Kim CH, et al. Wnt1-lmx1a forms a novel autoregulatory loop and controls midbrain dopaminergic differentiation synergistically with the SHH-FoxA2 pathway. Cell Stem Cell. 2009;5(6):646–58. doi:10.1016/j.stem.2009.09.015. PubMed PMID: 19951692, PubMed Central PMCID: PMC2788512.

85. Hoekstra EJ, von Oerthel L, van der Heide LP, Kouwenhoven WM, Veenvliet JV, Wever I, et al. Lmx1a encodes a rostral set of mesodiencephalic dopaminergic neurons marked by the Wnt/B-catenin signaling activator R-spondin 2. PLoS One. 2013;8(9):e74049. doi:10.1371/journal.pone.0074049. PubMed PMID: 24066094, PubMed Central PMCID: PMC3774790.

# 7

# Monocular enucleation alters retinal waves in the surviving eye

Samuel Wilson Failor[1,4*], Arash Ng[1] and Hwai-Jong Cheng[1,2,3*]

## Abstract

**Background:** Activity in neurons drives afferent competition that is critical for the refinement of nascent neural circuits. In ferrets, when an eye is lost in early development, surviving retinogeniculate afferents from the spared eye spread across the thalamus in a manner that is dependent on spontaneous retinal activity. However, how this spontaneous activity, also known as retinal waves, might dynamically regulate afferent terminal targeting remains unknown.

**Methods:** We recorded retinal waves from retinae ex vivo using multi-electrode arrays. Retinae came from ferrets who were binocular or who had one eye surgically removed at birth. Linear mixed effects models were used to investigate the effects of early monocular enucleation on retinal wave activity.

**Results:** When an eye is removed at birth, spontaneous bursts of action potentials by retinal ganglion cells (RGCs) in the surviving eye are shorter in duration. The shortening of RGC burst duration results in decreased pairwise RGC correlations across the retina and is associated with the retinal wave-dependent spread of retinogeniculate afferents previously reported in enucleates.

**Conclusion:** Our findings show that removal of the competing eye modulates retinal waves and could underlie the dynamic regulation of competition-based refinement during retinogeniculate development.

## Background

Developing nascent neural circuitry undergoes modifications in an activity-dependent manner [1–6]. Neural activity that is essential for early stages of visual system development originates from spontaneous processes [1, 4–6] and appears to facilitate circuit refinement by driving Hebbian-like competition for synaptic partners between innervating neurons [7–9]. This activity-dependent refinement results in the precise mapping of sensory areas, for example by establishing eye-specific laminae and fine-scale retinotopy across visual areas [1, 4].

Patterned spontaneous retinal activity (i.e. retinal waves) occurs primarily during periods of functional blindness [10–13] and is characterized by periodically occurring domains of retinal ganglion cell (RGC) activity that slowly propagate across the retina in a wave-like fashion. This spatiotemporal feature of retinal waves leads to a high level of correlated activity between neighboring RGCs and very little correlated activity between RGCs that are distant from each other. Retinal waves have been shown to play a critical role in the establishment of eye-specific laminae in the dorsal lateral geniculate nucleus (dLGN) [7, 8, 14–20], as well as fine-scale retinotopy [8, 21] and receptive field size [8, 22, 23] in the dLGN and superior colliculus. For example, when an eye is lost early in development, retinogeniculate afferents from the surviving eye spread across the dLGN in a retinal wave-dependent manner [8]. This study demonstrated that retinal waves drive both inter-eye [7] and intra-eye competition for synaptic space in the dLGN. However, it remains unclear how retinal waves might facilitate retinogeniculate expansion. One possibility is that the loss of the competing eye alters retinal waves to guide this process.

Here we show that in ferrets when we surgically remove a competing eye, retinal waves in the surviving eye were altered. Primarily, retinal wave associated bursts of action potentials by retinal ganglion cells in the surviving eye were shorter as were the number of spikes

---

* Correspondence: s.failor@ucl.ac.uk; hjcheng@ucdavis.edu
[1]Center for Neuroscience, University of California, Davis, 1544 Newton Court, Davis, CA 95618, USA
Full list of author information is available at the end of the article

contained in these bursts. The shortening of bursts also decreased levels of pairwise RGC correlation. Thus, a significant reduction in levels of correlated RGC activity during retinal waves is associated with removal of the competing eye.

Based on these data, we propose a model where the presence of the competing eye reduces intra-eye competition for synaptic space in the dLGN by increasing correlated RGC activity, which facilitates the formation of eye-specific laminae during inter-eye competition. Conversely, the absence of the competing eye promotes the expansion of retinogeniculate laminae by reducing pairwise RGC correlations and increasing intra-eye competition. In this way, adjustments to the duration of RGC bursts during retinal waves could dynamically optimise competition-based retinogeniculate refinement during the establishment of eye-specific laminae.

## Methods
### Animals
Time-pregnant fitch-coat ferrets were received at mid to late gestation, giving birth 2–3 weeks later (Marshall BioResources, NY, USA; RRID:SCR_015489). Food and water were provided ad libitum. All procedures were authorized by the University of California, Davis (RRID:SCR_012713) Institutional Animal Care and Use Committee (IACUC) and performed in accordance with national and international standards for humane animal research as set forth by the National Institutes of Health (RRID:SCR_011417), Institute of Laboratory Animal Research (RRID:SCR_006872), USDA (RRID:SCR_011486), and Assessment and Accreditation of Laboratory Animal Care, International (RRID:SCR_015496).

### Monocular enucleation
Neonatal ferrets of either sex were anesthetized with isoflurane at P1. After topical lidocaine was applied, the eyelids of one eye were separated, and the muscles and connective tissue of the eyeball were blunt dissected. Hemostats were used to clamp the optic nerve after which it was severed and the eyeball removed. Antibiotic ointment was applied to the orbit, and sterile gelfoam was inserted to stem any subsequent bleeding. A liquid suture was applied to seal the eyelids. Before the animal fully awakened a single dose of buprenex was administered intramuscularly (0.02 mg/kg) as a postoperative analgesic. The monocular enucleation procedure typically took under 5 min. Age-matched littermates served as controls.

### Multielectrode array recordings
Ferrets were euthanized with a lethal dose of pentobarbital (0.1–0.2 ml) via an inter-peritoneal injection. An eye was enucleated, and the retina was removed and stored in ice-cold buffered and oxygenated media (M7278, Sigma-Aldrich, USA; RRID:SCR_008988). A piece of the retina was placed RGC side down onto a 60-channel MEA (MEA2100 System, Multi-Channel Systems, Germany; RRID:SCR_014809), and held in place with a piece of dialysis membrane (Spectrapore 132,130, Spectrum Labs, USA; RRID:SCR_015488). The tissue was superfused with buffered media at 1–2 ml/min at 34 or 37 °C. The array electrodes were 30 μm in diameter and arranged in an 8 × 8 rectilinear grid with an interelectrode spacing of 200 μm. At this distance, the signal for a given cell appeared on only one electrode, so each isolated cell was assigned the spatial coordinates of the electrode on which it was recorded. Analog data were acquired at 20 kHz per channel simultaneously from each electrode. After the retina had been placed on the MEA, the tissue was allowed to acclimate for at least 45 min. When retinal waves appeared stable, recordings were performed for 20 min.

### Spike identification
Raw data were digitally filtered with a 125-Hz high-pass filter (four-pole Butterworth) for sorting spike events. A threshold of six STD was set for each channel and 1 ms of data before, and 4 ms after a threshold-crossing event were stored for each negative-slope event. These candidate spike waveforms were then sorted with Offline Sorter (Plexon, USA; RRID:SCR_000012) using the first three principal components of the spike waveforms. Coincident events within 0.5 ms of each other that were detected on at least 90% of the channels were attributed to perfusion noise and removed. Clusters were first identified using an EM cluster algorithm [24] then manually edited for clustering errors. Typically, each electrode recorded the activity of one to three cells.

### Analysis of RGC burst properties
RGC bursts were identified as previously described [25]. All burst analyses were carried out using custom scripts written in Matlab (Mathworks, USA; RRID:SCR_001622). The beginning of a burst was defined as the point in an RGC spike train when the inter-spike interval (ISI) was less than 0.1 s. Subsequent spikes with ISIs less than 1 s were included in the burst, whereas an ISI of greater than 1 s denoted the end of the burst. If two bursts occurred within 5 s of each other, they were merged.

The properties of bursts identified by this algorithm were then averaged for each cell. Firing rate, burst duration, the number of spikes within a burst, the percentage of spikes within bursts, burst frequency, burst ISI, the percentage of burst time above 10 spikes/s, the percentage of bursts in waves, and bursts per wave were all quantified.

### Analysis of wave properties
Retinal waves were identified in a similar way to that previously described [26]. All wave analyses were carried out using custom scripts written in Matlab (Mathworks, USA;

RRID:SCR_001622). MEA recordings were divided into 1 s time bins. The beginning of a retinal wave was defined as the time bin when greater than 5% of all cells were bursting and considered over when less than 2.5% were bursting.

The position of a wave over time was the center of mass of the cells participating in the wave in each time bin. Wave speed was defined as the average change in wave position over time. Wave spread was defined as the average percentage of new electrodes that detected bursting cells in each time bin. Waves that lasted for less than 3 s were not included in analyses of wave speed or spread.

The size of a wave was defined as the average percentage of electrodes that detected bursting cells across the duration of a wave.

## Correlation analysis

Correlation analyses were carried out using custom scripts written in Matlab (Mathworks, USA; RRID:SCR_001622). Pairwise correlations between RGC spike trains were measured by calculating the spike time tiling coefficient [27] (STTC), which is bounded and insensitive to firing rate. STTC is defined as

$$STTC = \frac{1}{2} \left( \frac{P_A - T_B}{1 - P_a T_B} + \frac{P_B - T_A}{1 - P_B T_A} \right)$$

where $T_A$ is the total recording time that lies within $\pm \Delta t$ of any spike from cell A. $T_B$ is calculated similarly for cell B. $P_A$ is the proportion of spikes from cell A which lie within $\pm \Delta t$ of any spike from cell B. $P_B$ is calculated similarly for cell B. For our calculations $\Delta t$ was defined as 0.1 s. STTC is 1 with autocorrelation and $-1$ when $P_A = 0$ and $T_B = 1$.

## Statistical analysis

All statistical analyses were carried out in Matlab (Mathworks, USA; RRID:SCR_001622). The sample sizes required for this study were estimated based on previous studies [22, 26]. For descriptive statistics, we used mean ± STD, or mean ± SEM where indicated. For box plots, the height of the boxes extended between the 25th and the 75th percentiles of the data. The horizontal bar and cross mark signified the median and mean, respectively. For plotting, outliers were defined as data points 1.5 times higher than or 1.5 times lower than the interquartile range and were shown as circles. The box plot whiskers extended to the most extreme data points that were not considered outliers. Outliers were not excluded from analyses. We considered $P$ values less than 0.05 as significant. Significance values for comparisons of burst property means were calculated by fitting hierarchical linear mixed-effects models to cell data where the condition (monocular or binocular) and recording temperature (34 or 37 °C) were the fixed-effects, and recording/retina was the random-effect

to correct for the non-independence of recorded cells. Significance values for comparisons of wave properties were also calculated by fitting linear mixed effects models as described above, except when comparing wave frequencies where the model only included terms for condition and temperature. In cases where samples were lognormal, we carried out a log transformation to bring samples to a normal distribution. In other cases, sample distributions had downward skews and were transformed with the exponential function. Comparing STTC values between enucleation conditions was similarly carried out using a hierarchical linear-mixed effects model where condition and temperature were fixed-effects, RGC pair distance was a covariate, and recording/retina was a random effect. STTC values were averaged for all RGC pairs by distance for each retina, resulting in a single value for each unique RGC pair distance. Before fitting the model, distance values were log transformed to improve linearity as shown in Fig. 6. All figures display data in their transformed state.

## Results

### Monocular enucleation has multiple effects on retinal waves

To investigate changes in the properties of retinal waves following the removal of a competing eye, we surgically removed one eye from newborn ferrets 1 day after birth (P1). Retinae were dissected away from the eyes of binocular and monocular ferrets between P5 and P6 and placed RGC layer side down on a 60-channel multielectrode array to record retinal wave activity ex vivo (Fig. 1a). We chose this time point as it has been previously shown that the expansion of the ipsilateral projection is retinal wave-dependent between P5 and P10 [8].

The waves recorded from the retinae of monocular and binocular ferrets appeared at first glance to be qualitatively similar (Fig. 1b). However, with further analysis, it was found that retinal waves were notably different in several ways following early monocular enucleation. The largest and most significant effects observed were those on RGC burst duration and the number of spikes within a burst (Fig. 1d-e). Compared to retinae from binocular ferrets, those from enucleates had RGCs whose bursts of action potentials were approximately 30% shorter in duration (binocular, 2.39 ± 1.32 s; monocular, 1.67 ± 0.99 s; mean ± STD; binocular, $N = 1178$ cells, 13 retinae; monocular, $N = 1001$ cells, 11 retinae; $T(2168) = 4.91$, $P = 9.9609 \times 10^{-7}$, linear mixed-effects model with log transformation) (Fig. 1d). The reduction in burst duration was for the most part consistent across retinae recorded at temperatures of either 34 °C (binocular, 2.76 ± 1.42; monocular, 1.82 ± 0.91; mean ± STD; binocular, $N = 731$, 7 retinae; monocular, $N = 592$, 6 retinae; $T(1317) = 3.90$, $P = 9.952 \times 10^{-5}$, linear mixed-effects model with log transformation) or 37 °C (binocular, 1.79 ± 0.83; monocular, 1.46 ± 1.07; mean ± STD; binocular, $N = 447$, 6 retinae; monocular, $N = 409$, 5 retinae; $T(850) = 3.37$, $P = 0.00078$, linear

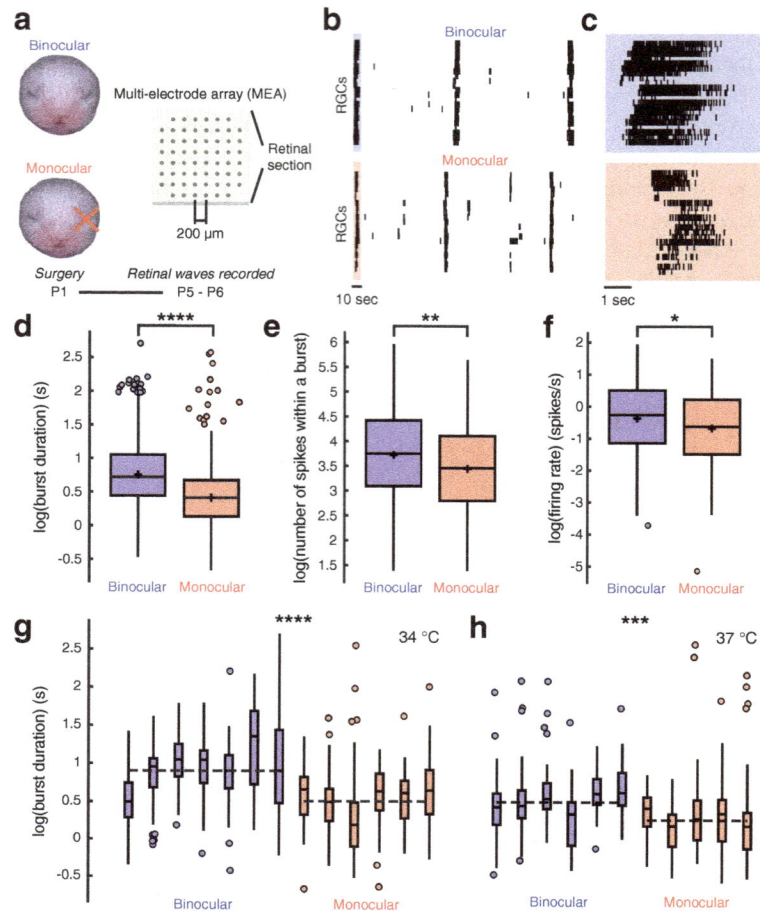

**Fig. 1** Effects of removing inter-eye competition on RGC activity. **a** An illustration of the enucleation protocol and MEA used for recording retinal waves. **b** Raster plots of wave activity from the retina of a binocular (**top**) and a monocular (**bottom**) ferret. **c** The RGC activity from highlighted periods shown in **b** on a finer time scale. **d-f**) Plots showing the difference in burst duration (s) (binocular, 2.39 ± 1.32; monocular, 1.67 ± 0.99; mean ± STD; T(2168) = 4.91, P = 9.9609 × 10⁻⁷, linear mixed-effects model with log transformation) (**d**), number of spikes within a burst (binocular, 60.16 ± 53.26; monocular, 44.87 ± 39.82; mean ± STD; T(2168) = 2.92, P = 0.0036, linear mixed-effects model with log transformation) (**e**), and firing rate (spikes/s) (binocular, 1.19 ± 1.19; monocular, 0.86 ± 0.84; mean ± STD; T(2176) = 2.49, P = 0.0128, linear mixed-effects model with log transformation) (**f**), between RGCs from retinae of binocular or monocular ferrets. **g - h** Plots of RGC burst duration for all retinae recorded at a temperature of 34 °C (binocular, 2.76 ± 1.42; monocular, 1.82 ± 0.91; mean ± STD; T(1317) = 3.90, P = 9.952 × 10⁻⁵, linear mixed-effects model with log transformation) (**g**) and 37 °C (binocular, 1.79 ± 0.83; monocular, 1.46 ± 1.07; mean ± STD; T(850) = 3.37, P = 0.00077, linear mixed-effects model with log transformation) (**h**). Dashed lines indicate group means. The heights of the box plots extend between the 25th and the 75th percentiles of the data. The horizontal bar and cross mark indicate the median and mean, respectively. Outliers are shown as circles and are data points that are 1.5 times higher than or 1.5 times lower than the interquartile range. The box plot whiskers extend to the most extreme data points that are not outliers. Binocular, N = 1178 cells, 13 retinae; Monocular, N = 1001 cells, 11 retinae. * = P < 0.05, ** = P < 0.01, *** = P < 0.001, **** = P < 0.0001

mixed-effects model with log transformation) (Fig. g-h). The impact on burst duration due to enucleation lead to the number of spikes within a burst to be reduced by approximately 25% (binocular, 60.16 ± 53.26; monocular, 44.87 ± 39.82; mean ± STD; binocular, N = 1178 cells, 13 retinae; monocular, N = 1001 cells, 11 retinae; T(2168) = 2.92, P = 0.00357, linear mixed-effects model with log transformation) (Fig. 1e). As expected, given that fewer spikes were contained within bursts, the overall firing rate of RGCs was reduced with enucleation (binocular, 1.19 ± 1.19 spikes/s; monocular, 0.86 ± 0.84 spikes/s; mean ± STD; binocular,

N = 1178 cells, 13 retinae; monocular, N = 1001 cells, 11 retinae; T(2176) = 2.49, P = 0.0128, linear mixed-effects model with log transformation) (Fig. 1f).

In most other ways retinal waves were generally unaffected by monocular enucleation. Bursts occurred at the same frequency in both conditions (binocular, 1.02 ± 0.56; monocular, 0.96 ± 0.52; mean ± STD; binocular, N = 1178 cells, 13 retinae; monocular, N = 1001 cells, 11 retinae; T(2168) = 1.36, P = 0.174, linear mixed-effects model with log transformation) (Fig. 2a), and the vast majority of RGC spikes were contained within bursts, although this

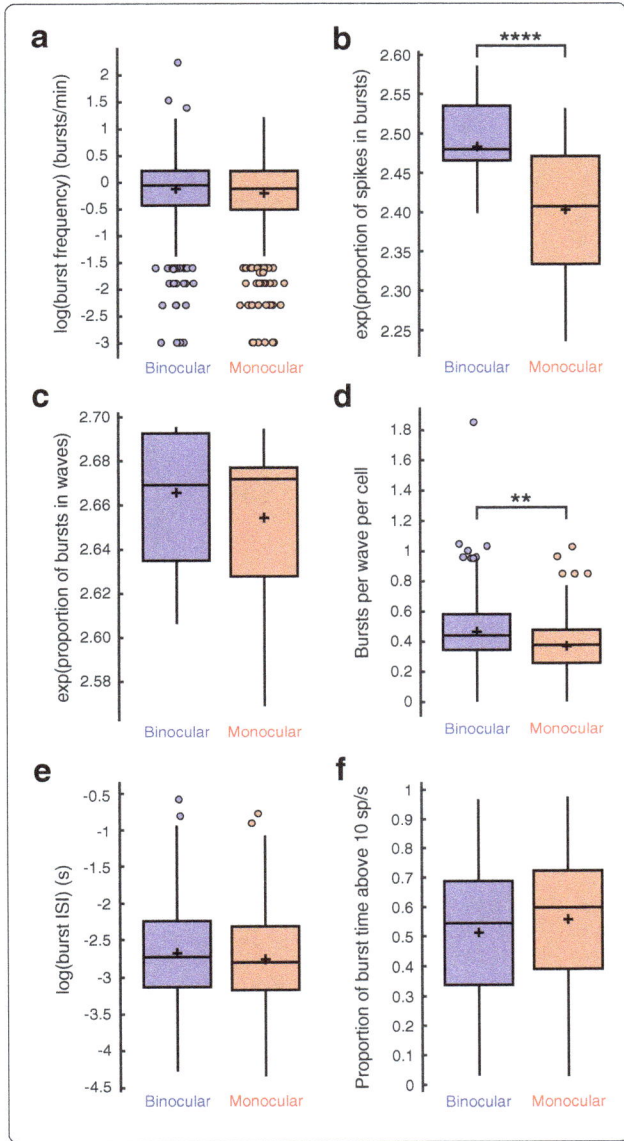

**Fig. 2** Other burst properties. **a** Burst frequency (bursts/min) (binocular, 1.02 ± 0.56; monocular, 0.96 ± 0.52; mean ± STD; T(2168) = 1.361, $P = 0.174$, linear mixed-effects model with log transformation), **b** proportion of spikes in bursts (binocular, 0.900 ± 0.155; monocular, 0.862 ± 0.186; mean ± STD; T(2168) = 5.44, $P = 5.814 \times 10^{-8}$, linear mixed-effects model with exponential transformation), **c** proportion of bursts in waves (binocular, 0.978 ± 0.068; monocular, 0.975 ± 0.057; mean ± STD; T(2168) = 1.744, $P = 0.0814$, linear mixed-effects model with exponential transformation), **d** bursts per wave per cell (binocular, 0.467 ± 0.191; monocular, 0.371 ± 0.159; mean ± STD; T(2168) = 2.66, $P = 0.0078$, linear mixed-effects model), **e** ISI for all bursts (s) (binocular, 0.086 ± 0.062; monocular, 0.078 ± 0.055; mean ± STD; T(2168) = 0.981, $P = 0.327$, linear mixed-effects model with log transformation), and **f** proportion of burst time firing above 10 spikes/s for all bursts (binocular, 0.512 ± 0.217; monocular, 0.557 ± 0.213; mean ± STD; T(2168) = 1.783, $P = 0.0747$, linear mixed-effects model) for each condition. The heights of the box plots extend between the 25th and the 75th percentiles of the data. The horizontal bar and cross mark indicate the median and mean, respectively. Outliers are shown as circles and are data points that are 1.5 times higher than or 1.5 times lower than the interquartile range. The box plot whiskers extend to the most extreme data points that are not outliers. Binocular, $N = 1178$ cells, 13 retinae; Monocular, $N = 1001$ cells, 11 retinae. ** = $P < 0.01$, **** = $P < 0.0001$

was slightly less so for the monocular condition (binocular, 0.900 ± 0.155 proportion of spikes in bursts; monocular, 0.862 ± 0.186 proportion of spikes in bursts; mean ± STD; binocular, $N = 1178$ cells, 13 retinae; monocular, $N = 1001$ cells, 11 retinae; T(2168) = 5.44, $P = 5.814 \times 10^{-8}$, linear mixed-effects model with exponential transformation) (Fig. 2b). Bursts occurred almost exclusively during waves regardless of condition (binocular, 0.978 ± 0.068 proportion of bursts in waves; monocular, 0.975 ± 0.057 proportion of bursts in waves; mean ± STD; binocular, $N = 1178$ cells, 13 retinae; monocular, $N = 1001$ cells, 11 retinae; T(2168) = 1.74, $P = 0.0814$, linear mixed-effects model with exponential transformation) (Fig. 2c) but for the monocular condition, the number of bursts per wave per cell was slightly reduced (binocular, 0.467 ± 0.191; monocular, 0.371 ± 0.159; mean ± STD; binocular, $N = 1178$ cells, 13 retinae; monocular, $N = 935$ cells, 11 retinae; T(2168) = 2.66, $P = 0.00777$, linear mixed-effects model) (Fig. 2d). Additionally, the burst ISI (binocular, 0.086 ± 0.062 s; monocular, 0.078 ± 0.055 s; mean ± STD; binocular, $N = 1178$ cells, 13 retinae; monocular, $N = 1001$ cells, 11 retinae; T(2168) = 0.98, $P = 0.327$, linear mixed-effects model with log transformation) (Fig. 2e) and the proportion of burst time above 10 spikes/s (binocular, 0.512 ± 0.217; monocular, 0.557 ± 0.213; mean ± STD; binocular, $N = 1178$ cells, 13 retinae; monocular $N = 935$ cells, 11 retinae; T(2168) = 1.78, $P = 0.0747$, linear mixed-effects model) (Fig. 2f) were unchanged with enucleation, further confirming that the reduction in the number of spikes in a burst was due to shorter burst durations. When analyses were constrained to only wave associated bursts, the differences between conditions were consistent with our general findings (Fig. 3a-d).

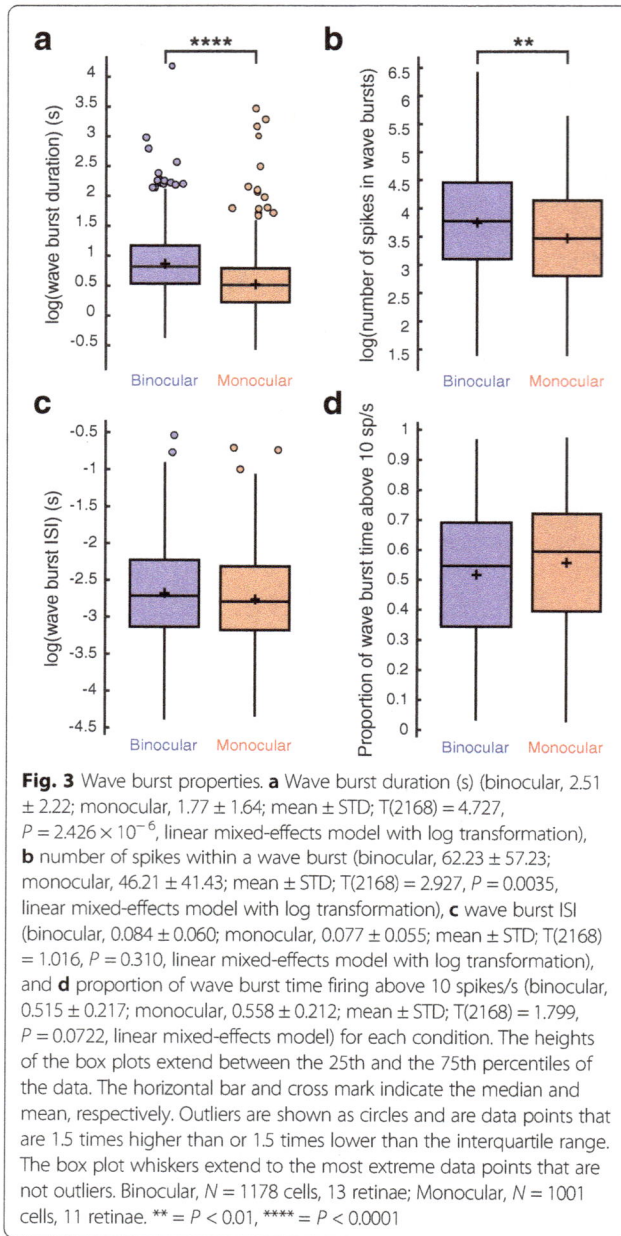

**Fig. 3** Wave burst properties. **a** Wave burst duration (s) (binocular, 2.51 ± 2.22; monocular, 1.77 ± 1.64; mean ± STD; T(2168) = 4.727, $P = 2.426 \times 10^{-6}$, linear mixed-effects model with log transformation), **b** number of spikes within a wave burst (binocular, 62.23 ± 57.23; monocular, 46.21 ± 41.43; mean ± STD; T(2168) = 2.927, P = 0.0035, linear mixed-effects model with log transformation), **c** wave burst ISI (binocular, 0.084 ± 0.060; monocular, 0.077 ± 0.055; mean ± STD; T(2168) = 1.016, P = 0.310, linear mixed-effects model with log transformation), and **d** proportion of wave burst time firing above 10 spikes/s (binocular, 0.515 ± 0.217; monocular, 0.558 ± 0.212; mean ± STD; T(2168) = 1.799, P = 0.0722, linear mixed-effects model) for each condition. The heights of the box plots extend between the 25th and the 75th percentiles of the data. The horizontal bar and cross mark indicate the median and mean, respectively. Outliers are shown as circles and are data points that are 1.5 times higher than or 1.5 times lower than the interquartile range. The box plot whiskers extend to the most extreme data points that are not outliers. Binocular, N = 1178 cells, 13 retinae; Monocular, N = 1001 cells, 11 retinae. ** = P < 0.01, **** = P < 0.0001

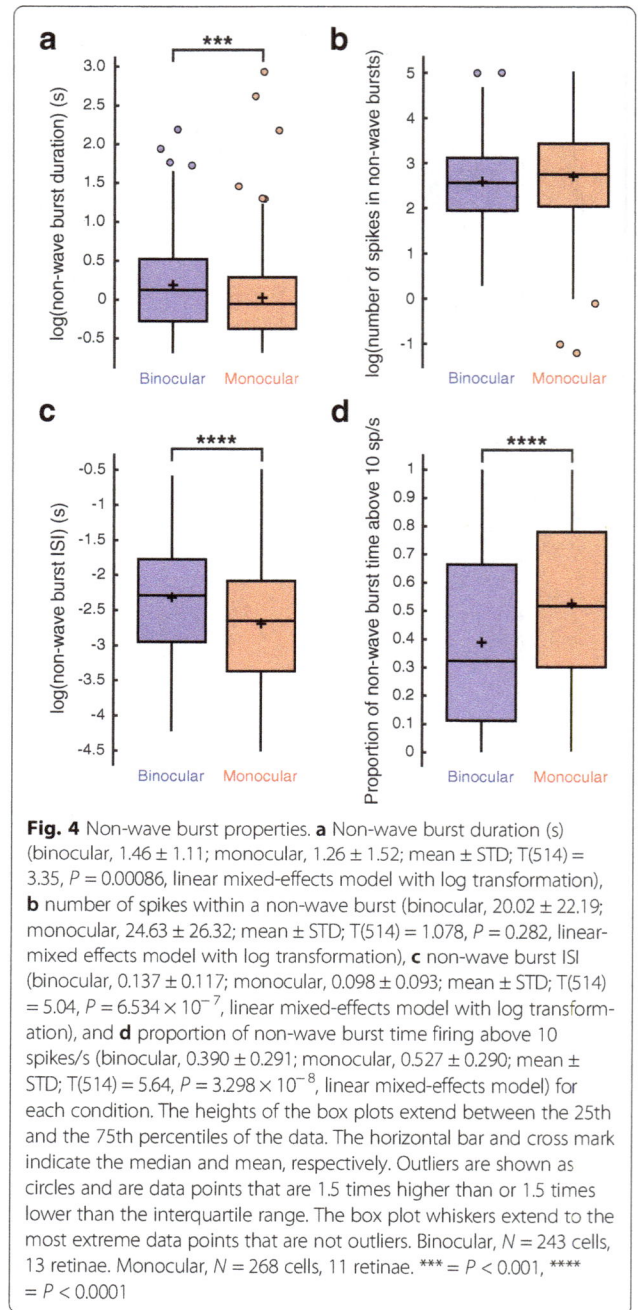

**Fig. 4** Non-wave burst properties. **a** Non-wave burst duration (s) (binocular, 1.46 ± 1.11; monocular, 1.26 ± 1.52; mean ± STD; T(514) = 3.35, P = 0.00086, linear mixed-effects model with log transformation), **b** number of spikes within a non-wave burst (binocular, 20.02 ± 22.19; monocular, 24.63 ± 26.32; mean ± STD; T(514) = 1.078, P = 0.282, linear-mixed effects model with log transformation), **c** non-wave burst ISI (binocular, 0.137 ± 0.117; monocular, 0.098 ± 0.093; mean ± STD; T(514) = 5.04, $P = 6.534 \times 10^{-7}$, linear mixed-effects model with log transformation), and **d** proportion of non-wave burst time firing above 10 spikes/s (binocular, 0.390 ± 0.291; monocular, 0.527 ± 0.290; mean ± STD; T(514) = 5.64, $P = 3.298 \times 10^{-8}$, linear mixed-effects model) for each condition. The heights of the box plots extend between the 25th and the 75th percentiles of the data. The horizontal bar and cross mark indicate the median and mean, respectively. Outliers are shown as circles and are data points that are 1.5 times higher than or 1.5 times lower than the interquartile range. The box plot whiskers extend to the most extreme data points that are not outliers. Binocular, N = 243 cells, 13 retinae. Monocular, N = 268 cells, 11 retinae. *** = P < 0.001, **** = P < 0.0001

Other observed effects on burst properties due to enucleation were unique to non-wave bursts, which were very rare in both conditions (Fig. 2c). Non-wave bursts, like wave bursts, were shorter in duration in the monocular condition (binocular, 1.46 ± 1.11 s; monocular, 1.26 ± 1.52 s; mean ± STD; binocular, N = 245 cells, 13 retinae. Monocular, N = 272 cells, 11 retinae; T(514) = 3.35, P = 0.00086, linear mixed-effects model with log transformation) (Fig. 4a), but had shorter burst ISIs (binocular, 0.137 ± 0.117 s; monocular, 0.098 ± 0.093 s; mean ± STD; binocular, N = 245 cells, 13 retinae. Monocular, N = 272 cells, 11 retinae; T(514) = 5.04,

$P = 6.534 \times 10^{-7}$, linear mixed-effects model with log transformation) (Fig. 4c) and spent a larger proportion of time firing at rates above 10 spikes/s (binocular, 0.390 ± 0.291; monocular, 0.527 ± 0.290; mean ± STD; binocular, N = 245 cells, 13 retinae. Monocular, N = 272 cells, 11 retinae; T(514) = 5.65, $P = 3.298 \times 10^{-8}$, linear mixed-effects model) (Fig. 4d). These combined effects resulted in non-wave bursts containing a similar number of spikes in both conditions (binocular, 20.02 ± 22.20; monocular, 24.63 ± 26.32; mean ± STD; binocular,

$N$ = 245 cells, 13 retinae. Monocular, $N$ = 272 cells, 11 retinae; T(514) = 1.08, $P$ = 0.282, linear-mixed effects model with log transformation) (Fig. 4b).

Lastly, we found small but significant effects on retinal wave size (binocular, 0.275 ± 0.158 proportion of electrodes active; monocular, 0.224 ± 0.130 proportion of electrodes active; mean ± STD; binocular, $N$ = 495 waves, 13 retinae. Monocular, $N$ = 485 waves, 11 retinae; T(977) = 2.58, $P$ = 0.00999, linear mixed-effects model) (Fig. 5c) and speed (binocular, 167.67 ± 77.63 μm/s; monocular, 199.39 ± 83.63 μm/s; mean ± STD; binocular, $N$ = 449 waves, 13 retinae. Monocular, $N$ = 409 waves, 11 retinae; T(855) = 2.22, $P$ = 0.0267, linear mixed-effects model) (Fig. 5d). However, the rate that waves spread to new electrodes was unchanged with enucleation (binocular, 0.060 ± 0.042 proportion of new electrodes active/s; monocular, 0.065 ± 0.045 proportion of new electrodes active/s; mean ± STD; binocular, $N$ = 449 waves, 13 retinae. Monocular, $N$ = 409 waves, 11 retinae; T(855) = 0.821, $P$ = 0.412, linear mixed-effects model) (Fig. 5e). Wave frequency was not significantly different with enucleation (binocular, 2.53 ± 1.26; monocular, 2.86 ± 1.64; mean ± STD; binocular, $N$ = 13 retinae; monocular, $N$ = 11 retinae; T(21) = 1.216, $P$ = 0.237, linear-mixed effects model) (Fig. 5f). However, there was a shortening of wave duration (binocular, 5.79 ± 3.15 s; monocular, 5.07 ± 7.60 s; mean ± STD; binocular, $N$ = 495 waves, 13 retinae. Monocular, $N$ = 485 waves, 11 retinae; T(977) = 5.744, $P$ = 1.233 × 10$^{-8}$, linear mixed-effects model with log transformation) (Fig. 5g) consistent with the shortening of RGC burst duration.

### Shortening RGC burst duration reduces pairwise RGC correlation levels

The effects on RGC bursts were intriguing, as bursts appear to play a critical role in retinofugal refinement [9, 17, 28, 29]. Due to the spatiotemporal properties of retinal waves, the bursting activity of neighboring RGCs is highly correlated but is largely uncorrelated between pairs of RGCs that are distant from each other [26, 30]. A large body of work has supported the hypothesis that correlated activity is critical for retinotopic refinement of RGC afferent terminals within the dLGN and superior colliculus [9, 26, 28, 31]. If the duration of bursts is shortened, the pairwise correlation between RGCs with offset burst times, as is the case during propagating waves, should be reduced (Fig. 6a).

Based on the hypothesis that a shortening of burst duration should reduce pairwise correlation levels between RGCs during waves (Fig. 6a), we carried out additional measurements to determine if levels of correlated activity decreased with enucleation. To quantify pairwise RGC correlations we calculated the "spike time tiling coefficient" (STTC) [27], which is a pairwise correlation measure that is bounded and insensitive to firing rate. Retinae from enucleates and binocular ferrets showed

pairwise RGC correlations that fell as a function of the distance between cell pairs consistent with what has been previously described [30] (Fig. 6b). However, as predicted, levels of correlated RGC activity during waves were reduced across RGC pair distances for retinae from enucleates (binocular, $N$ = 401 distances, 13 retinae; monocular, $N$ = 341 distances, 11 retinae; T(738) = 2.85, $P$ = 0.00452, linear mixed-effects model) (Fig. 6c).

The number of spikes within bursts and non-wave burst properties between retinae from binocular and monocular ferrets were different as described above. Although spikes outside bursts and non-wave bursts were rare, it may be the case that they had an impact on overall levels of correlated activity. For non-wave associated activity, pairwise RGC correlation levels were not significantly different between conditions (binocular, $N$ = 401 distances, 13 retinae; monocular, $N$ = 341 distances, 11 retinae; T(738) = 1.02, $P$ = 0.310, linear-mixed effects model) (Fig. 7b and d). However, when correlation levels were measured for all recorded RGC activity, a difference between conditions was still found (binocular, $N$ = 401 distances, 13 retinae; monocular, $N$ = 341 distances, 11 retinae; T(738) = 2.56, $P$ = 0.0106, linear mixed-effects model) (Fig. 7a and c) indicating that correlation levels are predominately determined by the properties of wave bursts.

### Discussion

We have previously shown that retinal waves are critical for the targeting of retinogeniculate afferents following the removal of competing inputs to the dLGN [8]. While this work demonstrated that aspects of afferent terminal targeting during retinogeniculate refinement are retinal wave-dependent, it remained unclear what retinal wave properties might be necessary for this process. This study aimed to elucidate what retinal wave properties could dynamically guide afferent terminal targeting when an eye is lost. We show that the removal of the competing eye alters the duration of retinal wave associated RGC bursts, which has impacts on RGC correlation. Since studies have shown that correlation plays a critical role in retinogeniculate refinement, our finding is consistent with the hypothesis that retinal wave activity can dynamically guide retinogeniculate refinement while taking into consideration the presence of inter-eye competition.

We should note that since monocular enucleation is the complete removal of an organ, there is essentially no sham surgery that can fully replicate its potential side effects. Thus, our study cannot authoritatively rule out effects on retinal waves due to stress the ferrets may have experienced due to the monocular enucleation procedure. However, there is data to suggest that noxious stimuli at this age are unlikely to have large impacts on the brain. Studies have shown that newborn mammals that undergo extended periods of brain development *ex utero*

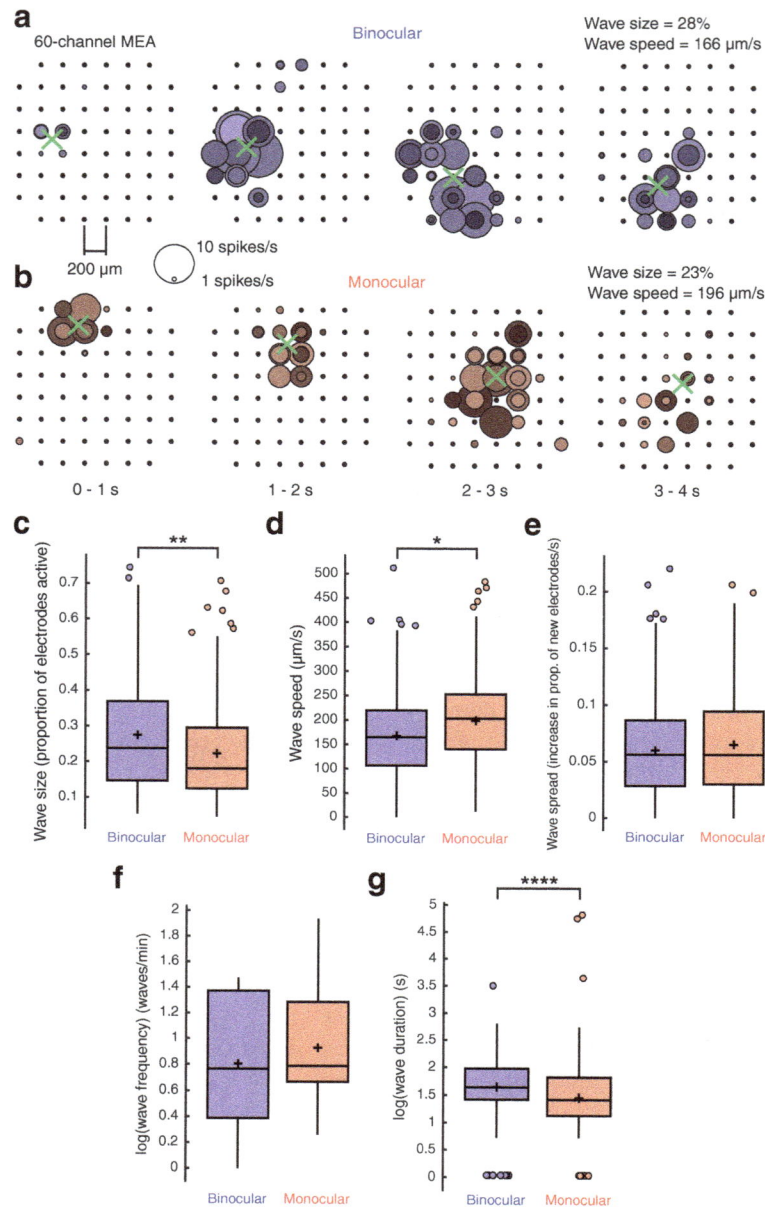

**Fig. 5** Effects of removing inter-eye competition on the spatiotemporal properties of retinal waves. **a-b**) Visualizations of representative waves recorded from the retina of a binocular (**a**) or and a monocular (**b**) ferret. Each colored circle represents an RGC active during the period designated on the bottom of (**b**). Circle size corresponds to RGC firing rate as shown by the legend between (**a**) and (**b**). The green cross indicates the center of the wave for each period. **c-g** Plots showing the difference in size (proportion of electrodes active) (binocular, 0.275 ± 0.158; monocular, 0.224 ± 0.130; mean ± STD; T(977) = 2.58, $P$ = 0.00999, linear mixed-effects model) (**c**), speed (μm/s) (binocular, 167.67 ± 77.63; monocular, 199.39 ± 83.63; mean ± STD; T(855) = 2.22, $P$ = 0.0267, linear mixed-effects model) (**d**), spread (proportion of new electrodes active/s) (binocular, 0.060 ± 0.042; monocular, 0.065 ± 0.045; mean ± STD; T(855) = 0.821, $P$ = 0.412, linear mixed-effects model) (**e**), frequency (waves/min) (binocular, 2.53 ± 1.26; monocular, 2.86 ± 1.64; mean ± STD; T(21) = 1.216, $P$ = 0.237, linear mixed-effects model with log transformation) (**f**), and duration (s) (binocular, 5.79 ± 3.15; monocular, 5.07 ± 7.60; mean ± STD; T(977) = 5.74, $P$ = 1.233 × 10$^{-8}$, linear mixed-effects model with log transformation) (**g**) of waves recorded from the retinae of binocular and monocular ferrets. The heights of the box plots extend between the 25th and the 75th percentiles of the data. The horizontal bar and cross mark indicate the median and mean, respectively. Outliers are shown as circles and are data points that are 1.5 times higher than or 1.5 times lower than the interquartile range. The box plot whiskers extend to the most extreme data points that are not outliers. Binocular, $N$ = 451 waves, 13 retinae. Monocular, $N$ = 408 waves, 11 retinae. * = $P$ < 0.05, ** = $P$ < 0.01, **** = $P$ < 0.0001

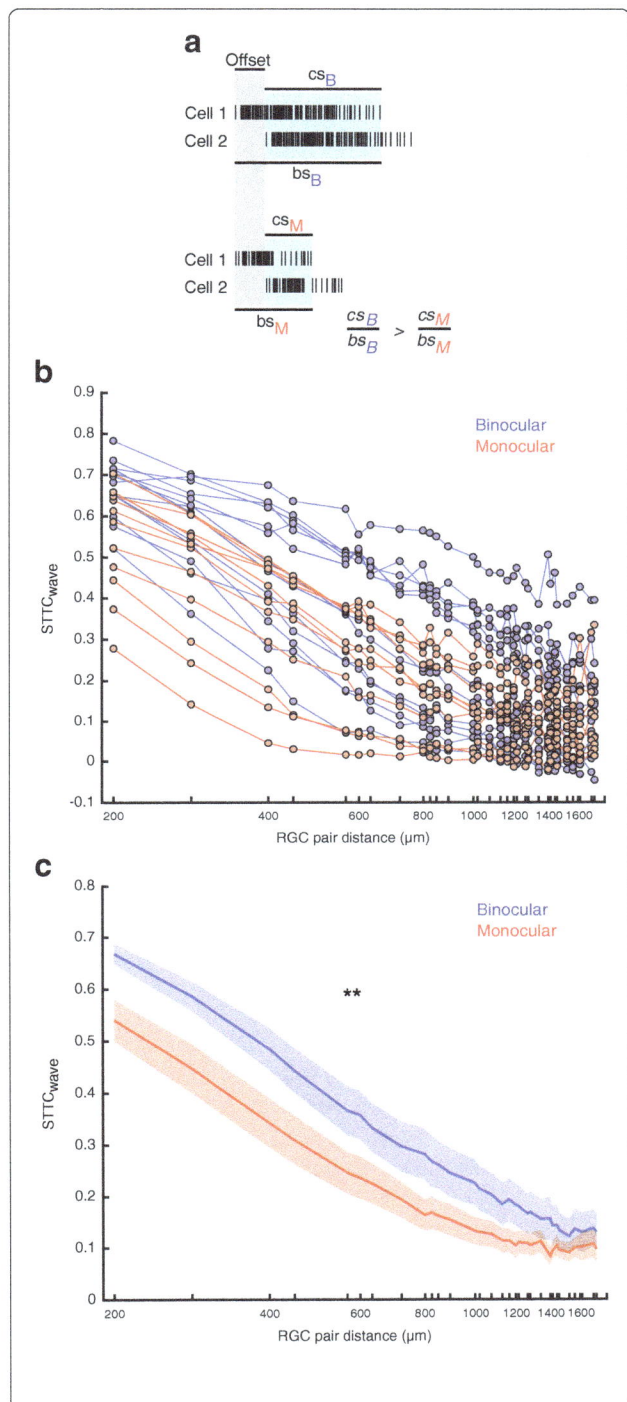

**Fig. 6** Removing inter-eye competition reduces levels of pairwise RGC correlation during waves. **a** Illustration of the hypothesized effects of shortening burst duration on pairwise RGC correlation levels during waves. The gray shading is the offset time between bursts due to the propagation speed of a retinal wave. bs = burst spikes. cs = correlated spikes. Subscripts M and B signify monocular or binocular spikes. **b** Plot of STTC over distance for all retinae recorded. **c** Plot of average STTC as a function of RGC pair distance for both conditions (T(738) = 2.85, P = 0.00452, linear mixed-effects model). Tick marks indicate cell pair distances included for STTC measures as constrained by the spatial organization of the MEA. Binocular, N = 401 distances, 13 retinae. Monocular, N = 341 distances, 11 retinae. Error bars are SEM. ** = P < 0.01

are hyporesponsive to noxious stimuli in the first two postnatal weeks [32]. Additionally, we found that newborn ferrets that underwent the short enucleation procedure healed quickly and did not display any developmental stunting or signs of distress. Ultimately, future experiments utilizing more targeted interventions are required to elucidate further how monocular enucleation affects retinal wave activity.

**The role of burst duration and RGC correlation**

RGC bursts are important for refinement of the retinogeniculate pathway [4, 9, 17, 28, 29]. Thus, the changes in RGC burst duration following monocular enucleation (Fig. 1) may indicate a role of the competing eye in influencing the refinement of the retinogeniculate pathway of the other. Additionally, we found that RGC burst duration scales RGC correlation (Fig. 6). Removal of an eye thus results in reductions in correlation level that are associated with the expansive targeting seen in the dLGN following monocular enucleation [8]. Since a large body of experimental and theoretical work has supported a role for pairwise RGC correlations in retinogeniculate refinement [8, 9, 18, 26, 28, 31, 33, 34], we believe this finding is unlikely to be coincidental. Based on the evidence that afferent terminal targeting is guided by competition [8], we propose a model where RGC burst duration scales RGC correlation to dynamically guide afferent targeting within the dLGN during visual system development:

In binocular ferrets, RGC burst duration is longer, which results in higher pairwise RGC correlation levels within an eye. Higher RGC correlation levels decrease intra-eye competition, which in the context of inter-eye competition between ipsilateral and contralateral inputs, is optimal for establishing eye-specific laminae (Fig. 8a and e). Conversely, in monocular ferrets, burst durations are shorter, RGC correlations are reduced, and intra-eye competition is increased. Increasing intra-eye competition facilitates the spread of afferents resulting in expanded ipsilateral laminae, thus utilizing more synaptic space within the dLGN when contralateral

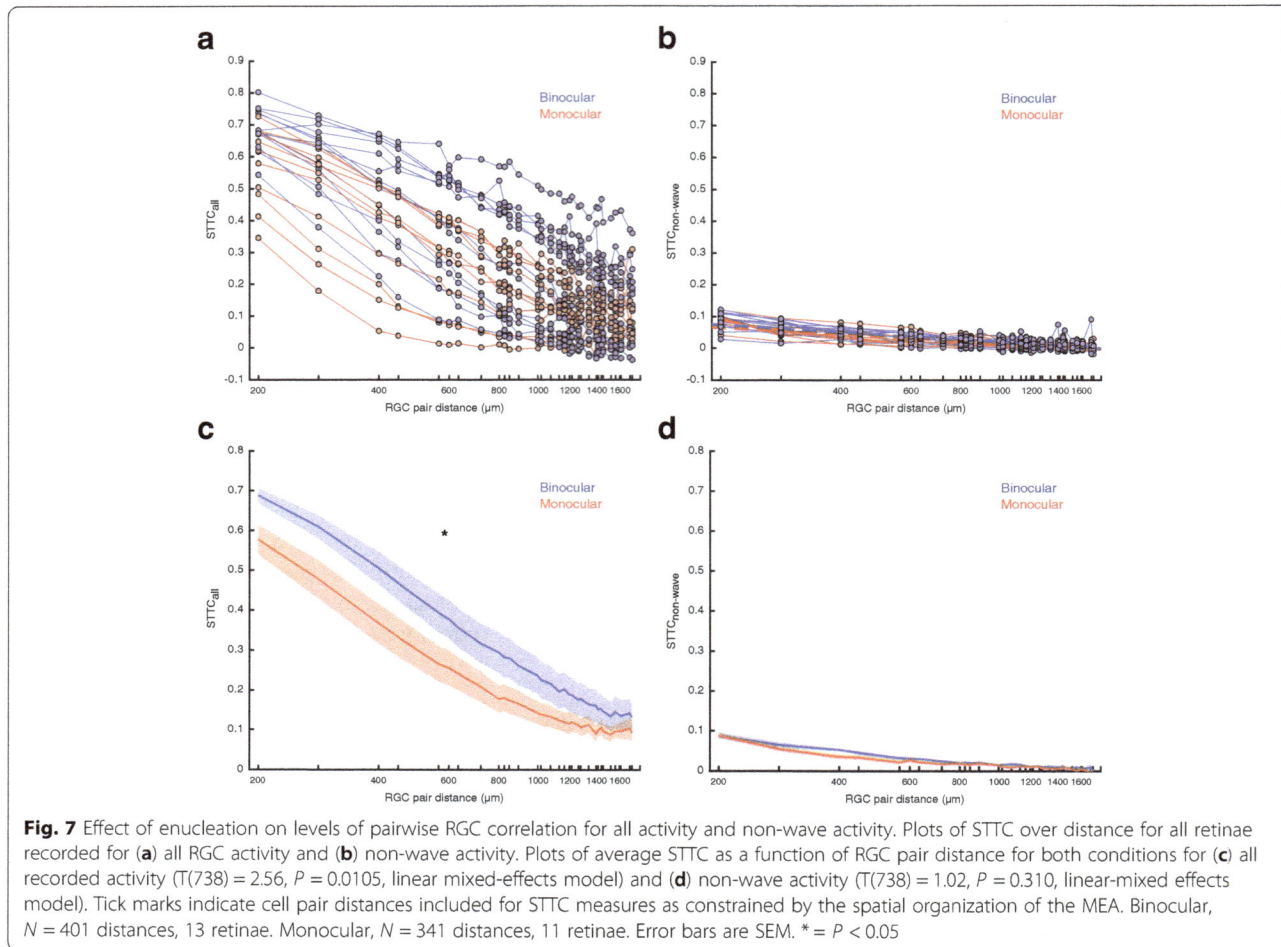

**Fig. 7** Effect of enucleation on levels of pairwise RGC correlation for all activity and non-wave activity. Plots of STTC over distance for all retinae recorded for (**a**) all RGC activity and (**b**) non-wave activity. Plots of average STTC as a function of RGC pair distance for both conditions for (**c**) all recorded activity (T(738) = 2.56, P = 0.0105, linear mixed-effects model) and (**d**) non-wave activity (T(738) = 1.02, P = 0.310, linear-mixed effects model). Tick marks indicate cell pair distances included for STTC measures as constrained by the spatial organization of the MEA. Binocular, N = 401 distances, 13 retinae. Monocular, N = 341 distances, 11 retinae. Error bars are SEM. * = P < 0.05

afferents from the competing eye are absent (Fig. 8b and f). Previous studies have effectively blocked retinal waves (i.e., spatiotemporal correlations) in ferrets by decorrelating the activity of neighboring RGCs with the cholinergic agonist epibatidine (EPI) [7, 8, 35]. Blocking retinal waves with EPI in binocular ferrets disrupts eye-specific segregation and lamination, and in enucleates, the lamination and expansion of retinogeniculate projections, resulting in ipsilateral projections of approximately the same size in binocular and monocular ferrets [8] (Fig. 8c-d). Thus, blocking retinal waves with EPI results in abnormal afferent competition in both the binocular and monocular condition, causing randomized afferent terminal targeting that is no longer being effectively guided by intra-eye and inter-eye competition (Fig. 8g-h).

Consistent with our model, the importance of low intra-eye competition for eye-specific segregation in binocular ferrets was recently demonstrated [36]. In this study, we used an immunotoxin to ablate starburst amacrine cells (SACs) that are responsible for retinal wave generation. This SAC ablation resulted in a reduction of RGC correlation similar to that seen following monocular enucleation,

with fewer SACs leading to less RGC correlation. In binocular ferrets where laminae appeared normal, SAC ablation levels were symmetric across eyes. However, in ferrets where one eye's retinogeniculate projection was larger, SAC ablation was lower in that eye (i.e., SAC ablation was asymmetric). This result demonstrated that when intra-eye competition is increased in one eye relative to the other due to asymmetric SAC ablation, the eye with increased intra-eye competition (less RGC correlation) is hindered in its ability to compete for synaptic space in the dLGN and loses territory to the eye with lower intra-eye competition (more RGC correlation). Similarly, recent studies in mice have used transgenic lines to investigate the role of retinal wave size in retinogeniculate refinement. In two different transgenic mouse lines, neighboring RGC correlation levels were reduced but not eliminated [33, 34]. Consistent with our model, these studies showed that reduced RGC correlation disrupted eye-specific segregation [33, 34] and resulted in an expanded ipsilateral projection in binocular transgenic mice [33]. Additionally, in transgenic enucleates where competing contralateral inputs were absent, fine-

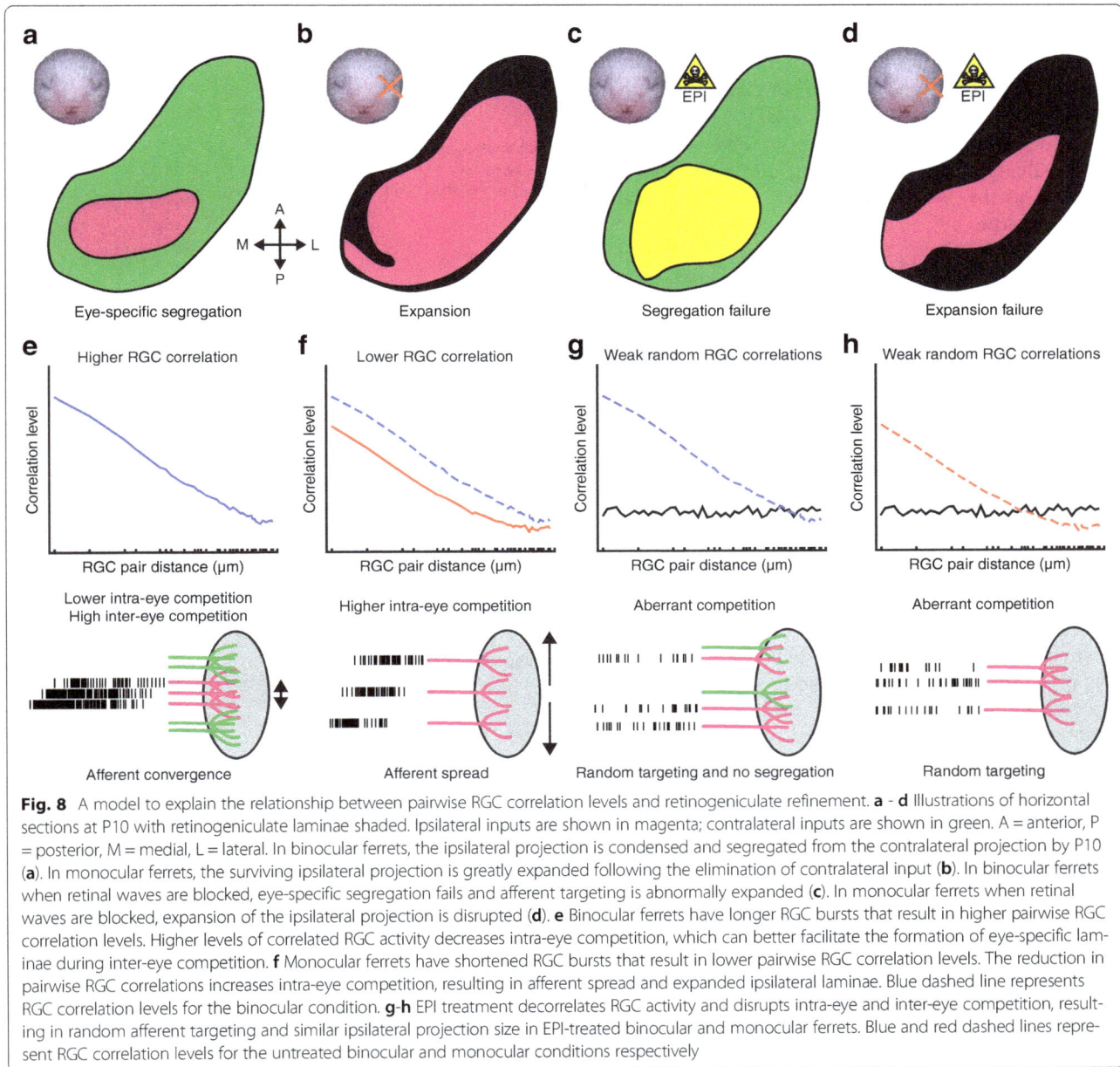

**Fig. 8** A model to explain the relationship between pairwise RGC correlation levels and retinogeniculate refinement. **a - d** Illustrations of horizontal sections at P10 with retinogeniculate laminae shaded. Ipsilateral inputs are shown in magenta; contralateral inputs are shown in green. A = anterior, P = posterior, M = medial, L = lateral. In binocular ferrets, the ipsilateral projection is condensed and segregated from the contralateral projection by P10 (**a**). In monocular ferrets, the surviving ipsilateral projection is greatly expanded following the elimination of contralateral input (**b**). In binocular ferrets when retinal waves are blocked, eye-specific segregation fails and afferent targeting is abnormally expanded (**c**). In monocular ferrets when retinal waves are blocked, expansion of the ipsilateral projection is disrupted (**d**). **e** Binocular ferrets have longer RGC bursts that result in higher pairwise RGC correlation levels. Higher levels of correlated RGC activity decreases intra-eye competition, which can better facilitate the formation of eye-specific laminae during inter-eye competition. **f** Monocular ferrets have shortened RGC bursts that result in lower pairwise RGC correlation levels. The reduction in pairwise RGC correlations increases intra-eye competition, resulting in afferent spread and expanded ipsilateral laminae. Blue dashed line represents RGC correlation levels for the binocular condition. **g-h** EPI treatment decorrelates RGC activity and disrupts intra-eye and inter-eye competition, resulting in random afferent targeting and similar ipsilateral projection size in EPI-treated binocular and monocular ferrets. Blue and red dashed lines represent RGC correlation levels for the untreated binocular and monocular conditions respectively

scale retinogeniculate refinement appeared normal [33]. We must note, however, that while the above studies demonstrated the importance high RGC correlation levels for the establishment of eye-specific laminae, the nature of the effects for ferrets and mice were different. In ferrets, moderate increases in relative intra-eye competition shrank eye-specific laminae and had minor effects on eye-specific segregation [36], while in transgenic mice ipsilateral projection size increased for both eyes and eye-specific segregation was disrupted [33, 34]. The difference can be explained by the high levels of RGC correlation found in ferrets relative to mice [35]. The reduction to the mouse's already relatively low RGC correlation levels in the above transgenic lines may have prevented effective inter-eye competition [33, 34] and resulted in expanded ipsilateral projections [33] like observed in monocular ferrets where no inter-eye competition is present [8, 37], or in binocular ferrets when EPI treatment completely blocks retinal waves [7, 8].

Surprisingly, bursts that occurred outside of waves were affected differently by monocular enucleation. For non-wave bursts, burst ISIs were shorter and the percentage of burst time above 10 spikes/s was greater (Fig. 4). However, it is important to note that non-wave bursts made up less than 3% of all bursts in either condition (Fig. 2) and do not appear to have any significant impact on overall levels of pairwise RGC correlation

(Fig. 7). For these reasons, the observed changes to non-wave burst properties are unlikely to be related to the altered retinogeniculate refinement in enucleates. It is hard to speculate on why these effects are observed for non-wave bursts and not wave bursts, but after additional studies are carried out, it may prove valuable in understanding the neurobiological mechanisms by which monocular enucleation alters burst properties.

### A signal for the presence of the competing eye?

Removing an eye alters retinal waves in the one that is spared. However, this study is unable to elucidate the neurobiological mechanism underlying such effects. It is important to note that we observe differences in retinal waves due to monocular enucleation ex vivo, indicating that the competing eye must be inducing relatively long-lasting effects in the opposing retina. One candidate mechanism is inputs from the competing eye onto neuromodulator releasing amacrine cells, which modify synaptic connectivity or other cell membrane properties [38]. Retino-retinal projecting retinal ganglion cells (rrRGCs) have been identified in several vertebrate species [39–41] and are greatest in number during early visual system development in rodents [39]. While a direct projection between the retinae to signal the presence of a competing eye is perhaps the most parsimonious explanation for the effects on retinal waves reported here, there is no direct evidence that rrRGCs modulate retinal wave activity. Future experiments to target these cells carefully, with either ablation or silencing, will be necessary to understand their role, if any, in visual system development.

### Conclusion

Our results demonstrate a novel phenomenon whereby the removal of a competing region of the central nervous system influences the patterned spontaneous neural activity of another. When the competing eye is absent, it shortens the RGC burst duration of the surviving eye. This effect on RGC burst duration scales the levels of RGC correlation in the developing retina, and reduced correlation levels coincide with the retinal wave-dependent spread of the retinogeniculate projection following the loss of an eye. Based on these novel findings and their association with the retinal-wave-dependent anatomical remodeling found in enucleates, we propose the hypothesis that the presence or absence of the competing eye dynamically scales afferent competition to guide retinogeniculate refinement during visual system development.

### Abbreviations

dLGN: Dorsal lateral geniculate nucleus; EPI: Epibatidine; ISI: Inter-spike interval; MEA: Multi-electrode array; RGC: Retinal ganglion cell; rrRGC: Retino-retinal projecting retinal ganglion cell; SAC: Starburst amacrine cell; STTC: Spike time tiling coefficient

### Acknowledgements

We would like to thank members of the Cheng lab for providing valuable scientific feedback over the course of the study.

### Funding

NIH National Eye Institute (RRID:SCR_011411) grants EY011369 (to H.-J.C.) and EY012576 (to J. S. Werner) supported this research.

### Authors' contributions

SWF and H-J C conceived the project. SWF performed surgical procedures, collected MEA data, and analyzed electrophysiological data. AN performed surgical procedures and collected MEA and anatomical data. SWF and H-JC wrote the manuscript. All authors read and approved the final manuscript.

### Competing interests

The authors declare that they have no competing interests.

### Author details

¹Center for Neuroscience, University of California, Davis, 1544 Newton Court, Davis, CA 95618, USA. ²Department of Neurobiology, Physiology, and Behavior, University of California, Davis, One Shields Avenue, Davis, CA 95616, USA. ³Department of Pathology and Laboratory Medicine, University of California, Davis, One Shields Avenue, Davis, CA 95616, USA. ⁴Wolfson Institute for Biomedical Research, University College London, Gower Street, London WC1E 6BT, UK.

### References

1.   Huberman AD, Feller MB, Chapman B. Mechanisms underlying development of visual maps and receptive fields. Annu Rev Neurosci. 2008; 31:479–509.
2.   Espinosa JS, Stryker MP. Development and plasticity of the primary visual cortex. Neuron. 2012;75:230–49.
3.   Levelt CN, Hübener M. Critical-period plasticity in the visual cortex. Annu Rev Neurosci. 2012;35:309–30.
4.   Kirkby LA, Sack GS, Firl A, Feller MB. A role for correlated spontaneous activity in the assembly of neural circuits. Neuron. 2013;80:1129–44.
5.   Cang J, Feldheim DA. Developmental mechanisms of topographic map formation and alignment. Annu Rev Neurosci. 2013;36:51–77.
6.   Ackman JB, Crair MC. Role of emergent neural activity in visual map development. Curr Opin Neurobiol. 2014;24:166–75.
7.   Penn AA, Riquelme PA, Feller MB, Shatz CJ. Competition in retinogeniculate patterning driven by spontaneous activity. Science (New York, NY). 1998; 279:2108–12.
8.   Failor S, Chapman B, Cheng HJ. Retinal waves regulate afferent terminal targeting in the early visual pathway. Proc Natl Acad Sci U S A. 2015; 112(22):E2957–66.

9. Butts DA, Kanold PO, Shatz CJ. A burst-based "Hebbian" learning rule at retinogeniculate synapses links retinal waves to activity-dependent refinement. PLoS Biol. 2007;5(3):e61.

10. Maffei L, Galli-Resta L. Correlation in the discharges of neighboring rat retinal ganglion cells during prenatal life. Proc Natl Acad Sci U S A. 1990;87:2861–4.

11. Warland DK, Huberman AD, Chalupa LM. Dynamics of spontaneous activity in the fetal macaque retina during development of retinogeniculate pathways. J Neurosci. 2006;26:5190–7.

12. Ackman JB, Burbridge TJ, Crair MC. Retinal waves coordinate patterned activity throughout the developing visual system. Nature. 2012;490(7419):219–25.

13. Meister M, Wong RO, Baylor DA, Shatz CJ. Synchronous bursts of action potentials in ganglion cells of the developing mammalian retina. Science. 1991;252(5008):939–43.

14. Chapman B. Necessity for afferent activity to maintain eye-specific segregation in ferret lateral geniculate nucleus. Science. 2000;287:2479–82.

15. Rossi FM, Pizzorusso T, Porciatti V, Marubio LM, Maffei L, Changeux JP. Requirement of the nicotinic acetylcholine receptor beta 2 subunit for the anatomical and functional development of the visual system. Proc Natl Acad Sci U S A. 2001;98:6453–8.

16. Huberman AD, Stellwagen D, Chapman B. Decoupling eye-specific segregation from lamination in the lateral geniculate nucleus. J Neurosci. 2002;22:9419–29.

17. Torborg CL, Hansen KA, Feller MB. High frequency, synchronized bursting drives eye-specific segregation of retinogeniculate projections. Nat Neurosci. 2005;8:72–8.

18. H-p X, Furman M, Mineur YS, Chen H, King SL, Zenisek D, Zhou ZJ, Butts DA, Tian N, Picciotto MR, et al. An instructive role for patterned spontaneous retinal activity in mouse visual map development. Neuron. 2011;70:1115–27.

19. Zhang J, Ackman JB, Xu H-P, Crair MC. Visual map development depends on the temporal pattern of binocular activity in mice. Nat Neurosci. 2012;15:298–307.

20. Burbridge TJ, Xu HP, Ackman JB, Ge X, Zhang Y, Ye MJ, Zhou ZJ, Xu J, Contractor A, Crair MC. Visual circuit development requires patterned activity mediated by retinal acetylcholine receptors. Neuron. 2014;84(5):1049–64.

21. Grubb MS, Rossi FM, Changeux JP, Thompson ID. Abnormal functional organization in the dorsal lateral geniculate nucleus of mice lacking the beta 2 subunit of the nicotinic acetylcholine receptor. Neuron. 2003;40:1161–72.

22. Davis ZW, Chapman B, Cheng HJ. Increasing spontaneous retinal activity before eye opening accelerates the development of geniculate receptive fields. J Neurosci. 2015;35(43):14612–23.

23. Chandrasekaran AR, Plas DT, Gonzalez E, Crair MC. Evidence for an instructive role of retinal activity in retinotopic map refinement in the superior colliculus of the mouse. J Neurosci. 2005;25(29):6929–38.

24. Shoham S, Fellows MR, Normann RA. Robust, automatic spike sorting using mixtures of multivariate t-distributions. J Neurosci Methods. 2003;127(2):111–22.

25. Warland DK, Huberman AD, Chalupa LM. Dynamics of spontaneous activity in the fetal macaque retina during development of retinogeniculate pathways. J Neurosci. 2006;26(19):5190–7.

26. Stafford BK, Sher A, Litke AM, Feldheim DA. Spatial-temporal patterns of retinal waves underlying activity-dependent refinement of retinofugal projections. Neuron. 2009;64:200–12.

27. Cutts CS, Eglen SJ. Detecting pairwise correlations in spike trains: an objective comparison of methods and application to the study of retinal waves. J Neurosci. 2014;34(43):14288–303.

28. Butts DA, Rokhsar DS. The information content of spontaneous retinal waves. J Neurosci. 2001;21:961–73.

29. Gjorgjieva J, Toyoizumi T, Eglen SJ. Burst-time-dependent plasticity robustly guides ON/OFF segregation in the lateral geniculate nucleus. PLoS Comput Biol. 2009;5:e1000618.

30. Wong RO, Meister M, Shatz CJ. Transient period of correlated bursting activity during development of the mammalian retina. Neuron. 1993;11:923–38.

31. Chandrasekaran AR, Plas DT, Gonzalez E, Crair MC. Evidence for an instructive role of retinal activity in retinotopic map refinement in the superior colliculus of the mouse. J Neurosci. 2005;25:6929–38.

32. Lupien SJ, McEwen BS, Gunnar MR, Heim C. Effects of stress throughout the lifespan on the brain, behaviour and cognition. Nat Rev Neurosci. 2009;10(6):434–45.

33. Xu HP, Burbridge TJ, Chen MG, Ge X, Zhang Y, Zhou ZJ, Crair MC. Spatial pattern of spontaneous retinal waves instructs retinotopic map refinement more than activity frequency. Dev Neurobiol. 2015;75(6):621–40.

34. Xu HP, Burbridge TJ, Ye M, Chen M, Ge X, Zhou ZJ, Crair MC. Retinal wave patterns are governed by mutual excitation among starburst Amacrine cells and drive the refinement and maintenance of visual circuits. J Neurosci. 2016;36(13):3871–86.

35. Sun C, Speer CM, Wang G-Y, Chapman B, Chalupa LM. Epibatidine application in vitro blocks retinal waves without silencing all retinal ganglion cell action potentials in developing retina of the mouse and ferret. J Neurophysiol. 2008;100:3253–63.

36. Speer CM, Sun C, Liets LC, Stafford BK, Chapman B, Cheng HJ. Eye-specific retinogeniculate segregation proceeds normally following disruption of patterned spontaneous retinal activity. Neural Dev. 2014;9:25.

37. Thompson ID, Morgan JE, Henderson Z. The effects of monocular enucleation on ganglion cell number and terminal distribution in the ferret's retinal pathway. Eur J Neurosci. 1993;5(4):357–67.

38. Marder E. Neuromodulation of neuronal circuits: back to the future. Neuron. 2012;76(1):1–11.

39. Muller M, Hollander H. A small population of retinal ganglion cells projecting to the retina of the other eye. Exp Brain Res. 1988;71:611–7.

40. Bunt SM, Lund RD. Development of a transient retino-retinal pathway in hooded and albino rats. Brain Res. 1981;211(2):399–404.

41. Toth P, Straznicky C. Retino-retinal projections in three anuran species. Neurosci Lett. 1989;104(1–2):43–7.

# 8

# Lacking of palladin leads to multiple cellular events changes which contribute to NTD

Juan Tan[1,2], Xue-Jiao Chen[1,2], Chun-Ling Shen[1], Hong-Xin Zhang[1], Ling-Yun Tang[1,2], Shun-Yuan Lu[1], Wen-Ting Wu[3], Ying Kuang[3], Jian Fei[3] and Zhu-Gang Wang[1,2,3*]

## Abstract

**Background:** The actin cytoskeleton-associated protein palladin plays an important role in cell motility, morphogenesis and adhesion. In mice, Palladin deficient embryos are lethal before embryonic day (E) 15.5, and exhibit severe cranial neural tube and body wall closure defects. However, the mechanism how palladin regulates the process of cranial neural tube closure (NTC) remains unknown.

**Methods:** In this paper, we use gene knockout mouse to elucidate the function of palladin in the regulation of NTC process.

**Results:** We initially focus on the expression pattern of *palladin* and found that in embryonic brain, *palladin* is predominantly expressed in the neural folds at E9.5. We further check the major cellular events in the neural epithelium that may contribute to NTC during the early embryogenesis. Palladin deficiency leads to a disturbance of cytoskeleton in the neural tube and the cultured neural progenitors. Furthermore, increased cell proliferation, decreased cell differentiation and diminished apical cell apoptosis of neural epithelium are found in palladin deficient embryos. Cell cycle of neural progenitors in *Palladin*[-/-] embryos is much shorter than that in wt ones. Cell adhesion shows a reduction in *Palladin*[-/-] neural tubes.

**Conclusions:** *Palladin* is expressed with proper spatio-temporal pattern in the neural folds. It plays a crucial role in regulating mouse cranial NTC by modulating cytoskeleton, proliferation, differentiation, apoptosis, and adhesion of neural epithelium. Our findings facilitate further study of the function of palladin and the underlying molecular mechanism involved in NTC.

**Keywords:** Palladin, Neural tube defect, Cytoskeleton, Proliferation, Differentiation, Apoptosis

## Background

Neurulation is the process that gives rise to the central nervous system, whereby the neural plate undergoes bending, elevating, fusion and remodeling to form the neural tube [1, 2]. In the mouse, neurulation is divided into two phases, primary and secondary neurulation. The brain and most of the spinal cord are created during primary neurulation, while the rest of the spinal cord is created during secondary neurulation. In primary neurulation, NTC is typically initiated at the midline of the hindbrain/cervical boundary, which is termed closure 1. Then neural tube fusion proceeds bi-directionally, toward both the hindbrain and the spinal cord. NTC also initiates at the midbrain/forebrain boundary and the rostral end of the forebrain, these two initiation points are designated closure 2 and closure 3, respectively. Then closure 2 proceeds caudally and rostrally, closure 3 proceeds caudally. After closure 2 meets closure 1 at the midbrain/hindbrain neuropore, and closure 3 meets closure 2 at the anterior neuropore, the whole neural tube closes completely [1, 3]. With the contribution of genetic and environmental factors, neural tube may fail to close, causing neural tube defects (NTDs) [4]. NTDs

* Correspondence: zhugangw@shsmu.edu.cn
[1]State Key Laboratory of Medical Genomics, Research Center for Experimental Medicine, Rui-Jin Hospital Affiliated to Shanghai Jiao Tong University School of Medicine (SJTUSM), Building 17, No. 197, Ruijin 2nd Rd, Shanghai 200025, China
[2]Model Organism Division, E-Institutes of Shanghai Universities, SJTUSM, Shanghai 200025, China
Full list of author information is available at the end of the article

are the second most common birth defects with an incidence of 1:1000 in human births, after congenital heart defects [3]. In terms of occurring at different axial levels, there are three types of NTDs: exencephaly, spina bifida and craniorachischisis, representing the cranial region NTDs, spinal cord NTDs and NTDs along the entire body axis, respectively [5].

Animal models ranging from flies to mice have been used to explore the mechanisms underlying NTC [6–10]. By 2009, the number of mouse mutants and strains with NTDs exceeds 240, including 205 specific genes, 30 unidentified genes, and 9 multifactorial strains. These genes encode many diverse proteins that participate in cellular functions and biochemical pathways [11]. With in toto live imaging of mouse morphogenesis technology, the NTC process can be observed intuitively [12, 13]. Cellular events involved in NTC have been clarified, including actin organization, proliferation, differentiation, apoptosis, adhesion and so on [9, 10, 14]. However the molecular mechanisms behind the complex process remain poorly understood.

*Palladin* was first found to be one of genes whose expressions were up-regulated in acute promyelocytic leukemia cell line NB4 with all-trans retinoic acid (ATRA) treatment [15]. Shortly thereafter, it was reported to colocalize with α-actinin in stress fibers [16]. To study the function of palladin in vivo, we previously generated *palladin* gene knockout mice through homologous recombination, and observed NTD in palladin deficient embryos which died before E15.5 [17]. We demonstrated that peripheral nerves were not significantly stunted and neurite outgrowth was not impaired in *Palladin*[-/-] embryos [18]. However the reason that deletion of palladin causes NTD was still unknown. Over the past years, research on palladin has been focused on its interacting proteins [19, 20], its role in tumorigenesis and tumor invasion [21–24]. There are no other but our previous reports on studying its role in NTC. With the gene knockout mouse model, we have the advantages to study the role that palladin plays during NTC process. In this article, we describe that *palladin* expresses predominantly in the neural folds at E9.5 in wt mouse embryonic brain. NTD caused by palladin deficiency exhibits normal neural tube closure 1 but defective closure 2 and closure 3. Deletion of palladin leads to disrupted cytoskeleton, increased cell proliferation, decreased differentiation apoptosis, and cell adhesion in the developing neural folds. These results may partially explain the causes of NTD in *Palladin*[-/-] embryos.

## Methods

### Mice

Mice containing a heterozygous deletion of palladin were generated previously [17], and maintained on an inbred 129/Sv background under specific pathogen-free (SPF) conditions.

### Genotyping

Embryos at E9.5 were collected at somite stage 17–21, embryos at E10.5 were collected at somite stage 32–36. All experiments were performed using somite matched wt and *Palladin*[-/-] embryos. Genotype analysis of embryos and adult mice was performed as previously described [17].

### Immunofluorescence staining

Embryos were dissected and fixed in 4% paraformaldehyde overnight at 4 °C, dehydrated by sucrose series, then frozen in a Tissue Tek O.C.T. compound (Sakura Finetek, Torrance, CA), and processed to generate 10 μm frozen sections. For immunofluorescence staining, sections were treated with frozen absolute acetone for 10 min, air dried, washed with PBS and blocked with 10% normal goat serum (Jackson ImmunoResearch Laboratories) in 5% BSA/PBS for 15 min at room temperature. After incubation overnight at 4 °C with primary antibodies listed in Additional file 4: Table S1, fluorescently labeled secondary antibodies (Invitrogen) were then used and incubated for 1 h at room temperature. After antibody staining, sections were counterstained with DAPI and mounted with fluorescent mounting medium (Dako). Imaging was performed on a Nikon Eclipse 80i.

### Neural progenitors preparation

E10.5 embryonic telencephalons were microscopically dissected to separate the neuroepithelium from the mesenchyme and non-neural ectoderm. The tissue was triturated and trypsinized into single-cell suspension. Single cells were then cultured in DMEM/F-12 medium, a neural progenitor culture medium, containing 20 ng/ml EGF (R&D systems) and 20 ng/ml bFGF (R&D systems) to maintain the pluripotency. Neural progenitor cells were identified by immunofluorescence with an antibody against Nestin.

### Whole mount in situ hybridization (WISH)

WISH probes corresponding to the open reading frame were performed as previously described [25]. WISH was performed according to a standard procedure with optimization [25]. Briefly, embryos were dissected and fixed in 4% paraformaldehyde overnight at 4 °C, dehydrated and rehydrated through a graded methanol series. Embryos were then permeabilized with 10 μg/ml proteinase K in PBS for 30 min at room temperature, hybridized with 1 μg/ml digoxigenin (DIG)-UTP-labeled antisense or sense riboprobes at 68 °C. After hybridization, embryos were washed and incubated with blocking reagent for 1 h at room temperature, and then incubated with Anti-DIG-AP Conjugate (Roche) overnight at 4 °C. Signals were detected using a DIG Nucleic Acid Detection Kit (Roche). Images were taken using a Nikon SMZ 800. Primer pairs for *Palladin* isoform 2 are: sense primer: CACACAC TCGGCGCACACGC; antisense primer: CAACTGGGC ACCAAATACGC.

### TUNEL assay
Apoptotic cells on sections were detected using an In Situ Cell Death Detection Kit (Roche) according to the manufacturer's protocol. Images were taken with a Nikon fluorescent microscope.

### Quantitative RT-PCR (qRT-PCR)
Total RNA was extracted from E9.5 and E10.5 embryonic brains using TriPure Isolation Reagent (Roche) according to the manufacturer's instructions. The RNA was immediately reverse transcribed into cDNA using PrimeScript RT reagent kit (Takara) according to the manufacturer's protocol. The process was performed under the following conditions: 37 °C for 15 min, followed by 85 °C for 5 s. SYBR Premix Ex Taq (Takara) was used for qRT-PCR with gene specific primers that amplified across exon-exon junctions. qRT-PCR was performed on an ABI Fast 7500 using the cycling conditions: 95 °C for 30 s, followed by 40 cycles of 95 °C for 5 s, 60 °C for 30 s. The transcript numbers were determined from the linear regression of the standard curves. Each qRT-PCR was performed in triplicate with normalization to *Gapdh* expression level.

### Western blot analysis
Embryonic brains were dissected and treated with radio immunoprecipitation assay (RIPA) lysis buffer (1% Nonidet P-40, 0.1% SDS and 0.5% sodium deoxycholate in PBS) with protease inhibitors mixture (Sigma). The protein concentration was assayed by BCA protein assay kit (Thermo). 50 μg of proteins were separated by SDS/PAGE. The following antibodies and dilutions were used: anti-Cyclin E polyclonal antibody (1:500, Santa cruz), anti-α-actinin monoclonal antibody (1:800, Sigma-aldrich), and anti-GAPDH monoclonal antibody (1:500, Santa cruz). The membranes were incubated with secondary antibodies (LI-COR), and then scanned with the LI-COR Odyssey imaging system.

### Cumulative BrdU Assay
Cumulative BrdU labeling in E10.5 embryos was performed as previously described [26, 27]. Briefly, pregnant female mice were intraperitoneally injected with BrdU (1 mg BrdU per 20 g body weight). A series of repeated BrdU injection was performed at an interval of two hours with the following time points: 30 min, 2 h 30 min, 4 h 30 min, 6 h 30 min, and 8 h 30 min.

Embryos ($n = 5$ at each time point) were fixed 30 min after the last injection, and processed to generate frozen sections. Samples were then treated with 2 N HCl at 37 °C for 30 min, washed with PBS, incubated with 20 μg/ml proteinase K for 10 min at room temperature, and treated with 0.1% Triton X-100 for 10 min at room temperature for cell permeabilization. Treated sections were incubated with an anti-BrdU antibody at 4 °C overnight. Signals were detected using an Alexa Fluor 488 conjugated antibody. The proportion of BrdU positive nuclei of neural progenitors was used to calculate Tc (total cell-cycle length) and Ts (S phase) as previously described [26].

### Statistical analysis
The Student's *t* test was used for statistical analyses. Standard deviation was used to measure deviation from the mean, for all experiments. For all of the statistical tests, *p* values less than 0.05 were considered statistically significant.

## Results
### Palladin deficient embryos exhibited severe cranial NTD
We have previously constructed *palladin* knockout mice. *Palladin*$^{-/-}$ embryos showed severe cranial NTD and died before E15.5 [17]. To further understand why palladin disruption causes cranial NTD, we collected embryos at E9.5 when *Palladin*$^{-/-}$ embryos can be distinguished from wt littermates by their failure to close the cranial neural tube. We found that cranial neural tube closure 1 initiated normally in *Palladin*$^{-/-}$ embryos, yet closure 2 and closure 3 could not occur. Therefore they displayed complete exencephaly from forebrain to hindbrain (Fig. 1A).

The embryonic central nervous system (CNS) is patterned along its left-right, dorsal-ventral, and antero-posterior axes [28]. Neural patterning is the process that provides regional identities in neural cells in accordance with their location in the neural tube. In order to investigate whether palladin deficiency impairs the neural patterning process, we used a brain mesenchyme molecular marker *Twist* and a fore/midbrain molecular marker *Otx2* to examine the development of certain parts of embryonic brain [29, 30]. The expression pattern of these two molecules was not obviously altered in *Palladin*$^{-/-}$ embryos at E9.5 (Additional file 1: Figure S1).

### *Palladin* was located predominantly in the neural folds at E9.5
We have previously determined that in E8.5 mouse embryo, *palladin* was mainly expressed in neural plate, while in E9.5 and E10.5 embryos, it showed ubiquitous expression [17]. However, the specific cell types in embryo where each isoform is expressed remain obscure.

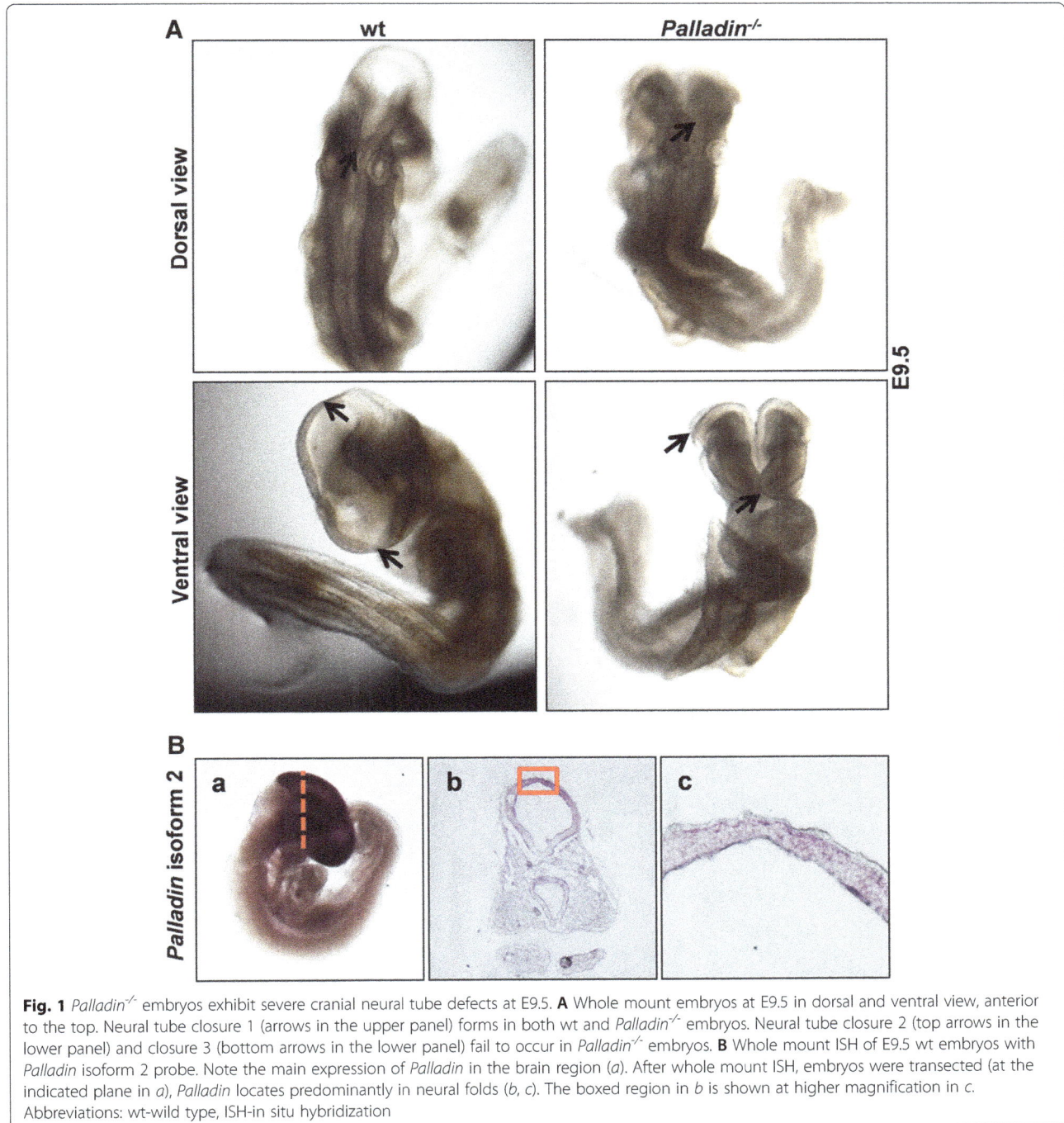

**Fig. 1** *Palladin*[-/-] embryos exhibit severe cranial neural tube defects at E9.5. **A** Whole mount embryos at E9.5 in dorsal and ventral view, anterior to the top. Neural tube closure 1 (arrows in the upper panel) forms in both wt and *Palladin*[-/-] embryos. Neural tube closure 2 (top arrows in the lower panel) and closure 3 (bottom arrows in the lower panel) fail to occur in *Palladin*[-/-] embryos. **B** Whole mount ISH of E9.5 wt embryos with *Palladin* isoform 2 probe. Note the main expression of *Palladin* in the brain region (*a*). After whole mount ISH, embryos were transected (at the indicated plane in *a*), *Palladin* locates predominantly in neural folds (*b*, *c*). The boxed region in *b* is shown at higher magnification in *c*. Abbreviations: wt-wild type, ISH-in situ hybridization

There are at least five *palladin* isoforms that produce proteins in mice due to alternative splicing and different promoter usage: isoform 1 encodes a 200 kDa protein, isoform 2 encodes a 140 kDa protein, isoform 3 and 4 encode 90–95 kDa proteins, isoform 5 encodes a 50 kDa protein [31]. Isoform 2 is the major isoform in mice brain. To identify the specific *palladin* isoforms that expressed in E9.5 mouse brains, we extracted total mRNA from E9.5 wt brains and conducted qRT-PCR using isoform-specific primers. Isoform 2 was detected to express at much higher level than the other four isoforms (Additional file 2: Figure S2). To further characterize the expression pattern of isoform 2 during cranial NTC at E9.5, WISH on E9.5 wt embryos were performed. Embryos were then processed to generate 10 μm frozen sections. We found that the expression of *Palladin* isoform 2 was restricted to the neural tube, with no expression detected in mesenchyme or non-neural ectoderm (Fig. 1B). Considering the complete exencephaly phenotype observed in *Palladin*<sup>-/-</sup> embryos, combined with the neural folds expression pattern of *palladin*, it would be reasonable to hypothesize that palladin might affect cranial NTC by regulating neural folds behavior. In order to confirm this hypothesis, we examined major cellular events that are essential for neural epithelium during cranial NTC. Cellular events have been inspected included cytoskeleton, proliferation, differentiation, apoptosis and adhesion.

### Cytoskeleton architecture was disturbed in palladin deficient neural folds and cultured neural progenitors

Palladin is an actin cytoskeleton-associated protein. We have previously reported that palladin deficiency resulted

in weakened actin stress fibers in mouse embryonic fibroblast (MEF) cells [17]. It is possible that cytoskeleton architecture in *Palladin*<sup>-/-</sup> neural folds might be affected. To verify this speculation, transverse cryosections at the presumptive mid/hindbrain region from wt and *Palladin*<sup>-/-</sup> embryos at E9.5 were stained with an F-actin marker FITC-phalloidin to visualize actin stress fibers. The actin stress fibers (phalloidin positive) in *Palladin*<sup>-/-</sup> neural tube were obviously fainter than those in somite matched wt counterpart (Fig. 2A, a and b). We also stained these sections with an antibody against cytoskeleton marker P-cofilin to confirm this observation. Conformably, actin cytoskeleton architecture was more obscure in *Palladin*<sup>-/-</sup> neural tube compared with wt neural tube (Fig. 2A, c and d).

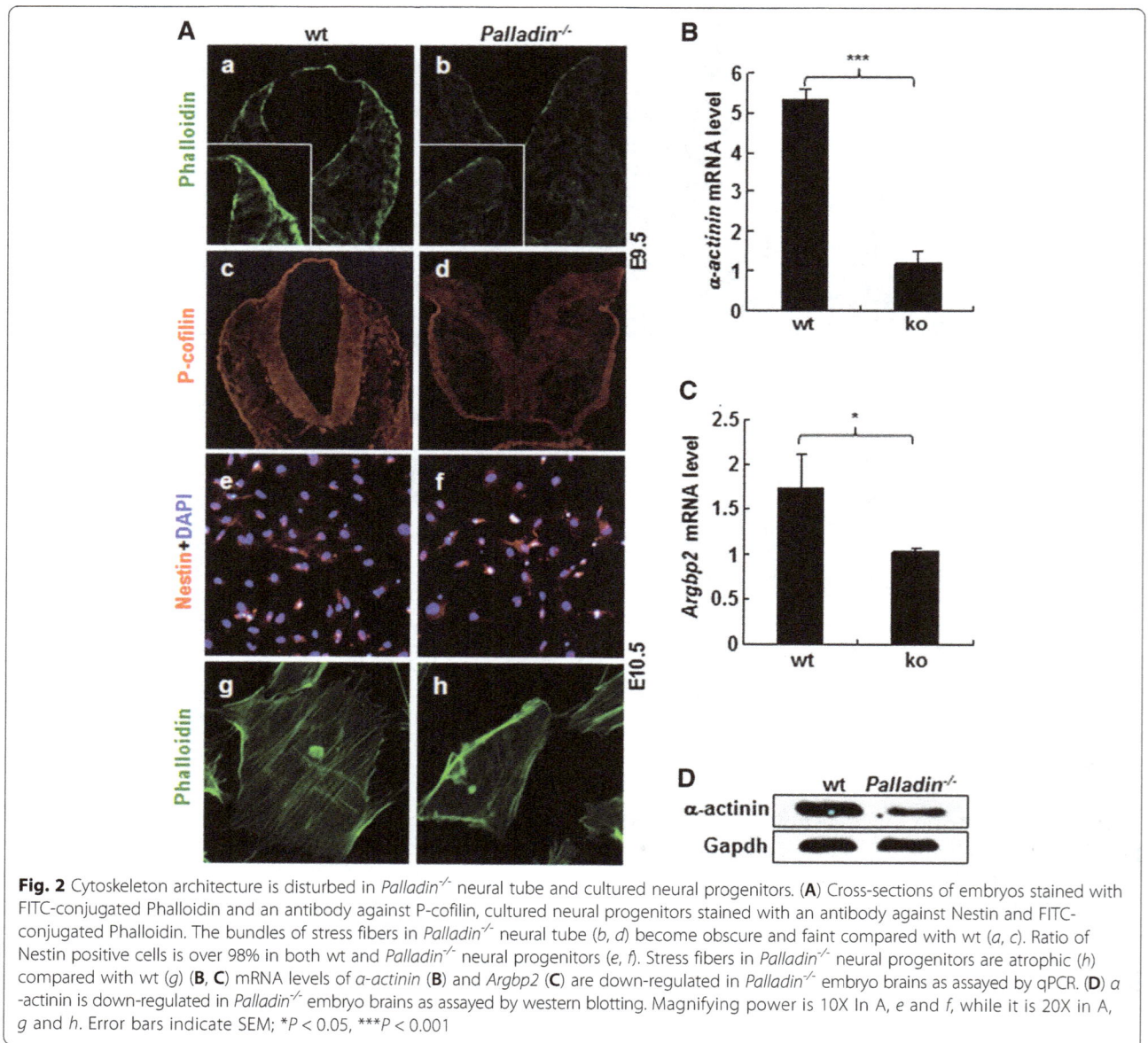

**Fig. 2** Cytoskeleton architecture is disturbed in *Palladin*<sup>-/-</sup> neural tube and cultured neural progenitors. (**A**) Cross-sections of embryos stained with FITC-conjugated Phalloidin and an antibody against P-cofilin, cultured neural progenitors stained with an antibody against Nestin and FITC-conjugated Phalloidin. The bundles of stress fibers in *Palladin*<sup>-/-</sup> neural tube (*b, d*) become obscure and faint compared with wt (*a, c*). Ratio of Nestin positive cells is over 98% in both wt and *Palladin*<sup>-/-</sup> neural progenitors (*e, f*). Stress fibers in *Palladin*<sup>-/-</sup> neural progenitors are atrophic (*h*) compared with wt (*g*) (**B**, **C**) mRNA levels of *a-actinin* (**B**) and *Argbp2* (**C**) are down-regulated in *Palladin*<sup>-/-</sup> embryo brains as assayed by qPCR. (**D**) *a*-actinin is down-regulated in *Palladin*<sup>-/-</sup> embryo brains as assayed by western blotting. Magnifying power is 10X In A, *e* and *f*, while it is 20X in A, *g* and *h*. Error bars indicate SEM; *P < 0.05, ***P < 0.001

To determine the phenotype of cytoskeleton in *Palladin*$^{-/-}$ neural tube in vitro, neural progenitors taken from E10.5 embryonic neuroepithelium were prepared and subjected to immunostaining with Nestin (a neural stem cell and neural progenitor marker). Results showed that both wt and *Palladin*$^{-/-}$ neural progenitors were more than 98% Nestin positive (Fig. 2A, e and f), which confirmed they were truly neural progenitors. Neural progenitors were then stained with FITC-phalloidin. F-actin showed a significant decrease in E10.5 *Palladin*$^{-/-}$ neuroepithelium-derived neural progenitors, compared to that in wt neural progenitors (Fig. 2A, g and h).

In order to understand the mechanism behind the decreased cytoskeleton in *Palladin*$^{-/-}$ neural tube, total RNAs were extracted from E9.5 wt and *Palladin*$^{-/-}$ embryonic brains, and reverse transcribed into cDNAs. The mRNA expression of cytoskeleton related proteins which can interact with palladin were then detected in these two genotypic cDNAs by qRT-PCR. Genes have been detected included α-actinin, Argbp2, Eps8, VASP, AKT1, Profilin, LASP1, Clp36, Spin90, Ezrin, ILKAP, LPP and Src [20, 31–41]. The expression of both α-actinin and Argbp2 showed a significant decrease in *Palladin*$^{-/-}$ embryonic brain-derived cDNAs compared to that in wt cDNAs (Fig. 2B-C). mRNA levels of Eps8, VASP, AKT1, Profilin, LASP1, Clp36, Spin90, Ezrin, ILKAP, LPP and Src showed no remarkable difference between wt and *Palladin*$^{-/-}$ brain at E9.5 (Additional file 3: Figure S3A). To confirm this finding, proteins from wt and *Palladin*$^{-/-}$ embryonic brains were prepared to perform western blot assay, α-actinin was remarkably down-regulated in *Palladin*$^{-/-}$ embryonic brains (Fig. 2D). The decreased expression of these two genes may contribute to the disturbed cytoskeleton in *Palladin*$^{-/-}$ neural tube.

### Loss of palladin resulted in increased proliferation and abnormal differentiation in neural folds

Cytoskeleton-associated proteins play a role in cell proliferation [42]. Previous studies noted that proper proliferation of neural progenitor cells is critical to NTC [43]. The observation that *Palladin*$^{-/-}$ embryos displayed NTD suggested that proliferation might be disrupted in *Palladin*$^{-/-}$ embryos. Therefore, transverse cryosections from wt and *Palladin*$^{-/-}$ embryos at E9.5 and E10.5 were stained with antibodies against phosphorylated-histone H3-Ser10 (PH3, a M phase marker, marking mitotic cells) and Ki67 (a late G1-M phase marker, marking all dividing cells). For PH3 staining, the number of PH3-positive cells was greatly increased in the region of neural tube at both E9.5 and E10.5 (Fig. 3A, a, b, e and f). PH3-positive cells in the neural tubes were quantitated for 3 sections of each embryo (five embryos from each genotype were stained). The average cell number was compared using unpaired two-tailed student's *t* test

between wt and *Palladin*$^{-/-}$ neural tube. It led to a significant difference in both E9.5 and E10.5 embryos (Fig. 3B). Results also showed that at E9.5, there were more PH3-positive cells in dorsal than ventral neural tube in wt embryos (Fig. 3A, a). However, in *Palladin*$^{-/-}$ embryos, the distribution of PH3-positive cells was more uniform between the dorsal and ventral aspect of the cranial neural tube (Fig. 3A, b). At E10.5, when the cranial NTC finished, proliferation was uniform along the dorso-ventral axis in both wt and *Palladin*$^{-/-}$ embryos (Fig. 3A, e and f). Moreover, at E9.5, PH3-positive cells specifically distributed at the first layer of neural epithelium at the duct edge in wt neural tube, while they could also been seen in the more internal area in *Palladin*$^{-/-}$ neural tube (arrows in Fig. 3A, a and b). The abnormal proliferation showed in *Palladin*$^{-/-}$ embryos was confirmed by Ki67 staining. Proliferation was enormously increased in *Palladin*$^{-/-}$ neural tube at both E9.5 and E10.5 (Fig. 3A, c, d, g and h).

The development of the nervous system is a very complicated process. It is not only spatially but also temporally regulated, depending on the production of functionally diverse neuronal cell types at their proper locations. Differentiation and proliferation of neural epithelium are related and interdependent. Considering the abnormally increased proliferation in *Palladin*$^{-/-}$ embryos, we speculated that differentiation might be disrupted. Therefore, we stained embryos at E9.5 and E10.5 with antibody against TuJ1 (also know as beta III Tubulin, a neuronal differentiation marker). At E9.5, in the ventral side of wt neural tube, neural progenitors began to exit the cell cycle, and gradually differentiate into neurons and glial cells, while no differentiation could be seen in *Palladin*$^{-/-}$ embryos at the same domain (Fig. 3A, c and d). Instead, differentiation was observed in the dorsal half of the neural tube in *Palladin*$^{-/-}$ embryos, which was not obvious in wt embryos (Fig. 3A, c and d). Interestingly, the area with decreased differentiation in the ventral side of neural tube was corresponding to the region of abnormally increased proliferation in *Palladin*$^{-/-}$ neural tube. Moreover, at E10.5, with more proliferation in *Palladin*$^{-/-}$ than wt embryos, differentiation declined in *Palladin*$^{-/-}$ embryos compared with wt counterparts (Fig. 3A, g and h). This unique correlated pattern of proliferation and differentiation is a confusing issue.

### Decreased cell-cycle length in palladin deficient neural progenitors

In order to further elucidate the defects of increased proliferation and decreased differentiation, cryosections from E10.5 wt and *Palladin*$^{-/-}$ embryos were stained with antibodies against Sox9 (a neural progenitor marker) and P27 (a differentiated neuron marker). The number of Sox9 positive cells and P27 positive cells in the ventral

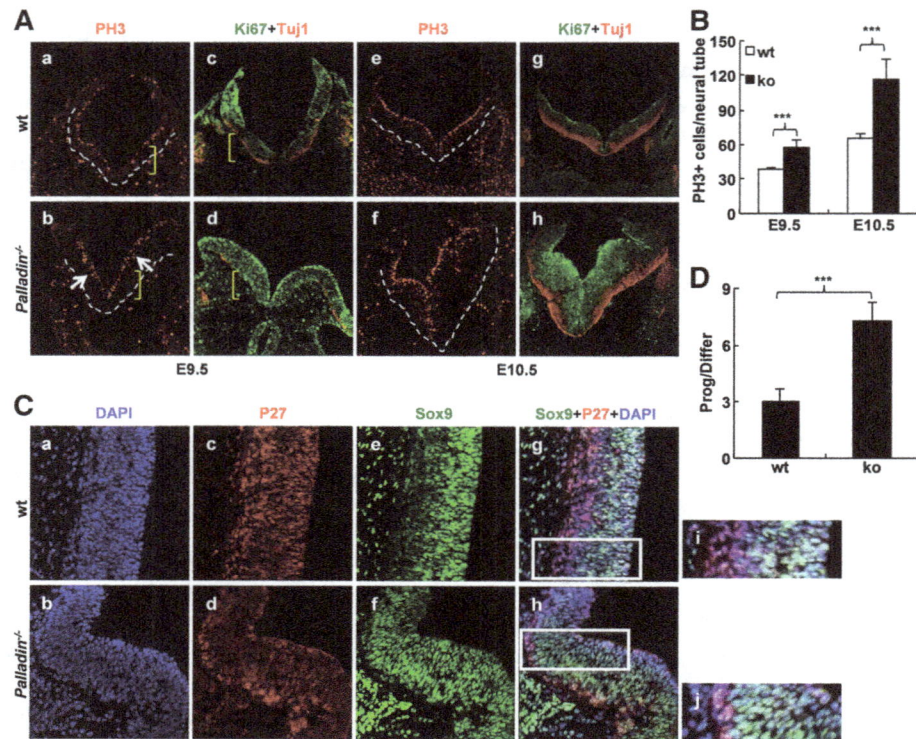

**Fig. 3** Proliferation is increased while differentiation is reduced in *Palladin*[-/-] neural tube. (**A**) Cross-sections of embryos are detected for PH3, Ki67 and Tuj1. Proliferation is increased in *Palladin*[-/-] neural tube at both E9.5 (*b, green in d*) and E10.5 (*f, green in h*). At E9.5, differentiation mainly occurs in the ventral side of wt neural tube (*red in c*) but dorsal side of *Palladin*[-/-] neural tube (*red in d*). Differentiation is decreased in the ventral side of neural tube in *Palladin*[-/-] at E10.5 (*red in g and h*). (**B**) Quantification of PH3-positive cells in the neural tube region at both E9.5 and E10.5. (**C**) E10.5 neural tubes are detected for Sox9 and P27. Neural progenitors (*green*) are increased and differentiated neurons (*red*) are reduced in *Palladin*[-/-] neural tube. The boxed region in *g and h* are shown at higher magnification in *i and j* respectively. (**D**) Quantification of the ratio of progenitors to differentiated neurons at E10.5. White dotted lines outline the neural tube, yellow brackets indicate ventral side of the neural tube, while arrows indicate abnormal proliferation in the internal area of neural tube. Error bars indicate SEM; ***$P < 0.001$

side of neural tube was quantitated respectively to represent the neural progenitors and the differentiated neurons. Results showed neural progenitors increased and differentiated neurons decreased in *Palladin*[-/-] neural tube (Fig. 3C). The ratio of proliferating neural progenitors to differentiated neurons was more than 2-fold increased in *Palladin*[-/-] embryos than that in wt controls (Fig. 3D). Also qPCR analysis of neural progenitor genes *Sox9*, *Nestin* and *Pax6* and differentiation genes *MAP2*, *Olig2* and *Neurogenin2* was performed to address the phonotype of increased proliferation and decreased differentiation, it turned out that the expression of *Sox9* increased in *Palladin*[-/-] embryos (Additional file 3: Figure S3B).

Change in cell proliferation is often related to a change in cell cycle length. Embryonic cell cycle process is mediated by cyclins, cyclin-dependent kinases (cdks) and cyclin-related proteins [44]. In order to verify whether the increase of neural progenitors in E10.5 *Palladin*[-/-] neural tube was due to a shortened cell cycle length, we first examined the expression of cyclin E (a key positive regulator of cell cycle phase G1/S), by western blotting on embryonic brain

proteins from E10.5. Cyclin E showed a significant increase in *Palladin*[-/-] embryonic brain (Fig. 4A). *Cdk2* (a cyclin E binding partner) was up-regulated and *wee1* (a negative regulator of phase G1/S) was down-regulated in E10.5 *Palladin*[-/-] brain, determined by qRT-PCR of E10.5 embryonic brain cDNA (Fig. 4B-C). Expression of *Cyclin A*, *Cyclin B* and *Cyclin D1* was also addressed by qRT-PCR, it showed no significant change in *Palladin*[-/-] brain (Additional file 3: Figure S3C). This data suggested a shortened G1/S length in cell cycle of neural progenitors in *Palladin*[-/-] embryos. To verify this speculation, a cumulative BrdU incorporation study was performed. At all the five time points, the proportion of BrdU positive cells was significantly higher in *Palladin*[-/-] neural tube than that in wt neural tube (Fig. 4D). In wt cranial neural tube, the total cell cycle length minus S phase length was 7.95 h, whereas in *Palladin*[-/-] siblings it was shortened to 6.83 h (Fig. 4E).

**Decreased apoptosis in neural folds after palladin disruption**

Apoptosis plays an important role in NTC, tips of dorsal neural folds undergo apoptosis process so that the

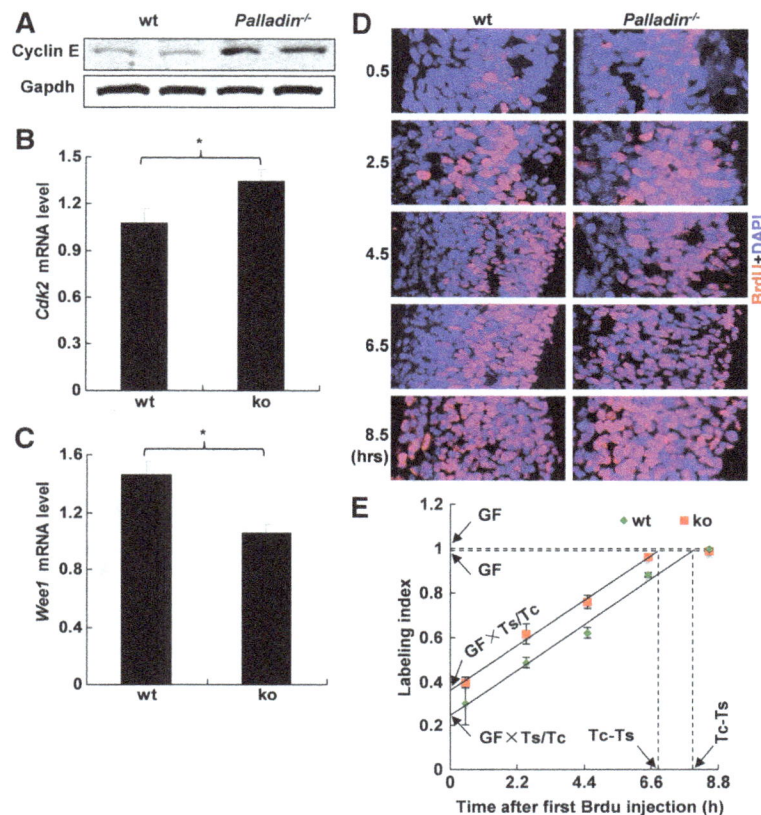

**Fig. 4** Cell cycle of *Palladin*<sup>-/-</sup> neural progenitors at E10.5 is shortened. **A** Expression of Cyclin E in *Palladin*<sup>-/-</sup> embryo brains is up-regulated at E10.5, as detected by western blotting. Expression of *Cdk2* (a cell cycle enhancer) is up-regulated (**B**) while expression of *Wee1* (a cell cycle suppressor) is down-regulated (**C**) in *Palladin*<sup>-/-</sup> embryo brain at E10.5, as assayed by qPCR. Error bars indicate SEM; *$P < 0.05$. **D** BrdU labeling of neural progenitors (*pink*) after indicated time of incubation. The proportion of BrdU-stained progenitors is higher in *Palladin*<sup>-/-</sup> neural progenitors at each time point (right panel) compared with wt (left panel). **E** Cell cycle of neural progenitors in wt and *Palladin*<sup>-/-</sup> at E10.5, Tc-Ts is 7.95 h in wt and 6.83 h in *Palladin*<sup>-/-</sup> neural progenitors ($n = 5$ at each time point). Error bars indicate SEM

neural folds can bend and both ends can meet and fuse [45]. To investigate whether NTD in *Palladin*<sup>-/-</sup> embryos was related to a change in apoptosis in the neural fold region, TUNEL assay was performed on E9.5 cryosections. It revealed that *Palladin*<sup>-/-</sup> neural folds had a lower level of apoptotic cells compared with that in wt neural folds (Fig. 5A). TUNEL positive cells were quantitated, and there was a significant decrease in *Palladin*<sup>-/-</sup> neural tube (Fig. 5B). To confirm this finding, IHC for the antibody of caspase 3 was performed. It turned out a reduction in *Palladin*<sup>-/-</sup> neural tubes (Fig. 5C).

To further explore the mechanism of decreased apoptosis, we detected key regulators of cell apoptosis by qRT-PCR on E9.5 embryonic brain cDNAs. Genes have been detected included *Bcl2*, *Bcl-xl*, *Bad* and *Bax*. *Bcl2*, a negative regulator of apoptosis, was significantly increased in *Palladin*<sup>-/-</sup> embryos (Fig. 5D, Additional file 3: Figure S3D).

## Reduced cell adhesion in *Palladin*<sup>-/-</sup> neural tubes

Cell adhesion is another important factor that regulates NTC. During the NTC process, after the formation of dorsolateral hinge point (DLHP), neural epithelium migrate from the lateral aspects of the neural tube towards the midline, neural folds then fuse at their dorsal tips to generate a closed neural tube [45]. We have previously observed that MEFs lacking of palladin showed decreased adhesion to fibronectin compared to wt MEFs [17], so we speculated that cell adhesion in *Palladin*<sup>-/-</sup> neural folds would be compromised. To assess whether palladin deficiency impaired cell adhesion on the tips of the neural folds, the expression of E-cadherin (a key component of cell adhesion) was first examined by immunofluorescence staining on E9.5 cryosections. A strong expression of E-cadherin could be detected on the tips of neural folds in both wt and *Palladin*<sup>-/-</sup> embryos, showing no significant difference (Fig. 6A).

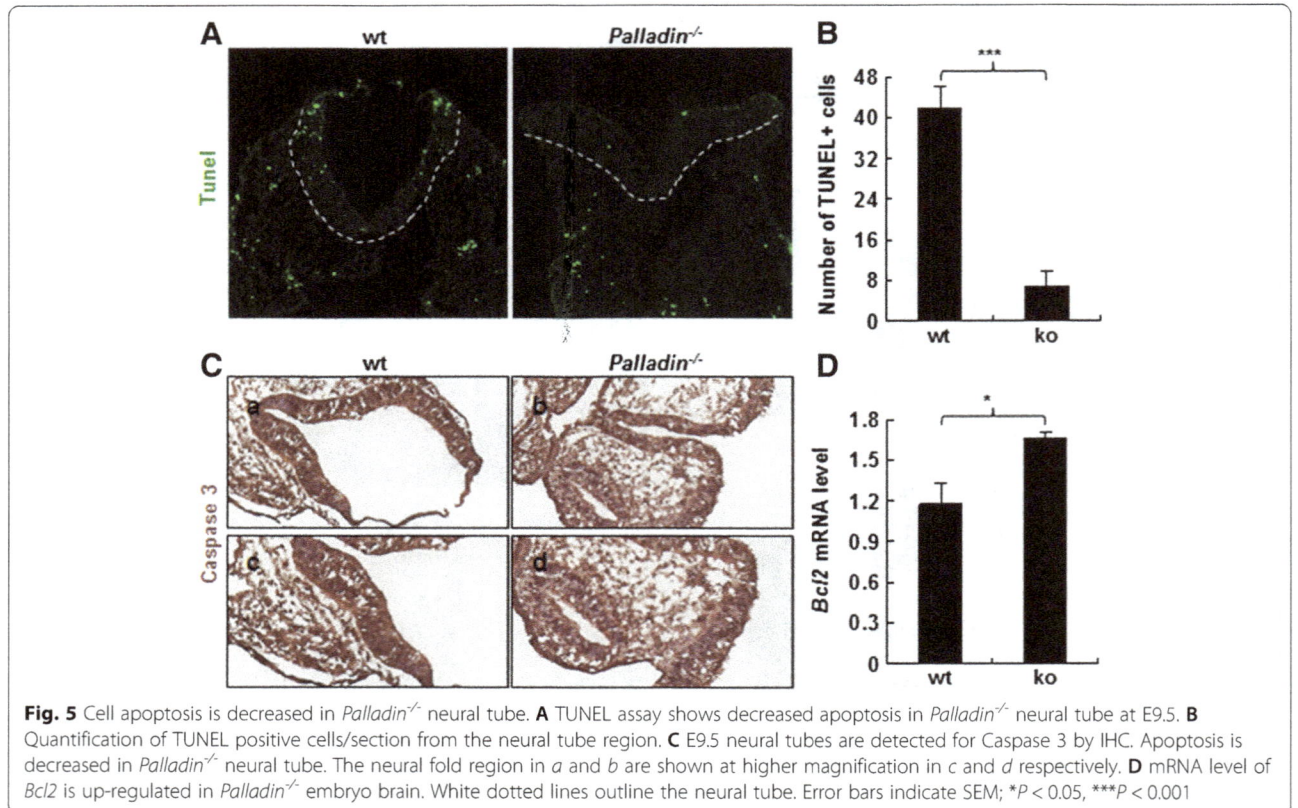

**Fig. 5** Cell apoptosis is decreased in *Palladin*−/− neural tube. **A** TUNEL assay shows decreased apoptosis in *Palladin*−/− neural tube at E9.5. **B** Quantification of TUNEL positive cells/section from the neural tube region. **C** E9.5 neural tubes are detected for Caspase 3 by IHC. Apoptosis is decreased in *Palladin*−/− neural tube. The neural fold region in *a* and *b* are shown at higher magnification in *c* and *d* respectively. **D** mRNA level of *Bcl2* is up-regulated in *Palladin*−/− embryo brain. White dotted lines outline the neural tube. Error bars indicate SEM; *$P < 0.05$, ***$P < 0.001$

We previously found that β1-integrin is significantly decreased in *Palladin*−/− MEFs [46]. Given that integrins are critical for cell adhesion and migration [47, 48], we had reasons to presume that β1-integrin might reduce in *Palladin*−/− neural tube. We checked the expression of β1-integrin on embryos at E9.5 by immunofluorescence staining, and it turned out to be a decreased β1-integrin in *Palladin*−/− neural tube (Fig. 6B).

## Discussion

Although the function of palladin on actin organization, cancer development and invasion has been described, also molecular associations of palladin have been identified one by one, little is known about the role palladin plays during NTC process. In this paper, we show how palladin regulates NTC in vivo. We found that deletion of palladin causes changes of multiple cellular events which are critical for NTC in the developing neural folds. Actin stress fibers within the neuroepithelium is fainter. Proliferation of neural epithelium is increased. Differentiation of neural progenitors is decreased and abnormal spatially. Apoptosis is decreased. Our results suggest that palladin may regulate NTC by modulating these cellular events in the developing neural folds. Hence a general genetic pathway from palladin to the control of NTC has been established. Moreover, we find expression changes of critical molecules for each

cellular events, it is absolutely useful for the establishment of direct biochemical pathway for palladin to control of NTC.

Research on expression analysis of *palladin* has been described [31], we also have investigated stage- and tissue-specific expression of *palladin* in early embryos [17], However, no reports indicate the specific cell types *palladin* is expressed during NTC, which is an important question for the study of palladin in NTC. Therefore, we perform qRT-PCR and WISH, and identify that the expression of *palladin* is highly restricted to the neural epithelium in the embryonic brain at E9.5. This indicates the particular and crucial role of palladin during NTC process. Therefore, our research focuses on the neural folds from E9.5 to E10.5.

Palladin is a cytoskeleton-associated protein. Research in vitro indicated that palladin plays a critical role in actin organization, our results confirmed this finding in vivo. Cytoskeleton is fundamental for many cellular processes, including cell proliferation and differentiation. Since loss of palladin weakens actin network in the developing neural folds, combined the phenotype of extensive outgrowth of neural epithelium in *Palladin*−/− embryos, it is an expected finding that proliferation is increased in palladin deficient embryos. Since proliferation is often related to cell cycle, shortened cell cycle

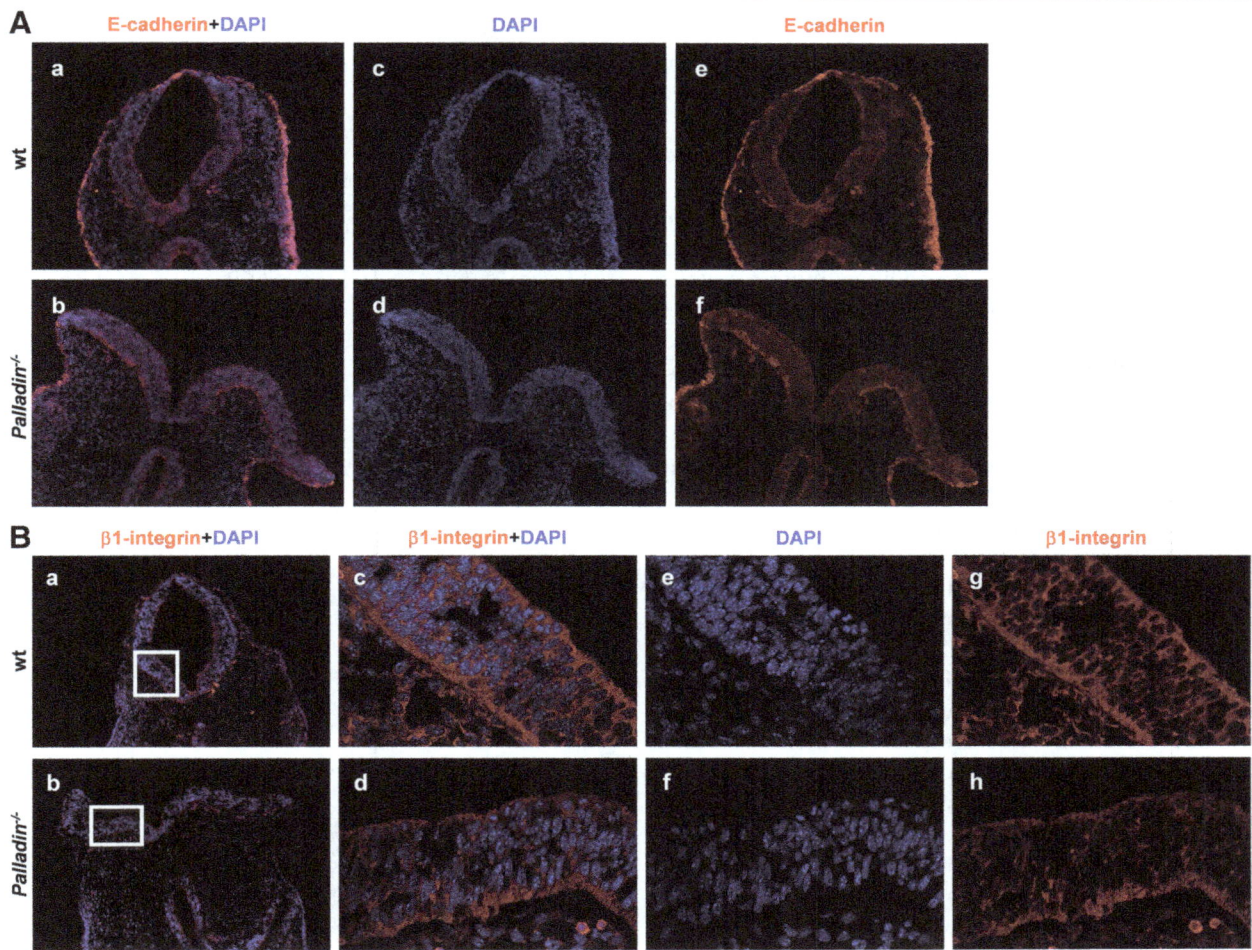

**Fig 6** Cell adhesion shows a reduction in *Palladin⁻/⁻* neural tube but not in non-neural ectoderm. (**A**) Cross-sections of wt and *Palladin⁻/⁻* embryos at E9.5 are stained with an antibody against E-cadherin to detect cell adhesion in the surface ectoderm. There is strong expression of E-cadherin at the edge of neural folds in both wt and *Palladin⁻/⁻* embryos. (**B**) Wt and *Palladin⁻/⁻* embryos at E9.5 are stained with an antibody against β1-integrin. Cell adhesion is reduced in *Palladin⁻/⁻* neural tubes (*a, c, g*) than that in wt ones (*b, d, h*). The boxed regions in *a* and *b* are shown at higher magnification in *c* and *d*, respectively

length is probably a reason of increased proliferation in neural epithelium, thus the cell cycle length was qualified in vivo by cumulative BrdU assay. It turns out a shorter cell cycle length in palladin deficient neural progenitors, which explains the phenomenon of increased proliferation. A report has showed that down-regulation of palladin enhances cell vitality and proliferation in vitro [49], which confirms our finding. However the mechanism of palladin involving in regulating proliferation and cell cycle has not yet been studied, a better understanding of this field is necessary.

The fates of neural progenitors in the ventral side of neural folds in the early embryogenesis are proliferation and differentiation. Since proliferation is increased in *Palladin⁻/⁻* neural progenitors, it is possible that differentiation in the corresponding location is decreased. To confirm this hypothesis, we quantify

the ratio of proliferating neural progenitors to differentiated neurons. It turns out a significant increased ratio in palladin deficient neural tube compared to that of wt. It should be noted that in the dorsal side of neural folds, differentiated neurons is increased in palladin deficient neural tube. This is probably a consequence of disturbed cytoskeleton within the neural tube, by differentiated neurons moving from the ventral side to the dorsal side. There is a report suggests that *palladin* knockdown may facilitate cell differentiation in vitro [49]. It is commonly accepted that dramatic cytoskeletal changes can trigger skeletal muscle differentiation. However, more research is needed to address whether the function of palladin in regulating differentiation is positive or negative.

In the dorsal side of neural folds, neural epithelium undergoes apoptosis to allow the two ends of neural folds to meet and fuse. However, proliferation is increased along the whole neural tube in palladin deficient embryos. So we examine apoptosis in the dorsal side of neural folds, it turns out a significant decreased apoptosis in palladin deficient neural folds. So far, little is known on the role palladin plays in cell apoptosis. For this reason, more research is needed to complete this field.

In our previous study, palladin plays an important role in regulating cell adhesion either in vivo or in vitro by stabilizing β1-integrin [17, 46]. In addition, other researches confirm this finding [50, 51]. So we examined the expression of β1-integrin in neural tube, and found it decreased slightly in palladin deficient neural tubes. Nevertheless, cell adhesion on the tips of neural folds is found to be normal in palladin deficient mouse embryos. It is possible that in surface ectoderm, the function of palladin in cell adhesion is compensated by other proteins in vivo during mouse NTC. Myotilin and myopalladin are members of the palladin/myotilin/myopalladin family [34]. Therefore, further study is needed to determine whether myotilin and myopalladin can functionally compensate for the loss of palladin in vivo during NTC.

NTC is an extremely complex process during embryogenesis. Other than proliferation, differentiation, apoptosis and adhesion, there are other events involved in NTC process. Correct head mesenchyme behaviors, correct cell division direction of non-neural ectoderm, intrinsic forces in neural plate are important for NTC [1, 52, 53]. Therefore, to better understand the mechanism of palladin regulating NTC, the function of palladin in these events requires further exploration.

## Conclusions

In conclusion, our results demonstrate that actin-associated protein palladin plays a role in cell proliferation, differentiation and apoptosis in the developing neural folds to regulate NTC process. Our work provides an evidence that palladin is a cell-cycle regulator spatially and temporally required for the neural epithelium proliferation. We believe our findings are helpful for further study of the function of palladin and a better understanding of the underlying molecular mechanism involved in NTC process.

## Additional files

**Additional file 1: Figure S1.** Neural patterning is normal in *Palladin*$^{-/-}$ embryos. Whole mount and section ISH of wt and *Palladin*$^{-/-}$ embryos for Twist and Otx2 at E9.5. (A) Twist is located in the head mesenchyme region in both wt (a, c, e) and *Palladin*$^{-/-}$ embryos (b, d, f). (B) Otx2 is located in the forebrain and midbrain region in both wt (a, c, e) and *Palladin*$^{-/-}$ embryos (b, d, f). The boxed regions in c and d are shown at higher magnification in e and f.

**Additional file 2: Figure S2.** Palladin isoform 2 is the main isoform expressed in E9.5 mouse brain. Detection of Palladin isoforms in E9.5 wt mouse brain by qRT-PCR using isoform-specific primers. Palladin isoform 2 is the main expressing isoform. Isoform 3 and 4 were detected in a much lower expression level. Isoform 1 and 5 were barely detected.

**Additional file 3: Figure S3.** mRNA level changes in *Palladin*$^{-/-}$ brain. mRNA levels of *Eps8, VASP, AKT1, Profilin, LASP1, Clp36, Spin90, Ezrin, ILKAP, LPP* and *Src* showed no remarkable difference between wt and *Palladin*$^{-/-}$ brain at E9.5 (A). mRNA levels of neural progenitor genes *Sox9, Nestin* and *Pax6* and differentiation genes *MAP2, Olig2* and *Neurogenin2*, expression of *Sox9* increased in *Palladin*$^{-/-}$ embryos at E10.5 (B). Expression of *Cyclin A, Cyclin B* and *Cyclin D1* showed no significant change in *Palladin*$^{-/-}$ brain at E10.5 as assayed by qPCR (C). mRNA expression of BCL-XL, Bax and Bad in wt and *Palladin*$^{-/-}$ embryonic brains. They show no significant differences between wt and *Palladin*$^{-/-}$. Error bars indicate SEM; *$P < 0.05$.

**Additional file 4: Table S1.** Antibody list.

## Abbreviations

ATRA: All-trans retinoic acid; CNS: Central nervous system; DIG: Digoxigenin; DLHP: Dorsolateral hinge point; E: Embryonic day; MEF: Mouse embryonic fibroblast; NTC: Neural tube closure; NTDs: Neural tube defects; SJTUSM: Shanghai Jiao Tong University School of Medicine; WISH: Whole mount in situ hybridization

## Acknowledgments

We thank Dr. Da Fu for critical comments and helpful suggestions on this manuscript.

## Funding

This work was partially supported by grants from the National Natural Science Foundation of China (81430028), the Ministry of Science and Technology of China (2011BAI15B02), the grants from the Science and Technology Commission of Shanghai municipality (15DZ2290800, 14ZR1425500, and 13DZ2280600), and the E-Institutes of Shanghai Municipal Education Commission (E03003).

## Authors' contributions

JT performed most of the experiments in the paper, including most of the immunofluorescence staining experiments, many of the whole mount in situ hybridization experiments and western blotting experiments, and all of the neural progenitors preparation and the cumulative BrdU assay; XC performed the genotyping, qRT-PCR and some of the immunofluorescence staining experiments; LT performed some of the whole mount in situ hybridization experiments; SL performed some of the western blotting experiments; WW performed all of the frozen sectioning experiments; ZW and JT designed the study; ZW directed the study, and obtained the funding; JT drafted the manuscript; CS and HZ revised of the manuscript; YK and JF directed the study. All authors read and approved the final manuscript.

## Competing interests

The authors declare that they have no competing interests.

## Author details

¹State Key Laboratory of Medical Genomics, Research Center for Experimental Medicine, Rui-Jin Hospital Affiliated to Shanghai Jiao Tong University School of Medicine (SJTUSM), Building 17, No. 197, Ruijin 2nd Rd, Shanghai 200025, China. ²Model Organism Division, E-Institutes of Shanghai

Universities, SJTUSM, Shanghai 200025, China. [3]Shanghai Research Center for Model Organisms, Shanghai 201203, China.

## References

1. Yamaguchi Y, Miura M. How to form and close the brain: insight into the mechanism of cranial neural tube closure in mammals. Cell Mol Life Sci. 2013;70:3171–86.
2. Sullivan-Brown J, Goldstein B. Neural tube closure: the curious case of shrinking junctions. Curr Biol. 2012;22:R574–6.
3. Copp AJ, Greene ND, Murdoch JN. The genetic basis of mammalian neurulation. Nat Rev Genet. 2003;4:784–93.
4. Kappen C. Modeling anterior development in mice: diet as modulator of risk for neural tube defects. Am J Med Genet C Semin Med Genet. 2013;163C:333–56.
5. Massarwa R, Ray HJ, Niswander L. Morphogenetic movements in the neural plate and neural tube: mouse. Wiley Interdiscip Rev Dev Biol. 2014;3:59–68.
6. Ting SB, Wilanowski T, Auden A, Hall M, Voss AK, Thomas T, Parekh V, Cunningham JM, Jane SM. Inositol- and folate-resistant neural tube defects in mice lacking the epithelial-specific factor Grhl-3. Nat Med. 2003;9:1513–9.
7. Chu CW, Gerstenzang E, Ossipova O, Sokol SY. Lulu regulates Shroom-induced apical constriction during neural tube closure. PLoS One. 2013;8:e81854.
8. Ueno N, Greene ND. Planar cell polarity genes and neural tube closure. Birth Defects Res C Embryo Today. 2003;69:318–24.
9. Pyrgaki C, Liu A, Niswander L. Grainyhead-like 2 regulates neural tube closure and adhesion molecule expression during neural fold fusion. Dev Biol. 2011;353:38–49.
10. Patterson ES, Waller LE, Kroll KL. Geminin loss causes neural tube defects through disrupted progenitor specification and neuronal differentiation. Dev Biol. 2014;393:44–56.
11. Harris MJ, Juriloff DM. An update to the list of mouse mutants with neural tube closure defects and advances toward a complete genetic perspective of neural tube closure. Birth Defects Res A Clin Mol Teratol. 2010;88:653–69.
12. Massarwa R, Niswander L. In toto live imaging of mouse morphogenesis and new insights into neural tube closure. Development. 2013;140:226–36.
13. Yamaguchi Y, Shinotsuka N, Nonomura K, Takemoto K, Kuida K, Yosida H, Miura M. Live imaging of apoptosis in a novel transgenic mouse highlights its role in neural tube closure. J Cell Biol. 2011;195:1047–60.
14. Okae H, Iwakura Y. Neural tube defects and impaired neural progenitor cell proliferation in Gbeta1-deficient mice. Dev Dyn. 2010;239:1089–101.
15. Liu TX, Zhang JW, Tao J, Zhang RB, Zhang QH, Zhao CJ, Tong JH, Lanotte M, Waxman S, Chen SJ, et al. Gene expression networks underlying retinoic acid-induced differentiation of acute promyelocytic leukemia cells. Blood. 2000;96:1496–504.
16. Parast MM, Otey CA. Characterization of palladin, a novel protein localized to stress fibers and cell adhesions. J Cell Biol. 2000;150:643–56.
17. Luo H, Liu X, Wang F, Huang Q, Shen S, Wang L, Xu G, Sun X, Kong H, Gu M, et al. Disruption of palladin results in neural tube closure defects in mice. Mol Cell Neurosci. 2005;29:507–15.
18. Shu RZ, Zhang F, Liu XS, Li CL, Wang L, Tai YL, Wu XL, Yang X, Liao XD, Jin Y, et al. Target deletion of the cytoskeleton-associated protein palladin does not impair neurite outgrowth in mice. PLoS One. 2009;4:e6916.
19. Hasegawa T, Ohno K, Funahashi S, Miyazaki K, Nagano A, Sato K. CLP36 interacts with palladin in dorsal root ganglion neurons. Neurosci Lett. 2010;476:53–7.
20. Zhou W, Cui S, Han S, Cheng B, Zheng Y, Zhang Y. Palladin is a novel binding partner of ILKAP in eukaryotic cells. Biochem Biophys Res Commun. 2011;411:768–73.
21. Goicoechea SM, Bednarski B, Stack C, Cowan DW, Volmar K, Thorne L, Cukierman E, Rustgi AK, Brentnall T, Hwang RF, et al. Isoform-specific upregulation of palladin in human and murine pancreas tumors. PLoS One. 2010;5:e10347.
22. Henderson-Jackson EB, Helm J, Strosberg J, Nasir NA, Yeatman TJ, Kvols LK, Coppola D, Nasir A. Palladin is a marker of liver metastasis in primary pancreatic endocrine carcinomas. Anticancer Res. 2011;31:2957–62.
23. Najm P, El-Sibai M. Palladin regulation of the actin structures needed for cancer invasion. Cell Adhes Migr. 2014;8:29–35.
24. Goicoechea SM, Garcia-Mata R, Staub J, Valdivia A, Sharek L, McCulloch CG, Hwang RF, Urrutia R, Yeh JJ, Kim HJ, et al. Palladin promotes invasion of pancreatic cancer cells by enhancing invadopodia formation in cancer-associated fibroblasts. Oncogene. 2014;33:1265–73.
25. Wilkinson DG, Nieto MA. Detection of messenger RNA by in situ hybridization to

tissue sections and whole mounts. Methods Enzymol. 1993;225:361–73.
26. Nowakowski RS, Lewin SB, Miller MW. Bromodeoxyuridine immunohistochemical determination of the lengths of the cell cycle and the DNA-synthetic phase for an anatomically defined population. J Neurocytol. 1989;18:311–8.
27. Kim TH, Goodman J, Anderson KV, Niswander L. Phactr4 regulates neural tube and optic fissure closure by controlling PP1-, Rb-, and E2F1-regulated cell-cycle progression. Dev Cell. 2007;13:87–102.
28. Altmann CR, Brivanlou AH. Neural patterning in the vertebrate embryo. Int Rev Cytol. 2001;203:447–82.
29. Dill KK, Thamm K, Seaver EC. Characterization of twist and snail gene expression during mesoderm and nervous system development in the polychaete annelid Capitella sp. I. Dev Genes Evol. 2007;217:435–47.
30. Puelles E, Acampora D, Lacroix E, Signore M, Annino A, Tuorto F, Filosa S, Corte G, Wurst W, Ang SL, et al. Otx dose-dependent integrated control of antero-posterior and dorso-ventral patterning of midbrain. Nat Neurosci. 2003;6:453–60.
31. Rachlin AS, Otey CA. Identification of palladin isoforms and characterization of an isoform-specific interaction between Lasp-1 and palladin. J Cell Sci. 2006;119:995–1004.
32. Boukhelifa M, Parast MM, Bear JE, Gertler FB, Otey CA. Palladin is a novel binding partner for Ena/VASP family members. Cell Motil Cytoskeleton. 2004;58:17–29.
33. Ronty M, Taivainen A, Moza M, Otey CA, Carpen O. Molecular analysis of the interaction between palladin and alpha-actinin. FEBS Lett. 2004;566:30–4.
34. Otey CA, Rachlin A, Moza M, Arneman D, Carpen O. The palladin/myotilin/myopalladin family of actin-associated scaffolds. Int Rev Cytol. 2005;246:31–58.
35. Ronty M, Taivainen A, Moza M, Kruh GD, Ehler E, Carpen O. Involvement of palladin and alpha-actinin in targeting of the Abl/Arg kinase adaptor ArgBP2 to the actin cytoskeleton. Exp Cell Res. 2005;310:88–98.
36. Boukhelifa M, Moza M, Johansson T, Rachlin A, Parast M, Huttelmaier S, Roy P, Jockusch BM, Carpen O, Karlsson R, et al. The proline-rich protein palladin is a binding partner for profilin. FEBS J. 2006;273:26–33.
37. Goicoechea S, Arneman D, Disanza A, Garcia-Mata R, Scita G, Otey CA. Palladin binds to Eps8 and enhances the formation of dorsal ruffles and podosomes in vascular smooth muscle cells. J Cell Sci. 2006;119:3316–24.
38. Jin L, Kern MJ, Otey CA, Wamhoff BR, Somlyo AV. Angiotensin II, focal adhesion kinase, and PRX1 enhance smooth muscle expression of lipoma preferred partner and its newly identified binding partner palladin to promote cell migration. Circ Res. 2007;100:817–25.
39. Ronty M, Taivainen A, Heiska L, Otey C, Ehler E, Song WK, Carpen O. Palladin interacts with SH3 domains of SPIN90 and Src and is required for Src-induced cytoskeletal remodeling. Exp Cell Res. 2007;313:2575–85.
40. Maeda M, Asano E, Ito D, Ito S, Hasegawa Y, Hamaguchi M, Senga T. Characterization of interaction between CLP36 and palladin. FEBS J. 2009;276:2775–85.
41. Chin YR, Toker A. The actin-bundling protein palladin is an Akt1-specific substrate that regulates breast cancer cell migration. Mol Cell. 2010;38:333–44.
42. May SF, Peacock L, Almeida Costa CI, Gibson WC, Tetley L, Robinson DR, Hammarton TC. The Trypanosoma brucei AIR9-like protein is cytoskeleton-associated and is required for nucleus positioning and accurate cleavage furrow placement. Mol Microbiol. 2012;84:77–92.
43. Yang SL, Yang M, Herrlinger S, Liang C, Lai F, Chen JF. MiR-302/367 regulate neural progenitor proliferation, differentiation timing, and survival in neurulation. Dev Biol. 2015;408:140–50.
44. Murray AW, Kirschner MW. Cyclin synthesis drives the early embryonic cell cycle. Nature. 1989;339:275–80.
45. Pai YJ, Abdullah NL, Mohd-Zin SW, Mohammed RS, Rolo A, Greene ND, Abdul-Aziz NM, Copp AJ. Epithelial fusion during neural tube morphogenesis. Birth Defects Res A Clin Mol Teratol. 2012;94:817–23.
46. Liu XS, Luo HJ, Yang H, Wang L, Kong H, Jin YE, Wang F, Gu MM, Chen Z, Lu ZY, et al. Palladin regulates cell and extracellular matrix interaction through maintaining normal actin cytoskeleton architecture and stabilizing beta1-integrin. J Cell Biochem. 2007;100:1288–300.
47. Jokinen J, Dadu E, Nykvist P, Kapyla J, White DJ, Ivaska J, Vehvilainen P, Reunanen H, Larjava H, Hakkinen L, et al. Integrin-mediated cell adhesion to type I collagen fibrils. J Biol Chem. 2004;279:31956–63.
48. Shafaq-Zadah M, Gomes-Santos CS, Bardin S, Maiuri P, Maurin M, Iranzo J, Gautreau A, Lamaze C, Caswell P, Goud B, et al. Persistent cell migration and adhesion rely on retrograde transport of beta(1) integrin. Nat Cell Biol. 2016;18:54–64.

49. Nguyen NU, Liang VR, Wang HV. Actin-associated protein palladin is required for migration behavior and differentiation potential of C2C12 myoblast cells. Biochem Biophys Res Commun. 2014;452:728–33.

50. Wan HT, Mruk DD, Li SY, Mok KW, Lee WM, Wong CK, Cheng CY. p-FAK-Tyr(397) regulates spermatid adhesion in the rat testis via its effects on F-actin organization at the ectoplasmic specialization. Am J Physiol Endocrinol Metab. 2013;305:E687–99.

51. Tay PN, Tan P, Lan Y, Leung CH, Laban M, Tan TC, Ni H, Manikandan J, Rashid SB, Yan B, et al. Palladin, an actin-associated protein, is required for adherens junction formation and intercellular adhesion in HCT116 colorectal cancer cells. Int J Oncol. 2010;37:909–26.

52. Schoenwolf GC, Smith JL. Mechanisms of neurulation: traditional viewpoint and recent advances. Development. 1990;109:243–70.

53. Levine AJ, Brivanlou AH. Proposal of a model of mammalian neural induction. Dev Biol. 2007;308:247–56.

# 9

# Ensheathing cells utilize dynamic tiling of neuronal somas in development and injury as early as neuronal differentiation

Evan L. Nichols[1], Lauren A. Green[1,2] and Cody J. Smith[1,2]* (iD)

## Abstract

**Background:** Glial cell ensheathment of specific components of neuronal circuits is essential for nervous system function. Although ensheathment of axonal segments of differentiated neurons has been investigated, ensheathment of neuronal cell somas, especially during early development when neurons are extending processes and progenitor populations are expanding, is still largely unknown.

**Methods:** To address this, we used time-lapse imaging in zebrafish during the initial formation of the dorsal root ganglia (DRG).

**Results:** Our results show that DRG neurons are ensheathed throughout their entire lifespan by a progenitor population. These ensheathing cells dynamically remodel during development to ensure axons can extend away from the neuronal cell soma into the CNS and out to the skin. As a population, ensheathing cells tile each DRG neuron to ensure neurons are tightly encased. In development and in experimental cell ablation paradigms, the oval shape of DRG neurons dynamically changes during partial unensheathment. During longer extended unensheathment neuronal soma shifting is observed. We further show the intimate relationship of these ensheathing cells with the neurons leads to immediate and choreographed responses to distal axonal damage to the neuron.

**Conclusion:** We propose that the ensheathing cells dynamically contribute to the shape and position of neurons in the DRG by their remodeling activity during development and are primed to dynamically respond to injury of the neuron.

**Keywords:** Development, Ensheathment, Neuronal soma, Tiling, Neural niche

## Background

Ensheathment of neuronal cells is essential for proper functioning of the nervous system. The role of ensheathment is diverse and ranges from functions such as myelination to aid neural transmission [1–3], to metabolic homeostasis and trophic support to maintain neuronal health [4, 5]. This ensheathment typically occurs at an early, yet largely undefined, time in the development of functional neural circuits and is consistently maintained following the initial ensheathment [3, 6, 7]. Disruption of ensheathment at any point can result in various pathologies depending on the cell types affected [5, 8]. Axonal ensheathment and myelination have been extensively studied, but an understanding of neuronal soma ensheathment in vertebrates remains elusive [1, 9, 10].

Studies in *C. elegans* and *Drosophila* have observed that glial subpopulations extend processes around the soma to completely ensheath the neuron [11, 12]. These soma-ensheathing glia play an important role in development. Studies in *C. elegans* demonstrate that glial association with neurons guides neuronal maturation and axonal outgrowth [13–15]. These ensheathing glia also are closely associated with the neurons and respond to changes within the cell [11]. For example, after neuronal injury these glia have been shown to respond and phagocytize debris [16]. Previous work also demonstrates that disruption of cortex glia, the cells ensheathing neuronal cell somas in *Drosophila*, leads to neuronal death, suggesting an important role of ensheathing glia

* Correspondence: csmith67@nd.edu
Department of Biological Sciences, University of Notre Dame, 015 Galvin Life Sciences Building, Notre Dame, IN 46556, USA
2Center for Stem Cells and Regenerative Medicine, University of Notre Dame, Notre Dame, IN, USA

in neuronal growth and survival [17]. Disruption to cortex glia also leads to the disorganization of neuronal and glial cell populations in the *Drosophila* CNS [17, 18]. In vertebrates, molecular communication between the neuronal soma and oligodendrocytes ensures the proper ensheathment of specific neuronal compartments, like axons [19]. Collectively, these studies point to tightly controlled and conserved interactions between ensheathing glia and sub-compartments of neurons on the macroscopic and microscopic level.

One organizational principle of glia that has emerged is cellular tiling. Tiling ensures comprehensive yet non-redundant coverage of a target area [11, 20, 21]. This principle appears to be largely universal across cell-types and phylogeny as retinal neurons [22], sensory neurons [20, 21, 23–25], oligodendrocytes [26, 27] and other ensheathing glia [17, 28] have all demonstrated tiling in numerous model systems. In glial cells, this tiling behavior has been shown to subdivide neural domains by creating a comprehensive sheathe around the target area without redundant commitment of cellular resources [29]. Disruption of glial tiling has been shown to disrupt the overall organization of neural compartments [17, 18, 30]. A hallmark of tiling is a space filling response from neighboring cells following perturbation [7, 27, 31]. For example, oligodendrocyte progenitor cells have been reported to exhibit tiling behavior following injury to mature oligodendrocytes [27]. During development, oligodendrocytes also exhibit tiling to space themselves in the spinal cord [26, 27]. Oligodendrocytes also tile with other cell types in the nervous system [28]. This tiling phenomenon with glia is likely more extensive given that both Drosophila astrocytes in the brain and cortex glia around cell somas in the CNS also exhibit tiling [18, 29]. However, the role of tiling in other glia, like those that ensheath neuronal cell somas has yet to be described in vertebrates.

During early development, neuronal populations are often associated with glial progenitors that tightly ensheath the differentiating neuron and its progenitors [32]. This ensheathment of progenitor populations has been shown to aid in strict compartmentalization of the nervous system which helps give rise to stereotyped neuronal topographies such as *Drosophila* brain lobes [11, 17, 30, 32]. The dorsal root ganglia of vertebrates (DRG) also exhibits a stereotyped sequestration of neuronal subtypes in a specific spatiotemporal manner. Mechanoreceptive and proprioceptive neurons develop first in the ventrolateral region of the DRG followed by nociceptive neurons in the dorsomedial region of the ganglion [33]. The DRG is also home to a subset of glial cells that ensheathe DRG neuronal somas: satellite glia [9, 10]. Throughout life, these cells serve as important precursors for a diverse set of cell types such as terminal glia and melanocytes that locate to the periphery [34]. During differentiation of these cells, resident precursors in the DRG

must migrate through the packed ganglia, exit and then travel along nerves to the periphery. This process of differentiation continues through adulthood.

It is currently unclear if and how satellite glia actively and continually contribute to the stereotyped topography of the DRG. However, genetic ablation of glial precursors or disruption of precursor migration to the nascent DRG has been shown to disturb proliferation and cell fate decisions, leading to an disorganized or absent DRG [23, 35, 36]. DRG neurons can also be ectopically located outside of their normal ganglia location when non-neuronal ganglia cells are disrupted [23]. These studies highlight the possibility that cellular mechanisms are constantly and dynamically employed within the ganglia to ensure neurons are stereotypically located while non-neuronal populations retain the capacity to translocate when needed.

Our understanding of these topics is limited because techniques to dynamically image and label glial progenitors distinctly from the neuron that they ensheath has been lacking. Moreover, the majority of studies that investigate ensheathment of neuronal cell somas has typically investigated the ensheathment of fully differentiated neurons. To address this, we used single cell photoconversion of glial progenitors within the nascent DRG in zebrafish. Using this approach, we visualized cells extending pericellular processes around neuronal progenitors. These sheaths were present throughout the life of the DRG, including during neurite initiation where they remodel to allow for neurite extension. We demonstrate these ensheathing cells exhibit cellular behaviors consistent with dynamic tiling in response to disruption of ensheathment of the neuronal soma in both normal development and disease states. Such pathological disruptions to the neuronal soma ensheathment also led to immediate changes in neuron size and shape, suggesting they could play an active role in restricting neuronal positioning in the ganglia. These ensheathing cells also exhibited a consistent and choreographed response to peripheral axonal injury. These data provide an important step-wise visualization of the neuronal soma ensheathment early in development and provide insight into how cell soma ensheathing glia dynamically ensure DRG neurons retain their stereotypical ganglia location.

## Methods

### Fish husbandry

All animal experiments were approved by the University of Notre Dame Institutional Animal Care and Use Committee. The zebrafish transgenic lines used in this study were *Tg(sox10:eos)* [37], *Tg(ngn1:gfp)* [38], and *Gt(foxd3:gfp)* [39]. All embryos were produced by pairwise mating and raised in egg water at 28 °C. Embryos of both sexes were used for all experiments. Stable, germline, transgenic lines were used for all experiments.

## In vivo imaging

All embryos were dechorionated at 48 hpf and anesthetized with 3-amino-benzoic acid ester. Anesthetized embryos were mounted in 0.8% low-melting point agarose and mounted on their right side in 35 mm Petri dishes with glass bottoms. For imaging, a spinning disk confocal microscope from 3i technology© was used. It is equipped with a Zeiss Axio Observer Z1 Advanced Mariana Microscope with X-cite 120LED White Light LED System and filter cubes for GFP and mRFP, a motorized X,Y stage, piezo Z stage, 20X Air (0.50 NA) objective with 2 mm working distance, 63X (1.15NA) water objective with 0.66 mm working distance, 40X (1.1NA) water objective with 0.62 mm working distance, CSU-W1 T2 Spinning Disk Confocal Head (50 uM) with 1X camera adapter, andor iXon3 1Kx1K EMCCD camera, dichroic mirrors for 446, 515, 561, 405, 488, 561, 640 excitation, laser stack containing 405 nm, 445 nm, 488 nm, 561 nm and 637 nm with laserstack FiberSwitcher that has 250 uS switch time, photomanipulation with vector© high speed point scanner ablations at diffraction limited capacity, Ablate!TM© Photoablation System (532 nm pulsed laser, pulse energy 60 J @ 200 HZ). Time lapse images were taken every 5 min over 24 h. Adobe Illustrator and ImageJ were used to process the images and enhance the brightness and contrast.

## Eos photoconversion

To label individual progenitor cells, we used Tg(sox10:eos) fish to express Eos, a photoconvertible protein in DRG cells. Upon exposure to ultraviolet light, Eos transitions from green to red emission. Using the laserstack system described above, single cells were exposed to a 405 nm laser through the z-stack [40]. This laser exposure resulted in the photoconversion of the targeted cell from green to red. Pre and post images were acquired to ensure photoconversion of single cells within the DRG was accomplished.

## Immunohistochemistry

Zebrafish were fixed and stained as previously reported [28]. Primary antibody Sox10 (rabbit, 1:5000) [28] and secondary antibody Alexa anti-mouse conjugated to 561 (Invitrogen, 1:600) was used. DAPI was also used (ThermoFisher, 1:1000).

## Focal lesioning

To create lesions of individual cells and axons, the Ablate!TM© Photoablation System described above was utilized. Adjacent, unablated DRG or axons were used as controls. One lesion at a DRG was performed in each animal. Following the lesion, time lapse images were taken as described above. Animals were placed 0.02% 3-aminobenzoic acid ester (Tricaine) in egg water with anesthetic and

mounted with 0.8% low-melting point agarose on a 10 mm glass-coverslip bottom petri dish. Confocal z-stack images of Tg(sox10:eos) at the appropriate age were taken pre-injury. A DRG cell or axon was chosen and brought into a focused ablation window. To ablate we utilized a double-clicked feature which creates an 8 um cursor tool to fire the ablate laser. All laser parameters used are specific to our confocal microscope. Specific parameters include: Laser Power (2), Raster Block Size (4), Double-Click Rectangle Size (8), Double-Click Repetitions (4).

## SU6656 treatment

A stock solution of SU6656 (Santa Cruz Biotechnology) was stored at $-20$ °C at a concentration of 375 µM in DMSO. Treated embryos were manually dechorionated at 36 hpf and incubated at 28 °C in 3 µM of SU6656 in egg water until imaging as previously described [41]. Control fish were incubated in 1.25% DMSO in egg water.

## Shape descriptors

The shape descriptors (circularity, aspect ratio, roundness, and solidity) were measured using ImageJ. They were calculated using the following formulas:

$$Circularity = \frac{4\pi \times area}{(perimeter)^2}$$

$$Aspect\ Ratio = \frac{major\ axis}{minor\ axis}$$

$$Roundness = \frac{4 \times area}{\pi \times (major\ axis)^2}$$

$$Solidity = \frac{area}{convex\ area}$$

## Quantification of approaching ensheathing processes

To create the intensity profiles found in Figs. 1g and 4b, sum z-projection frames from a 24-h timelapse were deconvolved using Autoquant Blind deconvolution in Slidebook software. Intensity profiles were created along a line that transected two approaching processes. These profiles were taken at 75 min intervals as the cellular processes approached to make a coherent sheathe around the neuron soma. All intensity values were normalized to the background intensity of the image. These graphs quantify the ensheathment of a single neuron.

## Quantification and statistical analysis

Slidebook software was used to create maximum and sum z-projections for all images used for analysis. Individual z-projections were sequentially reviewed to confirm accuracy. All data presented in graphs represent the mean of data. All error bars represent standard error of the mean. Cell tracking was performed using MTrackJ, a

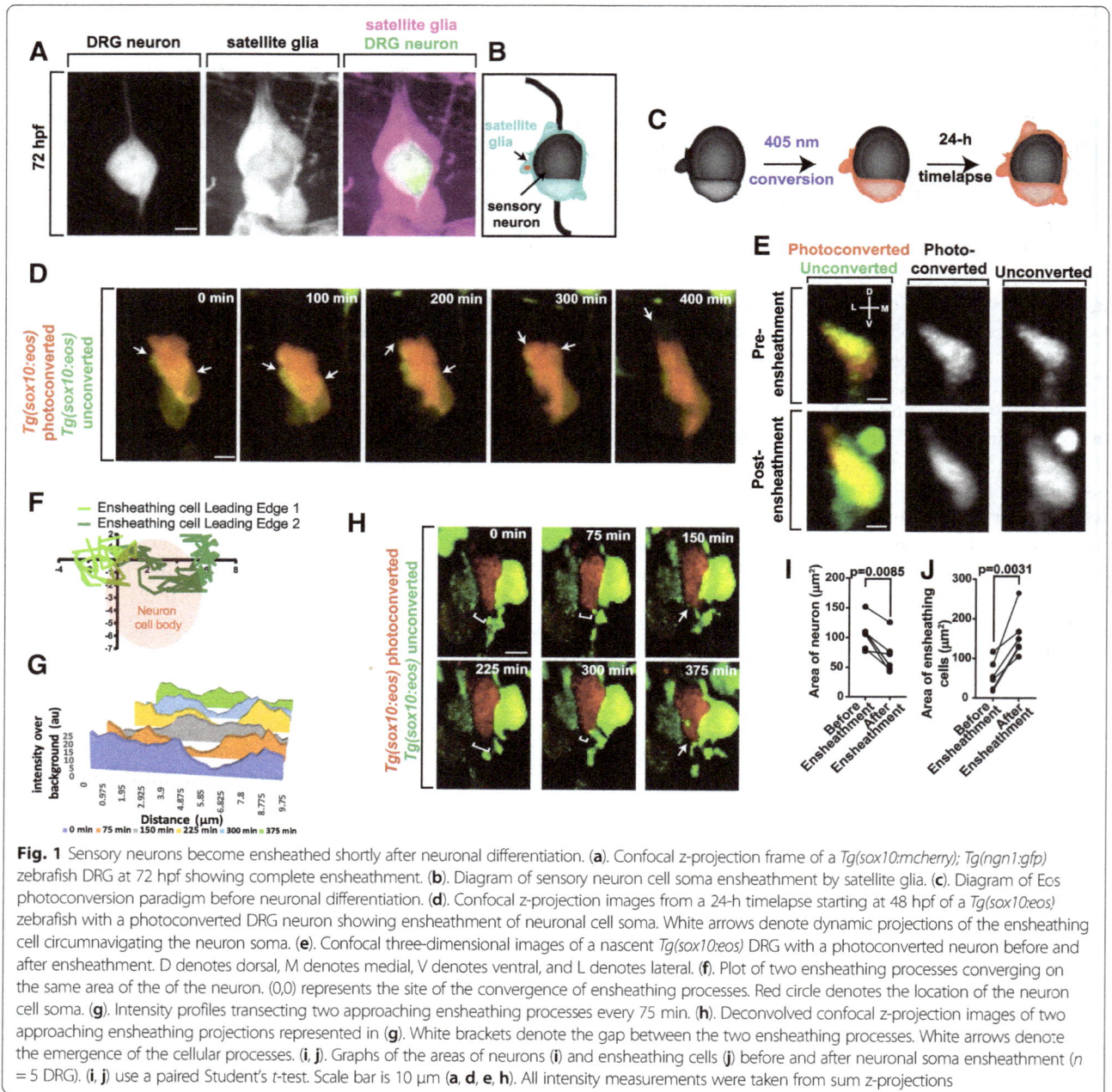

**Fig. 1** Sensory neurons become ensheathed shortly after neuronal differentiation. (**a**). Confocal z-projection frame of a *Tg(sox10:mcherry); Tg(ngn1:gfp)* zebrafish DRG at 72 hpf showing complete ensheathment. (**b**). Diagram of sensory neuron cell soma ensheathment by satellite glia. (**c**). Diagram of Eos photoconversion paradigm before neuronal differentiation. (**d**). Confocal z-projection images from a 24-h timelapse starting at 48 hpf of a *Tg(sox10:eos)* zebrafish with a photoconverted DRG neuron showing ensheathment of neuronal cell soma. White arrows denote dynamic projections of the ensheathing cell circumnavigating the neuron soma. (**e**). Confocal three-dimensional images of a nascent *Tg(sox10:eos)* DRG with a photoconverted neuron before and after ensheathment. D denotes dorsal, M denotes medial, V denotes ventral, and L denotes lateral. (**f**). Plot of two ensheathing processes converging on the same area of the of the neuron. (0,0) represents the site of the convergence of ensheathing processes. Red circle denotes the location of the neuron cell soma. (**g**). Intensity profiles transecting two approaching ensheathing processes every 75 min. (**h**). Deconvolved confocal z-projection images of two approaching ensheathing projections represented in (**g**). White brackets denote the gap between the two ensheathing processes. White arrows denote the emergence of the cellular processes. (**i, j**). Graphs of the areas of neurons (**i**) and ensheathing cells (**j**) before and after neuronal soma ensheathment (*n* = 5 DRG). (**i, j**) use a paired Student's *t*-test. Scale bar is 10 μm (**a, d, e, h**). All intensity measurements were taken from sum z-projections

plugin for ImageJ. All intensity measurements were taken from sum Z-projections and were normalized to background intensity. GraphPad Prism and Microsoft Excel were used to create all graphs and perform statistical analyses. Unpaired Student's *t*-tests, paired Student's *t*-test, and unpaired one-way ANOVAs with multiple comparisons (Tukey's Honest Significant Difference test) were used to calculate statistical significance as noted in the figure legends.

## Results

Differentiated dorsal root ganglia neurons (DRG) are encased by a perineuronal glial population known as satellite glia [9, 10]. We visualized this ensheathment in zebrafish using transgenic animals that express a fluorescent protein in glial populations using *sox10* regulatory sequences and expression of a different reporter in neuronal cells using *neurogenin1*, *ngn1*, regulatory sequences (Fig. 1a,b). We sought to identify how the progenitor populations envelop the neurons during the initial development of the neuron when it is morphologically plastic.

## Neurons are ensheathed during early neuronal differentiation

To dissect how these ensheathing cells develop in relation to the developing neuron, we devised an experimental paradigm that allowed us to mark individual cells of the nascent DRG before they expressed their differentiation markers. To do this we utilized $Tg(sox10:eos)$ animals which express the photoconvertible protein, Eos, in DRG precursors under the regulatory sequence of $sox10$ [37]. To label individual DRG cells we photoconverted single cells within the nascent DRG by directing UV laser light with our confocal microscope system to an 8 μm region in each DRG [40]. Since a typical DRG cell at this age in development is approximately 10 μm in diameter we could reliable photoconvert single cells within the DRG (Fig. 1c). Using this setup, we then could collect confocal z-stacks spanning the DRG every 5 min for 24 h and produce of movie of early DRG development. In zebrafish at 48 h post fertilization (hpf), the DRG is comprised of 2–4 cells.

We first hypothesized that the ensheathing progenitor would extend processes around the cell membrane of the developing neuron, like reported in axonal ensheathment by Schwann cells [42]. We further hypothesized that cell soma ensheathment likely occurs after axonal extensions are completed. To test these hypotheses we imaged $Tg(sox10:eos)$ animals every 5 min for 24 h from 48 to 72 hpf. At the start of these movies, we could reliably visualize two round cells within the ganglia (Fig. 1d, Additional file 1: Movie S1). Using cell tracking software, we determined that after 74.6 ± 21.4 min, one cell remains round (neuronal progenitor) and the other cell within the DRG extends cellular processes that guide along the edge of the other DRG cell ($n = 12$ ensheathing processes). These processes move at an average speed of 0.029 ± 0.0083 μm/min (n = 12 processes). The cellular extensions eventually encircle the entire round DRG cell completing the initial ensheathment of that cell. After ensheathment, the round DRG cell that is ensheathed adopts a more amoeboid-like morphology but continues to be enveloped by the other DRG cell even at these early stages (Fig. 1d,e). Within 24 h, the ensheathed cell produces a dorsally and ventrally projecting axon indicating its neuronal identity. We hypothesized that this ensheathment was occurring around the entire neuronal progenitor rather than just encircling it in a single dimension. To dissect this possibility, we rotated the images of the nascent DRG 90° before and after ensheathment so that the x-axis of the image would represent the lateromedial axis of the animal (Fig. 1e). These images show that the ensheathing progenitor completely surrounds the neuronal soma in all

three dimensions. Taken together, these results are consistent with hypothesis that the neuron is ensheathed even before neuronal projections are produced, indicating that they are ensheathed throughout the neuron's lifespan.

We next sought to gain a step-wise understanding of neuronal soma ensheathment. We hypothesized that this process is similar to axonal ensheathment where membranous sheets extend around the axon [19]. Alternatively, thin, finger-like projections could be initiated by the ensheathing progenitors, more similar to astrocyte processes [43]. To test this hypothesis, we used cell tracking software to determine the dynamic arrangement of ensheathing cells around the soma. In this analysis, we identified that early ensheathment occurs as two pericellular extensions independently migrate around the neuronal precursor until they converge and the entire soma is covered by a membrane. Figure 1f represents the ensheathment dynamics of a representative DRG by two distinct pericellular extensions. The ensheathing extensions travel variable speeds and total distances, as much as 55.6 μm or as little as 3.1 μm ($n = 6$ DRG, 12 ensheathing processes, mean ± SEM: 25.9 ± 6.3 μm). Ensheathing projections that traveled shorter distances still ensured that the entire round neuronal cell is covered by cell membrane. We did not observe the finger-like projections in this analysis but rather the extension of a migrating leading edge around the soma. These results are consistent with the model that neuronal ensheathment occurs by ensheathing cells initiating projections that wrap around the entirety of the neuronal soma.

Given that multiple projections lead to the ensheathment of the neuronal soma, we also sought to determine how a consistent ensheathment around the neuron is achieved. We hypothesized that the pericellular processes could: 1. halt their navigation immediately upon contact with a neighboring ensheathing cell, 2. overlap to form layers of ensheathing cells in the ganglia, or 3. stabilize with a gap between them. To distinguish these possibilities, we measured intensity profiles at 75 min intervals that transect the two ensheathing projections as they approach each other (Fig. 1g) as has previously been completed for oligodendrocyte sheathe formation [3]. If cellular processes overlapped, then we would expect a sharp increase (~ 2×) in the fluorescent intensity at the point of intersection. If there was a gap between cellular processes, then decreased intensity would be detected at the center point of the transection. Our data reveal that after two projections approach the same area, the level of fluorescence was measured as a single uniform platform that was not significantly larger than the individual extending peaks, consistent with the hypothesis that two projections could contact each other without measurable overlap. Additional time points showed a decrease in florescent intensity into two distinct platforms, consistent with a slight retraction of the processes of approximately 2.28 μm. Eventually, in all 5 DRG that were analyzed, the profiles return to a single platform (Fig. 1g,h). Unfortunately, because of the spatial resolution limits of light microscopy, homotypic contact cannot be definitively concluded. However, together these data are consistent with the hypothesis that ensheathing cells likely utilize a self-correction mechanism to completely, but non-redundantly cover their target – the neuronal cell soma.

To investigate if, in addition to changes in the ensheathment event, the neuronal soma also changed shape during ensheathment, we measured the area of the glia and neuron both before and after the ensheathment of the neuron. These measurements revealed that the glia greatly expand in size during ensheathment consistent with their organization to completely envelop the neuron (Fig. 1j, $p = 0.0031$, $n = 6$, mean difference ± SEM: $100.6 \pm 18.91$ $\mu m^2$). Conversely, the neuron decreases in area during ensheathment (Fig. 1i, $p = 0.0085$, $n = 6$, $-36.07 \pm 8.6$ $\mu m^2$). These data raise the possibility that early ensheathment event of the DRG neuron may be important for restricting the size, shape, and/or location of the developing neurons in the ganglia.

### Ensheathing progenitors remodel to cover neurons during neurite extension

Given that the DRG neuron must extend processes to the periphery and spinal cord, the complete ensheathment of the soma needs to change during the extension of these projections [44]. We reasoned that the ensheathing cells would rearrange to allow for this process to occur. To test this hypothesis we visualized DRG neuronal differentiation using $Tg(ngn1:gfp)$ [38] in combination with $Tg(sox10:eos)$. In these animals, GFP is expressed in newly differentiated neurons while Sox10 is expressed in DRG progenitor cells that ensheath the neurons. To distinguish the two transgenes we photoconverted Eos during each 5 min interval. We first hypothesized that the glia could undergo cell death to allow for process extension to occur. However, in our movies we did not visualize cell death during axonal extension. We therefore hypothesized that ensheathing cells dynamically remodel during axonal initiation. To test this we scored the rearrangement of ensheathing cells during axonal extension. In these movies, we visualized that these early neurons extend into an oval-like morphology before initiating an axon that extends dorsally toward the dorsal root entry zone (DREZ). As this extension is initiated, the ensheathed cell/s retracts two projections at the dorsal apex of the neuron (Fig. 2a). To measure this, we used cell tracking software to measure the location of these two projections at 5 min intervals. This allowed us to determine the distance between them throughout initiation of the axonal projection. These calculations revealed an increase in the distance between

the two ensheathing projections (~ 3 μm) during the period of axonal initiation (Fig. 2b, $n = 12$). We were also able to measure the length of the extending axon at each time point. These tracings reveal that length of the axon remains constant at $1.5 \pm 0.68$ μm for the initial period that the ensheathing cell rearranges and quickly increases after approximately $250 \pm 90.8$ min of ensheathing cell separation (Fig. 2b).

To examine the observed changes in the orientation of the DRG cells during the extension of the axon, we used four measures of shape: circularity, aspect ratio, roundness, and solidity. These measurements were taken of the shape of the ensheathing glia before, during, and after neurite extension. Circularity reflects how closely the shape reflects that of a perfect circle, so a mature, round neuronal soma would have a high circularity value. The circularity of the glia decreases during the process of neurite initiation (Fig. 2c, $p = 0.0016$, $n = 12$, before: $0.671 \pm 0.0214$, during: $0.492 \pm 0.0425$) and then increases to the original level after the extension of the projection is completed ($p = 0.6665$, $n = 12$, after: $0.652 \pm 0.0289$). This decrease in glial circularity during axonal extension reflects an irregularly shaped ensheathing glia to allow for the physical extension of neuronal processes. Aspect ratio and roundness are measures of the elongation of a shape. Both the aspect ratio (Fig. 2d, $p = 0.055$, $n = 12$, before: $1.946 \pm 0.139$, during: $2.278 \pm 0.240$, after: $2.113 \pm 0.173$) and roundness of the ensheathing cells (Fig. 2e, $p = 0.0827$, $n = 12$, before: $0.542 \pm 0.0406$, during: $0.490 \pm 0.0501$, after: $0.507 \pm 0.0410$) do not change during neurite extension. Last, solidity measures how symmetric and regular a shape is. During rearrangement of ensheathing cells during neurite extension, the solidity of the ensheathing cells decreases (Fig. 2f, $p = 0.025$, $n = 12$, before: $0.904 \pm 0.00486$, during: $0.841 \pm 0.0203$) and returns to a more solid shape following axon initiation ($p = 0.0008$, $n = 12$, after: $0.920 \pm 0.00704$). Taken together these data support the hypothesis that the ensheathing cells remodel during neurite extension which has lasting changes on the shape of the neuronal/ensheathing glia unit. These data demonstrate that ensheathment remains plastic as differentiation continues to ensure axonal projections can extend to their appropriate targets.

Previous studies have shown that pioneer axons are associated with Sox10[+] cells throughout their navigation [45]. To dissect the mechanistic relationship between ensheathment of the neuronal cell soma and association with growing axons we tracked the spatial relationship of the ensheathing cell with the extending nascent axon. We hypothesized that the soma ensheathing cells could rearrange their processes to extend with nascent axons. Conversely, cell divisions could produce a new ensheathing cell/s that associate with the axon. When distinguishing between these possibilities, we often visualized

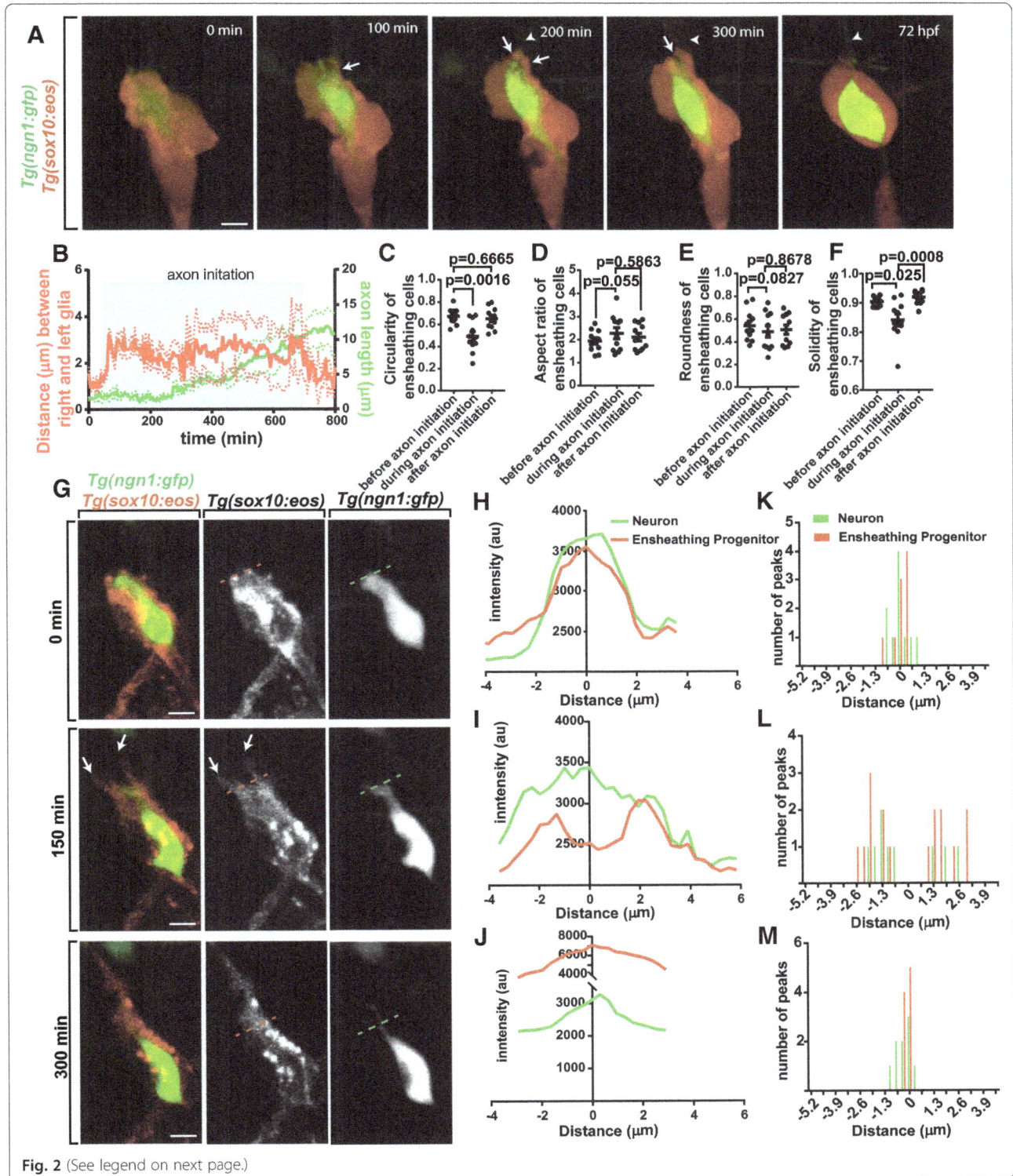

Fig. 2 (See legend on next page.)

(See figure on previous page.)
**Fig. 2** Ensheathing cells remodel during neurite outgrowth. (**a**). Confocal z-projection images from a 24-h timelapse starting at 48 hpf of *Tg(ngn1:gfp)*, *Tg(sox10:eos)* zebrafish with photoconverted ensheathing cells. White arrowheads denote the extending axon. White arrows denote glial horns. (**b**). Graph of the distance between the two dorsally located ensheathing projections (red) and the length of the extending axon (green). Shaded blue box denotes the period of axon initiation (n = 12 DRG). (**c-f**). Graphs of the circularity (**c**), aspect ratio (**d**), roundness (**e**), and solidity (**f**) of the ensheathing glia before, during, and after axon initiation (n = 12 DRG). (**g**). Confocal images of a *Tg(ngn1:gfp)*, *Tg(sox10:eos)* DRG before, during, and after axonal initiation showing glial horn formation. Dashed red and green lines denote the transecting lines used for the intensity profiles in (**h-j**). (**h-j**). Intensity profiles of *Tg(ngn1:gfp)* expression (green) and photoconverted *Tg(sox10:eos)* expression (red) through the dorsal apex of the DRG neuron before (**h**), during (**i**), and after (**j**) axon initiation. The line x = 0 represents the center of the neuron. (**k-m**). Histogram of the location of the *Tg(ngn1:gfp)* (green) and photoconverted *Tg(sox10:eos)* (red) intensity peaks before (**k**), during (**l**), and after (**m**) axon initiation (n = 12 DRG). X = 0 represents the center of the neuron. (**c-f**) use a Tukey's honest significant difference (HSD) test. Scale bar is 10 μm (**a, g**)

a rearrangement of the soma ensheathing processes where cells parted for neurites to extend resulting in two glial protrusions on each side of the extending axon (Fig. 2g). These protrusions are reminiscent "glial horns." Given this consistent morphology, we hypothesized that the extending axon may interact with one or both of these glial horns. To explore the potential relationship between the axon and the glial horns, we scored the interaction of the extending neurite with the glial horns by measuring intensity profiles for *Tg(ngn1:gfp)* and converted *Tg(sox10:eos)* that transected the two glial projections before, during, and after axon initiation. These profiles revealed that before and after axon initiation, the *Tg(ngn1:gfp)* and converted *Tg(sox10:eos)* intensities were represented with a single peak, suggesting that the glia are ensheathing the neuronal soma before and after neurite initiation (Fig. 2h,j). During the initiation of the axon, there are two peaks of converted *Tg(sox10:eos)* intensity, consistent with the observation that the ensheathing cells retract and extend two horns during axon initiation (Fig. 2i). In these profiles, the *Tg(ngn1:gfp)* intensity formed a single peak that was always associated with one of the converted *Tg(sox10:eos)* peaks. To ask if there was a preferential association with one of the glial horns we scored the axons that associate with either horn (Fig. 2k-m). However, these nascent axons did not show a preference for either the anterior or posterior glial horn. Interestingly, nascent axons initially extended and retracted along both horns before ultimately selecting a horn to extend along. The other, adjacent horn without an axon, then returned to the neuronal cell body. Taken together, these data are consistent with the hypothesis that the retraction of the ensheathing glial projections not only physically allows for axon initiation but may also provide a substrate for the developing neurite to stabilize on as it grows.

### Ensheathment of the cell body is independent of axonal ensheathment

With our data that the ensheathing cell of neuronal soma projects dorsally during axonal initiation, we sought to test whether inhibiting the ensheathment of the axon would affect the ensheathment of the cell soma. To do this, we utilized a drug, Src-family kinase inhibitor SU6656, that inhibits the ensheathment of the axonal projection (Nichols and Smith, unpublished data).

We hypothesized that axonal and neuronal ensheathment were two, distinct processes. However, if the cells that ensheath the axon originate as an ensheathing cell of the neuronal soma, disruption of axonal ensheathment could affect neuronal cell soma ensheathment. To test this, we molecularly manipulated axonal ensheathment and measured neuronal soma ensheathment. We treated *Tg(sox10:eos)* larvae with SU6656 or DMSO at 36 hpf and imaged them from 48 to 72 hpf, the period when axons navigate dorsally and become ensheathed (Fig. 3a). To distinguish between the neurons and the ensheathing glia, we photoconverted the neuron. We then quantified the ensheathment of the axonal projections by measuring the intensity profiles for both converted and unconverted *Tg(sox10:eos)* intensities that transect the axon and any associated glia (Fig. 3b, c). These intensity profiles revealed a decrease in the width of *Tg(sox10:eos)* unconverted[+] ensheathing cells around the *Tg(sox10:eos)* converted axon in SU6656 treated animals, suggesting a lack of axonal ensheathment in these animals (Nichols and Smith, unpublished data). To determine the ensheathment of the neuronal cell bodies in both DMSO and SU6656 treated animals we rotated the images of the ensheathed neurons 90° to visualize the association of ensheathing cells with neurons in three dimensions. These rotated images revealed that the entire ganglion was ensheathed in both treatment groups (Fig. 3d, e), suggesting that ensheathment of the cell body is not affected by SU6656 treatment. These data are consistent with the hypothesis that the ensheathment of the neuronal soma is independent of axonal ensheathment mechanisms.

We sought to further characterize the ensheathment of the neuronal soma and the axon by determining the width of ensheathment in both neuronal compartments. It is possible that the ensheathment of the axon and neuronal soma are entirely independent and exhibit two distinct forms of ensheathment. However, it is also possible that similar biological principles underlie both processes so that similar ensheathment profiles are present in both neuronal compartments. To do this, we used *Tg(sox10:mcherry)*; *Tg(ngn1:gfp)* animals to quantify intensity profiles transecting the axon and neuronal soma and calculated the ratios of the width of the *Tg(sox10:mcherry)* peak

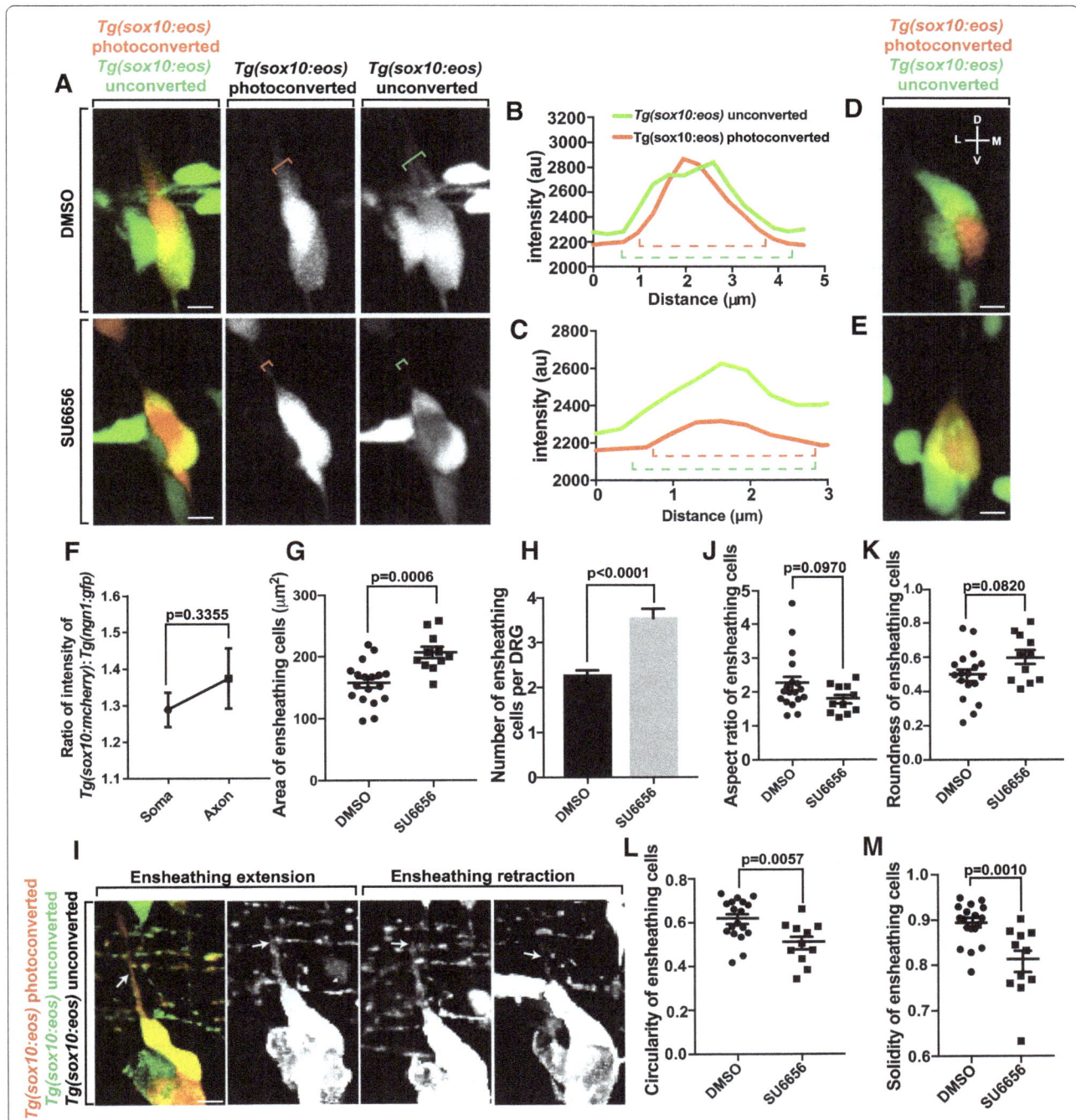

**Fig. 3** Neuronal cell soma ensheathment is distinct from axonal ensheathment. (**a**). Confocal z-projection images of a *Tg(sox10:eos)* zebrafish with a photoconverted neuron at 72 hpf. The top images were taken of an animal treated with DMSO. The bottom images were taken from an animal treated with SU6656. Red bracket denotes the width of the axon. Green bracket denotes the width of the ensheathing cells. (**b**, **c**). Intensity profiles of *Tg(sox10:eos)* unconverted (green) and *Tg(sox10:eos)* converted (red) transecting the axon from animals treated with DMSO (**b**) and SU6656 (**c**). Dashed red bracket denotes the width of the axon. Dashed green bracket denotes the width of the ensheathing cell. (**d**, **e**). Confocal three-dimensional images of a *Tg(sox10:eos)* DRG with a photoconverted neuron in DMSO and SU6656 treated animals. D denotes dorsal, M denotes medial, V denotes ventral, and L denotes lateral. (**f**). Ratio of the width of *Tg(sox10:mcherry); Tg(ngn1:gfp)* peaks taken from intensity profiles transecting the neuronal soma and axon ($n = 10$ DRG). (**g**). Area of the ensheathing cells in DMSO and SU6656 treated animals ($n = 18$ DMSO DRG, $n = 11$ SU6656 DRG). (**h**). Number of ensheathing cells per DRG at 72 hpf (n = 18 DMSO DRG, n = 11 SU6656 DRG). (**i**). Deconvolved confocal z-projections of a *Tg(sox10:eos)* DRG with a photoconverted neuron in a SU6656-treated animal. White arrow denotes the dorsal tip of an ensheathing cell on the DRG axon. (**j-m**). Graphs of the aspect ratio (**j**), roundness (**k**), circularity (**l**) and solidity (**m**) of the ensheathing cells before, during, and after axon initiation (n = 18 DMSO DRG, n = 11 SU6656 DRG). (**g**, **h**, **j-m**) use an unpaired Student's *t*-test. (**f**) uses a paired Student's *t*-test. Scale bar is 10 μm (**a**, **d**, **e**, **i**). All intensity measurements were taken from sum z-projections

(ensheathing cells) to the width of the *Tg(ngn1:gfp)* peak. These ratios showed no significant difference between the ensheathment widths of the axon and neuronal soma (Fig. 3f, $p = 0.3355$, $n = 10$ DRG, $0.0853 \pm 0.0839$). This data suggest that similar ensheathment profiles are shared between the axon and the soma during early development. Later, axonal ensheathment likely expands as myelination occurs.

### Inhibiting axonal ensheathment leads to increased glia ensheathing the neuron cell body

We reasoned that the observed increase in ensheathing glia coverage in SU6656 animals was due to an axon-ensheathing cell returning to the ganglion after failed axonal ensheathment. Alternatively, failed axonal ensheathment could lead to increased proliferation of ensheathing cells. To test this, we first measured the area of the ensheathing glia at 72 hpf in both DMSO and SU6656 treated animals. These measurements showed an increase in the area of the ensheathing cells in SU6656 treated animals (Fig. 3g, $p = 0.0006$, $n = 18$ DMSO, $n = 11$ SU6656, DMSO: $156.923 \pm 7.933$ $\mu m^2$, SU6656: $196.455 \pm 13.301$ $\mu m^2$). To determine if this increase was due to an increase in size of individual glial cells or in the number of glial cells, we counted the number of glial cells that were associated with the neuronal cell body in both treatments. The SU6656 treated animals had, on average, one extra glial cell present in the ganglia compared to DMSO treated animals (Fig. 3h, $p < 0.0001$, n = 18 DMSO, n = 11 SU6656, DMSO: $2.278 \pm 0.109$, SU6656: $3.545 \pm 0.207$). We were also able to visualize this phenomenon using time-lapse imaging of axonal ensheathment. In SU6656 treated animals, a *Tg(sox10:eos)* unconverted[+] cell (white arrow) travels dorsally along the nascent axon but returns to the soma before axonal ensheathment can occur (Fig. 3i). These two data sets are consistent with the hypothesis that if axonal ensheathment is inhibited during development, the glial cell that was to ensheath the axon returns back to the ganglia.

From these data, we hypothesized that the presence of an extra glial cell in the DRG could change the shape of entire ganglia. To do this, we determined the shape descriptors circularity, aspect ratio, roundness, and solidity for the ensheathing cells in both DMSO and SU6656 treated animals. We detected no significant change in the aspect ratio (Fig. 3j, $p = 0.0970$, n = 18 DMSO, n = 11 SU6656, DMSO: $2.249 \pm 0.200$, SU6656: $1.776 \pm 0.125$) or roundness (Fig. 3k, $p = 0.0820$, n = 18 DMSO, n = 11 SU6656, DMSO: $0.493 \pm 0.0344$, SU6656: $0.592 \pm 0.0312$) of the ensheathing cells, consistent with the conclusion that the extra cell did not lead to an elongation of the neuronal/ensheathing glia unit. However, both the circularity (Fig. 3l, $p = 0.0057$, n = 18 DMSO, n = 11 SU6656,

DMSO: $0.622 \pm 0.0244$, SU6656: $0.506 \pm 0.0290$) and solidity (Fig. 3m, $p = 0.0010$, n = 18 DMSO, n = 11 SU6656, DMSO: $0.891 \pm 0.0105$, SU6656: $0.807 \pm 0.0236$) decreased in SU6656-treated animals. These shape changes are consistent with the conclusion that the extra glial cell from failed axonal ensheathment leads to a larger glial unit and an irregularly shaped, bulky ganglion. It is worth noting that our experiments do not distinguish whether SU6656 impacted these measurements cell-autonomously.

### Ensheathing progenitors exhibit space filling potential

Our analysis thus far indicated that these ensheathing cells non-redundantly cover the neuronal cells in the DRG even despite considerable morphological changes. We hypothesized that these ensheathing cells could therefore exhibit continuous tiling potential which ensures cells' complete but non-redundant coverage of a target area. To first test this tiling hypothesis, we imaged the DRG during the proliferation of the ensheathing cells. In this experiment we observed that the individual neurons were continuously ensheathed. The only point where ensheathment was slightly disrupted was when an ensheathing cell divided and the neuron became momentarily and partially unensheathed (Fig. 4a). In this analysis over a 24-h period, we did not observe any neurons that became completely unensheathed. However, if these progenitors do exhibit continuous tiling behavior we would expect that even if a neuron becomes even momentarily unensheathed, the ensheathing cells would respond to eventually fully ensheath the neuron again. To test this, we imaged the projections of the ensheathing cells after partial unensheathment (Fig. 4a). In doing so, we were able to visualize ensheathing projections travel toward the unensheathed area of the soma. We further hypothesized that the stabilization of this re-ensheathment would recapitulate the first ensheathment paradigm where two ensheathing processes converged and retracted. To test this, we measured intensity profiles that transected the migrating processes as they approached each other every 75 min. These data showed cellular processes with a single intensity platform which 75 min later separated into two peaks (Fig. 4b, representative DRG chosen from 5 assayed DRG). These results are consistent with the hypothesis that these cells likely maintain continuous tiling behavior throughout life by recapitulating developmental ensheathment.

Given that multiple ensheathing cells and processes are present in the ganglia, it is possible that these cells exhibit this tiling behavior either equally or at different rates. To explore this possibility, we calculated the average velocity of each cell that responded to fill the empty space around the neuron. In responding to the partial unensheathment, responding processes within the same DRG exhibited differences in their speed at tiling the neuronal soma. These

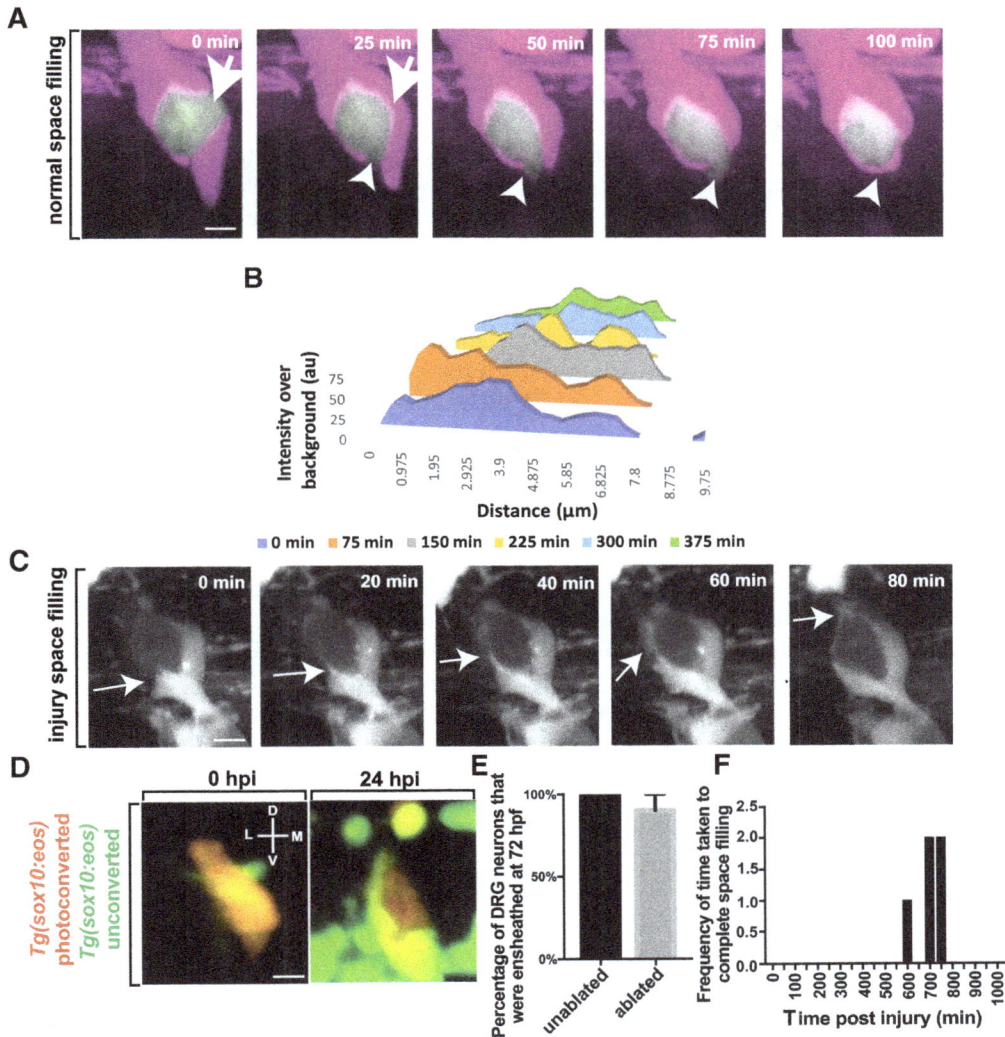

**Fig. 4** Cells ensheathing DRG neuron cell somas exhibit space filling throughout life. (**a**). Confocal z-projection images from a 24-h timelapse starting at 72 hpf of a *Tg(sox10:eos); Tg(ngn1:gfp)* with photoconverted ensheathing cells. White arrowhead and arrows denotes areas of neuronal soma that are re-ensheathed. (**b**). Intensity profiles transecting two approaching ensheathing processes every 30 min. (**c**). Confocal z-projection images from a 24-h timelapse starting at 48 hpf of a *Tg(sox10:eos)* zebrafish with a laser ablation of an ensheathing cell. White arrows denote the migrating ensheathing process. (**d**). Confocal 3D images of a *Tg(sox10:eos)* DRG with a photoconverted neuron and an ablated ensheathing cell at 0 and 24 hpi. D denotes dorsal, M denotes medial, V denotes ventral, and L denotes lateral. (**e**). Percent of DRG neurons that are ensheathed 24 hpi (*n* = 14 unablated DRG, n = 10 ablated DRG). (**f**). Histogram of the time after ablation that re-ensheathment of the neuron soma is completed (n = 5 DRG). Scale bar is 10 μm (**a**, **c**, **d**)

speeds ranged from 0.00515 μm/min to 0.0621 μm/min (mean ± SEM: 0.0286 ± 0.0059 μm/min). This data is consistent with the hypothesis that in normal tiling, the cells may not respond equally to partial unensheathment but instead one cell responds quickly and travels a further distance to fill space on the neuron.

To continue to provide mechanistic insight into the ability of these cells to tile the neuron we tested our hypothesis by manipulating the ensheathing cells experimentally to create an unensheathment event. Previous studies on tiling mechanisms have reported that the remaining ensheathing cells expand to cover the target area following cell ablation. To test the ability of DRG ensheathing cells to do this, we ablated one of the ensheathing cells and visualized the behavior of the remaining cells. To do this we created small ablations of individual ensheathing cells using our laser ablation system. In this paradigm, we created a 4 μm region of interest to ablate individual cells and then captured images every 5 min for 24 h (Fig. 4c, Additional file 2: Movie

S2). First, we confirmed that the ablation resulted in an unensheathment event in the DRG by rotating the image of the ablated DRG 90° to view the ensheathment along the lateromedial axis of the animal at 0 and 24 h post injury (hpi). The resulting images revealed a neuron with little glial ensheatment following ablation (Fig. 4d), consistent with the idea that the ablation resulted in an unensheathment event. The same DRG 24 h later exhibited complete, three-dimensional ensheathment of the neuron (Fig. 4d). This change demonstrated that the remaining ensheathing cells responded to the ablation by filling the area on the neuron where the ablated cell existed. We scored that 90% of all DRG with an ablated glia had been re-ensheathed 24 hpi (Fig. 4e, $n = 10$ DRG).

Many possibilities, including cell divisions, glial volume expansion and rearrangement, could be responsible for the observed re-ensheathment. We hypothesized that re-ensheathment following injury recapitulated the developmental mechanism and resulted in the rearrangement of the remaining ensheathing glia. To test this hypothesis we visualized the movement of the ensheathing cells into the ablated site with time-lapse imaging. These movies showed that responding glia initiated projections that migrated to the ablated area where they converged, just as in developmental space filling. To further compare this experimentally induced space filling to that observed in development, we calculated the velocities of the responding glia. Just as in the developmental context, the injury-induced glial response led to asymmetric responses from the ensheathing cells where cells within the same DRG responded to the unensheathment with a wide variability of speeds ranging from 0.00493 μm/min to 0.0206 μm/min (mean ± SEM: 0.0149 ± 0.00155 μm/min). To gain a temporal understanding of the re-ensheathment events following injury, we recorded the times that the ensheathing cells required to re-ensheath the neuron following experimentally induced unensheathment. We found that the ensheathing cells required 679 ± 27.386 min after the injury event to re-ensheath the cell body (Fig. 4f, $n = 5$ DRG). Taken together, these data provide an understanding of ensheathment demonstrating re-ensheathment is performed by existing rearrangement of cells within the neuron/ensheathing cell unit. This is consistent with the hypothesis that ensheathing cells in the DRG exhibit continuous tiling capacity throughout life.

**Lack of ensheathment perturbs neuronal cell soma shape**
Neurons in the DRG exhibit a stereotypical round cell soma morphology and are positioned with precise topography in the ganglia [23, 33]. Due to their close association, these ensheathing cells have the potential to

continuously impact neurons morphologically and physiologically. Previous research has demonstrated their physiological role [4, 5]. To investigate their potential role in neuronal morphology or spatial location in the ganglia we first investigated how neuronal shape changed in response to modulations in ensheathing cells. We hypothesized that if these ensheathing cells do continuously impact neuronal shape then even short perturbations to the ensheathment would impact neuronal shape. We first tested this possibility by visualizing neurons and ensheathing cells in *Tg(ngn1:gfp)*; *Tg(sox10:eos)* animals from 48 to 72 hpf that have already extended processes. We specifically scored events in which the ensheathing cells proliferate, causing a partial unensheathment event, and then visualized the morphological behavior of the neurons (Fig. 5a). These images revealed a bulging of the neuronal soma during a partial unensheathment. To quantify this, we measured the area of the neuronal soma before, during, and after proliferation of the ensheathing cells. These measurements showed a dynamic decrease in area of the neuron during the perturbation of its glial sheath (Fig. 5b, $p = 0.0136$, $n = 11$ neurons, before: $71.51 ± 6.24$ μm$^2$, during: $59.94 ± 4.89$ μm$^2$) which then immediately increased back to its normal level following re-ensheathment ($p = 0.0011$, after: $76.43 ± 5.78$ μm$^2$). Using the shape descriptors for the neuron cell body, we were able to quantify the neuronal morphology before, during, and after proliferation of the ensheathing cells. The aspect ratio (Fig. 5c, $p = 0.1400$, $n = 11$ neurons, before: $1.78 ± 0.131$, during: $2.174 ± 0.124$, after: $1.82 ± 0.046$) and the roundness (Fig. 5d, $p = 0.1656$, $n = 11$ neurons, before: $0.585 ± 0.0330$, during: $0.478 ± 0.0323$, after: $0.565 ± 0.0287$) of neurons did not change during the proliferation of ensheathing cells. However, the circularity (Fig. 5e, $p = 0.0194$, $n = 11$ neurons, before: $0.722 ± 0.0315$, during: $0.585 ± 0.0341$) and solidity (Fig. 5f, $p = 0.0024$, $n = 11$ neurons, before: $0.924 ± 0.00575$, during: $0.826 ± 0.0214$) of the neuron decreased during glial proliferation. Both measurements (circularity: $p = 0.0058$, after: $0.766 ± 0.0256$; solidity: $p = 0.0011$, after: $0.937 ± 0.00444$) returned to their normal levels following the completion of glial proliferation, consistent with an overall decrease in area and the observed bulging of the neuron during a short perturbation of its glial sheath. These results are consistent with the conclusion that ensheathing cells may continuously provide a physical, restrictive force on DRG neurons.

To provide further mechanistic insight into this, we continued to test this hypothesis experimentally by ablating individual ensheathing cells and visualizing the morphological changes of the neuron. In these experiments, ablation of the ensheathing glia caused neurons to alter their morphology similar to the partial unensheathment from the proliferation of ensheathing cells (Fig. 5g). First,

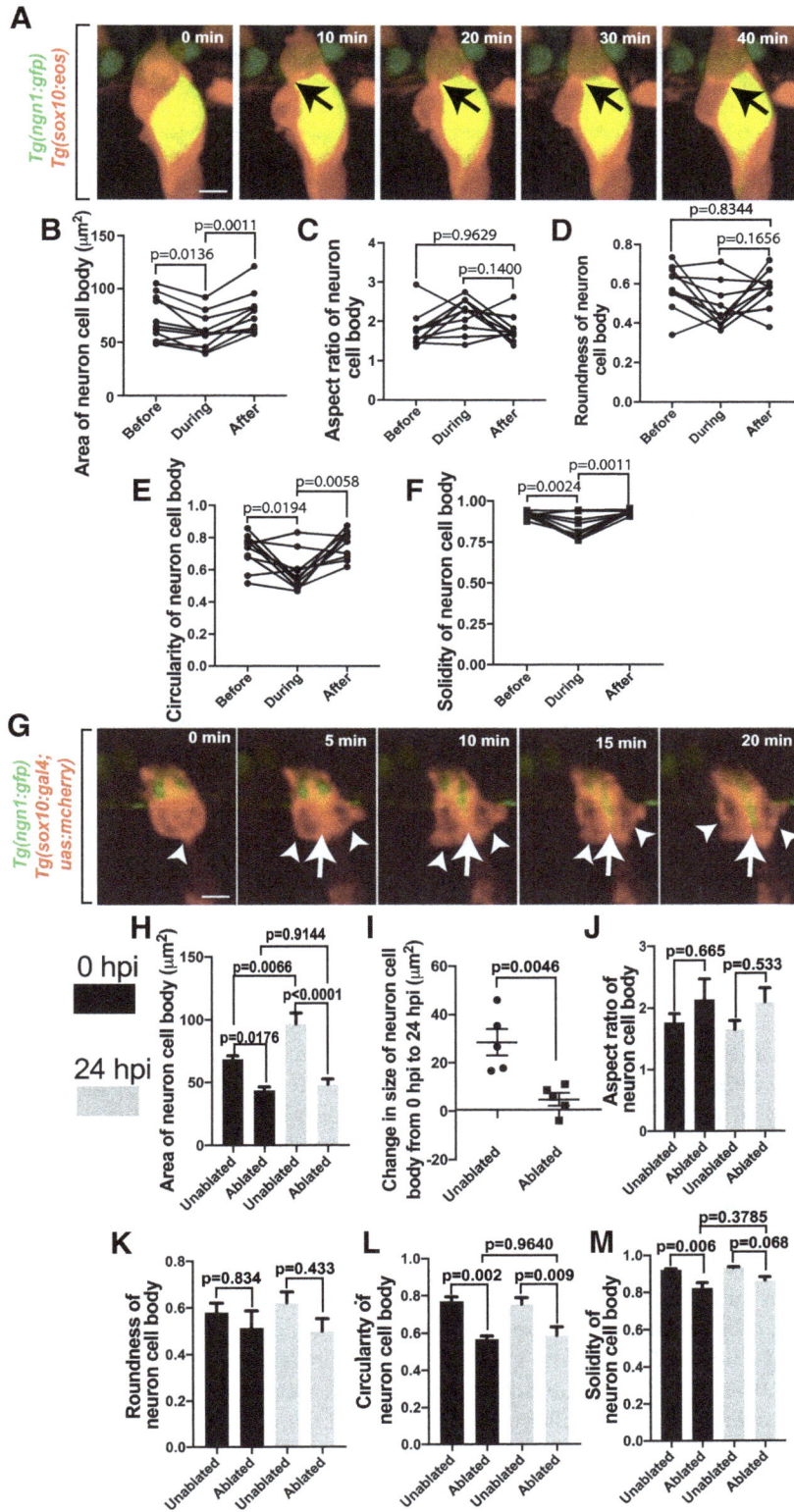

**Fig. 5** (See legend on next page.)

**Fig. 5** Perturbation of ensheathment impacts DRG neuron shape. (**a**). Confocal z-projection images from a 24-h timelapse starting at 72 hpf of a *Tg(ngn1:gfp), Tg(sox10:eos)* zebrafish with photoconverted *sox10⁺* cells. Black arrows denote change in neuronal shape. (B-F). Graphs of area (**b**), aspect ratio (**c**), roundness (**d**), circularity (**e**), and solidity (**f**) of the neuron soma before, during, and after the division of an ensheathing cell (n = 11 neurons). (**g**). Confocal z-projection images from a 24-h timelapse starting at 48 hpf of a *Tg(ngn1:gfp), Tg(sox10:gal4; uas:mcherry)* zebrafish with photoconverted *sox10⁺* cells and with an ablated ensheathing cell. White arrowheads denote responding ensheathing cells. White arrows denote the change in neuronal shape. (**h**). Area of the neuronal soma of DRG with ablated and unablated ensheathing cells at 0 hpi (black) and 24 hpi (gray) (n = 5 unablated DRG, n = 5 ablated DRG). (**i**). Change in the area of the neuronal soma in ablated and unablated DRG from 0 hpi and 24 hpi (n = 5 unablated DRG, n = 5 ablated DRG). (**j-m**). Graphs of the aspect ratio (**j**), roundness (**k**), circularity (**l**), and solidity (**m**) of the neuronal soma in ablated and unablated DRG at 0 hpi (black) and 24 hpi (gray) (n = 5 unablated DRG, n = 5 ablated DRG). (**b-f**) use a paired Tukey's HSD test. (**h,j-m**) use an unpaired Tukey's HSD test. (**i**) uses an unpaired Student's *t*-test. Scale bar is 10 μm (**a, g**)

the ablation of an ensheathing cell led to a decrease in the area of the neuron shortly after the ablation compared to neighboring unablated control ganglia (Fig. 5h, $p$ = 0.0176, $n$ = 5 unablated DRG, n = 5 ablated DRG, ablated: 43.52 ± 2.97 μm², unablated: 68.47 ± 3.01 μm²). This decrease in neuron size persisted following re-ensheathment and was still present 24 hpi ($p$ < 0.0001 unablated DRG, n = 5 ablated DRG, ablated: 48.29 ± 4.56 μm², unablated: 69.99 ± 8.34 μm²). To further explore this injury-induced perturbation of neuronal soma size, we quantified the change in the size of the soma from 0 to 24 hpi. Unablated control DRG neurons increased 26.53 ± 5.52 μm² (Fig. 5i, n = 5 neurons) during that time period, while the neurons with an ablated glial cell increased only 4.77 ± 2.63 μm² (n = 5 neurons, $p$ = 0.0046). To continue to examine the neuronal morphological changes resulting from an unensheathment event, we quantified the shape descriptors for the neuronal cell bodies in DRG with ablated and with unablated ensheathing glia. Just as in the normal developmental partial unensheathment, the aspect ratio (Fig. 5j, $p$ = 0.665, n = 5 neurons, unablated at 0 hpi: 1.767 ± 0.145, ablated at 0 hpi: 2.139 ± 0.336, unablated at 24 hpi: 1.654 ± 0.146, ablated at 24 hpi: 2.097 ± 0.230) and roundness (Fig. 5k, $p$ = 0.834, n = 5 neurons, unablated at 0 hpi: 0.579 ± 0.0405, ablated at 0 hpi: 0.513 ± 0.0744, unablated at 24 hpi: 0.621 ± 0.0469, ablated at 24 hpi: 0.500 ± 0.0527) were not affected by unensheathment, suggesting that the neurons did not elongate. However, the circularity (Fig. 5l, p = 0.002, n = 5 neurons, unablated at 0 hpi: 0.769 ± 0.0245, ablated at 0 hpi: 0.567 ± 0.0188) and solidity (Fig. 5m, $p$ = 0.006, n = 5 neurons unablated at 0 hpi: 0.921 ± 0.00662, ablated at 0 hpi: 0.822 ± 0.0298) both decreased in neurons with an ablated glia. The circularity of neurons with ablated ensheathing cells remained depressed 24 hpi ($p$ = 0.009, unablated at 24 hpi: 0.756 ± 0.0330, mean ablated at 24 hpi ± SEM: 0.588 ± 0.0445). The solidity of these neurons slightly recovered to levels similar to that of DRG neurons without ablated cells ($p$ = 0.068, unablated at 24 hpi: 0.933 ± 0.00530, ablated at 24 hpi: 0.864 ± 0.0185). The simplest explanation for this is that a larger unensheathment event following an injury to the ensheathing cells results in a persistent change to both the size and shape to the DRG neuron. Overall, these changes

in neuron morphology in both the developmental and injury contexts are consistent with the hypothesis that ensheathing cells could provide continuous structural forces to maintain the morphology of individual DRG neurons.

When DRG glial precursors are genetically ablated, the developing DRG becomes mislocalized at inconsistent locations along the dorsoventral axis of the animal [23]. Based on this observation and our data above that injury to ensheathing cells resulted in prolonged alterations in neuron size and shape, we hypothesized that prolonged unensheathment of neurons could have an impact on the location of the neuron within the ganglia. To address this possibility, we ablated multiple ensheathing cells and traced any movement of the neuron that they once surrounded. This quantification was done by measuring the center point of the neuron before and after the cells were ablated. In these experiments, we visualized that ablation of ensheathing glia first caused an immediate ectopic shifting of the neuron toward the area that was ablated (Fig. 6a, b). To determine if these neurons displayed a consistent direction of movement, we quantified the trajectory of the neurons following ablation and observed that neurons typically shifted either ventrally or dorsally (Fig. 6c). In these movements, the neurons did not move with a consistent velocity. Adjacent neurons without any ablated glia moved less. To further explore this injury-induced neuronal movement, we quantified the total displacement and velocities in these neurons. Neurons with ablated glia were displaced 8.476 ± 0.699 μm at a speed of 0.0077 μm/min (Fig. 6d, n = 5 neurons). These measurements were both greater than neurons in unablated DRG which traveled an average distance of 6.0 ± 0.776 μm at a speed of 0.0054 μm/min (Fig. 6d, $p$ = 0.0429, $n$ = 5 neurons). These tracings are consistent with the possibility that prolonged unensheathment of DRG neurons could cause not only momentary morphological changes (Fig. 5) but also shifting of the neurons within the ganglia.

Given that ablation of ensheathing cells resulted in misplaced DRG neurons, we next tested if ablation of ensheathing cells resulted in axonal pathfinding defects. However, we did not observe any obvious pathfinding defects. The axon initiated and traveled dorsally, entering the spinal cord at a typical DREZ location (Fig. 6e).

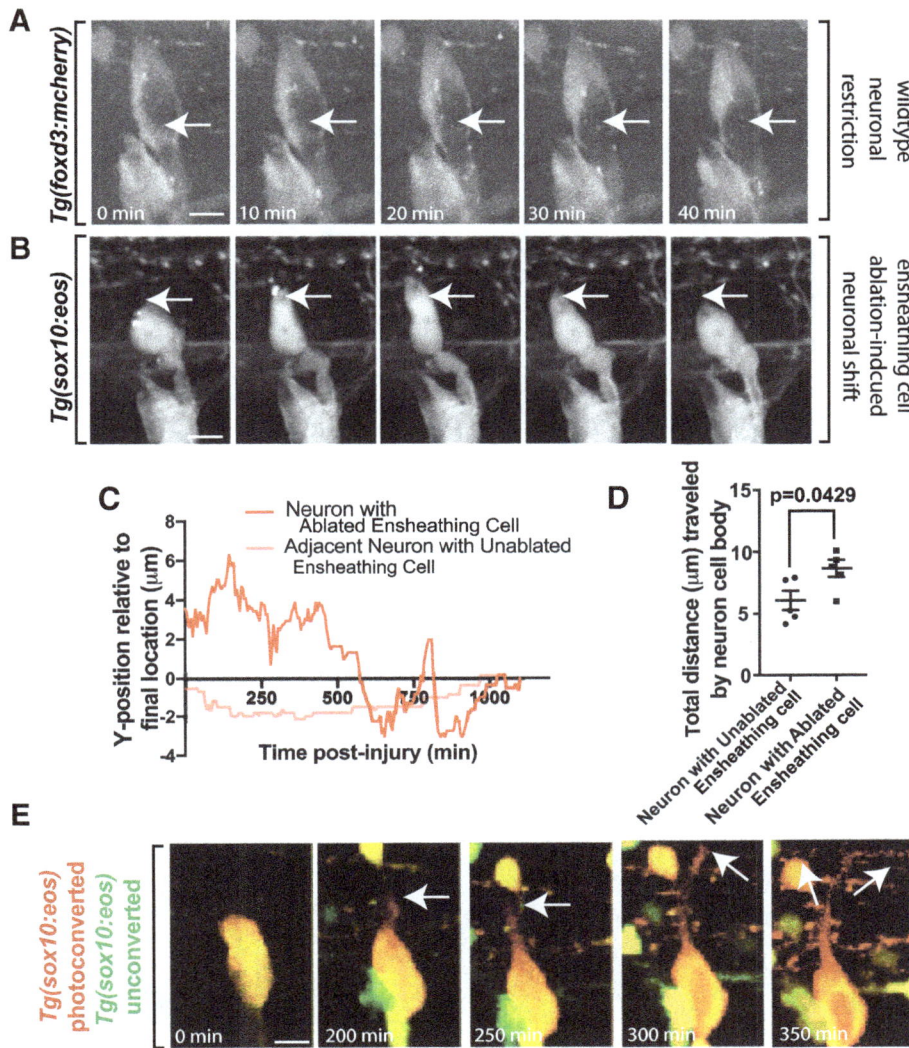

**Fig. 6** Extended perturbations of soma-ensheathing cells results in misplaced neurons. (**a**). Confocal z-projection images from a 24-h timelapse starting at 48 hpf of a *Tg(foxd3:mcherry)* zebrafish. White arrows denote the center of the neuronal soma. (**b**). Confocal z-projection images from a 24-h timelapse starting at 72 hpf of a *Tg(sox10:eos)* zebrafish with a laser ablation of multiple ensheathing cells. White arrows denote the original location of the dorsal apex of the DRG neuron. (**c**). Change in the y-position over time of a neuron in an ablated and unablated DRG. Y = 0 denotes the final location of the neuronal soma. (**d**). Total distance traveled by the DRG neuronal soma in an ablated and unablated DRG (n = 5 neurons). (**e**). Confocal z-projection images from a 24-h timelapse starting at 48 hpf of a *Tg(sox10:eos)* zebrafish with a photoconverted neuron and ablated ensheathing cell. White arrows denote the migration of the nascent axon. (**d**) use an unpaired Student's *t*-test. Scale bar is 10 µm (**a**, **b**, **e**)

## Proliferation of neurons corresponds with expansion of progenitors

Since these ensheathing cells are present during early ganglia development, we sought to identify if they represented a terminally defined cell-type or if they were a progenitor population. To first test the progenitor possibility of these ensheathing cells, we imaged *Tg(sox10:eos)* animals at 2 dpf and photoconverted a single ensheathing cell. Twenty-four hours later, we observed multiple *Tg(sox10:eos)* photoconverted cells in the DRG, suggesting that the ensheathing cells actively divide like a progenitor population (Fig. 7a, b)

as previously described [37]. To further explore this possibility, we quantified whether they expanded as the neuron number increased. To do this, we imaged the DRG in *Tg(ngn1:gfp); Tg(sox10:eos)* animals at two, three, and four dpf and photoconverted the Eos in the entire animal (Fig. 7c). In these images, we quantified the ratio of *sox10*[+] cells and neurons at each time point. The ratios steadily decreased at each time point (Fig. 7d). To further expand this analysis, we quantified the number of ensheathing cells and neurons present in the DRG at each time point (Fig. 7e). From 2 to 4 dpf, the number of neurons increased by one

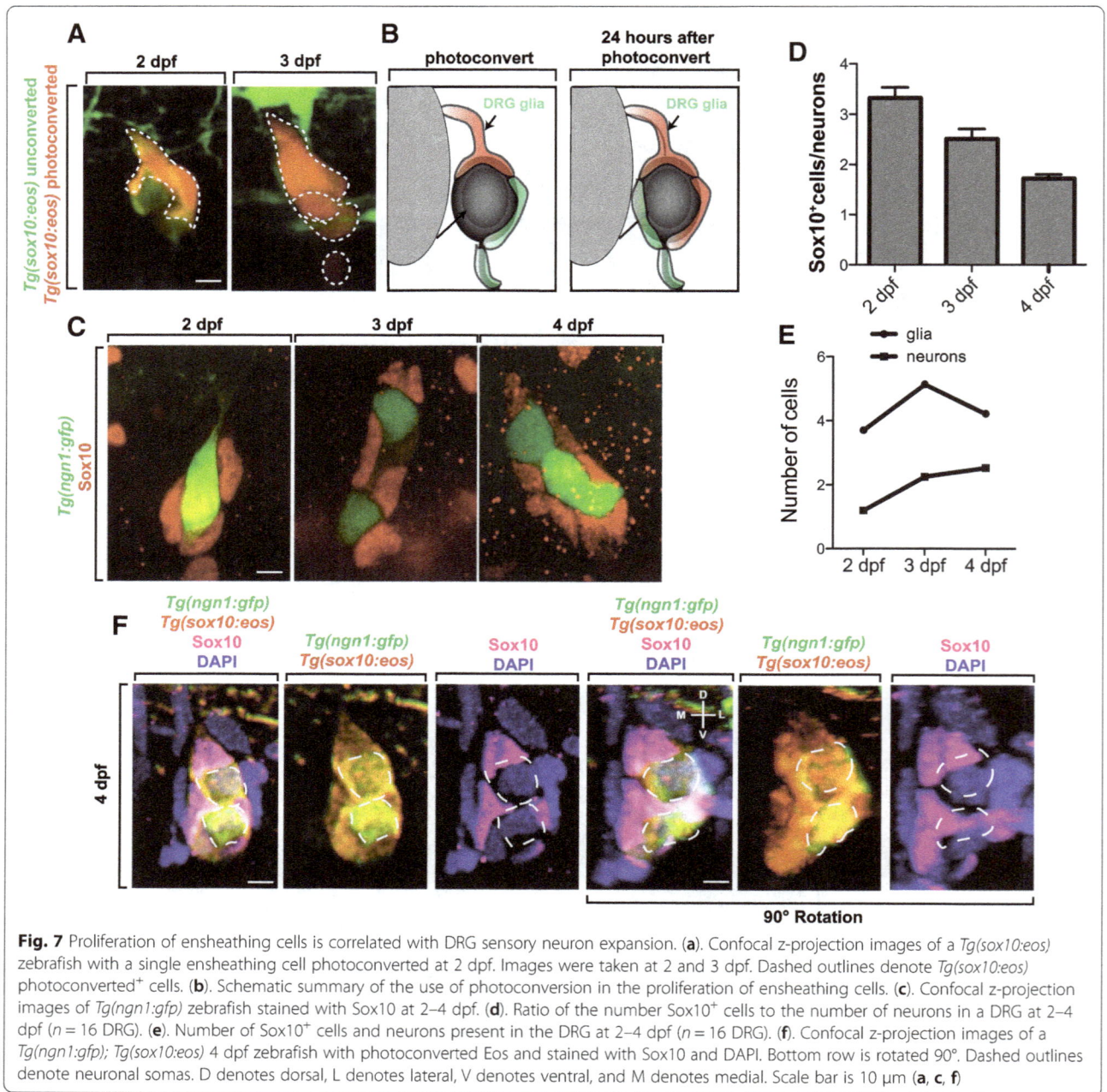

**Fig. 7** Proliferation of ensheathing cells is correlated with DRG sensory neuron expansion. (**a**). Confocal z-projection images of a *Tg(sox10:eos)* zebrafish with a single ensheathing cell photoconverted at 2 dpf. Images were taken at 2 and 3 dpf. Dashed outlines denote *Tg(sox10:eos)* photoconverted[+] cells. (**b**). Schematic summary of the use of photoconversion in the proliferation of ensheathing cells. (**c**). Confocal z-projection images of *Tg(ngn1:gfp)* zebrafish stained with Sox10 at 2–4 dpf. (**d**). Ratio of the number Sox10[+] cells to the number of neurons in a DRG at 2–4 dpf (*n* = 16 DRG). (**e**). Number of Sox10[+] cells and neurons present in the DRG at 2–4 dpf (*n* = 16 DRG). (**f**). Confocal z-projection images of a *Tg(ngn1:gfp); Tg(sox10:eos)* 4 dpf zebrafish with photoconverted Eos and stained with Sox10 and DAPI. Bottom row is rotated 90°. Dashed outlines denote neuronal somas. D denotes dorsal, L denotes lateral, V denotes ventral, and M denotes medial. Scale bar is 10 μm (**a, c, f**)

on average. The number of glia increased by one from 2 to 3 dpf but then decreased by one by 4 dpf. Overall, these data are consistent with the idea that the proliferation of the ensheathing cells corresponds with an increase in sensory neurons and that the new neurons could arise from *sox10*[+] ensheathing progenitor cells.

We next sought to gain a spatial understanding of DRG expansion. We hypothesized that ensheathing cells could ensheath multiple neurons during DRG expansion. However, it is also possible that neurons could be individually encased by individual cells. To test these possibilities, we used *Tg(ngn1:gfp); Tg(sox10:eos)* fish and photoconverted Eos at 4 dpf. After photoconverstion, animals were fixed and stained for Sox10 and DAPI. Images of these animals revealed that each neuron was individually encased by multiple ensheathing cells (Fig. 7f). While it is difficult to determine exactly how many cells participate in the ensheathment of an individual neuron, more than one cell nuclei that associated with processes that ensheath individual neurons at 4 dpf can be visualized, a result that is consistent with recent investigations into adult DRG ensheathment by mature satellite glia [9].

## Ensheathing cells respond to neuronal injury

Since these ensheathing cells are closely associated with sensory neurons from as early as we can visualize, we hypothesized that they would quickly respond to changes in neuronal homeostasis [10]. Although this phenomenon has been demonstrated, the temporal dynamics of this have not been thoroughly examined. To test this, we imaged DRG neurons that were axotomized distally in the periphery and visualized the response of the ganglia cells to that injury. Using *Tg(sox10:eos)* animals which label cells that ensheath the DRG neurons we performed an 8 μm axotomy injury approximately 100 μm from the ganglia and then collected images every 5 min for 10 h. In each image, we had an experimental-injured and a control non-injured sensory nerve (Fig. 8a). We first confirmed that our laser parameters created a complete transection of the peripheral nerve by imaging *Tg(sox10:eos)* intensity profiles of the length of the lesioned axon 1 h following injury and visualized a lack of fluorescent signal along the nerve (Fig. 8c).

In these animals we visualized that 100% of ganglia with injured peripheral nerves responded by re-arranging ensheathing cells around the neuronal soma (Fig. 8b, Additional file 3: Movie S3, Additional file 4: Movie S4). In control, non-injured, ganglia that were adjacent to the injured nerves we did not visualize this dynamic; within the 10-h period of imaging, 0% of ganglia associated with non-injured nerves re-arranged. We took this analysis further to dissect the dynamics of re-arrangement in order to investigate the speed of ganglia response to peripheral injury. Injured nerves induced a ganglia cell re-arrangement in 72.6 ± 48.22 min with the majority responding within the first hour (Fig. 8d, $n = 5$). These responses occurred in the ganglia 100 μm from the injury site. These results are consistent with the hypothesis that the ensheathing cells of the ganglia can respond rapidly to peripheral injury of those neurons.

To expand our understanding of the injury response, we traced the movements of the responding glia in

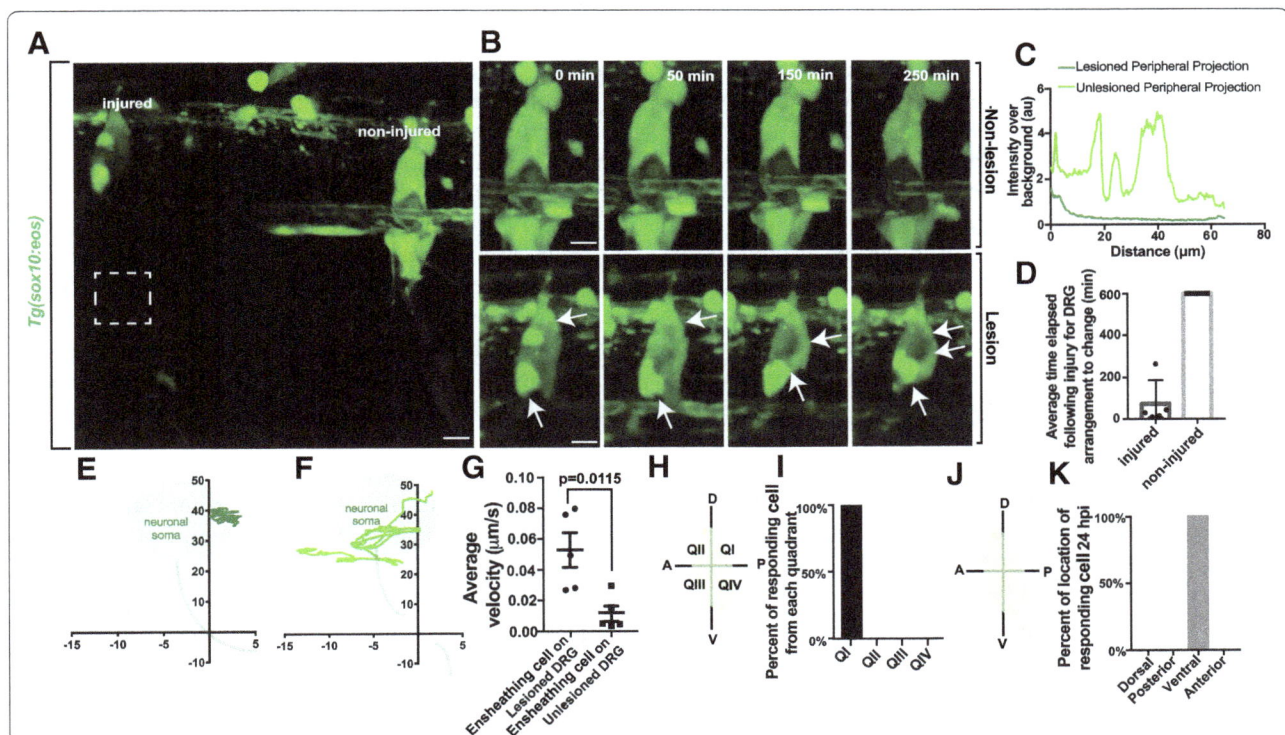

**Fig. 8** Ensheathing cells respond to peripheral neuronal injury. (**a**). Confocal z-projection image of a *Tg(sox10:eos)* zebrafish with a DRG with a peripheral lesion and an adjacent non-lesion DRG. White box denotes site of lesion. (**b**). Confocal z-projection image of a 24-h timelapse starting at 72 hpf in a *Tg(sox10:eos)* zebrafish. Top images denote a non-lesion DRG, and bottom images denote a DRG with a peripheral lesion. White arrows denote the movement of ensheathing cells. (**c**). Intensity profile of lesioned and non-lesioned peripheral axons. (**d**). Time elapsed after lesion for rearrangement of ensheathing cells in lesioned and non-lesioned DRG (n = 5 lesion DRG, n = 5 non-lesion DRG). (**e-f**). Plots of ensheathing cells following axonal lesion on non-lesioned (**e**) and lesioned (**f**) neurons. Shaded gray areas denote location of the neuron. (0,0) denotes the center of the peripheral axon. (**g**). Average velocity of ensheathing cells following injury on lesioned and non-lesioned neurons (n = 5 lesion DRG, n = 5 non-lesion DRG). (**h**). Schematic compass of DRG neuron into quadrants. D denotes dorsal, P denotes posterior, V denotes ventral, A denotes anterior. (**i**). Percentage of responding cells that originate in each quadrant of the neuron (n = 5 DRG). (**j**). Schematic compass of DRG neuron by anatomical descriptor. D denotes dorsal, P denotes posterior, V denotes ventral, A denotes anterior. (**k**). Percentage of responding cells that stabilize in each portion of the neuron (n = 5 DRG). (**g**) uses an unpaired Student's *t*-test. Scale bar is 10 μm (**a**, **b**)

DRG with lesioned axons as well as adjacent unlesioned DRG. Ensheathing cells in lesioned DRG dynamically traversed the entire ganglia, while ensheathing cells in unlesioned DRG remained in their original location (Fig. 8e, f). Further, we calculated the velocities of the ensheathing cell projections in both lesioned and unlesioned DRG. These cells responded to the lesion with a velocity of $0.0519 \pm 0.0113$ µm/min (Fig. 8g, n = 5 DRG), while cells on unlesioned ganglia were largely stationary (n = 5 DRG, $p = 0.0115$, $0.0117 \pm 0.00492$). Since the injury was consistently created in the same portion of the neuron, we hypothesized that the glial response may be similar following each injury. To do this, we determined the location of the cells that respond to the peripheral injury by quantifying which quadrant of the ganglia the responding cell originated. We found that 100% of the responding cells on lesioned DRG originated in the dorsal, posterior quadrant of the ganglia (Fig. 8h, i, n = 5 DRG). Given this highly consistent spatial response to the injury, we also quantified the final location of the responding cell. We hypothesized that the responding cell may travel to the sight of the injury. Instead, 100% of the responding cells eventually ended their migration at the ventral apex of the neuron cell body where the injured neurite originated (Fig. 8j, k, n = 5 DRG). These data suggest that ensheathing cells have a strikingly consistent and choreographed response to peripheral axonal injury; they migrate to the extension site of initiation of the injured axon.

Given the effects of unensheathment can have on the neuron and the apparent rearrangement of cells in the ganglia following injury, we next asked if neuronal soma shape was momentarily altered during the injury response. To ask this, we measured the area and shape descriptors for the neuronal cell bodies shortly after the injury and 24 h later. We did not detect any changes in area ($p = 0.6830$, n = 5 unlesioned neurons, n = 5 lesioned neurons, unlesioned at 0 hpi: $61.199 \pm 9.688$ µm$^2$, lesioned at 0 hpi: $73.937 \pm 15.863$ µm$^2$, unlesioned at 24 hpi: $76.472 \pm 12.843$ µm$^2$, lesioned at 24 hpi: $83.465 \pm 13.101$ µm$^2$), circularity ($p = 0.8453$, n = 5 unlesioned neurons, n = 5 lesioned neurons, nonlesioned at 0 hpi: $0.775 \pm 0.0600$, lesioned at 0 hpi: $0.768 \pm 0.0325$, nonlesioned at 24 hpi: $0.765 \pm 0.0595$, lesioned at 24 hpi: $0.796 \pm 0.0380$), aspect ratio ($p = 0.2491$, n = 5 unlesioned neurons, n = 5 lesioned neurons, nonlesioned at 0 hpi: $1.438 \pm 0.188$, lesioned at 0 hpi: $1.868 \pm 0.125$, nonlesioned at 24 hpi: $1.536 \pm 0.131$, lesioned at 24 hpi: $1.713 \pm 0.168$), roundness ($p = 0.2040$, n = 5 unlesioned neurons, n = 5 lesioned neurons, nonlesioned at 0 hpi: $0.739 \pm 0.0857$, lesioned at 0 hpi: $0.545 \pm 0.0357$, nonlesioned at 24 hpi: $0.671 \pm 0.0571$, lesioned at 24 hpi: $0.608 \pm 0.0650$), or solidity ($p = 0.6562$, n = 5 unlesioned neurons,

n = 5 lesioned neurons, nonlesioned at 0 hpi: $0.914 \pm 0.143$, lesioned at 0 hpi: $0.930 \pm 0.0106$, nonlesioned at 24 hpi: $0.918 \pm 0.185$, lesioned at 24 hpi: $0.921 \pm 0.0172$). These measurements suggest that the ensheathing glia exhibit a highly-coordinated response throughout the ganglia following peripheral injury that mirrors developmental expansion to ensure continued ensheathment of the neuronal cell body as one cell migrates across the ganglion. Only during longer pathological unensheathment events does neuronal morphology become altered. Together, these data support the hypothesis that during the lifespan of the DRG, the neuron and its dynamic ensheathing cells are intimately connected and plastic.

## Discussion

Ensheathment of neuronal cells is critical to proper formation and function of complete nerves. Using single-cell photoconversion and time lapse imaging in intact living vertebrates, we demonstrate that the ensheathment of DRG neuronal cell somas occurs during neuronal differentiation, a distinct event from axonal ensheathment. We show that these ensheathing cells must rearrange to allow for the initiation of neurites. During development they also exhibit tiling behavior. Perturbations of the soma ensheathment causes changes in neuronal soma morphology and positioning. Using laser induced lesions of the distal peripheral axon, we show that these ensheathing cells respond quickly to neuronal injury in a choreographed manner. Together, our data suggest that ensheathing cells of the DRG neuronal cell soma are closely associated with the neuron starting shortly after initial neuronal differentiation and persist throughout the life of the neuron to maintain stereotypical ganglia positions.

### DRG cells exhibit a neural niche

The proliferation of neural progenitor populations is necessary for the establishment and creation of a complete neuronal circuit [46]. These progenitor populations are often confined to small areas, called neural niches, where the production of neural precursors can be tightly controlled and regulated [47]. Previous studies have shown that cortex glia, a *Drosophila* cell type that ensheathes neuronal cell somas in adult brains, ensheath distinct neural progenitor populations in neural niches [32]. This ensheathment persists throughout the proliferation of the neural progenitors. Our data suggest that the development of the dorsal root ganglia can serve as an analogous model for such neural niches. We demonstrate that ensheathment of the DRG neuronal cell soma occurs shortly after neuronal differentiation and persists throughout the expansion of the DRG. Further, these data demonstrate that the ensheathing cells of the DRG serve as a progenitor population for DRG neurons [37], consistent with neuronal progenitor differentiation in classical neural niches. In fact, the fate of progenitor populations in neural niches and the DRG may even depend on the level of ensheathment of a daughter cell by dictating expression of neuronal markers. As a result, future studies on the precise development of the DRG in the context of ensheathing cells may yield valuable insights into the dynamics of neural niches and neuronal differentiation.

In addition, glial ensheathment of distinct portions of a mature neuron is critical to the establishment of a functional nervous system [10, 48]. While many previous studies have examined the mechanism of axonal ensheathment, few have explored the process of neuronal cell soma ensheathment. Our data helps fill this gap by visualizing the ensheathment of DRG neuronal somas in vertebrates. We elucidate the close association between the ensheathing cells and the neuron throughout its maturation. Studies in *Drosophila* have demonstrated the potential for cells ensheathing the cell soma to interact with and support the neuron which they ensheath. For example, expression of a (DE)-cadherin dominant negative in *Drosophila* cortex glia, which ensheath neuronal cell bodies, have been shown to lead to misplaced neural progenitors and neuronal somas as well as disrupt neuron morphology and neurite trajectories [18]. Here, we provide a step wise visualization of the ensheathment of such vertebrate neuronal somas.

### Soma ensheathing cells interact with axons

In a mature DRG, differentiated satellite glial cells ensheath the sensory neurons located in the ganglia [10]. Interestingly, co-cultures of mature satellite glial cells and neurons lead to inhibited dendrite formation [49]. Our data suggests that the precursors to satellite glial cells are intimately involved in neuronal maturation and morphology, including neurite extension. Given this and the formation of "glial horns" during neurite initiation, the ensheathment of the neuron cell body is likely critical to maturation of the neuron and its neurites. Coupled with increasing evidence for the role of glia in the initiation of neurites [15], our data suggest that rearrangement of the ensheathing DRG cells may provide a substrate to allow for the initiation or extension of axonal projections. Further, we demonstrate that the initial ensheathing cell of the sensory pioneer axon are produced in the ganglia by cells that ensheath the cell soma. This finding complements recent investigations seeking to characterize satellite glia which identified myelinogenic capabilities of mouse satellite glia in culture as well as robust transciptomic similarities between satellite glia and mature Schwann cells [9]. Our imaging of DRG development in zebrafish are consistent with these hypotheses. The intimate associations of the ensheathing cells with the DRG neurons from as early as we can delineate

suggests they could have a profound influence on neuronal development and homeostasis. But to date, neuronal development and homeostasis are often investigated in the absence of ensheathing cells. Future studies testing these hypotheses may yield important insights in axonal morphology, nerve assembly, and axonal compartmentalization.

### Forces that dictate neuronal cell shape and location

Further, our data suggest that neuronal soma ensheathment likely plays a conserved function in dictating the size and shape of the soma in development. In zebrafish mutants of Sox10, a gene required for glial differentiation, ensheathing cells of the DRG are absent and the DRG are mislocalized [23]. These data are consistent with the hypothesis that ensheathing cells also contribute to the positioning of the DRG. We also observe that the neuronal soma immediately bulges and shifts toward a site of disrupted ensheathment. The totality of these data, in conjunction with previous studies, point to a conserved role of continuous mechanical forces on the neuronal soma from the ensheathing cell membranes imposing a circular shape and potentially precise position on the neuron within the ganglia [17, 18, 23, 32]. The release of this restraining force in unensheathment events likely causes the neuron to accelerate toward ablated area much like a compressed spring.

The DRG has a precise and stereotypical spatial and temporal arrangement of neurons where specific neuronal subtypes localize to distinct regions within the ganglia [33]. In addition to neurons, ensheathing cells in the DRG must also continuously produce other cell types such as Schwann cells and melanocytes which then traverse around the ganglia to leave for their respective target areas [34, 50, 51]. Throughout each of these proliferation events, DRG neurons retain their precise location in both development and adulthood. As a result, a continuous mechanism must be employed in the ganglia to anchor DRG neurons in their locations throughout cell proliferation events while allowing differentiating cells to migrate away from the DRG. The data presented here suggest that the tiling behavior of soma-ensheathing cells could continuously help maintain precise shape and arrangement of DRG neurons by providing forces on the neuronal soma. Following a prolonged, injury-induced unensheathment event, the DRG neuron immediately bulges and becomes displaced from its original position, like an expanding spring. However, during homeostatic proliferation of ensheathing cells and partial unensheathment events, the neuronal movement is less pronounced. A greater mislocalization of DRG neurons was caused by complete, genetic ablations of ensheathing progenitors [23]. Together, this is consistent with continuous role of ensheathing cells to physically provide forces on DRG neurons throughout paradigmatic development. In addition, physical contacts between DRG cell types have been suggested as regulators of cell fate decisions between glia and neurons as well as between different types of neuronal subtypes [23, 33, 50]. Taken together with our data, this suggests that the precise forces on neurons by ensheathing cells may aid in the development of the diversity of somatosensory cell types.

Unfortunately, the physiological effects of changes to the shape of neuronal somas are currently unknown. Data comparing the morphology and electrophysiology of CA1 and CA2 hippocampal neurons in *Proechimys* rodents suggests that smaller cell somas are correlated with decreased electrical resistance and a longer latency period [52]. However, these recordings were taken from healthy and fully differentiated neuron populations. Cell soma size also correlates with axonal caliber [53]. Studies show axonal caliber impacts ensheathment and myelination, pointing to a hypothesis that neuronal size is important in the nervous system [54, 55]. Regardless, given that our data indicate that re-ensheathment itself is not sufficient to restore neuronal morphology following prolonged unensheathment, the importance of soma shape in neuron electrophysiology, although beyond the scope of this paper, should be investigated, especially given the possibility of unensheathment in disease states.

### Ensheathing cells respond to injury

Given the close proximity of ensheathing cells to axonal injury, they represent an important cell type that could respond to neural injury. Previous studies have shown that many ensheathing glial subtypes exhibit tiling behavior to maintain neuronal ensheathment following injury [16]. Our analysis of the space filling behavior by ensheathing processes in both normal development and injury states consistently demonstrated an asymmetric response to unensheathment by individual cells (Fig. 4). This response suggests that specific subpopulations of ensheathing glia, at least during development, may be hypervigilant to unensheathment events. We also demonstrate that ensheathing cells respond to modulated ensheathment through tiling behavior throughout the life of the DRG. Further, we show that neuronal soma-ensheathing cells display a consistent and choreographed response to neuronal injury to the distal axonal segment by migrating to the initiation site of the injured neurite. This response does not disrupt the ensheathment or morphology of the neuron, suggesting a coordinated space-filling response by all ensheathing cells following neuronal injury. As a result, our data point to DRG ensheathing glia as a population that can detect and respond to neural injury, a behavior also seen in mature satellite glial cells [10]. This observation is also consistent with previous reports in *Drosophila* where cortex glia respond to injury and phagocytize neural debris

[16]. Previous studies have also demonstrated that some DRG cell types are pluripotent stem cells that can differentiate into terminal glia, or even skin melanocytes, after migrating down the peripheral nerve to the skin [34]. Given the specific choreographed response by ensheathing glia from a consistent and specific neuronal domain following neural injury, it is possible that the responding cell we identified retains a stem-like quality in order to coordinate a cellular response to neuronal injury. Coupled with the hypervigilance of some cells to unensheathment, the cells that ensheath DRG neurons could form a heterogeneous population with specific cells primed to respond to various, yet specific disruptions to neuronal homeostasis. Future research will dissect this important topic.

### Conclusions

While many studies have been devoted to the mechanisms of axonal ensheathment and its role in neuronal homeostasis, mechanisms of ensheathment of neuronal somas has remained elusive. Here we used single-cell photoconversion to visualize the process of soma ensheathment in zebrafish dorsal root ganglia. Taken together, our data point to the importance of neuronal soma ensheathment in nerve development as early as neuronal differentiation. The close association of the ensheathing cells with the maturing neuron point to cross-talk as a possible important facet of nerve assembly. Elucidating these associated cues, as demonstrated by recent studies, could yield valuable insight into neural niches, neural injury responses and the diversity of soma-ensheathing cells.

### Additional files

**Additional file 1: Movie S1.** Ensheathment of neuronal progenitors occurs soon after neuronal differentiation. Excerpt from a 24-h time lapse of a *Tg(sox10:eos)* animal with a photoconverted neuronal progenitor from 48 to 72 hpf. (Left) A *Tg(sox10:eos)* unconverted cell wraps projections around the neuronal progenitor before neurite extension. (Right) Merged image of *Tg(sox10:eos)* converted (neuronal progenitor) and unconverted (ensheathing cell). Green arrows denote ensheathing projections. Dark green arrow denotes merged ensheathing projections. Frames in the video were captured every 5 min, and the video plays at 10 frames per second. Supplements Fig. 1d.

**Additional file 2: Movie S2.** Soma-ensheathing cells exhibit tiling behavior during injury. Excerpt from a 24-h time lapse of a *Tg(sox10:eos)* animal with a photoconverted neuronal progenitor from 48 to 72 hpf following a laser ablation of an ensheathing cell. (Left) *Tg(sox10:eos)* unconverted cells respond to the unensheathment of the neuronal soma by sending projections to restore soma ensheathment. (Right) Merged image of *Tg(sox10:eos)* converted (neuron) and unconverted (ensheathing cell). Green arrows denote ensheathing projections. Dark green arrow denotes merged ensheathing projections. Frames in the video were captured every 5 min, and the video plays at 10 frames per second. Supplements Fig. 4e.

**Additional file 3: Movie S3.** Ensheathing cells are stationary in the absence of neuronal injury. Excerpt from a 24-h time lapse of a *Tg(sox10:eos)*

animal from 72 to 96 hpf. The imaged DRG is adjacent to a DRG neuron with peripheral axonal injury at 72 hpf. Red arrow denotes an ensheathing cell. Frames in the video were captured every 5 min, and the video plays at 10 frames per second. Supplements Fig. 8b.

**Additional file 4: Movie S4.** Ensheathing cells dynamically remodel following distal axonal injury. Excerpt from a 24-h time lapse of a *Tg(sox10:eos)* animal from 72 to 96 hpf. The imaged DRG neuron suffered distal axonal injury at 72 hpf. Red arrow denotes an ensheathing cell. Frames in the video were captured every 5 min, and the video plays at 10 frames per second. Supplements Fig. 8b.

## Abbreviations
CNS: Central nervous system; DMSO: Dimethyl sulfoxide; dpf: Days post fertilization; DREZ: Dorsal root entry zone; DRG: Dorsal root ganglia; hpf: Hours post fertilization; hpi: Hours post injury

## Acknowledgements
We thank members of the Smith lab and Sarah Kucenas for their helpful comments, Sam Connell and Brent Redford of 3i for fielding imaging questions and Deborah Bang and Karen Heed for zebrafish care. This work was supported by the University of Notre Dame, the Elizabeth and Michael Gallagher Family, the Alfred P. Sloan Foundation, Center for Zebrafish Research at the University of Notre and Center of Stem Cells and Regenerative Medicine at the University of Notre Dame.

## Funding
This work was supported by the University of Notre Dame and the Elizabeth and Michael Gallagher Family, Center for Zebrafish Research at the University of Notre, Center of Stem Cells and Regenerative Medicine at the University of Notre Dame and the Alfred P. Sloan Foundation.

## Authors' contributions
ELN, LAG and CJS conducted the experiments. ELN analyzed all the experiments and quantified the data. LAG and CJS created injuries in sensory neurons. CJS conceived the project and ELN and CJS wrote the manuscript with input from LAG. All authors read and approved the final manuscript.

## Competing interests
The authors declare that they have no competing interests.

## References
1. Donaldson HH. 1902. The relation of myelin to the loss of water in the mammalian nervous system with advancing age. Proc Phil Soc Phil mag Wellisch, Amer J Sci Lattey proc R Soc, a Kovarick physic rev * Chaffee 209.
2. Hines JH, Ravanelli AM, Schwindt R, Scott EK, Appel B. Neuronal activity biases axon selection for myelination in vivo. Nat Neurosci. 2015;18:683–9.
3. Snaidero N, Molbius W, Czopka T, Hekking LHP, Mathisen C, Verkleij D, Goebbels S, Edgar J, Merkler D, Lyons DA, Nave KA, Simons M. Myelin membrane wrapping of CNS axons by PI(3,4,5)P3-dependent polarized growth at the inner tongue. Cell. 2014;156:277–90.
4. Brown AM, Ransom BR. Astrocyte glycogen and brain energy metabolism. Glia. 2007;55:1263–71.
5. Nave KA. Myelination and the trophic support of long axons. Nat Rev Neurosci. 2010;11:275–83.
6. Jessen KR, Mirsky R. Embryonic Schwann cell development: the biology of Schwann cell precursors and early Schwann cells. J Anat. 1997;191:501–5.
7. Wang H, Moyano AL, Ma Z, Deng Y, Lin Y, Zhao C, Zhang L, Jiang M, He X, Ma Z, Lu F, Xin M, Zhou W, Yoon SO, Bongarzone ER, Lu QR. miR-219 cooperates with miR-338 in myelination and promotes myelin repair in the CNS. Dev Cell. 2017;40:566–82. e5
8. Bin JM, Rajasekharan S, Kuhlmann T, Hanes I, Marcal N, Han D, Rodrigues SP, Leong SY, Newcombe J, Antel JP, Kennedy TE. Full-length and fragmented netrin-1 in multiple sclerosis plaques are inhibitors of oligodendrocyte precursor cell migration. Am J Pathol. 2013;183:673–80.
9. George D, Ahrens P, Lambert S. Satellite glial cells represent a population of developmentally arrested Schwann cells. Glia. 2018; Available from: http://doi.wiley.com/10.1002/glia.23320
10. Hanani M. Satellite glial cells in sensory ganglia: from form to function. Brain Res Rev. 2005;48:457–76.
11. Freeman MR. Drosophila central nervous system glia. Cold Spring Harb Perspect Biol. 2015;7
12. Oikonomou G, Shaham S. The glia of caenorhabditis elegans. Glia. 2011;59:1253–63.
13. Heiman MG, Shaham S. DEX-1 and DYF-7 establish sensory dendrite length by anchoring dendritic tips during cell migration. Cell. 2009;137:344–55. Available from: https://ac.els-cdn.com/S0092867409001597/1-s2.0-S0092867409001597-main.pdf?_tid=8bdd010c-feec-11e7-8c3f-00000aacb361&acdnat=1516567937_54b3b51834e8491ad68f0c8e91752af6
14. Procko C, Lu Y, Shaham S, Horvitz HR, Bargmann CI. Glia delimit shape changes of sensory neuron receptive endings in C. Elegans. Development. 2011;138:1371–81.
15. Rapti G, Li C, Shan A, Lu Y, Shaham S. Glia initiate brain assembly through noncanonical Chimaerin-Furin axon guidance in C. Elegans. Nat Neurosci. 2017;20:1350–60.
16. MacDonald JM, Beach MG, Porpiglia E, Sheehan AE, Watts RJ, Freeman MR. The Drosophila cell corpse engulfment receptor Draper mediates glial clearance of severed axons. Neuron. 2006;50:869–81.
17. Coutinho-Budd JC, Sheehan AE, Freeman MR. The secreted neurotrophin spätzle 3 promotes glial morphogenesis and supports neuronal survival and function. Genes Dev. 2017;31:2023–38.
18. Dumstrei K, Wang F, Hartenstein V. Role of DE-cadherin in neuroblast proliferation, neural morphogenesis, and axon tract formation in Drosophila larval brain development. J Neurosci. 2003;23:3325–35.
19. Redmond SA, Mei F, Eshed-Eisenbach Y, Osso LA, Leshkowitz D, Shen YAA, Kay JN, Aurrand-Lions M, Lyons DA, Peles E, Chan JR. Somatodendritic expression of JAM2 inhibits oligodendrocyte myelination. Neuron. 2016;91:824–36.
20. Gao FB, Kohwi M, Brenman JE, Jan LY, Jan YN. Control of dendritic field formation in Drosophila: the roles of flamingo and competition between homologous neurons. Neuron. 2000;28:91–101.
21. Grueber WB, Jan LY, Jan YN. Dendritic tiling in Drosophila. Development. 2002;129:2867–78. Available from: https://pdfs.semanticscholar.org/651e/308ef39e23a221b50b49aeb0e66fbf1be88d.pdf
22. Huckfeldt RM, Schubert T, Morgan JL, Godinho L, Di Cristo G, Huang ZJ, Wong ROL. Transient neurites of retinal horizontal cells exhibit columnar tiling via homotypic interactions. Nat Neurosci. 2009;12:35–43.
23. Carney TJ, Dutton KA, Greenhill E, Delfino-Machin M, Dufourcq P, Blader P, Kelsh RN. A direct role for Sox10 in specification of neural crest-derived sensory neurons. Development. 2006;133:4619–30. Available from: http://dev.biologists.org/cgi/doi/10.1242/dev.02668
24. Sagasti A, Guido MR, Raible DW, Schier AF. Repulsive interactions shape the morphologies and functional arrangement of zebrafish peripheral sensory arbors. Curr Biol. 2005;15:804–14. Available from: http://www.ncbi.nlm.nih.gov/pubmed/15886097
25. Smith CJ, Watson JD, Spencer WC, O'Brien T, Cha B, Albeg A, Treinin M, Miller DM III. Time-lapse imaging and cell-specific expression profiling reveal dynamic branching and molecular determinants of a multi-dendritic nociceptor in C. Elegans. Dev Biol. 2010;345:18–33. Available from: http://www.ncbi.nlm.nih.gov/pubmed/20537990
26. Hughes EG, Kang SH, Fukaya M, Bergles DE. Oligodendrocyte progenitors balance growth with self-repulsion to achieve homeostasis in the adult brain. Nat Neurosci. 2013;16:668–76.
27. Kirby BB, Takada N, Latimer AJ, Shin J, Carney TJ, Kelsh RN, Appel B. In vivo time-lapse imaging shows dynamic oligodendrocyte progenitor behavior during zebrafish development. Nat Neurosci. 2006;9:1506–11.

28. Smith CJ, Morris AD, Welsh TG, Kucenas S. Contact-mediated inhibition between oligodendrocyte progenitor cells and motor exit point glia establishes the spinal cord transition zone. PLoS Biol. 2014;12:e1001961. Available from: http://dx.plos.org/10.1371/journal.pbio.1001961

29. Pereanu W, Kumar A, Jennett A, Reichert H, Hartenstein V. Development-based compartmentalization of the drosophila central brain. J Comp Neurol. 2010;

30. Pereanu W, Spindler S, Cruz L, Hartenstein V. Tracheal development in the Drosophila brain is constrained by glial cells. Dev Biol. 2007;302:169–80.

31. Radtke C, Wewetzer K, Reimers K, Vogt PM. Transplantation of olfactory ensheathing cells as adjunct cell therapy for peripheral nerve injury. Cell Transplant. 2011;20:145–52.

32. Doyle SE, Pahl MC, Siller KH, Ardiff L, Siegrist SE. Neuroblast niche position is controlled by phosphoinositide 3-kinase-dependent DE-cadherin adhesion. Development. 2017;144:820–9. Available from: http://dev.biologists.org/lookup/doi/10.1242/dev.136713

33. Marmigère F, Ernfors P. Specification and connectivity of neuronal subtypes in the sensory lineage. Nat Rev Neurosci. 2007;8:114–27.

34. Gresset A, Coulpier F, Gerschenfeld G, Jourdon A, Matesic G, Richard L, Vallat JM, Charnay P, Topilko P. Boundary caps give rise to neurogenic stem cells and terminal glia in the skin. Stem Cell Reports. 2015;5:278–90.

35. Honjo Y, Kniss J, Eisen JS. Neuregulin-mediated ErbB3 signaling is required for formation of zebrafish dorsal root ganglion neurons. Development. 2008;135:2993. Available from: http://dev.biologists.org/cgi/doi/10.1242/dev.027763

36. Prendergast A, Linbo TH, Swarts T, Ungos JM, McGraw HF, Krispin S, Weinstein BM, Raible DW. The metalloproteinase inhibitor Reck is essential for zebrafish DRG development. Development. 2012;139:1141–52. Available from: http://dev.biologists.org/cgi/doi/10.1242/dev.072439

37. McGraw H, Snelson CD, Prendergast A, Suli A, Raible DW. Postembryonic neuronal addition in zebrafish dorsal root ganglia is regulated by notch signaling. Neural Dev. 2012;7:23. Available from: http://neuraldevelopment.biomedcentral.com/articles/10.1186/1749-8104-7-23

38. McGraw HF, Nechiporuk A, Raible DW. Zebrafish dorsal root ganglia neural precursor cells adopt a glial fate in the absence of neurogenin1. J Neurosci. 2008;28:12558–69. Available from: http://www.ncbi.nlm.nih.gov/pubmed/19020048

39. Hochgreb-Agele NT, Bronner ME. A novel FoxD3 gene trap line reveals neural crest precursor movement and a role for FoxD3 in their specification. Dev Biol. 2013;374:1–11. Available from: https://ac.els-cdn.com/S0012160612006549/1-s2.0-S0012160612006549-main.pdf?_tid=031708e6-feff-11e7-ad57-00000aab0f6b&acdnat=1516575868_f47a2848eebf488a04a7ee7c36adde09

40. Green L, Smith CJ. Single-cell Photoconversion in living intact zebrafish. J Vis Exp. 2018:e57024–4. Available from: https://www.jove.com/video/57024/single-cell-photoconversion-in-living-intact-zebrafish

41. Murphy DA, Diaz B, Bromann PA, Tsai JH, Kawakami Y, Maurer J, Stewart RA, Izpisúa-Belmonte JC, Courtneidge SA. A Src-Tks5 pathway is required for neural crest cell migration during embryonic development. PLoS One. 2011;6:e22499. Available from: http://dx.plos.org/10.1371/journal.pone.0022499

42. Woodhoo A, Sommer L. Development of the schwann cell lineage: from the neural crest to the myelinated nerve. Glia. 2008;56:1481–90.

43. Perez-Alvarez A, Navarrete M, Covelo A, Martin ED, Araque A. Structural and functional plasticity of astrocyte processes and dendritic spine interactions. J Neurosci. 2014;34:12738–44. Available from: http://www.jneurosci.org/cgi/doi/10.1523/JNEUROSCI.2401-14.2014

44. Basbaum AI, Bautista DM, Scherrer G, Julius D. Cellular and molecular mechanisms of pain. Cell. 2009;139:267–84.

45. Smith CJ, Wheeler MA, Marjoram L, Bagnat M, Deppmann CD, Kucenas S. TNFa/TNFR2 signaling is required for glial ensheathment at the dorsal root entry zone. PLoS Genet. 2017;13

46. Florio M, Huttner WB. Neural progenitors, neurogenesis and the evolution of the neocortex. Development. 2014;141:2182–94. Available from: http://dev.biologists.org/cgi/doi/10.1242/dev.090571

47. Preston M, Sherman LS. Neural stem cell niches: roles for the hyaluronan-based extracellular matrix. Front Biosci (Schol Ed). 2011;3:1165–79. Available from: http://www.ncbi.nlm.nih.gov/pubmed/21622263%5Cn. http://www.pubmedcentral.nih.gov/articlerender.fcgi?artid=PMC3256127

48. Donaldson. 1916.

49. De Koninck P, Carbonetto S, Cooper E. NGF induces neonatal rat sensory neurons to extend dendrites in culture after removal of satellite cells. J Neurosci. 1993;13:577–85.

50. Delfino-Machín M, Madelaine R, Busolin G, Nikaido M, Colanesi S, Camargo-Sosa K, Law EWP, Toppo S, Blader P, Tiso N, Kelsh RN. Sox10 contributes to the balance of fate choice in dorsal root ganglion progenitors. PLoS One. 2017;12:1–29.

51. Marol GS, Vermeren M, Voiculescu O, Melton L, Cohen J, Charnay P, Topilko P. Neural crest boundary cap cells constitute a source of neuronal and glial cells of the PNS. Nat Neurosci. 2004;7:930–8.

52. Scorza CA, Araujo BHS, Leite LA, Torres LB, Otalora LFP, Oliveira MS, Garrido-Sanabria ER, Cavalheiro EA. Morphological and electrophysiological properties of pyramidal-like neurons in the stratum oriens of Cornu ammonis 1 and Cornu ammonis 2 area of Proechimys. Neuroscience. 2011;177:252–68.

53. Sloper JJ, Powell TP. A study of the axon initial segment and proximal axon of neurons in the primate motor and somatic sensory cortices. Philos Trans R Soc Lond B Biol Sci. 1979;285:173–97.

54. Hildebrand C, Remahl S, Persson H, Bjartmar C. Myelinated nerve fibres in the CNS Prog Neurobiol. 1993;40:319–384.

55. Baumann N, Pham-Dinh D. Biology of Oligodendrocyte and Myelin in the Mammalian Central Nervous System. Physiol Rev. 2001;81:871–927.

# 10

# Contralateral migration of oculomotor neurons is regulated by Slit/Robo signaling

Brielle Bjorke[1], Farnaz Shoja-Taheri[1], Minkyung Kim[1], G. Eric Robinson[1], Tatiana Fontelonga[1], Kyung-Tai Kim[2], Mi-Ryoung Song[2] and Grant S. Mastick[1]* [iD]

## Abstract

**Background:** Oculomotor neurons develop initially like typical motor neurons, projecting axons out of the ventral midbrain to their ipsilateral targets, the extraocular muscles. However, in all vertebrates, after the oculomotor nerve (nIII) has reached the extraocular muscle primordia, the cell bodies that innervate the superior rectus migrate to join the contralateral nucleus. This motor neuron migration represents a unique strategy to form a contralateral motor projection. Whether migration is guided by diffusible cues remains unknown.

**Methods:** We examined the role of Slit chemorepellent signals in contralateral oculomotor migration by analyzing mutant mouse embryos.

**Results:** We found that the ventral midbrain expresses high levels of both Slit1 and 2, and that oculomotor neurons express the repellent Slit receptors Robo1 and Robo2. Therefore, Slit signals are in a position to influence the migration of oculomotor neurons. In Slit 1/2 or Robo1/2 double mutant embryos, motor neuron cell bodies migrated into the ventral midbrain on E10.5, three days prior to normal migration. These early migrating neurons had leading projections into and across the floor plate. In contrast to the double mutants, embryos which were mutant for single Slit or Robo genes did not have premature migration or outgrowth on E10.5, demonstrating a cooperative requirement of Slit1 and 2, as well as Robo1 and 2. To test how Slit/Robo midline repulsion is modulated, we found that the normal migration did not require the receptors Robo3 and CXCR4, or the chemoattractant, Netrin 1. The signal to initiate contralateral migration is likely autonomous to the midbrain because oculomotor neurons migrate in embryos that lack either nerve outgrowth or extraocular muscles, or in cultured midbrains that lacked peripheral tissue.

**Conclusion:** Overall, our results demonstrate that a migratory subset of motor neurons respond to floor plate-derived Slit repulsion to properly control the timing of contralateral migration.

**Keywords:** Oculomotor, Motor neuron, Migration, Floor plate, Slit/Robo

## Background

The oculomotor neurons are the most anterior motor neurons in the CNS, forming the oculomotor nerve (nIII). Their axons emerge from the ventral midbrain and innervate four of the six extraocular muscles. Development of the oculomotor system must occur with spatial and temporal accuracy to properly position the motor neuron cell bodies and to guide their axons to corresponding extraocular muscles. Errors in development can lead to abnormal eye movements or alignment, termed strabismus, and may result in partial blindness reviewed

in [1]. The mechanisms that guide the development of the oculomotor system remain poorly understood.

Early in embryonic development, clusters of oculomotor neurons project axons ipsilaterally toward muscle targets, similar to most motor neurons. However, during extraocular muscle innervation, a subset of neurons in the oculomotor nucleus repolarize to send a second process into and across the midline. This subset of motor neuron cell bodies then migrate across the ventral midbrain with axons trailing to join the contralateral oculomotor nucleus [2–7]. This process generates the oculomotor commissure and connects motor neurons located in the caudal half of the oculomotor nucleus to the contralateral superior (dorsal) rectus muscle.

* Correspondence: gmastick@unr.edu
[1]Department of Biology, University of Nevada, Reno, NV 89557, USA
Full list of author information is available at the end of the article

Contralateral innervation of the superior rectus muscle is highly conserved among vertebrates [8, and references within].

Oculomotor neurons navigate across the embryonic midline independent of an identifiable glial scaffold, and it was suggested that a "diffusible substance" guides the migrating neurons across the midline [3]. The embryonic ventral midline, consisting of specialized floor plate tissue, is a source of diffusible guidance factors [9]. However, it is unknown whether floor plate guidance cues guide oculomotor neurons. We have focused on two diffusible guidance factors that regulate midline crossing of commissural axons, the Slit proteins and Netrin1. In the developing spinal cord and hindbrain, Slits and Netrin1 mediate migration across the floor plate by their opposing chemotactic actions. The Slit proteins repel both navigating axons and migrating neuron cell bodies reviewed in [10, 11]. In vertebrates, there are three Slit proteins, of which Slit1 and 2 act at the midline to repel axons that express the Slit receptor Robo1 or 2 [12–14]. The third Slit receptor, Robo3 may either counteract the repellent activity of Robo1 and 2 [15] or facilitate Netrin1 attraction [16]. In contrast with Slit signaling, Netrin1 attracts both axons and neurons toward the midline thorough the receptor Deleted in Colorectal Cancer (DCC) [17–21]. Importantly, prior studies in hindbrain showed that these midline guidance signals are important for positioning other cranial neurons, including cranial axon repulsion by Netrin1 [22], and facial branchiomotor migration defects in Slit and Robo mutants and Netrin mutants [23, 24]. Both Slits and Netrin1 are expressed at the ventral midline in the midbrain during early developmental stages [25, 26]. The expression of both Slits and Netrin1 in the developing midbrain, coupled with their role in guiding midline crossing of axons, suggests a role for these cues in guiding the midline migration of oculomotor neurons.

Here we describe how Slit, but not Netrin, acts to gate migration of oculomotor cell bodies into the floor plate. We show that the initial clusters of motor neurons are in fact not static, but have considerable migratory potential, which is demonstrated by abnormal early migration across the floor plate when Slit/Robo signaling is disrupted.

## Methods
### Mouse embryos
#### Ethics approval
Animal experiments were approved by the UNR IACUC, following NIH guidelines, with the approved protocol #2015-00435. DCC embryos are previously described [27]. Robo, Slit and Netrin1 mutant mice were a kind gift from Marc Tessier-Lavigne (Rockefeller), and Frederic Charron (ICMR, Montreal CA). Mating to obtain various

Slit mutant combinations was previously described [13]). Robo, Slit and Netrin1 PCR genotyping were performed as previously described [12, 27–29]. CXCR4 mutant embryos were a gift from John Rubenstein (UCSF). Pitx2 mutant embryos were a kind gift from Philip J Gage (University of Michigan, Ann Arbor). Images of Robo3 mutant embryos were provided by Alain Chedotal (INSERM, Paris). Wild type CD-1 mice were purchased from Charles River Laboratories (Wilmington, MA USA). Embryos were collected in the afternoon of day 10.5, 13.5, or 16.5 with embryonic day 0.5 designated as the day of the vaginal plug. Embryos were fixed with 4 % paraformaldehyde (PFA) overnight or for several days. E16.5 embryos were fixed via cardiac perfusion, and fixed overnight in 4 % PFA.

### In situ hybridization
Whole mount in situ hybridization was previously described [30]. Probes for *Slit1,Slit2, Slit3, Robo1, Robo2, Robo3* were a kind gift from Marc Tessier-Lavigne, (Rockefeller).

### Immunohistochemistry
CD1 E10.5 and E13.5 embryos were dissected in cold 0.4 M phosphate buffer, and fixed with 0.4 % PFA for 1 day. Embryos were then embedded for cryostat sectioning as described [13]. 20 um cryostat sections were rinsed in warm 0.4 % phosphate buffer, and washed with PBS with 0.1 % TritonX-100, and 10 % normal goat serum (PBST). Primary antibodies were diluted in PBST and were applied overnight at room temperature. Primary antibodies included Robo3 (anti-rabbit, Abcam) 1:200, β-galactosidase (Jackson) 1:10,000, Islet1/2 ( DHSB, 39.4D5) 1:200, Robo1 and Robo2 antibodies (kind gift from Elke Stein, Yale; validated in [31]) 1:10,000. Sections were washed several times in PBST and Secondary antibody was applied. Secondary antibodies (Alexa 488, Alexa 555) were diluted in PBST and used at 1:200 for one hour at room temperature. For whole mount labeling of Islet1/2, tissue was placed in primary antibody for 4 days diluted in PBST. The biotin-avidin system (Invitrogen) was used for Islet1/2 amplification, biotin (donkey anti-mouse, 1:100 in PBST) was applied overnight at 4°, washed overnight in PBST, and followed by avidin555 or 488 (1:200in PBST) overnight at 4°.

### Axon tracing
To back-label the oculomotor nucleus and midline crossing fibers, the lipophilic dye, DiI, red, or DiO, green, was crushed onto the oculomotor nerve. First, the skin and mesenchymal tissue was carefully removed from the cephalic flexure ventral to the midbrain to reveal the nIII nerve, then forceps were used to pinch a small crystal of dye onto the nerve. Embryos were placed in 4 %

PFA with .1 % EDTA at 37 °C overnight (E10.5) or up to 3 days (E13.5, E16.5) to allow dye to travel. To visualize the labeled oculomotor nucleus, a 200 um coronal section was cut with a vibratome, and imaged with a confocal microscopy. To visualize the anterior-posterior axis of the CM nucleus, the embryo was cut along the dorsal edge to reveal the midline (open book preparation).

## Quantification of motor neurons in the floorplate

E10.5 midbrains were dissected from various combinations of Slit and Robo mutant mice and antibody labeled for Islet1/2 in open book or sectioned preparations. Islet-positive cells that were located in the space between the two defined oculomotor nuclei were quantified. The average number of cells was graphed with standard deviation indicated by error bars. Significance was determined by Tukey HSD one-way-ANOVA.

## Explant cultures of isolated midbrain tissue

E11.5 mouse midbrain tissues were dissected away from peripheral tissues as an open book preparation, and were cultured in a three-dimensional collagen gel matrix. The cultured tissues were fixed in 4 % PFA after 0, 24, 48, and 72 h of incubation. To label the migrated neurons, explant tissues were washed in PBS containing 10 % FBS and 1 % Triton for several hours (PBST). Primary antibody (1:200 mouse anti-Islet1/2, DSHB) in PBST was applied for 3-4 days. After washing the tissues for several hours, secondary antibody (1:200 Cy3 anti-rabbit (Invitrogen)) in PBST was applied for 2-3 days. The tissues were washed again and mounted on the slides for image acquisition under the confocal microscope (Olympus FV10-ASW).

## Results

### A subset of oculomotor neurons migrate across the midline of the midbrain

To investigate contralateral migration of oculomotor neurons in wild type mice, we first determined the time course of normal migration. To distinguish cell bodies and projections that originate from the left or right oculomotor nuclei, we back-labeled the right and left nucleus with DiI and DiO crushed onto the right and left nIII, respectively. We refer to cells and axons labeled through nIII in this manner as oculomotor, although we note that the embryonic nIII also includes visceral motor fibers from the closely-associated Edinger-Westphal nucleus. To determine the location of oculomotor neuron cell bodies, we labeled the ventral midbrain with Islet1/2 antibody, a general motor neuron marker [32].

On E10.5, oculomotor neurons reside ipsilateral to their respective peripheral nerves (Fig. 1A, B), clustered at the edge of the floor plate (Fig. 1B). Later in development, on E12.5 and 13.5, cell bodies located within the caudal half of the oculomotor nucleus extended labeled processes toward the midline (Fig. 1C, D). In agreement with previous findings in chick and rat, the leading tips of these processes were generally compact with one leading tip [2, 6]. These processes initially projected toward the ventricular surface of the neural tube, then curved slightly down toward the ventral midline and crossed the floor plate to the contralateral oculomotor nucleus (Fig. 1C). By E13.5, leading processes reached the ventrolateral region of the contralateral nucleus and numerous cell bodies were outlined by the lipophilic dye in the floorplate, with a concentration in the midline. By E14.5 leading fibers intercalated into the contralateral nucleus with cell bodies reaching the ventromedial aspect of the nucleus (arrow heads in Fig. 1F'). While the cell bodies accumulated at this ventromedial position, surprisingly many leading processes extended through and past the contralateral nucleus, suggesting that the trailing cell bodies encounter stop cues distinct from the leading processes. The commissure linking the bilateral oculomotor nuclei appeared complete by E16.5, with crossing axons forming the commissure but no cell bodies visible within it (Fig. 1G and schematic Fig. 1H).

To define the anterior-posterior organization of midline crossing on E13.5, transverse sections through the oculomotor nucleus were labeled with the motor-neuron specific marker Islet1/2. In sections taken through the anterior portion of the oculomotor nucleus, motor neurons bundled in discrete nuclei adjacent to the floor plate (Fig. 2A). However, in sections ranging from the middle to caudal oculomotor nucleus, several motor neuron cell bodies were separated from the nuclei, and found within the floor plate (Fig. 2B, C). Cell bodies in the floor plate did not contact the existing ventral tecto-tegmental commissure at the pial surface (brackets in Fig. 2A-D). Instead, the neurons migrated in the ventricular half of the tissue to pioneer a distinct commissure. Interestingly, cell bodies were also observed within fibers that project from the oculomotor nucleus toward the nerve exit points (arrow in Fig. 2C, D, E). Previous research noted cell bodies located within the peripheral oculomotor nerve [33]. We found that cells located within the peripheral oculomotor nerve expressed Islet1/2 (arrow heads point to nIII fibers, arrows point to Islet1/2 + cells in Fig. 2F). These images suggest that Islet1/2 positive cells migrating away from the oculomotor nucleus make their way into the peripheral nerve. Carpenter (1906) hypothesized that cells located in the peripheral nerve will migrate to join the ciliary ganglion [33].

### The Slit family of guidance cues and their receptors are in position to inhibit migration into the floor plate on E10.5

During axon guidance, Slits derived from the floor plate act as repulsive signals via the Robo1 and Robo2

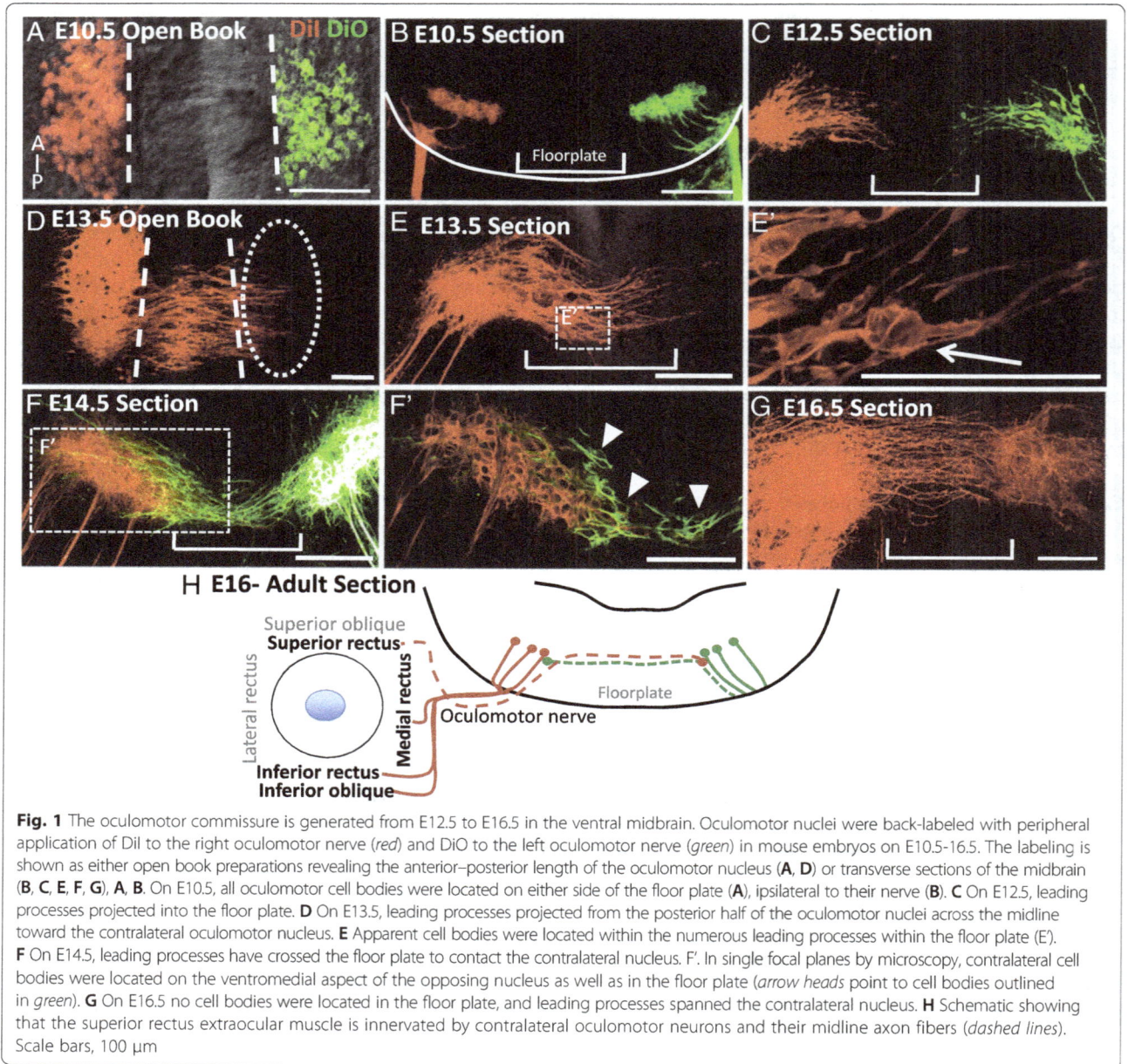

**Fig. 1** The oculomotor commissure is generated from E12.5 to E16.5 in the ventral midbrain. Oculomotor nuclei were back-labeled with peripheral application of DiI to the right oculomotor nerve (*red*) and DiO to the left oculomotor nerve (*green*) in mouse embryos on E10.5-16.5. The labeling is shown as either open book preparations revealing the anterior–posterior length of the oculomotor nucleus (**A, D**) or transverse sections of the midbrain (**B, C, E, F, G**), **A, B**. On E10.5, all oculomotor cell bodies were located on either side of the floor plate (**A**), ipsilateral to their nerve (**B**). **C** On E12.5, leading processes projected into the floor plate. **D** On E13.5, leading processes projected from the posterior half of the oculomotor nuclei across the midline toward the contralateral oculomotor nucleus. **E** Apparent cell bodies were located within the numerous leading processes within the floor plate (**E'**). **F** On E14.5, leading processes have crossed the floor plate to contact the contralateral nucleus. **F'**. In single focal planes by microscopy, contralateral cell bodies were located on the ventromedial aspect of the opposing nucleus as well as in the floor plate (*arrow heads* point to cell bodies outlined in *green*). **G** On E16.5 no cell bodies were located in the floor plate, and leading processes spanned the contralateral nucleus. **H** Schematic showing that the superior rectus extraocular muscle is innervated by contralateral oculomotor neurons and their midline axon fibers (*dashed lines*). Scale bars, 100 µm

receptors. In this system, Robo receptors expressed on migrating cell bodies or neurites bind Slit ligands to signal repulsion away from the ventral midline see review on neural guidance in [34]. The Slit/Robo system was shown in the hindbrain to keep dorsal-projecting motor neuron axons out of the midline [23]. We considered whether floor plate-derived Slit may be in position to guide midline crossing of oculomotor cell bodies. Previous research in chick shows expression of *Robo*2 mRNA co-localized with the oculomotor nucleus early in development [35]. To determine the expression of Robo1 and 2 in mouse, we used immunofluorescence labeling on E10.5 for Robo1 and 2. Using primary antibodies against

Robo1 or 2, we detected Robo1 and Robo2 antibody labeling co-localized to Islet1/2 positive cell bodies in the ventral midbrain, with varying levels of labeling throughout the nucleus (Fig. 3A, B). This indicates that both Robo1 and Robo2 are expressed by cells in the oculomotor nucleus. We also noted Robo1 and 2 antibody labeling of the exiting nIII axons (not shown), consistent with the cell body labeling.

Slit1 and 2 expression was previously shown to be prominent in ventral midbrain in E12 rat embryos [23], and in E10.5 mouse embryos [13]. To more specifically determine whether Slits are in a position to act as midline repellents prior to E13.5 in mouse, we examined the

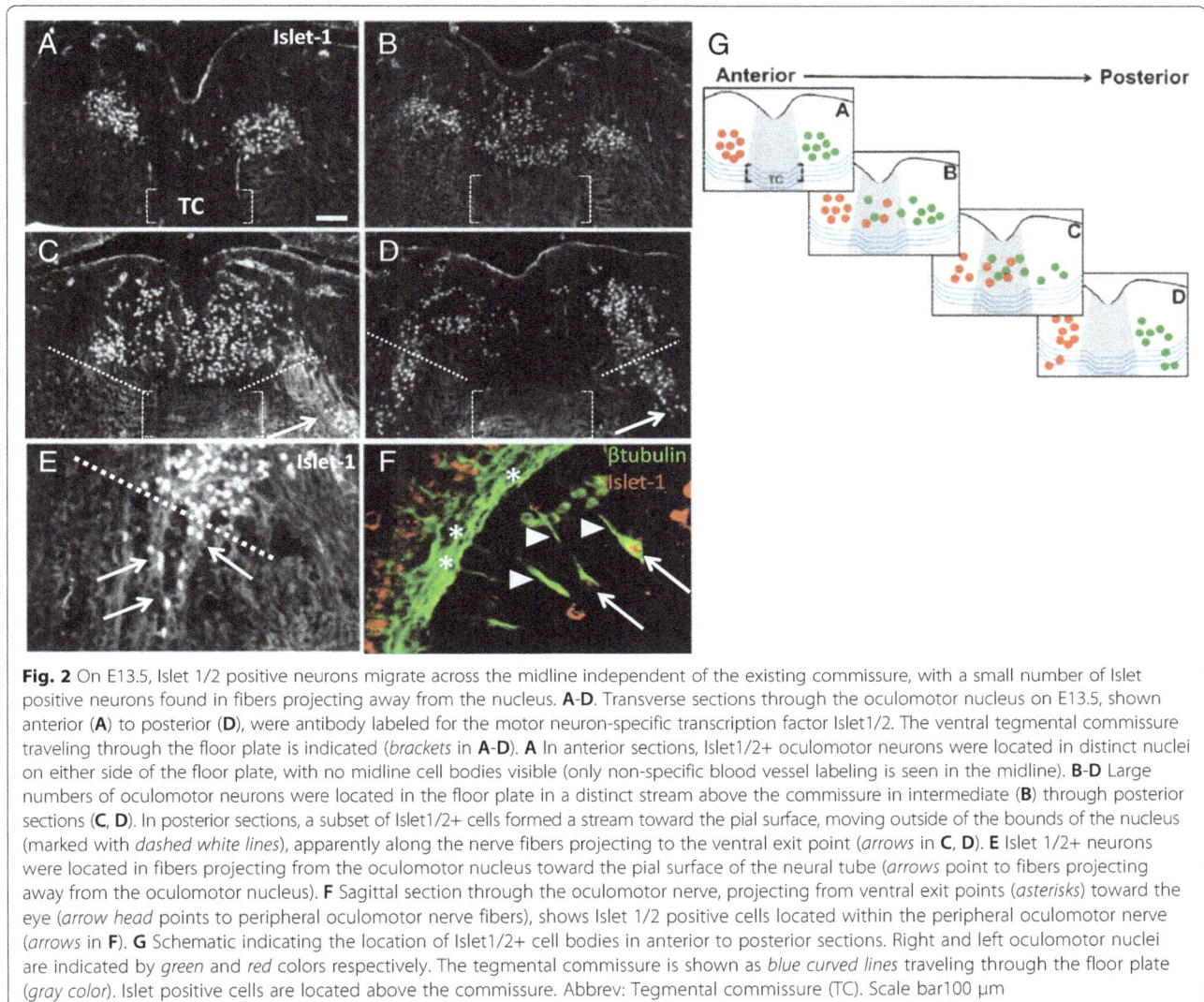

**Fig. 2** On E13.5, Islet 1/2 positive neurons migrate across the midline independent of the existing commissure, with a small number of Islet positive neurons found in fibers projecting away from the nucleus. **A-D**. Transverse sections through the oculomotor nucleus on E13.5, shown anterior (**A**) to posterior (**D**), were antibody labeled for the motor neuron-specific transcription factor Islet1/2. The ventral tegmental commissure traveling through the floor plate is indicated (*brackets* in **A-D**). **A** In anterior sections, Islet1/2+ oculomotor neurons were located in distinct nuclei on either side of the floor plate, with no midline cell bodies visible (only non-specific blood vessel labeling is seen in the midline). **B-D** Large numbers of oculomotor neurons were located in the floor plate in a distinct stream above the commissure in intermediate (**B**) through posterior sections (**C**, **D**). In posterior sections, a subset of Islet1/2+ cells formed a stream toward the pial surface, moving outside of the bounds of the nucleus (marked with *dashed white lines*), apparently along the nerve fibers projecting to the ventral exit point (*arrows* in **C**, **D**). **E** Islet 1/2+ neurons were located in fibers projecting from the oculomotor nucleus toward the pial surface of the neural tube (*arrows* point to fibers projecting away from the oculomotor nucleus). **F** Sagittal section through the oculomotor nerve, projecting from ventral exit points (*asterisks*) toward the eye (*arrow head* points to peripheral oculomotor nerve fibers), shows Islet 1/2 positive cells located within the peripheral oculomotor nerve (*arrows* in **F**). **G** Schematic indicating the location of Islet1/2+ cell bodies in anterior to posterior sections. Right and left oculomotor nuclei are indicated by *green* and *red* colors respectively. The tegmental commissure is shown as *blue curved lines* traveling through the floor plate (*gray color*). Islet positive cells are located above the commissure. Abbrev: Tegmental commissure (TC). Scale bar100 μm

three Slits in the ventral midbrain on E10.5 by *in situ* hybridization of mRNA. We found *Slit 1, 2* and *3* mRNA was expressed in the ventral floor plate medial to the oculomotor nuclei, as well as a strip of cells in the underlying ventricular zone (Fig. 3C-E) on E10.5. Complementary expression of Robo receptors by oculomotor neurons and Slit expression in the floor plate supports a role for Slit repulsion from the floor plate, and may act to inhibit oculomotor migration prior to E13.5. The ventricular zone expression of Slits suggests a potential role in hemming the neurons into the marginal zone. We also found *Slit2* and *3* expression overlaps with the region of the Islet1/2-positive oculomotor neurons (Fig. 3D, E). This is consistent with Slit2 and 3 expression found in spinal motor neurons [36].

During oculomotor migration on E14.5, Robo1 and 2 protein remained expressed in the oculomotor nucleus (Fig. 4A, B). Although the expression levels appeared to vary across the nucleus, there was no clear pattern of different levels in lateral vs. medial/ventral areas of the nucleus (not shown). Robo1 and 2 labeling also appeared on oculomotor neurons migrating in the midline, although Robo2 levels were low and variable (Fig. 4C, D). To further confirm Robo expression during the migration phase, Robo1 and 2 mRNA domains also overlapped with the oculomotor nucleus in the ventral-caudal midbrain (Fig. 4E, F). Similarly, *Slit1* and *2* mRNA continued to be expressed in the ventral floor plate and ventricular zone tissue on E14.5 (Fig. 4G, H). In addition, Slit2 and 3 was expressed in a region that overlapped with the Islet1/2-positive oculomotor nucleus, including overlapping with the migrating population positioned in the midline (Fig. 4H, I). Thus, Slit1 and Slit2 are in position to act as midline repellents at the early stages of stationary motor neurons on E10.5, and are also maintained during migration on E14.5.

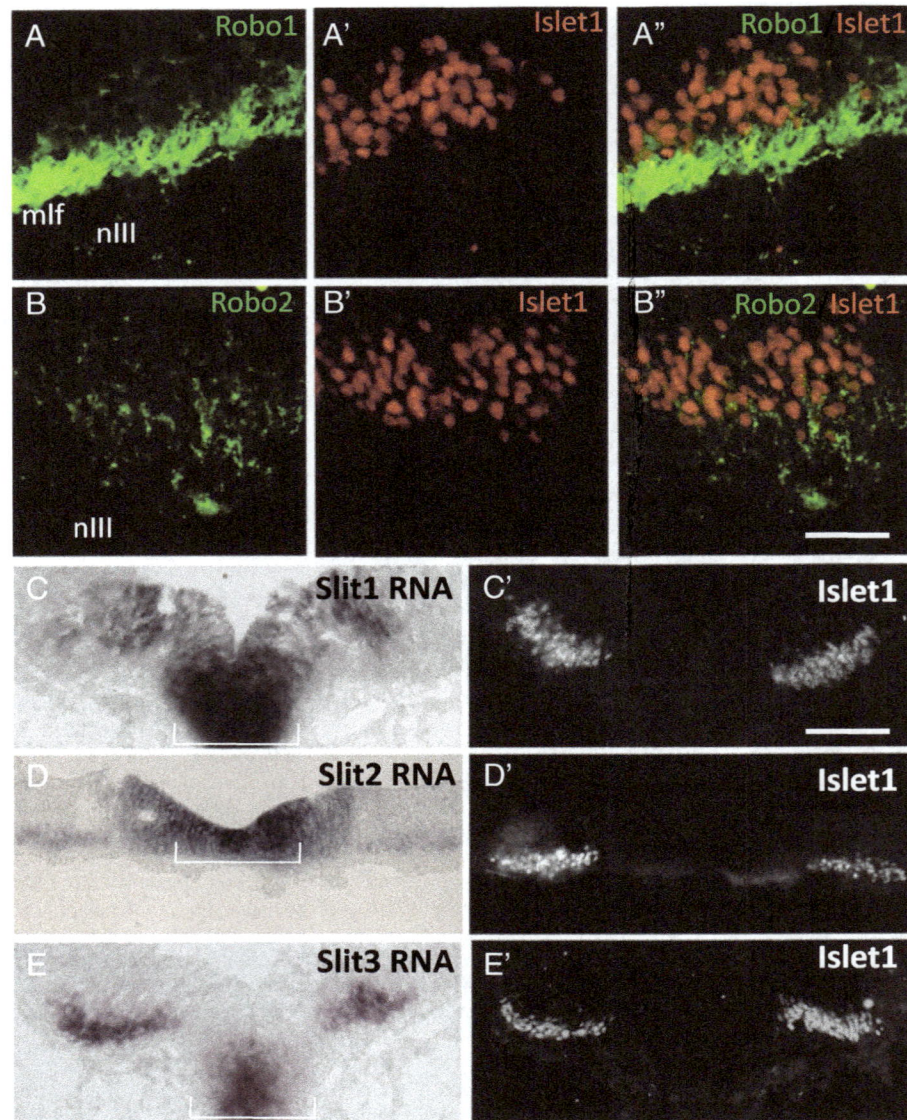

**Fig. 3** The guidance cues Slit1 and 2, and receptors Robo1 and 2, are in position to prevent oculomotor migration across the floor plate on E10.5. Coronal sections were taken through the posterior midbrain on E10.5 to determine Slit and Robo expression. Following protein (Robos) or mRNA (Slits) labeling, the same or adjacent section was labeled for Islet1/2 to co-localize expression to oculomotor neurons (A'-B', A", B"). **A, B** Robo1 and 2 protein was found in the ventral midbrain and in the oculomotor nerve fibers (nIII). Expression was co-localized with Islet1/2 indicating Robo1 and Robo2 expression in oculomotor neurons (A",B"). Robo1 antibody also strongly labels the adjacent medial longitudinal fasciculus (mlf). **C-E** In situ hybridization for *Slit1, 2*, and *3* mRNA. Slit 1, 2 and 3 expression was localized to the floor plate. Expression of *Slit2* and *3* co-localized to Islet 1/2+ neurons (D', E'). Scale bars: B", 50 μm, applies to Robo antibody labels; C', 100 μm, applies to Slit in situs

### Oculomotor cell bodies migrate prematurely in *Slit* and *Robo* mutant mice

Slit expression in the ventral floor plate and Robo expression in oculomotor cell bodies suggests a function for floor plate-derived Slit in oculomotor migration. To determine whether Slit signaling mediates contralateral migration, oculomotor cell bodies were back-labeled from the oculomotor nerve(s) in Slit 1/2 or Robo1/2 double mutants and compared with wild type controls.

In wild type controls on E10.5, three days prior to normal migration, the oculomotor nuclei were constrained to their location adjacent to the floor plate and ipsilateral to their corresponding nerve (Fig. 5A, C). Interestingly, in some control embryos on E10.5, rare cellular processes projected from the oculomotor nucleus, into the midline but did not appear to reach the contralateral nucleus (asterisk in Fig. 5A, C). These observations suggest a phase in normal development in which transient

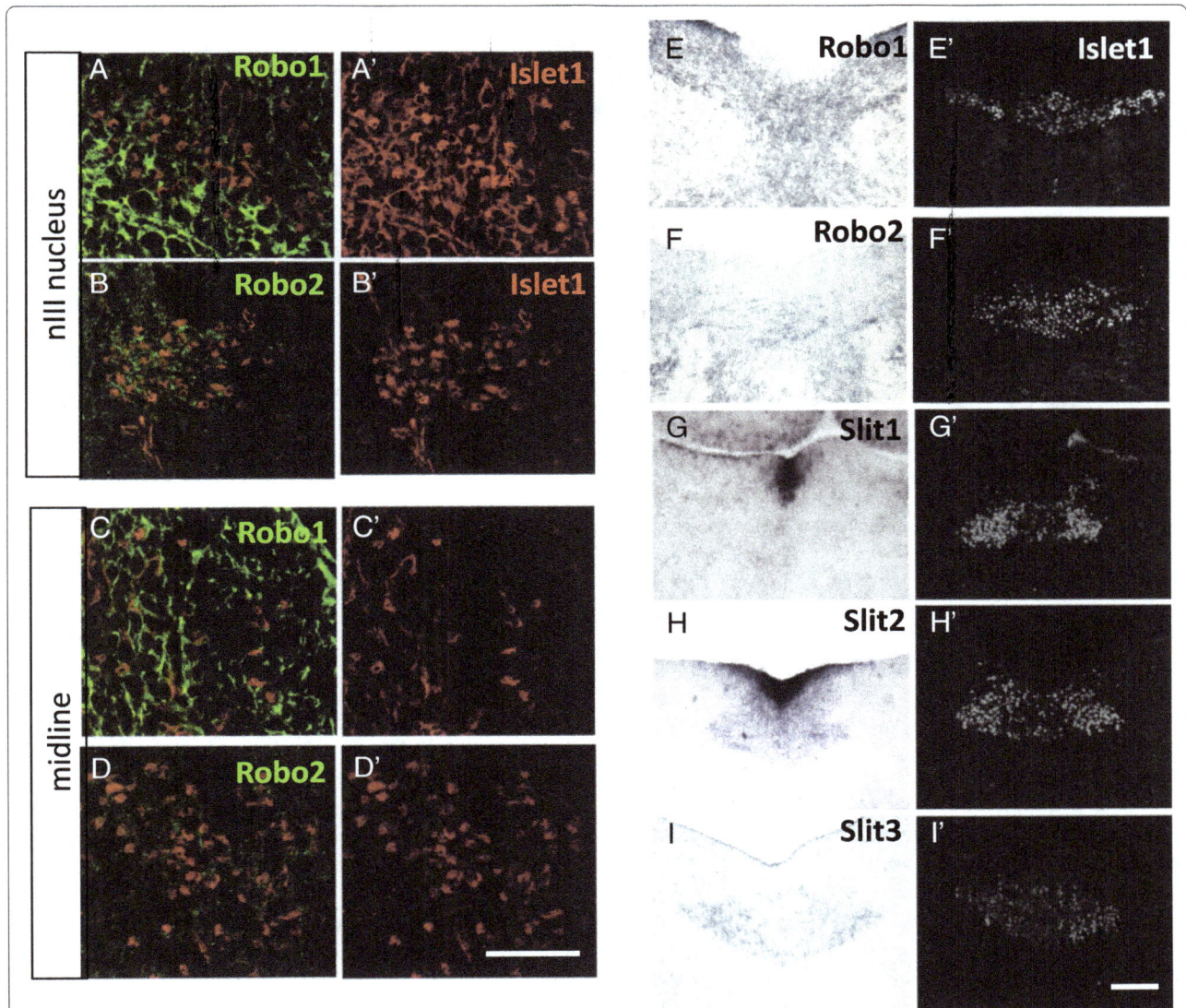

**Fig. 4** Slit and Robo remain in position to regulate floor plate crossing on E14.5. Coronal sections through the caudal oculomotor nucleus on E14.5 were labeled with Robo1 or 2 antibodies, or hybridized to Robo or Slit mRNA probes, followed by antibody labeling for Islet1/2 of the same section (for Robo antibodies), or adjacent sections (for in situ hybridization). **A**, **B** Within the nucleus, Robo1 and Robo2 was localized to Islet1/2+ cells indicating Robo expression by oculomotor neurons. **C-D**. In the midline of the caudal midbrain, Robo1 antibody labeling could be seen on some migrating neurons, while Robo2 labeling was less intense and variable. **E**, **F** In situ hybridization for Robo1 and 2 mRNAs showed labeling that overlapped with the nuclei, and also bridged across the midline in the area of migrating neurons. **G-I**. Slit mRNA expression by in situ hybridization, compared to Islet antibody labeling in adjacent sections. Slit1 and 2 continued to be expressed by floor plate cells on E14.5, while there was very little Slit3. *Slit2* and *Slit3* transcript was localized to the oculomotor nuclei as well as overlapping with the motor neurons migrating across the midline (**H**, **I**). Scale bars: D', 50 μm, applies to Robo antibody labels; I', 100 μm, applies to in situs

secondary processes are produced by early oculomotor neurons but are retracted and do not support the migration of cell bodies. However, in Slit1/2 or Robo1/2 double mutant embryos, numerous leading processes projected out from the nucleus reaching into the floor plate, with some reaching the contralateral nucleus (Fig. 5B, D). The path traveled by these processes was not linear, and frequently the processes curved back toward the nucleus of origin (Fig. 5B"). In Slit1/2 mutant

embryos, we noted imprecise navigation by the leading processes, including looping and zig-zag patterns. Similar, but less numerous, loops were observed in Robo1/2 mutant embryos (Fig. 5D"). Therefore, the disruption of Slit/Robo signaling caused leading processes to project into and across the floor plate three days prior to normal migration.

Labeled neuron cell bodies in the ventromedial aspect of the contralateral nucleus as well as within several leading

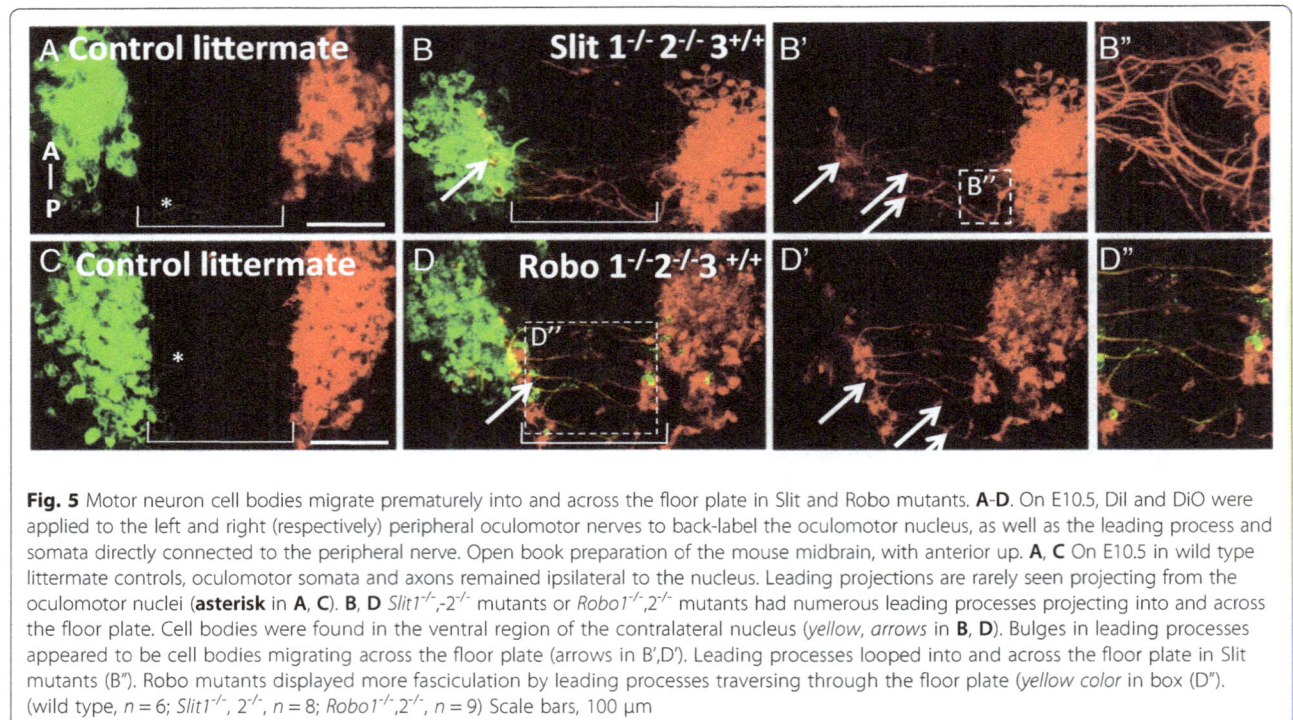

**Fig. 5** Motor neuron cell bodies migrate prematurely into and across the floor plate in Slit and Robo mutants. **A**-**D**. On E10.5, DiI and DiO were applied to the left and right (respectively) peripheral oculomotor nerves to back-label the oculomotor nucleus, as well as the leading process and somata directly connected to the peripheral nerve. Open book preparation of the mouse midbrain, with anterior up. **A**, **C** On E10.5 in wild type littermate controls, oculomotor somata and axons remained ipsilateral to the nucleus. Leading projections are rarely seen projecting from the oculomotor nuclei (**asterisk** in **A**, **C**). **B**, **D** Slit1−/−,-2−/− mutants or Robo1−/−,2−/− mutants had numerous leading processes projecting into and across the floor plate. Cell bodies were found in the ventral region of the contralateral nucleus (*yellow, arrows* in **B**, **D**). Bulges in leading processes appeared to be cell bodies migrating across the floor plate (arrows in B',D'). Leading processes looped into and across the floor plate in Slit mutants (B"). Robo mutants displayed more fasciculation by leading processes traversing through the floor plate (*yellow color* in box (D"). (wild type, $n = 6$; Slit1−/−, 2−/−, $n = 8$; Robo1−/−,2−/−, $n = 9$) Scale bars, 100 µm

processes in Slit and Robo mutants on E10.5 suggest that cell bodies have crossed over from the opposing nucleus (arrow pointing to yellow color in Fig. 5B, D, arrows in Fig. 5B', D'). To identify and quantify migrating cells, we labeled midbrain tissue for Islet1/2. In wild type controls, Islet1/2-positive cell bodies were rarely seen between the bilateral oculomotor nuclei (Fig. 6A). Conversely, in Slit and Robo mutant embryos, several Islet1/2-positive cells separated from the compact oculomotor nuclei, with several located within the floor plate (Fig. 6B, C). To determine the contribution of single or double Slit or Robo genes in midline crossing, we examined embryos mutant for single Slit or Robo genes (Fig. 6D). There was very little premature crossing observed in embryos homozygous mutant for Slit1, or embryos homozygous mutant for Slit2, in contrast to the strong crossing in Slit1/2 double homozygous mutants. Similarly, we found that a loss of one copy of *Robo1* did not increase Islet1/2 -positive cells in the floor plate. However, loss of Robo2 was sufficient to allow migration into the midline (Fig. 6D). Thus, early midline migration can be prevented by single functional Slit genes or a single functional Robo2 gene, suggesting redundant functions in midline crossing. The strongest effect was found in Robo 1/2 mutants, followed by Slit1/2 mutants. Interestingly, Robo1/2 mutant mice have twice as many Islet1/2 positive cells in the floor plate than Slit1/2 mutants. A more severe phenotype in Robo1/2 mutants compared to Slit1/2 mutant mice is consistent with previous suggestions of Slit-independent repulsive functions for Robo receptors [37].

### Loss of Slit 2 in motor neurons does not cause premature migration

From the initial discovery of mammalian Slit2 expression in the spinal cord floor plate, it was noted that spinal motor neurons also have cell-autonomous expression of Slit2 [36]. However, a cell-autonomous role for Slit2 in cell migration has not been examined. We also found Slit2 expressed by the oculomotor nucleus and midbrain floor plate cells on E10.5-E14.5 (Figs. 3 and 4). Because a global loss of *Slit* allows oculomotor neurons to migrate across the floor plate on E10.5 (Fig. 5), we wanted to separate the function of Slit2 derived from floor plate from Slit2 derived from the motor neurons. To determine whether Slit2 derived from oculomotor neurons plays a role in preventing premature migration on E11.5, we examined mice mutant for the gene Islet 1 (Isl1) that display a significant loss of *Slit2* in motor neurons [38]. We first confirmed a loss of *Slit2* in the oculomotor nucleus. In mice mutant for Isl1, there was little to no Slit2 transcript detected co-localized to the oculomotor nucleus, as counter-labeled with the alternative motor neuron marker, Phox2b (Fig. 7B). However, the strong midline Slit2 expression was retained. In mice mutant for Isl1, oculomotor neurons do not migrate across the midline prematurely (Fig. 7D). In addition, we confirmed in whole mount embryos that the oculomotor nerve forms its initial projections to the eye (data not shown). Thus, a loss of Isl1 and subsequently a loss of Slit2 (and potentially perturbed expression of other Islet-regulated genes) in

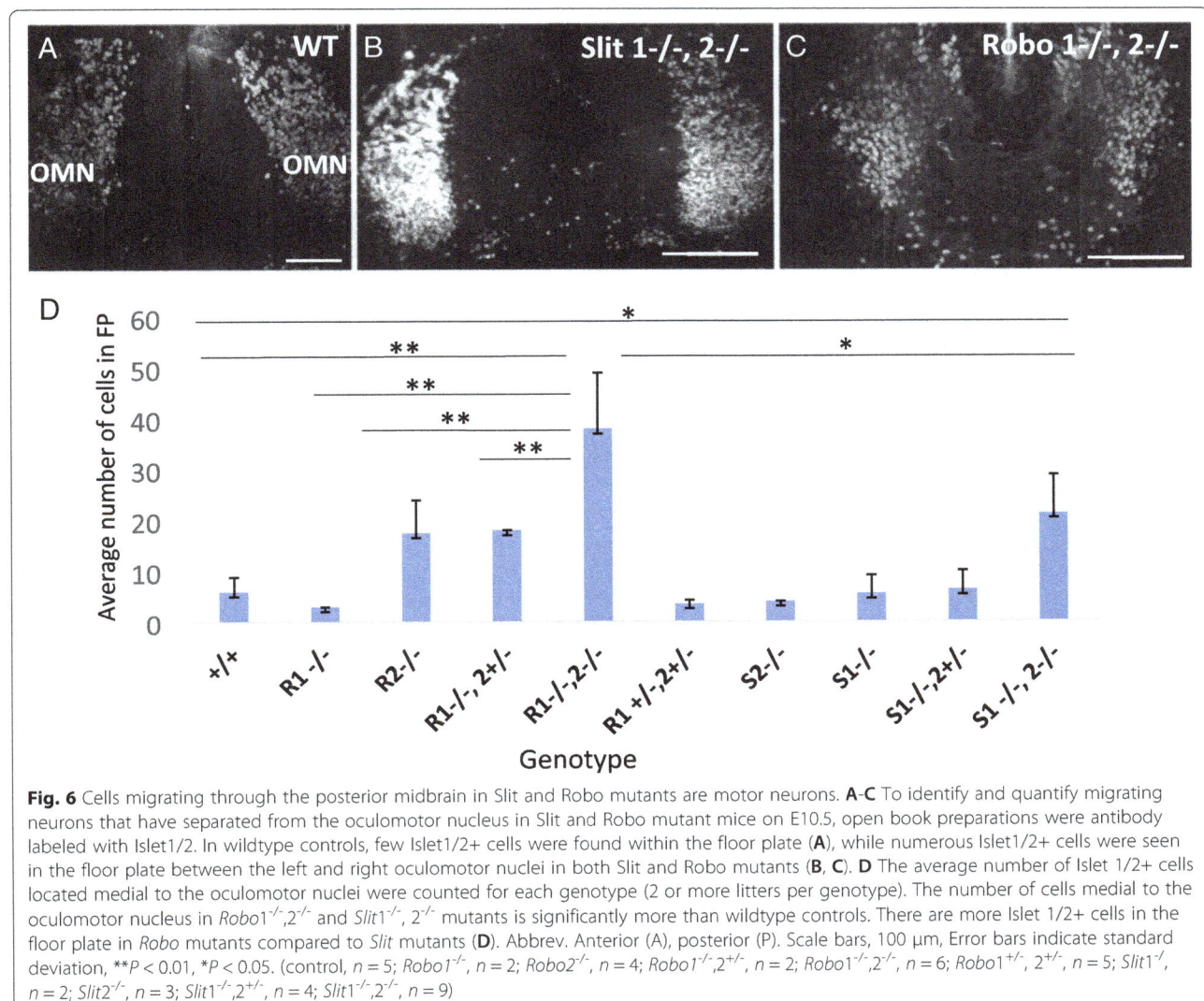

**Fig. 6** Cells migrating through the posterior midbrain in Slit and Robo mutants are motor neurons. **A-C** To identify and quantify migrating neurons that have separated from the oculomotor nucleus in Slit and Robo mutant mice on E10.5, open book preparations were antibody labeled with Islet1/2. In wildtype controls, few Islet1/2+ cells were found within the floor plate (**A**), while numerous Islet1/2+ cells were seen in the floor plate between the left and right oculomotor nuclei in both Slit and Robo mutants (**B**, **C**). **D** The average number of Islet 1/2+ cells located medial to the oculomotor nuclei were counted for each genotype (2 or more litters per genotype). The number of cells medial to the oculomotor nucleus in $Robo1^{-/-},2^{-/-}$ and $Slit1^{-/-}, 2^{-/-}$ mutants is significantly more than wildtype controls. There are more Islet 1/2+ cells in the floor plate in $Robo$ mutants compared to $Slit$ mutants (**D**). Abbrev. Anterior (A), posterior (P). Scale bars, 100 µm, Error bars indicate standard deviation, **$P < 0.01$, *$P < 0.05$. (control, $n = 5$; $Robo1^{-/-}$, $n = 2$; $Robo2^{-/-}$, $n = 4$; $Robo1^{-/-},2^{+/-}$, $n = 2$; $Robo1^{-/-},2^{-/-}$, $n = 6$; $Robo1^{+/-}, 2^{+/-}$, $n = 5$; $Slit1^{-/-}$, $n = 2$; $Slit2^{-/-}$, $n = 3$; $Slit1^{-/-},2^{+/-}$, $n = 4$; $Slit1^{-/-},2^{-/-}$, $n = 9$)

oculomotor neurons does not result in premature migration. This is indirect evidence that suggests that premature migration in Slit or Robo mutant mice on E11.5 is due to a loss of Slit signals derived from the floor plate.

### The oculomotor commissure forms properly in Slit and Robo mutant mice

Oculomotor neuron migration across the midline on E10.5 in Slit and Robo mutant mice could be non-specifically affecting the entire nucleus, or could represent a premature but specific migration of those that normally migrate, that is, the superior rectus subset. Unfortunately, we were unable to identify a molecular marker for the superior rectus neurons in mouse embryos. However, we predicted that the oculomotor commissure would be larger if another population of cells migrated across the floor plate and joined the contralateral nucleus to augment the usual superior rectus commissural axon projection.

We examined Slit and Robo null mutant embryos during leading process extension and cell migration on E13.5, and on E16, after migration ceased. In wild type embryos on E13.5, leading processes projected into and across the floor plate. Midline crossing was restricted to the caudal half of the nucleus. Migrating oculomotor cells could be seen in the midline, and approaching the ventral region of the contralateral oculomotor nucleus (Fig. 8A). Both Slit and Robo mutant mice had oculomotor neurons that appear similar to wild type, with leading processes and cell bodies located within the floor plate on E13.5 (Fig. 8B, C). However, we note that Robo1/2 mutant commissures had a more disordered appearance than Slit1/2 mutant commissures. It appeared in some cases that the Slit double mutant commissure may contain more axon fibers, and possibly extend further rostrally. However, because of the inability to quantify the inherently variable back-labeling tracing strategy, and the lack of a specific molecular

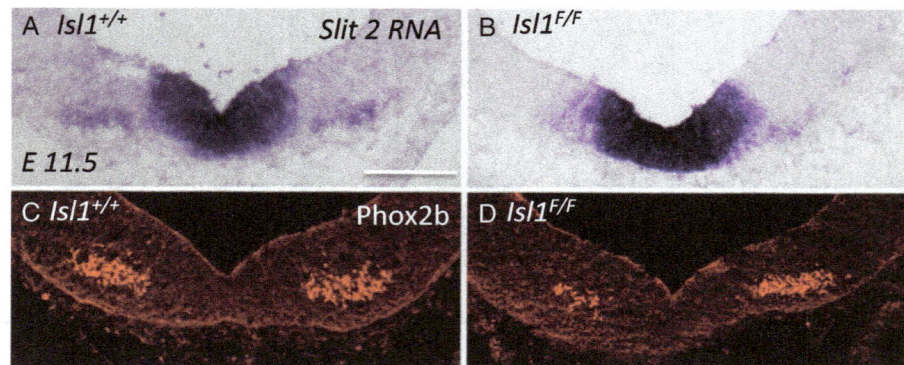

**Fig. 7** Loss of slit 2 in motor neurons is not sufficient to cause premature migration. **A**, **B** To confirm a loss of *Slit2* expression in the oculomotor nucleus in Islet1 mutant embryos, in situ hybridization was performed in the ventral midbrain on E11.5. **C**, **D**. Location of the oculomotor nucleus was determined by Phox2b expression (an Islet-independent transcription factor expressed in motor neurons). **A** In control embryos, *Slit2* RNA is found in the floor plate and co-localized to Phox2b positive cells (**C**). **B** In the Islet1 mutant midbrain, *Slit2* expression is retained in the floor plate, but is lost from the oculomotor nucleus (**D**). Phox2b positive neurons were clustered on either side of the floor plate, but not within the floor plate in both control and Islet1F/F mutants (**B**) indicating oculomotor cell bodies have not migrated into the floor plate (*n* = 4). Scale bar, 100 μm

marker for superior rectus neurons, we could not definitively distinguish whether ectopic oculomotor neurons were recruited to cross the midline.

To determine if Slit and Robo influence the final development of the commissure on E16.5, DiI-labeled oculomotor nuclei were sectioned across a coronal plane through the commissure. In controls, the oculomotor commissure was fully developed with leading processes, spanning the floor plate (Fig. 8D). DiI-labeled processes intercalated throughout the contralateral nucleus. No cell bodies were seen within the floor plate, suggesting that the contralateral migration was complete by E16.5 (Fig. 8D). In E16.5 Slit1/2 and Robo1/2 mutants, the

oculomotor commissure was positioned caudally, as in controls, with a similar size of the commissure (Fig. 8E, F). Together, this data suggests that premature migration on E10.5 does not appear to influence normal migration at later stages.

### Regulators of Slit signaling are not required for contralateral migration

Migration of oculomotor cells on E10.5 in Slit and Robo mutant embryos suggests a mechanism in which wild type oculomotor neurons are initially trapped in position by Slit/Robo repulsion, but later, on E13.5, suppression of Slit/Robo signals allow for migration into and across

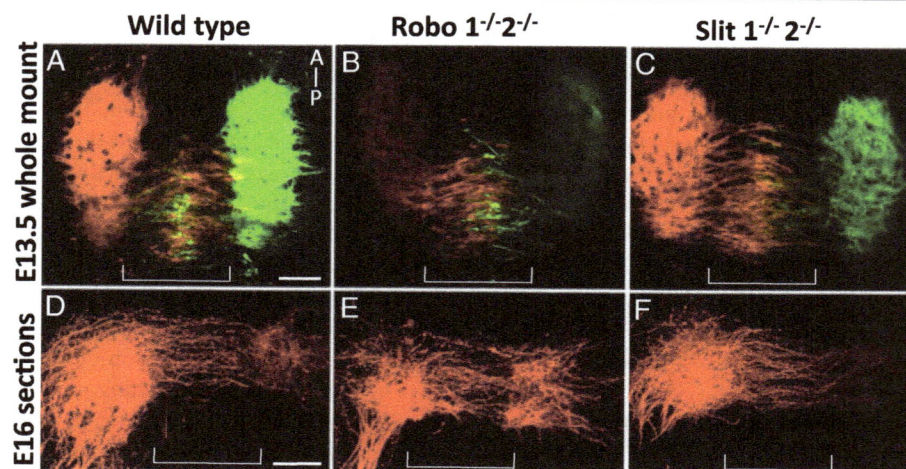

**Fig. 8** Slit and Robo mutants generate a normal oculomotor commissure. **A-C** Open book preparation of DiI and DiO back-labeled oculomotor nuclei. On E13.5, leading processes reached the contralateral nucleus. Neuron cell bodies, seen as bulges in the leading process, were in the midline (**A**, wild type control, Slit littermate). Loss of Slits or Robos (**B**, **C**) did not appear to reduce the number of leading processes or cells migrating through the floor plate. **D-F**. DiI back-label of the oculomotor nucleus on E16. 200 um coronal sections along the plane of the oculomotor nerve were compared by z-stacked confocal images. The oculomotor commissure was similar in thickness to wild type (**D**) in Slit and Robo mutants (**E**, **F**). (*n* = 3; control, Robo and Slit mutants) Scale bars, 100 μm

the midline. We considered and tested three mechanisms that suppress Robo repulsive signaling in other systems.

In the first Slit/Robo suppression mechanism, we examined Robo3. Robo3 has been proposed to act as a negative regulator of Slit repulsion via dominant negative action on Robo1 and Robo2. In the spinal cord, Robo1 and 2-expressing pre-crossing spinal cord commissural axons are allowed to approach the floor plate when Robo3 is co-expressed allowing these axons to enter an area of high Slit expression [15, 39]. Alternatively, Robo3 may potentiate Netrin attraction to counteract Slit repulsion [16]. We therefore hypothesized that Robo3 might be expressed on oculomotor neurons on E13.5 to negate Slit repulsion from the floor plate. *In situ* hybridization against *Robo3* mRNA on E13.5 showed that *Robo3* expression was restricted to a subset of neurons found just dorsal to the OM nucleus (Fig. 9A). To formally rule out a requirement for Robo3, we examined whether oculomotor neurons migrated across the floor plate in mouse embryos lacking Robo3, and found Islet-positive cells in the midline on E13.5 (Fig. 9C). This suggests that Robo3 activity is not required for oculomotor migration into or across the floor plate.

A second potential antagonist of Slit signaling is the receptor CXCR4. In chick, the binding of SDF-1 to CXCR4 suppresses the repellent activity of Slit2, Semaphorin3A, and 3C on axons cultured in vitro [40]. In zebrafish retinal ganglion cells, SDF-1 antagonizes Slit/Robo2 signaling in vivo [41]. CXCR4 is expressed in the mouse ventral midbrain where it is required for the exit of oculomotor and other cranial nerves [42]. We confirmed CXCR4 expression in the oculomotor nucleus by *in situ* hybridization (Fig. 9B). Therefore, we were interested in whether floor plate CXCR4 may antagonize Slit signaling in migrating oculomotor neurons to allow for midline crossing. However, in E13.5 CXCR4 mutant embryos, Islet1/2-positive cells were found in the midline (Fig. 9D). This suggests that CXCR4 signaling is not required to antagonize the repellent activity of the floor plate.

### Netrin1 attraction is not required for oculomotor migration into the floor plate

Rather than blocking a repulsive signal, the prematurely migrating cell bodies could be activating a response to a floor plate-derived attractant. In chick, overexpression of the N-terminal domain of the actin-binding protein Drebrin caused leading processes to orient toward the trochlear nucleus instead of the contralateral oculomotor nucleus [6]. This study suggests that leading processes are initially attracted toward the floor plate. The classical attractant found in the floor plate is Netrin1. In the hindbrain, Netrin1 is required to attract precerebellar neurons toward the floor plate [17]. Netrin/DCC signaling also attracts basal pontine neurons toward the ventral midline [43]. Interestingly, a previous study showed that rat ventral midbrain explants produced neurites that were repelled by floor plate tissue, but were unresponsive to Netrin1-secreting cell aggregates, although the experiment did not distinguish whether the responding neurites were primary motor axons or midline crossing leading processes [22]. We therefore examined *Netrin1* expression on E13.5. We find *Netrin1* expression in the ventricular

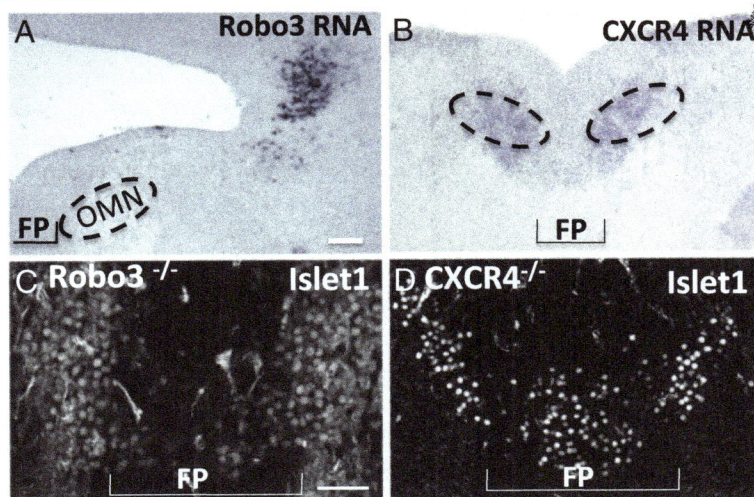

**Fig. 9** Robo3 or CXCR4 function is not required for oculomotor migration into the floor plate. **A**, **B**. To determine if Robo3 or CXCR4 are in position to repress Slit/Robo signaling in situ hybridization of RNA was performed on E14.5 midbrain sections. Robo3 was not expressed in the ventral midbrain on E14.5 (**A**). However, CXCR4 was expressed in the ventral midbrain in both the floor plate and regions lateral to the floor plate (**B**). **C**, **D** To identify migration patterns of oculomotor neurons on E13.5 in Robo3 and CXCR4 mutants, sections of the posterior midbrain were antibody labeled with Islet1/2. Islet1/2+ cells migrated into the floor plate in both Robo3 (**C**) and CXCR4 mutants (**D**) indicating neither Robo3 nor CXCR4 are required for migration oculomotor migration across the floor plate. (Robo3, $n = 2$; CXCR4, $n = 4$) Scale bar, 100 μm

surface and floor plate in the midbrain (Fig. 10A). However, in Netrin1 mutant mice, we find Islet1/2-positive cells in the floor plate on E13.5 (Fig. 10B), as well as normal projections toward the contralateral nucleus (Fig. 10C). Therefore, Netrin1 signaling is not required to attract oculomotor neurons or their leading processes toward the floor plate.

### Contralateral OM migration is regulated by signals intrinsic to the ventral midbrain

The initiation of contralateral migration coincides with the time when the oculomotor axons reach the superior

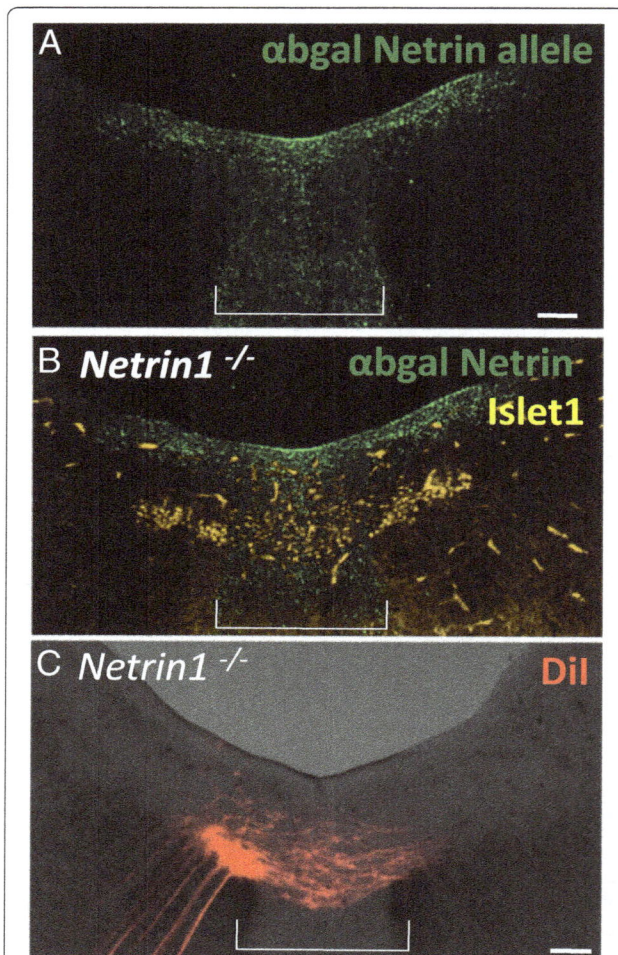

**Fig. 10** Netrin1 is not required for oculomotor migration into the floor plate. **A**, **B** To locate Netrin expression during oculomotor migration, the mutant allele Netrin1$^{lacZ}$ was labeled with anti beta-gal in Netrin1-/- (i.e. lacZ/lacZ) mutant mice. On E13.5, Netrin1 was expressed by the floor plate and ventricular layer of cells in ventral midbrain (**A**), adjacent to Islet1/2+ motor neurons located in the nucleus and in the floor plate (**B**). **C**. DiI back-label from nIII in a Netrin1$^{-/-}$ embryo on E13.5. A 200 um coronal section along the plane of the oculomotor nerve was imaged by z-stacked confocal images. Leading processes projected from the oculomotor nucleus toward the contralateral nucleus ($n = 3$). Scale bar, 100 µm

rectus extraocular muscle primordia in chick [5, 44, 45]. It has therefore been proposed that a signal from a peripheral target may initiate migration [44]. To determine whether a signal is transported from the developing extraocular muscles back to the cell body to initiate migration, we utilized three techniques to eliminate interaction between the oculomotor nerve and the peripheral tissue, and examined oculomotor neuron migration.

In the first approach, we examined mice mutant for the transcription factor *Pitx2*, where extraocular muscle precursors undergo apoptosis prior to the nerve reaching the precursor cells [46]. We first confirmed that Pitx2 mutant mice lacked muscles on E14 in both sagittal and coronal sections (data not shown). To determine whether an oculomotor commissure develops in mice lacking extraocular muscles, we back-labeled both left and right oculomotor nuclei with DiI from nIII. The oculomotor commissure is apparent in these mice and originates from the posterior half of the nucleus (Fig. 11A). Therefore, signals derived from the extraocular muscles are not required to initiate migration.

To eliminate the possibility that peripheral signals derived from tissue other than the extraocular muscles initiate midline migration, we utilized a second in vitro technique where the midbrain was dissected away from the oculomotor nerve and peripheral tissues on E11.5. The midbrain, devoid of peripheral tissue, was cultured for 72 h in vitro, then oculomotor neurons were labeled. At the starting point on E11.5 (0 h), all oculomotor neurons reside on the edge of the floor plate with no Islet1/2-positive neurons in the floor plate (Fig. 11B). Following 72 h in vitro, Islet1/2-positive neurons were found throughout the floor plate, particularly in the posterior half of the nucleus where migration normally occurs in vivo (Fig. 11C). Therefore, isolated midbrain cultures provided sufficient cues to initiate and guide migration, and demonstrate that removal of the peripheral nerve does not appear to restrict oculomotor migration.

A caveat to the explant culture strategy was that the initial outgrowth of the nerve toward the eye occurs on E9.5. Therefore, a signal to activate migration could be transported back to the oculomotor nucleus prior to E11.5, although it must remain latent until overt migration begins on E13.5. To test the possibility that a signal is transported during the initial outgrowth of nIII, we examined a mutant mouse where the oculomotor nerve outgrowth into the periphery is absent. In CXCR4 mutant mice, axons projecting from the oculomotor nucleus wander dorsally within the neuroepithelium instead of toward the peripheral mesenchyme where the attractive CXCR4 ligand, SDF-1, is expressed [42]. These mutants have an oculomotor nerve that aberrantly projects within the neuroepithelium, or is much smaller in size [42]; therefore, nIII would be unable to obtain or transport peripheral

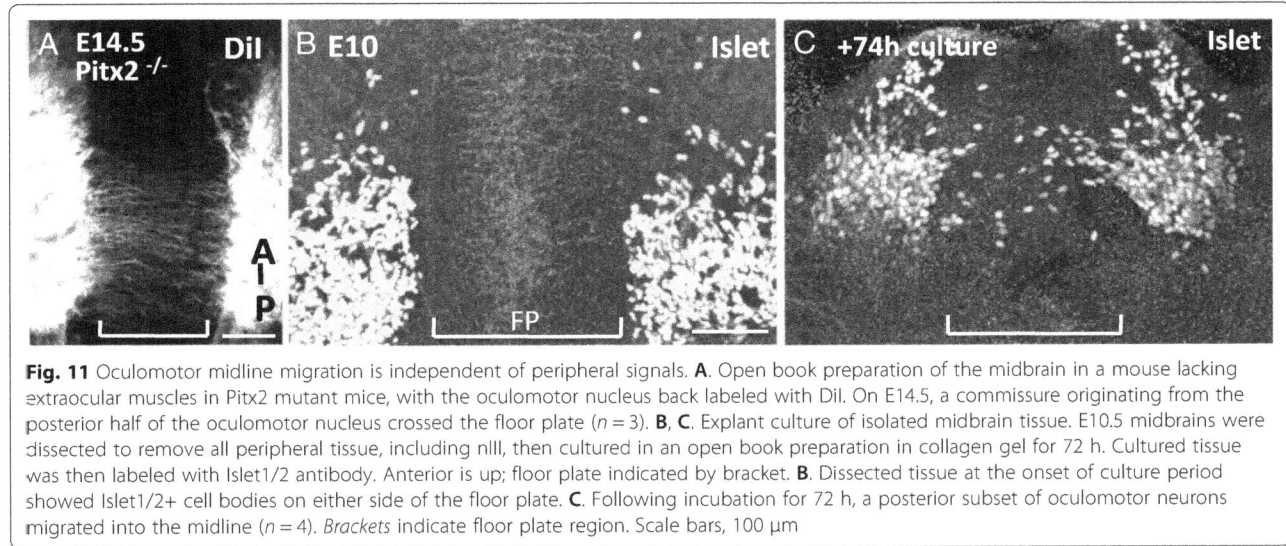

**Fig. 11** Oculomotor midline migration is independent of peripheral signals. **A**. Open book preparation of the midbrain in a mouse lacking extraocular muscles in Pitx2 mutant mice, with the oculomotor nucleus back labeled with DiI. On E14.5, a commissure originating from the posterior half of the oculomotor nucleus crossed the floor plate ($n = 3$). **B**, **C**. Explant culture of isolated midbrain tissue. E10.5 midbrains were dissected to remove all peripheral tissue, including nIII, then cultured in an open book preparation in collagen gel for 72 h. Cultured tissue was then labeled with Islet1/2 antibody. Anterior is up; floor plate indicated by bracket. **B**. Dissected tissue at the onset of culture period showed Islet1/2+ cell bodies on either side of the floor plate. **C**. Following incubation for 72 h, a posterior subset of oculomotor neurons migrated into the midline ($n = 4$). *Brackets* indicate floor plate region. Scale bars, 100 μm

signals back to the nucleus to initiate migration. We first verified that the oculomotor nerve in CXCR4 mutant mice was missing, both by visual inspection during dissection and axon antibody labeling in whole mount embryos. We were unable to identify a peripheral oculomotor nerve emerging from the midbrain (data not shown), confirming the previous report, and suggesting that a signal from a peripheral intermediate target was unlikely to be transported back to the nucleus in CXCR4 mutant mice. As previously stated, we found Islet1/2-positive cell bodies in the floor plate of the midbrain in CXCR4 mutant mice (Fig. 9D), indicating that contralateral oculomotor migration can occur independent of nerve-derived signals obtained from outside of the neural tube. This suggests that signals to initiate migration are intrinsic to the oculomotor nucleus and nearby tissues within the ventral midbrain.

## Discussion

Biondi first observed a group of neurons that separate from the developing oculomotor column and migrate toward the opposing oculomotor nucleus [47]. Later, through a series of Golgi labels, Puelles proposed that "diffusible factors" are likely responsible for guiding migration [3]. Until our study, the identity of such factors remained unknown.

To initiate and guide the several steps involved in migration across the midline, we speculate that a combination of diffusible extrinsic signals and intrinsic factors are required. The migration of a subset of oculomotor neurons appears to involve multiple steps: 1) the superior rectus motor neurons receive extracellular or intracellular signals to initiate and extend a secondary leading process; 2) leading processes receive guidance signals to attract them toward the midline and eventually toward the

contralateral nucleus; 3) the neuron cell bodies lose cell adhesion to the ipsilateral oculomotor nucleus and follow their secondary leading processes across the floor plate; 4) neurons must move to and integrate into the contralateral nucleus.

Here we show that Slit signaling is necessary to inhibit the initiation of oculomotor migration. Slits may function to gate migration, such that the suppression of Slit/Robo repulsion on E13.5 would allow a subset of oculomotor neurons to turn on migratory processes. Our data suggest a range of potential roles for Slit signaling in migratory OM neurons including; blocking extension of leading processes, promoting cell adhesion to ipsilateral nucleus, and blocking migration of the neuronal cell bodies across the floor plate.

### Migrating oculomotor neurons pioneer an independent path across the midline via leading axon-like processes

Oculomotor neurons initially make a conventional axon projection that exits the CNS out toward their peripheral targets. However, then a subset undergo a remarkable transition to produce second axon-like fibers (leading processes) oriented toward and across the ventral midline, followed soon after by translocation of the neuronal cell bodies [5]. We confirmed this time course in the mouse: all migrating oculomotor neurons possess a leading process that projects toward the midline, with a trajectory that is perpendicular to the radially-oriented ventricular cells in the floor plate on E13.5. The leading processes originate only from neurons in the caudal half of the nucleus, and can extend to reach the opposing oculomotor nucleus. These processes appear similar to leading processes found in migrating pontine neurons [43]: leading processes are long, branching, and fasciculate with other processes.

Similar to pontine neurons, the guidance of oculomotor leading processes does not depend upon pre-existing glial structures [2] or the existing tecto- tegmental commissure located in the floor plate. A distinct gap between the existing tecto-tegmental commissure and migrating motor neurons can be found in every section through the oculomotor nucleus. Therefore, oculomotor leading projections must navigate using other environmental cues to reach their target, and suggests that they pioneer a path through a permissive corridor across the midline, independent of the tegmental commissure. The potential molecular and cellular substrates for the oculomotor commissure remain undefined.

The observation in the midline of both cell bodies and secondary leading processes suggested that contralateral cell bodies were not the result of their primary axons making midline crossing errors. The number of migrating motor neurons is surprisingly large, as in posterior sections they outnumber the remaining non-migratory neurons. Interestingly, a large degree of cell death in the ventromedial aspect of the chick oculomotor nucleus was previously noted [48]. This suggests a large proportion of migratory neurons initiate migration but later succumb to cell death.

### Slit signals prevent premature migration of oculomotor neurons

Guidance cues of the Slit family have emerged as repulsive regulators of midline crossing of axons and, more recently, in neuron cell bodies in both vertebrates and invertebrates reviewed by [49]. In the ventral midbrain on E10.5, both Slit1 and 2 are expressed in the floor plate, and the Slit receptors, Robo1 and 2, expressed by the oculomotor neurons. Slit1 and 2 signals from the floor plate may actively repel the leading process, and hence oculomotor neurons, away from the floor plate via the Robo receptors. Consistent with this idea, we show significant premature outgrowth of leading processes in Slit1/2 or Robo1/2 mutants on E10.5. This is coupled with oculomotor cell migration across the floor plate in a subset of cells in the posterior region of the oculomotor nucleus. Previous research describes a similar role for Slit midline repulsion in the hindbrain where Slit1 and 2 are required to keep dorsally projecting motor neurons, but not ventrally projecting nerves, out of the floor plate [23]. We also find that Slits are not required to guide the ventrally projecting nerve fibers, but are required to inhibit the growth of leading processes and migration of cell bodies across the floor plate. In chick, outgrowth of leading processes depends upon the actin-binding protein Drebrin [6]. Therefore, Slit signaling may inhibit Drebrin activity to repress leading process outgrowth prior to E11.5. However, an interaction between Slit/Robo and Drebrin has yet to be described.

We found Slit2 and Slit3 transcripts in the oculomotor nucleus on E10.4 and E14.5. Slit2 and Slit3 also appear to be expressed by other motor neurons [36]. In motor neurons, it is suggested that Slit2 and Slit3 act cell autonomously to modulate their own Robo receptor responsiveness [36], or are transported to the axon to promote nerve fasciculation [50]. Our data from Isl1 mutant mice suggests that motor neuron-derived Slit2 does not participate in repelling oculomotor neurons from the floor plate on E11.5. However, Slit2 cell autonomous functions in the oculomotor nucleus remain to be clarified by future experiments with motor neuron-specific knockouts.

We find an increased number of cell bodies migrating across the midline in Robo mutants compared to Slit mutants on E10.5. This suggests that Robo may have additional ligands that mediate cell adhesion or inhibit cell migration. Signaling from the Robo receptor modulates cell adhesion by N-cadherin [51], and acts to either increase or decrease adhesion [52]. However, cell adhesion in these systems is dependent upon the Slit ligand. Future research may give insight into how the Robo receptor differentiates between mediating cell adhesion and signaling repulsion.

Taken together, we propose that Slit/Robo signals keep leading processes away from the floor plate, and also possibly inhibit neural translocation within the processes. In a similar case, precerebellar neurons of the inferior olive (IO) respond to repulsive Slit signals from the floor plate. IO neurons normally project a leading process across the midline, but their cell body stops just prior to entering the floor plate in the hindbrain. In Robo1/2 mutant mice, IO cell bodies migrate across the floor plate, indicating that Slits are acting as midline repellents via the Robo1/2 receptors [53, 54]. The leading processes in the IO are not normally repelled from the midline, indicating that these two actions—leading process guidance and neural translocation— are independent of each other, with neural translocation being susceptible to repellent Slit signals in IO neurons. However, in the oculomotor system, both leading process outgrowth and neural translocation appear equally responsive to repellent Slit signals.

Migration into the floor plate on E10.5 in Slit and Robo mutants is seen in only a subset of oculomotor neurons. These neurons emanate from the caudal half of the ipsilateral nucleus and are competent to cross the floor plate to reside in the contralateral nucleus. Wild type migration of superior rectus motor neurons occurs similarly, starting with a leading process projecting from the caudal half of the ipsilateral nucleus toward the contralateral nucleus, neuronal migration, and finally integration into the contralateral nucleus. The caudal location and size of the commissure suggests that oculomotor neurons that migrate on E10.5 in Slit and Robo mutants are superior rectus motor neurons that migrate prematurely. Premature projection of retinal ganglion cell axons also occurs in Slit1 and 2 mutant mice [12]. Premature migration suggests that superior rectus motor neurons are responsive to Slit repulsion at the floor plate prior to E13.5 and that Slit/Robo repulsion keeps the motor neurons in their initial ipsilateral positions until this later time point. However, a method to specifically label superior rectus motor neurons is not currently available, so we were not able to distinguish which sub-populations of oculomotor neurons were recruited to cross the midline in Slit or Robo mutants.

### Factors that regulate the timing of Slit repulsion of motor neurons

We suggest that Slits initially repel superior rectus motor neurons on E10.5. Later, on E13.5, this subset must become insensitive to Slit repulsion to enter the floor plate. This could occur by blocking the repulsive activity of floor plate-derived Slit, or increasing oculomotor attraction to the floor plate. Turning off the Slit signal could occur by a general decrease of Robo on the surface of migrating neurons. For example, in *Drosophila*, the cytoplasmic protein Commissureless acts to reduce Robo receptors at the cell surface thereby inhibiting repulsive Slit signaling [55, 56]. However, Commissureless homologues have not yet been identified in vertebrates, so it remains unclear whether an analogous mechanism might be involved with vertebrate Robos.

Activating receptors that compete with, or block Slit/Robo signaling, may be another strategy to release neurons to migrate into Slit positive territory. We tested the possibilities that receptors Robo3 or CXCR4 may interfere with Slit signaling allow for Robo-expressing oculomotor neurons to migrate into zones of high Slit expression. Although some evidence suggested that oculomotor neurons express Robo3 and CXCR4, we found that these receptors are not required for midline crossing. We also found that Netrin1 expressed by the ventral floor plate is not required for migrating oculomotor neurons. This may indicate that other attractive proteins function to attract oculomotor neurons either in concert with Netrin1 or independently. Other signals that block Slit/Robo signaling include NPN1. NPN1 interacts with Robo1 to reduce the repulsive effects of Semaphorin3A in cortical interneurons [57]. In chick, class 3 Semaphorins are expressed in the oculomotor nucleus as well as in the ventral floor plate, while NPN1 is found in migrating oculomotor neurons [44]. Therefore, NPN1 receptors may interact with Robo receptors on superior rectus motor neurons to allow for migration. However, we were unable to detect NPN1 antibody labeling in the oculomotor nucleus (data not shown). Future work may investigate the contribution of Semaphorin and Neuropilin signaling in mediating oculomotor migration.

### Oculomotor migration does not rely on signals from target tissues

The coincidental timing of superior rectus extraocular muscle innervation and motor neuron migration suggests that a signal obtained from the muscle or intermediate target may be transported from peripheral tissue to the cell body to initiate migration [44]. However, we found that oculomotor neurons migrate in the absence of extraocular muscles, peripheral tissue, and the peripheral nIII itself. These results agree with previous findings that superior rectus motor neurons migrate in Phox2b knock-in mice that lack the oculomotor nerve [58]. Signals from within the neural tube therefore provide the signal to initiate migration. For example, the idea that the tecto-tegmental commissural axons traveling from the dorsal midbrain toward and across the floor plate may initiate oculomotor migration [59] was tested by ablation of the commissural axons during chick development. However, oculomotor neuron migration was not altered [60]. Likewise, it was suggested that dopamine generated by midline cells that later generate the substantia nigra and ventral tegmentum may attract oculomotor neurons [3]. However, there is no evidence thus far that monoamines have chemoattractant properties.

Therefore, other signals from within the neural tube, likely in conjunction with intrinsic properties such as cell surface receptors, specific to superior rectus motor neurons, may initiate the outgrowth of the leading projection and subsequent neural migration.

### Conclusion

Migration of superior rectus motor neurons across the ventral midline to the contralateral oculomotor nucleus likely requires tight regulation by a number of extrinsic cues and intrinsic responses. Mice lacking *Slit1* and *2* or *Robo1* and *2* have motor neurons that migrate to the contralateral nucleus on E10.5, three days prior to the normal migration on E13.5. This suggests active Slit/Robo repulsion from the midline is required, at least at early stages, to maintain the ipsilateral position of oculomotor neurons. Neurons that migrate on E10.5 in Slit1/2 or Robo1/2 mutants are positioned in the caudal half of the nucleus, suggesting these neurons are superior rectus motor neurons migrating prematurely. Migration across the midline at E10.5 requires competency to interpret midline attraction, as well as attraction toward the contralateral nucleus. The classic midline attractant Netrin1, or its receptor DCC, does not appear to be required for successful superior rectus motor neuron migration. However, other attractive signals working independently of, or redundant to, Netrin1 are available as early as E10.5 to promote midline crossing in *Slit* and *Robo* mutant mice. Furthermore, the ability to respond to and initiate migration across the midline is intrinsic to the neural tube, and does not require signals obtained from the peripheral tissue.

## Abbreviations

DCC: Deleted in cortical cancer; DiI,DIO: Long Chain Dialkylcarbocyanine, Lipophilic Dyes; E: Embryonic day; IO: Inferior olive; Isl1: Islet 1; mlf: Medial longitudinal fasciculus; mRNA: Messenger ribonucleic acid; nIII: Cranial nerve three; NPN1: Neuropilin 1; OMN: Oculomotor nucleus; PBS: Phosphate buffered saline; PBST: Phosphate buffered saline with triton detergent; SHH: Sonic hedge hog; TC: Tegmental commissure

## Acknowledgements

We thank Marc Tessier-Lavigne (Rockefeller) for Slit1;2;3 and Robo1 and 2 mutant mouse lines, and *in situ* probes. We thank Marc Tessier-Lavigne and Fred Charron (IRCM, Montreal) for Netrin1 and DCC mutant mouse lines, John Rubenstein and Daniel Vogt (UCSF) for CXCR4 embryos, Alain Chedotal (INSERM, Paris) for providing Robo3 mutant mouse embryos and Robo3 expression data, Philip Gage and Lisheng Chen (U Michigan) for Pitx2 embryos, and Elke Stein (Yale) for providing Robo1 and 2 antibodies. We thank Andrew Roesener for providing images of emigrating neurons. We thank Katie Weller and Christine Schlemmer for assistance with experiments, insights and helpful comments.

## Funding

Funding sources included NIH grants NS054740, NS077169, and EY025205 to GSM, and NRF of Korea (NRF-2013R1A1A2058548), Integrative Aging Research Center of Gwangju Institute of Science and Technology and Korea Health Industry Development Institute (HI14C3484) to MRS. Further support for core facilities at the University of Nevada was provided by NIH COBREs RR024210, GM103650, GM103554, and the Nevada INBRE 8 P20 GM103440-11, P20 GM103554, with use of the Nevada Genomics Center supported by INBRE (NCRR) P20 RR-016464. The funding bodies had no roles in the study, collection, analysis, interpretation of data, nor in writing the manuscript.

## Authors' contributions

BB and GSM developed the project. TF, ER, and BB performed in situ hybridization, FST performed explants, and BB performed nerve tracing, antibody labeling and analysis. MKK performed Robo antibody labeling. KTK and MRS performed the analysis of Islet mutant embryos. BB and GSM wrote the paper. All authors read and approved the manuscript.

## Competing interests

The authors declare they have no competing interests.

## Author details

[1]Department of Biology, University of Nevada, Reno, NV 89557, USA. [2]School of Life Sciences, Gwangju Institute of Science and Technology, Oryong-dong, Buk-gu, Gwangju 500-712, Republic of Korea.

## References

1. Granet DB, Khayali S. Amblyopia and strabismus. Pediatr Ann. 2011;40:89–94.
2. Puelles L, Privat A. Do oculomotor neuroblasts migrate across the midline in the retal rat brain? Anat Embryol (Berl). 1977;150:187–206.
3. Puelles L. A Golgi-study of oculomotor neuroblasts migrating across the midline in chick embryos. Anat Embryol (Berl). 1978;152:205–15.
4. Hogg ID. Observations of the development of the nucleus of Edinger-Westphal in man and the albino rat. J Comp Neurol. 1966;126:567–84.
5. Puelles-Lopez L, Malagon-Cobos F, Genis-Galvez JM. The Migration of Oculomotor Neuroblasts Across the Midline in Chick Embryo. Exp Neurol. 1975;47:459–69.
6. Dun XP, Bandeira de Lima T, Allen J, Geraldo S, Gordon-Weeks P, Chilton JK. Drebrin controls neuronal migration through the formation and alignment of the leading process. Mol Cell Neurosci. 2012;49:341–50.
7. Cheng L, Desai J, Miranda CJ, Duncan JS, Qiu W, Nugent AA, Kolpak AL, Wu CC, Drokhlyansky E, Delisle MM, et al. Human CFEOM1 mutations attenuate KIF21A autoinhibition and cause oculomotor axon stalling. Neuron. 2014;82:334–49.
8. Naujoks-Manteuffel C, Sonntag R, Fritzsch B. Development of the amphibian oculomotor complex: evidences for migration of oculomotor motorneurons across the midline. Anat Embryol. 1991;183:545–52.
9. Colamarino SA, Tessier-Lavigne M. The role of the floor plate in axon guidance. Annu Rev Neurosci. 1995;18:497–529.
10. Dickson BJ, Gilestro GF. Regulation of commissural axon pathfinding by slit and its Robo receptors. Annu Rev Cell Dev Biol. 2006;22:651–75.
11. Wong K, Park H, Wu J, Rao Y. Slit proteins: molecular guidance cues for cells ranging from neurons to leukocytes. Curr Opin Genet Dev. 2002;12:583–91.
12. Plump AS, Erskine L, Sabatier C, Brose K, Epstein CJ, Goodman CS, Mason CA, Tessier-Lavigne M. Slit1 and Slit2 cooperate to prevent premature midline crossing of retinal axons in the mouse visual system. Neuron. 2002;33:219–32.
13. Farmer WT, Altick AL, Nural HF, Dugan JP, Kidd T, Charron F, Mastick GS. Pioneer longitudinal axons navigate using floor plate and Slit/Robo signals. Development. 2008;135:3643–53.
14. Long H, Sabatier C, Ma L, Plump A, Yuan W, Ornitz DM, Tamada A, Murakami F, Goodman CS, Tessier-Lavigne M. Conserved roles for Slit and Robo proteins in midline commissural axon guidance. Neuron. 2004;42:213–23.
15. Sabatier C, Plump AS, Le M, Brose K, Tamada A, Murakami F, Lee EY, Tessier-Lavigne M. The divergent Robo family protein rig-1/Robo3 is a negative regulator of slit responsiveness required for midline crossing by commissural axons. Cell. 2004;117:157–69.
16. Zelina P, Blockus H, Zagar Y, Peres A, Friocourt F, Wu Z, Rama N, Fouquet C, Hohenester E, Tessier-Lavigne M, et al. Signaling switch of the axon guidance receptor Robo3 during vertebrate evolution. Neuron. 2014; 84:1258–72.
17. Bloch-Gallego E, Ezan F, Tessier-Lavigne M, Sotelo C. Floor plate and netrin-1 are involved in the migration and survival of inferior olivary neurons. J Neurosci. 1999;19:4407–20.
18. Causeret F, Danne F, Ezan F, Sotelo C, Bloch-Gallego E. Slit antagonizes netrin-1 attractive effects during the migration of inferior olivary neurons. Dev Biol. 2002;246:429–40.
19. Kennedy TE, Serafini T, de la Torre JR, Tessier-Lavigne M. Netrins are diffusible chemotropic factors for commissural axons in the embryonic spinal cord. Cell. 1994;78:425–35.
20. Keino-Masu K, Masu M, Hinck L, Leonardo ED, Chan SS, Culotti JG, Tessier-Lavigne M. Deleted in Colorectal Cancer (DCC) encodes a netrin receptor. Cell. 1996;87:175–85.
21. Shoja-Taheri F, DeMarco A, Mastick GS. Netrin1-DCC-Mediated Attraction Guides Post-Crossing Commissural Axons in the Hindbrain. J Neurosci. 2015;35:11707–18.
22. Varela-Echavarría A, Tucker A, Püschel AW, Guthrie S. Motor axon subpopulations respond differentially to the chemorepellents netrin-1 and semaphorin D. Neuron. 1997;18:193–207.
23. Hammond R, Vivancos V, Naeem A, Chilton J, Mambetisaeva E, Andrews W, Sundaresan V, Guthrie S. Slit-mediated repulsion is a key regulator of motor axon pathfinding in the hindbrain. Development. 2005;132:4483–95.
24. Murray A, Naeem A, Barnes SH, Drescher U, Guthrie S. Slit and Netrin-1 guide cranial motor axon pathfinding via Rho-kinase, myosin light chain kinase and myosin II. Neural Dev. 2010;5:15.
25. Lin L, Rao Y, Isacson O. Netrin-1 and slit-2 regulate and direct neurite growth of ventral midbrain dopaminergic neurons. Mol Cell Neurosci. 2005;28:547–55.
26. Dugan JP, Stratton A, Riley HP, Farmer WT, Mastick GS. Midbrain dopaminergic axons are guided longitudinally through the diencephalon by Slit/Robo signals. Mol Cell Neurosci. 2011;46:347–56.
27. Fazeli A, Dickinson SL, Hermiston ML, Tighe RV, Steen RG, Small CG, Stoeckli ET, Keino-Masu K, Masu M, Rayburn H, et al. Phenotype of mice lacking functional Deleted in colorectal cancer (Dcc) gene. Nature. 1997;386:796–804.
28. Serafini T, Colamarino SA, Leonardo ED, Wang H, Beddington R, Skarnes WC, Tessier-Lavigne M. Netrin-1 is required for commissural axon guidance in the developing vertebrate nervous system. Cell. 1996;87:1001–14.
29. Grieshammer U, Le M, Plump AS, Wang F, Tessier-Lavigne M, Martin GR. SLIT2-mediated ROBO2 signaling restricts kidney induction to a single site. Dev Cell. 2004;6:709–17.

30. Mastick GS, Davis NM, Andrew GL, Easter Jr SS. Pax-6 functions in boundary formation and axon guidance in the embryonic mouse forebrain. Development 1997, 124:1985-1997

31. Kim M, Roesener AP, Mendonca PR, Mastick GS. Robo1 and Robo2 have distinct roles in pioneer longitudinal axon guidance. Dev Biol. 2011;358:181-8.

32. Ericson J, Thor S, Edlund T, Jessell TM, Yamada T. Early stages of motor neuron differentiation revealed by expression of homeobox gene Islet-1. Science. 1992;256:1555-60.

33. Carpenter F. The development of the oculomotor nerve, the ciliary ganglion, and the abducent nerve in the chick. Cambridge: Bulletin of the museum of comparative zoology; 1906.

34. Chedotal A, Richards LJ. Wiring the brain: the biology of neuronal guidance. Cold Spring Harb Perspect Biol. 2010;2:a001917.

35. Hasan KB, Agarwala S, Ragsdale CW. PHOX2A regulation of oculomotor complex nucleogenesis. Development. 2010;137:1205-13.

36. Brose K, Bland KS, Wang KH, Arnott D, Henzel W, Goodman CS, Tessier-Lavigne M, Kidd T. Slit proteins bind Robo receptors and have an evolutionarily conserved role in repulsive axon guidance. Cell. 1999;96:795-806.

37. Ricano-Cornejo I, Altick AL, Garcia-Pena CM, Nural HF, Echevarria D, Miquelajauregui A, Mastick GS, Varela-Echavarria A. Slit-Robo signals regulate pioneer axon pathfinding of the tract of the postoptic commissure in the mammalian forebrain. J Neurosci Res. 2011;89:1531-41.

38. Lee H, Kim M, Kim N, Macfarlan T, Pfaff SL, Mastick GS, Song MR. Slit and Semaphorin signaling governed by Islet transcription factors positions motor neuron somata within the neural tube. Exp Neurol. 2015;269:17-27.

39. Chen Z, Gore BB, Long H, Ma L, Tessier-Lavigne M. Alternative splicing of the Robo3 axon guidance receptor governs the midline switch from attraction to repulsion. Neuron. 2008;58:325-32.

40. Chalasani SH, Sabelko KA, Sunshine MJ, Littman DR, Raper JA. A chemokine, SDF-1, reduces the effectiveness of multiple axonal repellents and is required for normal axon pathfinding. J Neurosci. 2003;23:1360-71.

41. Chalasani SH, Sabol A, Xu H, Gyda MA, Rasband K, Granato M, Chien CB, Raper JA. Stromal cell-derived factor-1 antagonizes slit/robo signaling in vivo. J Neurosci. 2007;27:973-80.

42. Lerner O, Davenport D, Patel P, Psatha M, Lieberam I, Guthrie S. Stromal cell-derived factor-1 and hepatocyte growth factor guide axon projections to the extraocular muscles. Dev Neurobiol. 2010;70:549-64.

43. Yee KT, Simon HH, Tessier-Lavigne M, O'Leary DM. Extension of long leading processes and neuronal migration in the mammalian brain directed by the chemoattractant netrin-1. Neuron. 1999;24:607-22.

44. Chilton JK, Guthrie S. Development of oculomotor axon projections in the chick embryo. J Comp Neurol. 2004;472:308-17.

45. Fritzsch B, Nichols DH, Echelard Y, McMahon AP. Development of midbrain and anterior hindbrain ocular motoneurons in normal and Wnt-1 knockout mice. J Neurobiol. 1995;27:457-69.

46. Zacharias AL, Lewandoski M, Rudnicki MA, Gage PJ. Pitx2 is an upstream activator of extraocular myogenesis and survival. Dev Biol. 2011;349:395-405.

47. Biondi G. Osservaxioni sullo sviluppo e sulla struttura dei nuclei d'origine dei nervi oculomotore e trocleare nel pollo. Rivista Italiana Neuropathia. 1910;3:302-403.

48. Steljes TP, Kinoshita Y, Wheeler EF, Oppenheim RW, von Bartheld CS. Neurotrophic factor regulation of developing avian oculomotor neurons: differential effects of BDNF and GDNF. J Neurobiol. 1999;41:295-315.

49. Ypsilanti AR, Zagar Y, Chedotal A. Moving away from the midline: new developments for Slit and Robo. Development. 2010;137:1939-52.

50. Jaworski A, Tessier-Lavigne M. Autocrine/juxtaparacrine regulation of axon fasciculation by Slit-Robo signaling. Nat Neurosci. 2012;15:367-9.

51. Rhee J, Buchan T, Zukerberg L, Lilien J, Balsamo J. Cables links Robo-bound Abl kinase to N-cadherin-bound beta-catenin to mediate Slit-induced modulation of adhesion and transcription. Nat Cell Biol. 2007;9:883-92.

52. Shiau CE, Bronner-Fraser M. N-cadherin acts in concert with Slit1-Robo2 signaling in regulating aggregation of placode-derived cranial sensory neurons. Development. 2009;136:4155-64.

53. Marillat V, Sabatier C, Failli V, Matsunaga E, Sotelo C, Tessier-Lavigne M, Chedotal A. The slit receptor Rig-1/Robo3 controls midline crossing by hindbrain precerebellar neurons and axons. Neuron. 2004;43:69-79.

54. Di Meglio T, Nguyen-Ba-Charvet KT, Tessier-Lavigne M, Sotelo C, Chedotal A. Molecular mechanisms controlling midline crossing by precerebellar neurons. J Neurosci. 2008;28:6285-94.

55. Kidd T, Brose K, Mitchell KJ, Fetter RD, Tessier-Lavigne M, Goodman CS, Tear G. Roundabout controls axon crossing of the CNS midline and defines a novel subfamily of evolutionarily conserved guidance receptors. Cell. 1998;92:205-15.

56. Tear G, Harris R, Sutaria S, Kilomanski K, Goodman CS, Seeger MA. commissureless controls growth cone guidance across the CNS midline in Drosophila and encodes a novel membrane protein. Neuron. 1996;16:501-14.

57. Hernandez-Miranda LR, Cariboni A, Faux C, Ruhrberg C, Cho JH, Cloutier JF, Eickholt BJ, Parnavelas JG, Andrews WD. Robo1 regulates semaphorin signaling to guide the migration of cortical interneurons through the ventral forebrain. J Neurosci. 2011;31:6174-87.

58. Coppola E, Pattyn A, Guthrie SC, Goridis C, Studer M. Reciprocal gene replacements reveal unique functions for Phox2 genes during neural differentiation. EMBO J. 2005;24:4392-403.

59. Goldberg S. Studies on the mechanics of development of the visual pathways in the chick embryo. Dev Biol. 1974;36:24-43.

60. Heaton MB, Moody SA, Coultas PL. Oculomotor neuroblast migration in the chick embryo in the absence of tecto-tegmental fibers. Dev Biol. 1979;68:304-10.

# 11

# Characterization of primary cilia during the differentiation of retinal ganglion cells in the zebrafish

Paola Lepanto[1], Camila Davison[2,3], Gabriela Casanova[4], Jose L. Badano[1*] and Flavio R. Zolessi[2,3*]

## Abstract

**Background:** Retinal ganglion cell (RGC) differentiation in vivo is a highly stereotyped process, likely resulting from the interaction of cell type-specific transcription factors and tissue-derived signaling factors. The primary cilium, as a signaling hub in the cell, may have a role during this process but its presence and localization during RGC generation, and its contribution to the process of cell differentiation, have not been previously assessed in vivo.

**Methods:** In this work we analyzed the distribution of primary cilia in vivo using laser scanning confocal microscopy, as well as their main ultrastructural features by transmission electron microscopy, in the early stages of retinal histogenesis in the zebrafish, around the time of RGC generation and initial differentiation. In addition, we knocked-down *ift88* and *elipsa*, two genes with an essential role in cilia generation and maintenance, a treatment that caused a general reduction in organelle size. The effect on retinal development and RGC differentiation was assessed by confocal microscopy of transgenic or immunolabeled embryos.

**Results:** Our results show that retinal neuroepithelial cells have an apically-localized primary cilium usually protruding from the apical membrane. We also found a small proportion of sub-apical cilia, before and during the neurogenic period. This organelle was also present in an apical position in neuroblasts during apical process retraction and dendritogenesis, although between these stages cilia appeared highly dynamic regarding both presence and position. Disruption of cilia caused a decrease in the proliferation of retinal progenitors and a reduction of neural retina volume. In addition, retinal histogenesis was globally delayed albeit RGC layer formation was preferentially reduced with respect to the amacrine and photoreceptor cell layers.

**Conclusions:** These results indicate that primary cilia exhibit a highly dynamic behavior during early retinal differentiation, and that they are required for the proliferation and survival of retinal progenitors, as well as for neuronal generation, particularly of RGCs.

**Keywords:** Retina, Cilia, Retinal ganglion cell, Neurogenesis

## Background

Developmental processes are carried out based on a complex interaction between information inherited from the parent cell and time/tissue-specific environmental cues. The vertebrate retina is one of the most organized tissues in the body. To achieve this unique organization, dividing neuroepithelial cells must give rise to differentiating neuroblasts in a highly controlled and orderly fashion. Even though retinal ganglion cells (RGCs) are the first neuroblasts to be born, how these cells arise and differentiate into the correct neuronal type, with its corresponding morphology and connections, is still not completely understood.

Both cell type-specific expression of transcription factors and tissue-derived positional and trophic factors are likely to interact to achieve a mature and fully functional retina. Several signals from the environment have been shown to influence cell position and differentiation. For example, Notch signaling in relation to interkinetic

* Correspondence: jbadano@pasteur.edu.uy; fzolessi@fcien.edu.uy
[1]Human Molecular Genetics Laboratory, Institut Pasteur de Montevideo, Mataojo 2020, Montevideo 11400, Uruguay
[2]Cell Biology of Neural Development Laboratory, Institut Pasteur de Montevideo, Mataojo 2020, Montevideo 11400, Uruguay
Full list of author information is available at the end of the article

nuclear migration has been linked to cell cycle withdrawal, the first step in the differentiation process [1]. The basal lamina of the neuroepithelium (the "inner limiting membrane") has also been shown to play a critical role as RGC axon extension and orientation depends on the presence of Laminin [2]. Another contributing signaling molecule is Sonic Hedgehog (Shh), which is needed for spreading the wave of RGC and amacrine cell differentiation across the retina, as well as later on for photoreceptor cell differentiation [3–7]. Importantly, during RGC differentiation in vivo, neuroepithelial polarity is transiently maintained: it has been shown that polarity determinants are apically-positioned during the initial stages of differentiation, while in vitro these determinants show an erratic behavior [8]. Therefore, the tissue impinges constraints on the inherited differentiation program, guiding it to achieve the mature functional structure.

In recent years it has been shown that one of the main signaling hubs in cells, which has a critical role during development, is the primary cilium. Primary cilia are microtubule-based organelles that extend from a modified centriole, the basal body, protruding as an extension of the plasma membrane. Cilia are enriched in moieties required for sensing and transducing a number of signaling cascades that have been shown to rely on this particular cellular structure, including Wnt and Shh [9]. These findings, coupled with the ubiquitous presence of primary cilia in different cell types, explain why defects in the formation, maintenance and function of this organelle result in a range of clinical manifestations that have been grouped under the term ciliopathies [10, 11]. Importantly, central nervous system associated phenotypes, including structural defects, mental retardation and retinal degeneration, are hallmark phenotypes of several ciliopathies [12].

Primary cilia have been studied in the context of neuronal differentiation in different regions of the central nervous system. It has been shown for example that this organelle plays a role in progenitor cell proliferation in the cerebellum [13, 14], proliferation of progenitors and integration of neurons in the hippocampus [15, 16], and in the migration of neuroblasts in the mouse developing cortex [17, 18]. Early electron microscopy studies have shown that both neural tube and retinal neuroepithelial cells have an apically localized primary cilium, and that RGC neuroblasts of the mouse developing retina have a primary cilium that also displays a polarized localization, being positioned at the tip of the retracting apical process [19, 20]. Therefore, it is possible that the primary cilium is playing a role in RGC differentiation.

In this work we performed an in-depth characterization of the presence and localization of cilia during the differentiation of RGCs in the zebrafish retina combining electron and confocal microscopy with time-lapse video microscopy in live embryos. As an in vivo marker for cilia, we used a zebrafish transgenic line expressing EGFP fused to the carboxy-terminus of the small GTPase Arl13b (Arl13b-GFP; [21]). Arl13b, which belongs to the Arl/Arf family of GTPases involved in microtubule dynamics and membrane traffic, is specifically localized to the ciliary axoneme and is an essential protein for cilia maintenance in zebrafish and mice [22, 23]. In addition, we evaluated retinal development in conditions where cilia integrity was compromised. Our data show that RGCs primary cilia are highly dynamic organelles, changing in size and position during the differentiation process. The double knockdown of *ift88* and *elipsa*, two genes important for cilia formation and maintenance, shows that this organelle plays a role both during progenitor cell proliferation and maintenance, as well as during neurogenesis. Thus, our data provide important information that will help in achieving a more complete understanding of the role of primary cilia in RGC differentiation.

## Methods

### Fish breeding and care

Zebrafish were maintained and bred in a stand-alone system (Tecniplast), with controlled temperature (28 °C), conductivity (500 μS/cm2) and pH (7.5), under live and pellet dietary regime. Embryos were raised at temperatures ranging from 28.5 to 32 °C and staged in hours post-fertilization (hpf) according to Kimmel and collaborators [24]. We used wild-type (SAT; [25]) and different previously established transgenic lines in this work: Tg(actb2:Arl13b-GFP)hsc5 (Arl13b-GFP, kindly provided by B. Ciruna; [21]), Tg(atoh7:gap43-EGFP)cu1 (atoh7:gap-GFP; [8]), Tg(atoh7:gap43-RFP)cu2 (atoh7:-gap-RFP; [8]), SoFa1 (atoh7:gap-RFP/ptf1a:cytGFP/crx:gap-CFP; [26]). In addition, we generated a double transgenic line crossing atoh7:gap-RFP and Arl13b-GFP. All the manipulations were carried out following the approved local regulations (CEUA-Institut Pasteur de Montevideo, and CNEA).

### Morpholino treatment

The morpholino oligomers (MOs) used in this study were obtained from Gene Tools (Philomath, USA) and included those previously used to target zebrafish *elipsa* and *ift88* translational initiation: *elipsa*-ATG (GGCTACCGATTCGTTCATGGCATCA; [27]) and *ift88*-ATG (GCCTTATTAAACAGAAATACTCCCA; IFT88 MO3, [28]). We also used newly designed morpholinos to target the splicing of *ift88* and *elipsa* mRNA: *ift88*-SP (AACAGCAGATGCAAAATGACTCACT) which targets the exon 3 - intron 3 boundary; *elipsa*-SP (CTGTTTTAATAACTCACCTCGCTGA) which targets the exon 1 - intron 1 boundary. All MOs were injected in the yolk of 1–4 cell-stage embryos, at a maximum volume of 4 nL. As control, we used matching doses of a standard MO (CCTCTTACCTCAGTTACAATTTATA) from Gene Tools (Philomath, USA). When considered necessary, we co-injected a double amount per embryo of the standard anti-p53 MO [29].

To test the effectiveness of splice-blocking morpholinos we performed RT-PCR (primers sequences are available upon request). Total RNA was extracted from 30 morphant or wild-type embryos using TRIzol reagent (Invitrogen) and cDNA was prepared using the SuperScript First-Strand Synthesis System for RT-PCR (Invitrogen).

### Blastomere transplantation

Blastula stage embryos were used for transplantation experiments. Cells from the donor embryos were transplanted into the animal pole of hosts, following standard procedures. After transplantation embryos were incubated in E3 medium (5 mM NaCl, 0.17 mM KCl, 0.33 mM CaCl$_2$, 0.33 mM MgSO$_4$) plus 10 mM Hepes pH 7.4, 0.00005 % methylene blue and Penicillin/Streptomycin (Sigma) at 32 °C.

### Immunofluorescence

Embryos were grown in 0.003 % phenylthiourea (Sigma) from 10 hpf onwards to delay pigmentation, and fixed overnight at 4 °C, by immersion in 4 % paraformaldehyde in phosphate saline buffer (PBS; pH 7.4).

For whole-mount immunostaining all subsequent washes were performed in PBS containing 1 % Triton X-100. Further permeability was achieved by incubating the embryos in 0.25 % trypsin-EDTA for 10–15 min at 0 °C. Blocking was for 30 min in 1 % bovine serum albumin (BSA), 1 % Triton X-100 in PBS. The primary antibodies, diluted in the blocking solution, were used as follows: zn8 (ZIRC, Oregon), 1/100; anti-activated Caspase 3 (AbCam), 1/500; anti-histone H3 pSer10 (Santa Cruz), 1/300, anti-acetylated tubulin (Sigma), 1/750; anti-γ tubulin (Sigma), 1/500. The secondary antibodies used were: anti-rabbit IgG-TRITC (Life Technologies), 1/1000; anti-mouse IgG-Alexa 488 (Life Technologies), 1/1000; anti-mouse IgG1-Alexa 488 (Life Technologies), 1/1000; anti-mouse IgG2b-Alexa 568 (Life Technologies), 1/1000. When necessary, TRITC-conjugated phalloidin (Sigma) was mixed with the secondary antibody. Nuclei were fluorescently counterstained with methyl green [30]. All antibody incubations were performed overnight at 4 °C. Embryos were mounted in 70 % glycerol in 20 mM Tris buffer (pH 8.0) and stored at 4 °C or –20 °C.

Five day-old embryos were fixed as described above, washed in PBS and cryoprotected in 30 % sucrose in PBS overnight at 4 °C. They were then embedded in OCT (Tissue-Tek) and quickly frozen in liquid N$_2$.

Transverse cryosections (10 µm) were made on a Reichert-Jung Cryocut E cryostat and adhered to gelatin subbed slides. Mounting was made using 70 % glycerol in 20 mM Tris buffer (pH 8.0).

Observation of whole embryos or cryosections was performed using a Leica TCS-SP5 (for all in vivo and some fixed material imaging) or a Zeiss LSM800 (for some fixed material imaging) laser confocal microscopes, with 63x 1.4 NA oil immersion or 20x 0.7 NA and 63x 1.3 NA glycerol:water (80:20) or water immersion objectives.

### In vivo confocal microscopy

Around 30 hpf embryos were selected, anesthetized using 0.04 mg/mL MS222 (Sigma) and mounted in 0.8 % low melting-point agarose (Sigma) over n° 0 glass bottom dishes (MaTek). After agarose solidification and during overnight image acquisitions, embryos were kept in Ringer's solution (116 mM NaCl, 2.9 mM KCl, 1.8 mM CaCl$_2$, 5 mM HEPES pH 7.2) with 0.04 mg/mL MS222. Live acquisitions were made using a Leica TCS-SP5 laser confocal microscope with a 20x 0.7 NA objective and glycerol:water (80:20) immersion medium. Stacks around 60 µm-thick were acquired in bidirectional mode, at 1 µm spacing and 512 × 512 pixel resolution every 10 or 15 min (the acquisition time for each embryo was approximately 45 s).

### Transmission electron microscopy

Embryos were fixed at 26, 35 and 48 hpf by immersion in fixative solution (4 % paraformaldehyde, 2.5 % glutaraldehyde in PBS, pH 7.2–7.4). Then the head was dissected and incubated overnight at 4 °C. The fixed material was washed in PBS, post-fixed in 1 % osmium tetroxide in distilled water for 1 h, and washed in distilled water. Samples were dehydrated through a graded (25, 50, 75, 95, 100 %) ethanol-water series, transferred to acetone for 2 × 20 min, and infiltrated with araldite resin through a series of steps (2:1 acetone:araldite for 30 min, 1:1 acetone:araldite for 30 min, 1:2 acetone:araldite for 30 min, 100 % araldite overnight at 4 °C). On the next day, the material was transferred into flat-embedding molds with freshly made araldite resin and oriented as desired. The embedded samples were cured at 60 °C for 48 h. Blocks were semi-thin sectioned at 500 nm using a RMC MT-X ultramicrotome, stained with boraxic methylene blue and examined in a light microscope. Once the area of interest was reached, ultra-thin 70 nm sections were obtained and mounted on formvar-coated copper grids. Sections were stained for 2 h in 2 % aqueous uranyl acetate followed by staining in Reynold's lead citrate for 10 min. Observation and acquisition was performed using a Jeol JEM 1010 transmission electron microscope operated at 100 kV, equipped with a Hamamatsu C4742-95 digital camera.

## Image analysis

Images were analyzed using Fiji [31]. Primary cilia length in Kupffer's vesicle was measured manually in maximum intensity z-projections of the confocal stacks. Volume measurements (whole retina and zn8-positive region) were performed using intensity-based thresholding aided by manual selection. After that, the volume was obtained using 3D Roi Manager and 3D Objects Counter plugins [32, 33]. Cell counting (pH3 and activated Caspase 3-positive cells) was also done manually on the confocal stacks with the aid of the MTrackJ plugin [34]. For the fluorescence profile analysis of the retina in SoFa transgenic embryos, confocal planes from a 10 µm-deep stack were projected using intensity average and then a 100 µm-long and 20 µm-wide line selection was drawn across the retina. The fluorescence intensity along this line was measured for each channel using the Intensity Toolset from Imperial College of London FILM facility (http://www.imperial.ac.uk/medicine/facility-for-imaging-by-light-microscopy/equipment/software—fiji/). In some cases, bleed-through from the GFP signal into the CFP and RFP channel was detected. In these cases we processed the images as follows: 1) we calculated a normalization factor for the GFP channel = maximum GFP intensity / (maximum RFP intensity due to bleed-through – (minus) average RFP intensity in RGC layer); 2) we divided the GFP channel over this ratio generating a new image that corresponded to the bleed-through signal, 3) we subtracted this new image from the RFP channel. The same procedure was implemented for the CFP channel when necessary. In order to quantify the integrated fluorescence intensity from each layer, the boundaries of the region below the fluorescence curve corresponding to that layer were set to the point corresponding to the 50 % of the peak intensity (see Fig. 11b). The percentage of the signal corresponding to each cell type was calculated as the ratio between the area under the plot corresponding to each cell type layer and the area under the plot corresponding to that channel as a whole.

## Statistical analysis

In all cases, box plots represent the 25–75 % quartiles, the horizontal lines represent the median, and the short horizontal lines are the minimal and maximal values. All statistical analyses were performed as previously described [35, 36] using Past software [37]. As a routine, the datasets were checked for normality using Shapiro-Wilk normality test and for homogeneity of variances using Levene's test. In the case of normal and homogeneous data, we performed a Student's $t$-test for media comparison. If homogeneity requirement was not met, we performed a rank transformation [38]. In the case of non-normal data, we performed a Mann–Whitney test.

## Results

### Characterization of primary cilia in early stages of retina differentiation

We first analyzed the presence, localization and ultrastructure of primary cilia in the differentiating zebrafish neural retina by confocal and transmission electron microscopy (TEM) of 26 and 35 hpf (hours post-fertilization) embryos, just before and some time after RGC generation has started, respectively. We used double transgenic atoh7:gap-RFP/Arl13b-GFP (see Methods) embryos that allowed us to visualize the RGCs via a membrane form of mRFP under the control of an RGC progenitors/neuroblasts promoter, and cilia through the expression of Arl13b, a protein that localizes to the ciliary axoneme fused to GFP. Confocal analysis of Arl13b-GFP embryos at 26 hpf showed that all detectable cilia in the retinal neuroepithelium were localized apically (Fig. 1a), and that Arl13b-GFP signal coincided with the acetylated tubulin labeling, a general-use marker for cilia (Fig. 1c). As neurons start differentiating after 28 hpf, this latter marker loses its specificity, as tubulin acetylation extends to the whole cytoplasm of neuroblasts and neurons. Hence, all further description on cilia localization by confocal microscopy was achieved using Arl13b-GFP as a marker. At 35 hpf, when neurogenesis has spread through the ventronasal region of the retina, we observed that most cilia were still present at the apical border of the neuroepithelium (Fig. 1b). Some cells bearing an apical primary cilium also expressed low levels of the gap-RFP construct (Fig. 1d), suggesting that both cycling progenitors and early neuroblasts present an apically-localized primary cilium.

Likewise, our TEM analysis showed that in 35 hpf retinas most of the primary cilia are localized to the apical surface of the neuroepithelium, extending into the subretinal space (Fig. 1e-h). These cilia displayed different angles with respect to the neuroepithelial surface, albeit no correlation was evident between this angle and the region of the retina being examined. At the ultrastructural level, all these apical cilia had a 9 + 0 axoneme (Fig. 1i) and most (69/94) were immerse in a deep ciliary pocket (Fig. 1e), although in a few cases this structure was either incomplete (7/94; Fig. 1f) or absent (18/94; Fig. 1g-h). Some of the observed cilia projected into invaginations of retinal pigment epithelium (RPE) cells (Fig. 1h). Figure 1j presents a quantification of morphometric parameters of these apical cilia. Less frequently, we also observed basal bodies in close association with the plasma membrane but without a visible axoneme (Fig. 1k). In order to ascertain if these features were also present in a completely undifferentiated retinal

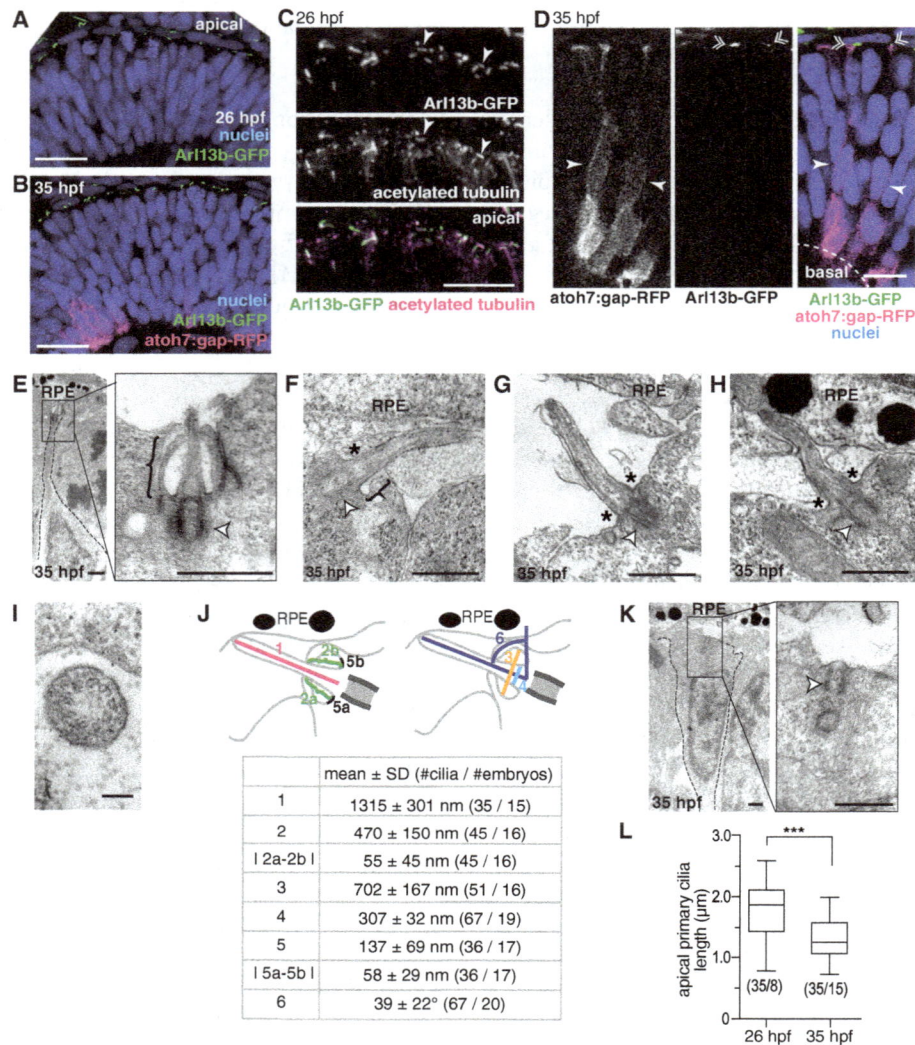

**Fig. 1** Main features of apical primary cilia in the early differentiating retinal neuroepithelium. The embryonic zebrafish retinal neuroepithelium was analyzed using confocal microscopy and TEM. **a-b** 26 hpf embryos expressing Arl13b-GFP (localized to primary cilia) (**a**) or double transgenic 35 hpf embryos expressing Arl13b-GFP and atoh7:gap-RFP (expressed in progenitors during the last cell cycle and in RGC neuroblasts) (**b**) were fixed and analyzed in toto using confocal microscopy. A 3D maximum intensity projection of a 3 μm-thick confocal stack is shown. **c** 26 hpf embryos expressing Arl13b-GFP were immunolabeled with anti-acetylated tubulin antibody. A maximum intensity projection of a 3 μm-thick stack of the apical region of the neuroepithelium is shown. The arrowheads show primary cilia with Arl13b-GFP and acetylated tubulin labeling. **d** Single confocal plane with a detail of the stack shown in **b**. It is possible to observe cells bearing a primary cilium (*double arrowhead*) and expressing low levels of gap-RFP (*full arrowheads*). **e-h** TEM micrographs showing examples of apical primary cilia, either with a complete (**e**, *bracket*), incomplete (**f**, *bracket - asterisk*) or absent ciliary pocket (**g** and **h**, *asterisks*). Primary cilia in close contact with RPE cells were also observed (**h**). The basal body is indicated with a white arrowhead. **i** Cross section of an apically localized primary cilium. **j** Morphological parameters of apical primary cilia of 35 hpf embryos obtained from measurements performed on TEM micrographs. Measured features are summarized in the upper diagrams, and values (mean ± standard deviation) shown in the lower table. **k** TEM micrograph showing a basal body (white arrowhead) associated with the apical plasma membrane but lacking an axoneme. **l** Comparison of apically-localized primary cilia length at 26 and 35 hpf. The numbers in brackets represent the number of cilia / embryos measured in each case. (***) $p < 0.001$, Student's $t$ test. RPE: retinal pigment epithelium. Scale bars: A-B, 20 μm; C-D, 10 μm; E, 1 μm; F-H, 0.5 μm; I, 0.1 μm; K, 1 μm. For a high resolution image of Fig. 1 please see Additional file 12

neuroepithelium, we also analyzed apical primary cilia ultrastructure in 26 hpf embryos using TEM. Interestingly, we found that these cilia were morphologically similar to those from 35 hpf embryos, except for their length: cilia were significantly longer in 26 hpf retinas (Fig. 1l).

In addition to cilia emerging from the apical membrane, we found that around 10 % of total cilia in 35 hpf embryos (15/153; 23 embryos) were clearly located subapically, protruding from the basolateral cell membrane (Fig. 2a). Although their basal bodies were localized

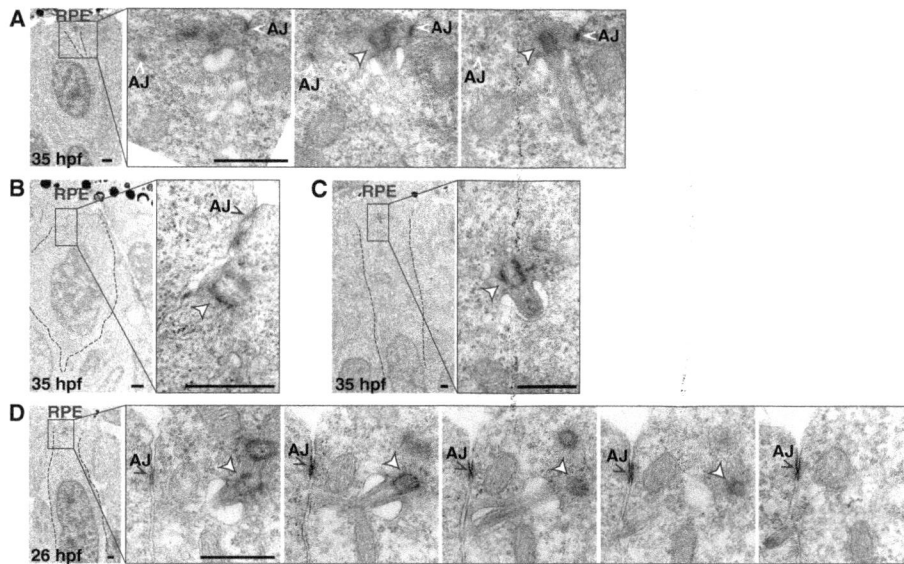

**Fig. 2** Primary cilia emerging from the basolateral membrane of retinal neuroepithelial cells. TEM micrographs of retinas from 26 and 35 hpf embryos. **a** Low magnification (*left*) and high magnification serial sections (*right*) of a retina from a 35 hpf embryo. A primary cilium emerges from the basolateral membrane, as evidenced by the presence of adherent junctions (AJ). **b** Basal body without an axoneme, but closely associated with the basolateral membrane. **c** Basal body with a short axoneme inside a cytoplasmic vesicle. **d** Low magnification (*left*) and high magnification serial sections (*right*) of a retina from a 26 hpf embryo showing a primary cilium emerging from the basolateral membrane. White arrowhead: basal body; RPE: retinal pigment epithelium. Scale bars: A-D, 1 μm. For a high resolution image of Fig. 2 please see Additional file 13

close to the apical border of neuroepithelial cells, these cilia emerged basally to the adherent junction belts and pointed towards the basal side of the neuroepithelium. We also observed some basal bodies docked to the basolateral membrane, without a visible axoneme (Fig. 2b) and small primary cilia inside cytoplasmic vesicles, with a short axoneme, pointing in a basal or basolateral direction (Fig. 2c). Basally oriented primary cilia have been previously observed in the mouse developing cortex, where they were present in neuroepithelial cells committed to delamination, so as to generate basal progenitors [39]. In the case of the neural retina, delamination only occurs in postmitotic cells, such as differentiating RGCs. To test if these retinal neuroblasts showed the same behavior as cortical progenitors, we analyzed 26 hpf embryos, in which progenitors have not yet become postmitotic. In these early embryos we also found a considerable number of basally oriented primary cilia (8 %, 10/123; 7 embryos; Fig. 2d).

## Cilia dynamics in early neuroblasts

To study the dynamics of primary cilia we performed live confocal microscopy on mosaic embryos resulting from the transplant of cells from double transgenic embryos (atoh7:gap-RFP/Arl13b-GFP) to unlabeled wild type embryos at the blastoderm stage. Transplanted embryos were imaged through time-lapse confocal microscopy from early developmental stages (30 hpf). In these movies, we were able to observe gap-RFP low-expressing cells bearing apically-localized Arl13b-labeled primary cilia. Some of these cells eventually divided, indicating that they were progenitors. As expected, dividing cells lost their cilia just before the onset of mitosis (Fig. 3a, Movie in Additional file 1).

After the last cell division, the neuroblast cell body moves towards the basal side of the neuroepithelium and the apical process detaches and begins to retract [8]. Some of the elongated atoh7-positive cells did not divide, but eventually retracted their apical processes and/ or extended an axon on the basal surface, indicating that they were post-mitotic neuroblasts (Fig. 3b). In a few cases (6 cells) it was possible to observe an apically localized primary cilium previous to apical detachment. In four of these cells the primary cilium seemed to disappear before the onset of detachment (Fig. 3b; Movie in Additional file 2; Fig. 4, denoted as ●), while in the other two cells it did not disappear but moved basally, towards the cell body, before the beginning of the apical retraction process (Movie in Additional file 3; Fig. 4, denoted as ○). In these latter cases, the apical process detached and eventually reached the position of the cilium, which then regained an apical localization.

A primary cilium usually re-appeared during the retraction of the apical process, localizing to its tip, and remaining visible until the end of the retraction (Fig. 3b; Movie in Additional file 2; Fig. 4, denoted as ■). The

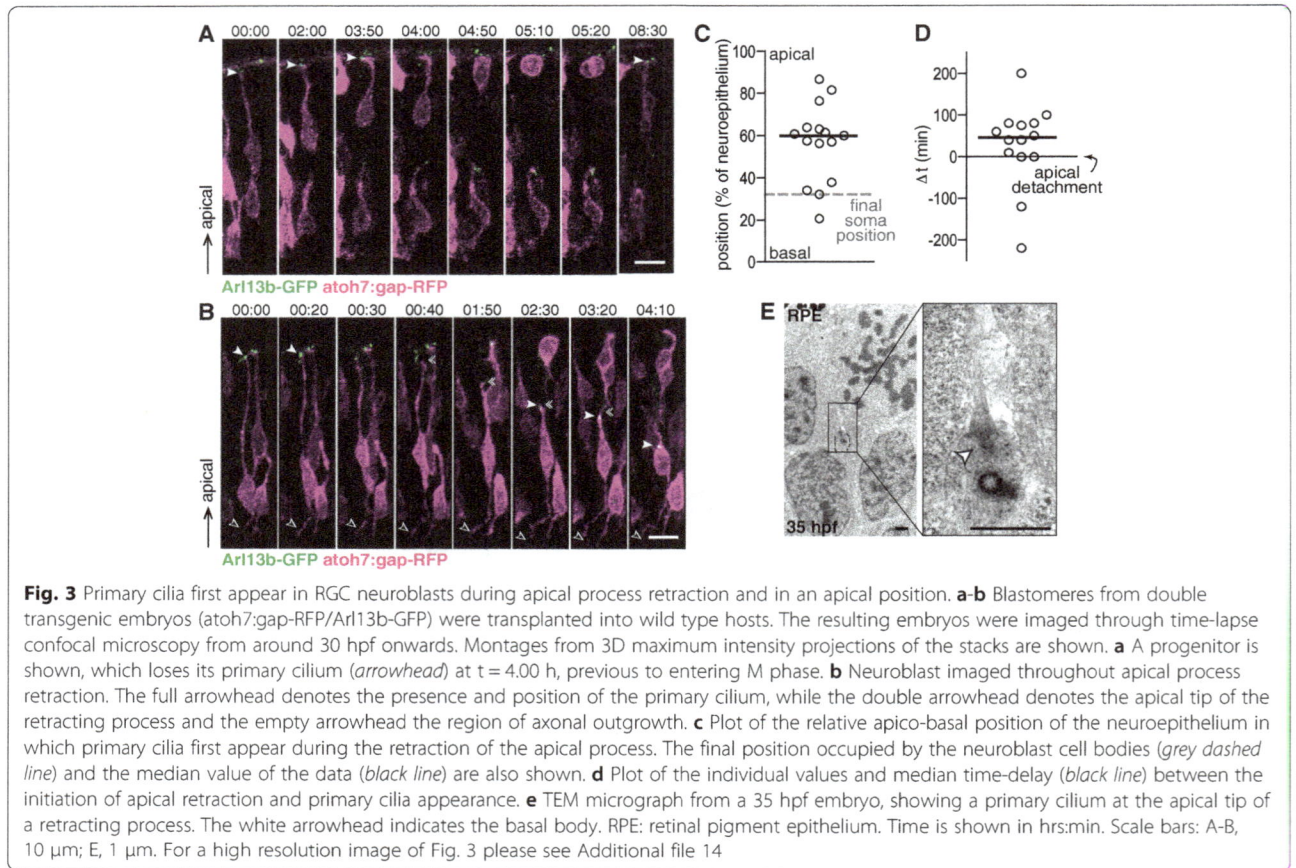

**Fig. 3** Primary cilia first appear in RGC neuroblasts during apical process retraction and in an apical position. **a-b** Blastomeres from double transgenic embryos (atoh7:gap-RFP/Arl13b-GFP) were transplanted into wild type hosts. The resulting embryos were imaged through time-lapse confocal microscopy from around 30 hpf onwards. Montages from 3D maximum intensity projections of the stacks are shown. **a** A progenitor is shown, which loses its primary cilium (*arrowhead*) at t = 4.00 h, previous to entering M phase. **b** Neuroblast imaged throughout apical process retraction. The full arrowhead denotes the presence and position of the primary cilium, while the double arrowhead denotes the apical tip of the retracting process and the empty arrowhead the region of axonal outgrowth. **c** Plot of the relative apico-basal position of the neuroepithelium in which primary cilia first appear during the retraction of the apical process. The final position occupied by the neuroblast cell bodies (*grey dashed line*) and the median value of the data (*black line*) are also shown. **d** Plot of the individual values and median time-delay (*black line*) between the initiation of apical retraction and primary cilia appearance. **e** TEM micrograph from a 35 hpf embryo, showing a primary cilium at the apical tip of a retracting process. The white arrowhead indicates the basal body. RPE: retinal pigment epithelium. Time is shown in hrs:min. Scale bars: A-B, 10 μm; E, 1 μm. For a high resolution image of Fig. 3 please see Additional file 14

position along the neuroepithelium where these primary cilia became evident again was variable among different cells, but most frequently we first detected the cilium in the central region of the neuroepithelium (i.e.,: halfway in the retraction process; Fig. 3c). The time of appearance of the primary cilium relative to the initiation of apical process retraction was also highly variable, although in most cases it happened within the following 1.5 h (Fig. 3d). Given the possibility that resolution constraints of our time-lapse experiments could hinder the visualization of cilia at early stages of retraction, we also analyzed the process by TEM. Cilia, both with and without a ciliary pocket, were observed on retracting apical processes either in close proximity to the apical surface of the neuroepithelium or in more basal positions, always pointing towards the apical surface (Fig. 3e). Importantly, this analysis allowed us to confirm the presence of apically localized primary cilia in retracting processes and showed that, at least in some cells, a primary cilium is present during the early stages of apical retraction. A summary of the behavior of all cells analyzed by time-lapse microscopy is shown in Fig. 4.

## Characterization of cilia in differentiating RGCs

Towards the end of the apical process retraction, the differentiating RGC cell bodies have reached a basal position in the neuroepithelium. Once there, they generate an axon that grows adjacent to the basal lamina towards the optic nerve exit and dendritogenesis starts at the apical pole of these neuroblasts [8]. Early neuroblasts and RGCs express the surface adhesion protein Neurolin/DM-Grasp (labeled by the monoclonal antibodies zn5 or zn8), which can be used as a cell-type specific marker [40]. Arl13b-GFP embryos, fixed and labeled with either of these antibodies at 35 hpf, showed neuroblasts in the final stages of retraction with prominent cilia in an apical position (Fig. 5a). Cilia in similar positions were also observed in TEM micrographs (Fig. 5b). We further analyzed cilia dynamics at these later stages of neuronal differentiation in transplanted embryos using time-lapse confocal microscopy. We found that the primary cilium usually remained visible after apical retraction was completed, but it disappeared at least transiently during the initial steps of filopodial activity that leads to dendritogenesis (Fig. 5c, d; Movie in Additional file 4; Fig. 4, denoted as Δ) [41]. Only two cells showed a primary

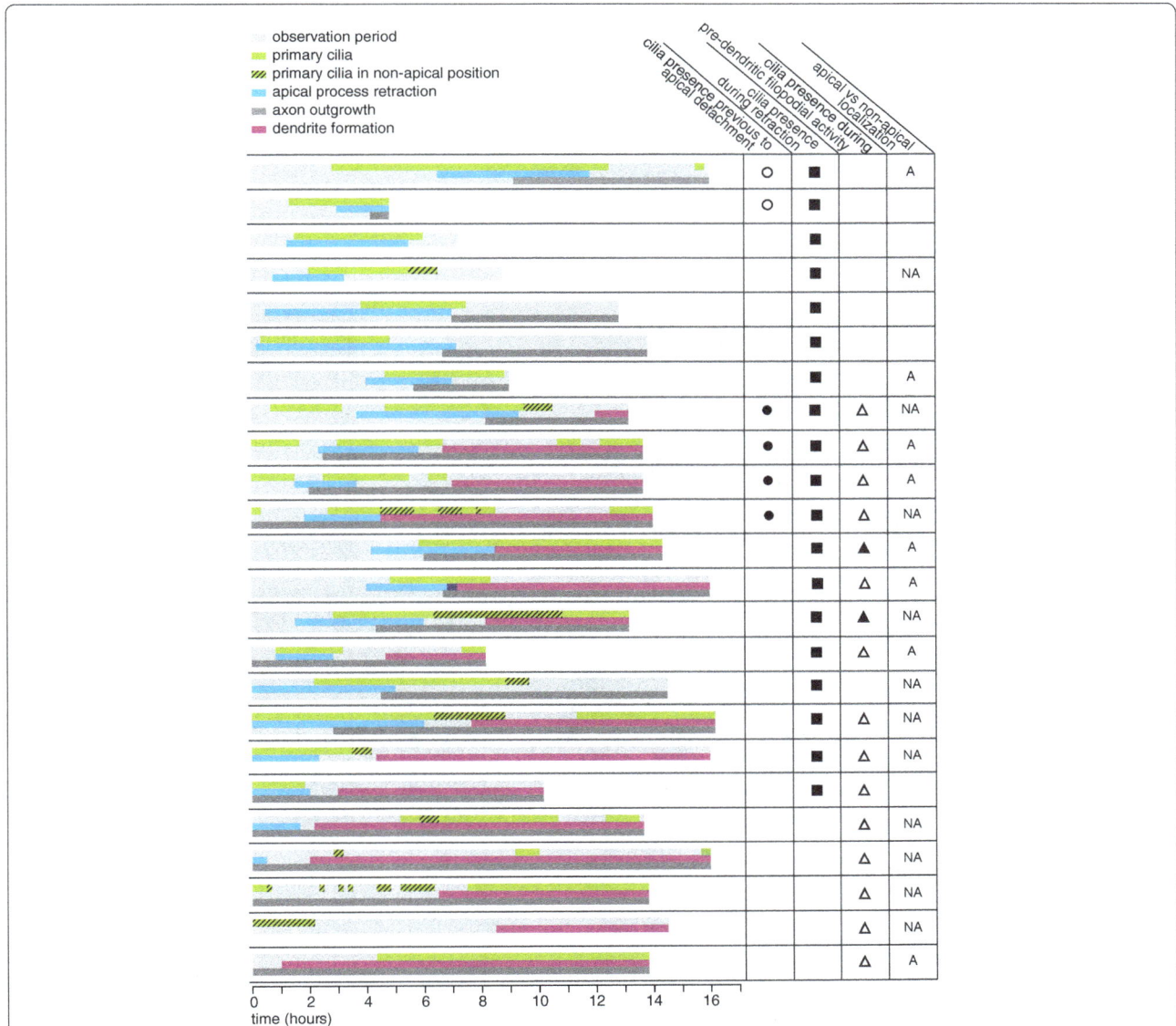

**Fig. 4** Primary cilia dynamics in relation to RGC differentiation events. Schematic representation and summary of the observations made in the time-lapse experiments. A single cell is represented in each row. For each cell, the presence of its primary cilium (*green*) is plotted in relation to the different events during RGC differentiation: apical process retraction (*cyan*), axon outgrowth (*dark grey*) and dendrite formation (*magenta*). The cells that show similar behaviors are indicated in the different columns: cells that show a primary cilium before apical detachment (●: cilium disappears previous to detachment; ○: cilium remains visible and moves basally previous to detachment); cells that show a primary cilium during the retraction of the apical process (■); cells that continuously show a primary cilium through the period from apical retraction to pre-dendritic filopodial activity/dendritogenesis (▲), and those in which the cilium disappears at least for a short time during this period (△). The dashed regions in the diagrams indicate the time interval in which the primary cilium was localized to non-apical positions. Cells that showed this behavior are indicated as "NA", and those in which the primary cilium remained apical after the retraction of the apical process are indicated as "A". A total of 24 cells from 14 embryos in 12 different experiments were analyzed. For a high resolution image of Fig. 4 please see Additional file 15

cilium throughout apical retraction and until the initiation of dendrite outgrowth (Fig. 4, denoted as ▲).

If we consider only those cells that showed a primary cilium after completion of apical process retraction and/or during the initial steps of dendrite formation, the primary cilium remained in the apical side of the cell during the imaging period in half of them (Fig. 4, denoted as "A"). Surprisingly, in the other half, primary cilia transiently lost their apical localization, occupying apparently random positions around the cell body, and rapidly moving from one position to another (Fig. 5e; Movie in Additional file 5; Fig. 4, denoted as "NA"). In TEM studies of 35 hpf embryos, fully formed cilia were rarely found in basally localized neuroblasts without an apical

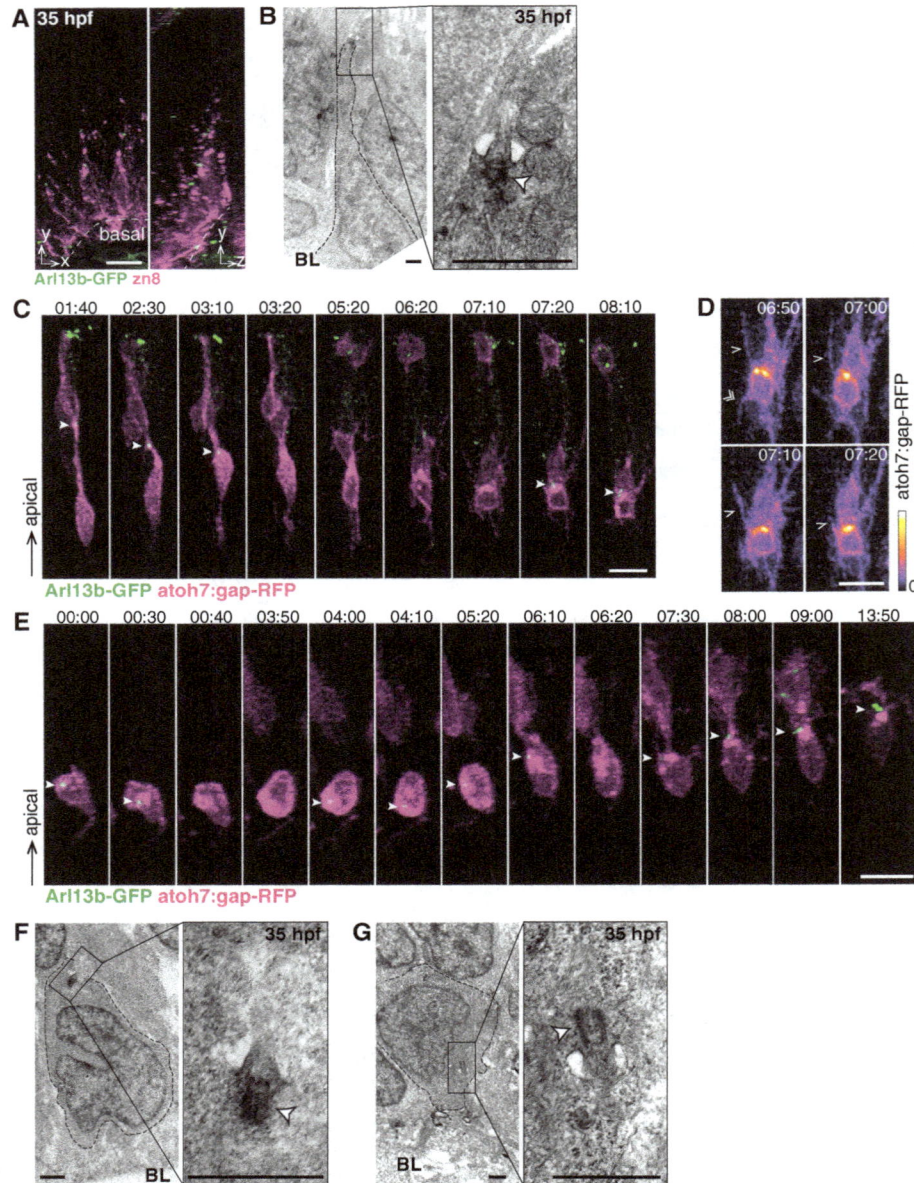

**Fig. 5** Upon completion of apical retraction, primary cilia may transiently disappear or lose their apical localization. **a** 3D maximum intensity projections of a region of the retina of a 35 hpf transgenic embryo expressing Arl13b-GFP and immunolabaled with zn8 antibody to identify RGCs. Primary cilia are observed colocalizing with the apical tip of cells finishing retraction. **b** TEM micrograph from a 35 hpf embryo showing a primary cilium at the tip of an apical process. The white arrowhead indicates the basal body. **c-e** Blastomeres from transgenic embryos (atoh7:gap-RFP/Arl13b-GFP) were transplanted into wild type hosts. The resulting embryos were imaged by time-lapse confocal microscopy from around 30 hpf onwards. Montages from 3D maximum intensity projections of the stacks are shown. (**d**) Detail of the cell shown in (**c**), where initial filopodial activity (*arrowheads*) previous to dendrite formation is observed; in order to highlight atoh7:gap-RFP signal intensity, a color ramp is used. The full white arrowheads indicate the presence and position of the primary cilium in **c** and **e**. **f-g** TEM micrographs from 35 hpf embryos, showing cells located in the basal region of the neuroepithelium (RGC neuroblasts) with primary cilia both in apical (**f**) and basal (**g**) positions. The white arrowhead indicates the basal body. BL: basal lamina. Scale bars: A, 10 μm; B, 1 μm; C-E, 10 μm; F-G, 1 μm. For a high resolution image of Fig. 5 please see Additional file 16

process. However, short cilia were eventually visualized, which exhibited different localizations and orientations around the cell (Fig. 5f and g). Interestingly, our time-lapse experiments showed that in cells bearing a primary cilium at the onset of dendritogenesis, the cilium was invariably localized to the base of the protrusion that finally branched to form the dendrites. This was the case even when cilia moved around the cell body before eventually reaching that position (Fig. 5e, Movie in Additional file 5).

By 48 hpf, all the RGCs in the central part of the retina have been born, their axons have exited the retina, and the synaptic connections have begun to form in the inner plexiform layer [42]. When we imaged Arl13b-GFP embryos fixed at 48 hpf, we were able to detect only a few primary cilia in the ganglion cell layer (Fig. 6a). A similar situation was observed at 5 days post fertilization (dpf) (Fig. 6b). After thorough TEM analysis of retinas from 48 hpf embryos, we observed a relatively small proportion of membrane-associated centrosomes in the ganglion cell layer (92/405, 22.7 %), of which nearly half (44/92, 48 %) did not nucleate visible axonemes, albeit they localized next to an electron-dense region of the plasma membrane (Fig. 6c and f). The rest of the centrosomes were acting as basal bodies of primary cilia of variable length. We found evident axonemes in only 19.5 % of the cases (18/92; Fig. 6d and f), and invariably, these cilia were positioned at the base of the RGC dendritic tree, where most were pointing basally. In 14 % of the cases (13/92) we could observe short cilia associated with basal bodies (Fig. 6e and f). These cilia presented dilated tips containing a granular, irregular material and without a visible axoneme or microtubules, although their proximal region appeared normal. The rest of the membrane-associated centrioles nucleated axonemes that could not be completely visualized in the section, and hence, of undefined length (17/92, 18.5 %) (Fig. 6f).

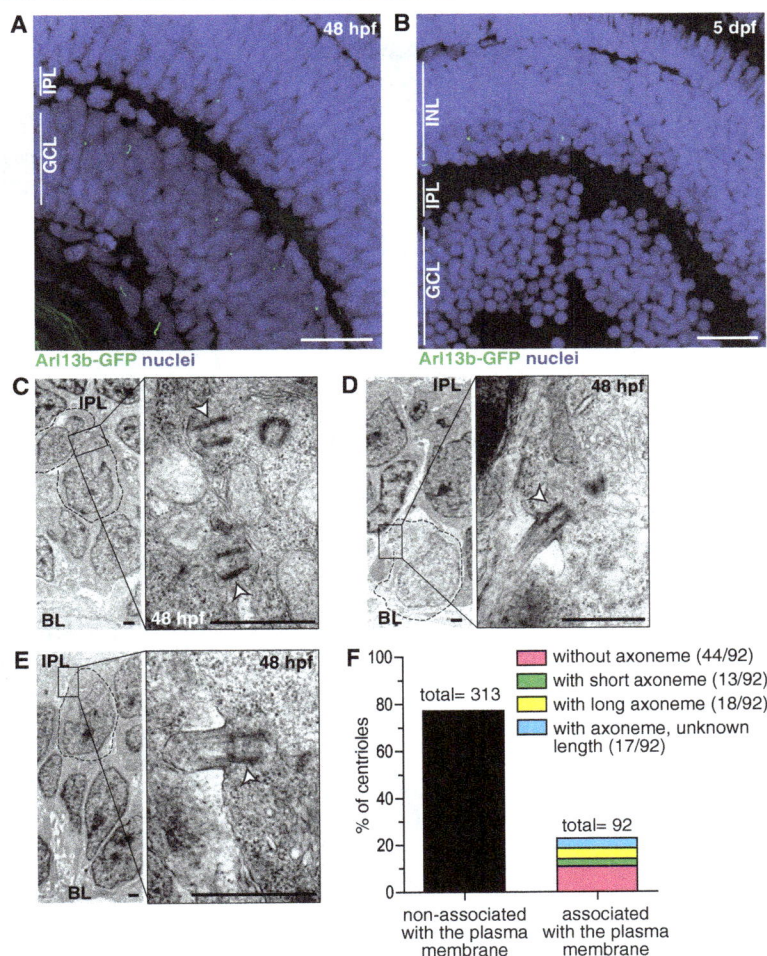

**Fig. 6** Primary cilia in maturing RGCs. **a-b** Arl13b-GFP transgenic embryos were fixed and imaged through confocal microscopy as whole-mounts (**a**, 48 hpf) or as cryosections (**b**, 5 dpf). Images shown are maximum intensity Z-projections of 1.5 μm (**a**) and 15 μm (**b**) confocal microscopy stacks. **c-e** TEM micrographs from retinas of 48 hpf embryos. In most of the cases we observed membrane-docked basal bodies without visible axonemes (**c**). Some cells showed basal bodies associated to long axonemes (**d**) or short axonemes with dilated tips (**e**). The white arrowhead indicates the basal body. **f** Comparison between the number of plasma membrane-associated and non-associated centrioles/centrosomes in the RGC layer of 48 hpf embryos (a total of 6 embryos were used in the quantification). The former were further classified in subtypes illustrated in the micrographs C, D and E. GCL: ganglion cell layer; IPL: inner plexiform layer; INL: inner nuclear layer; BL: basal lamina. Scale bars: A-B, 20 μm; C-E, 1 μm. For a high resolution image of Fig. 6 please see Additional file 17

## Cilia dysfunction leads to early retinal differentiation defects

To evaluate the possible function of primary cilia during the early stages of retinal development and RGC differentiation, we tested different previously described morpholino oligomers (MOs), targeting ciliary-specific genes and known to generate typical ciliary phenotypes. A translation-blocking MO to *ift88* [28] was able to generate a recognizable but relatively weak ciliary phenotype at low doses (3 ng/embryo) in the genetic background of

our fish lines. At slightly higher doses (4 ng/embryo), however, it caused generalized embryo mortality and severe defects that were not reverted by p53 MO co-injection (Fig. 7a). Another translation-blocking MO, in this case against *elipsa* [27], was not able to generate a marked ciliary phenotype, even at extremely high doses, such as 20 ng/embryo (Fig. 7b). Hence, we decided to design two splice-blocking MOs directed against these two genes (*ift88*-SP and *elipsa*-SP), with the intention of allowing the embryos to develop normally until

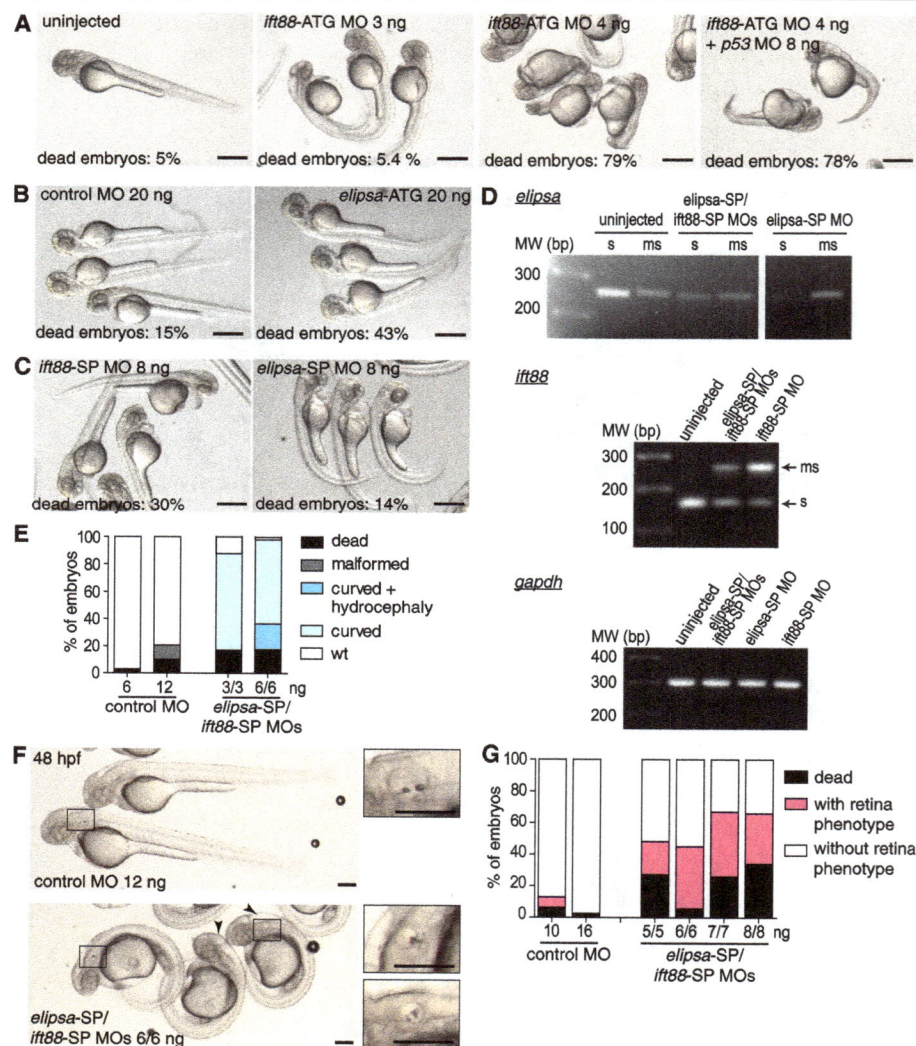

**Fig. 7** Evaluation of different morpholino oligomers for *elipsa* and *ift88* knock-down. **a-c** External phenotype of 48 hpf embryos injected with different morpholinos targeting the ciliary proteins *ift88* and *elipsa*; translational-blocking morpholinos: *ift88*-ATG MO (**a**), *elipsa*-ATG MO (**b**); splice-blocking morpholinos: *ift88*-SP or *elipsa*-SP (**c**). **d** RT-PCR analysis of *elipsa* and *ift88* mRNA levels in 35 hpf embryos either injected with *ift88*-SP (6 ng) or *elipsa*-SP (6 ng) alone or as a combination (6 ng each) ("s": spliced mRNA form; "ms": mis-spliced mRNA form). *Gapdh* mRNA was used as a control. **e** Evaluation of the external phenotype of 48 hpf embryos injected with different amounts of the combination of splice-blocking morpholinos (*elipsa*-SP/*ift88*-SP MOs), where "malformed" refers to morphological alterations not compatible with a classic "ciliary phenotype". **f** Main characteristics of the external phenotype of double morphants at the dose used in the rest of the study. The black rectangle marks the position of the otic vesicle in the low magnification images, magnified in the insets. The arrowheads indicate embryos with enlarged brain ventricles. **g** Quantification of the percentage of atoh7:gap-GFP embryos injected with different amounts of control MO or *elipsa*-SP/*ift88*-SP MOs displaying reduced size of the RGC layer ("retina phenotype"), at 48 hpf. Scale bars: A-C, 500 μm; F, 200 μm. For a high resolution image of Fig. 7 please see Additional file 18

gastrulation. Although the *ift88*-SP MO caused less embryo mortality or cell death than the translation-blocking one, even at 8 ng/embryo, phenotypes appeared too weak or absent (Fig. 7c). The *elipsa*-SP MO, on the other hand, produced very little embryo death and a recognizable ciliary phenotype, which was nevertheless still relatively weak (Fig. 7c). In spite of these results, both MOs were able to generate significant amounts of mis-spliced RNAs at the tested doses (6 ng each, Fig. 7d). Finally, a combination of these two splice-blocking MOs, at lower doses each, allowed us to obtain robust and reproducible ciliary phenotypes, with relatively little embryo or cell death (Fig. 7e). At 48 hpf, these double morphants (6 ng of each MO) displayed a ventrally-curved body and, in some cases, enlarged brain ventricles and abnormal otolith number (arrows and insets in Fig. 7f). This phenotype was reproduced in atoh7:gap-GFP transgenic embryos, where we observed an important reduction on the extent of the RGC layer at 48 hpf when compared to controls. We used this phenotypic

feature to assay the ideal MO working doses for further experiments, confirming that a combination of 6/6 ng of the *elipsa*-SP/*ift88*-SP MOs gave the highest proportion of embryos with phenotype, while maintaining low levels of embryo death (Fig. 7g).

To further confirm the effectiveness of this MO combination, we examined cilia in different ciliated organs (neural tube, otic vesicle, pronephros and nasal pit) and, in all cases, found them to be reduced in number as well as shorter and more disorganized in morphant embryos in comparison to control embryos (Fig. 8a). We also quantified cilia length in the Kupffer's vesicle at the eight-somite stage (around 12 hpf), observing a significant shortening of these organelles in morphant embryos (Fig. 8b and c). Finally, by using TEM, we evaluated the effect of the MOs in the differentiating neural retina, where we observed a significant reduction in apical primary cilia length (Fig. 8d). Overall, our results show that using a combination of *elipsa*-SP/*ift88*-SP MOs resulted in defective cilia formation and/or

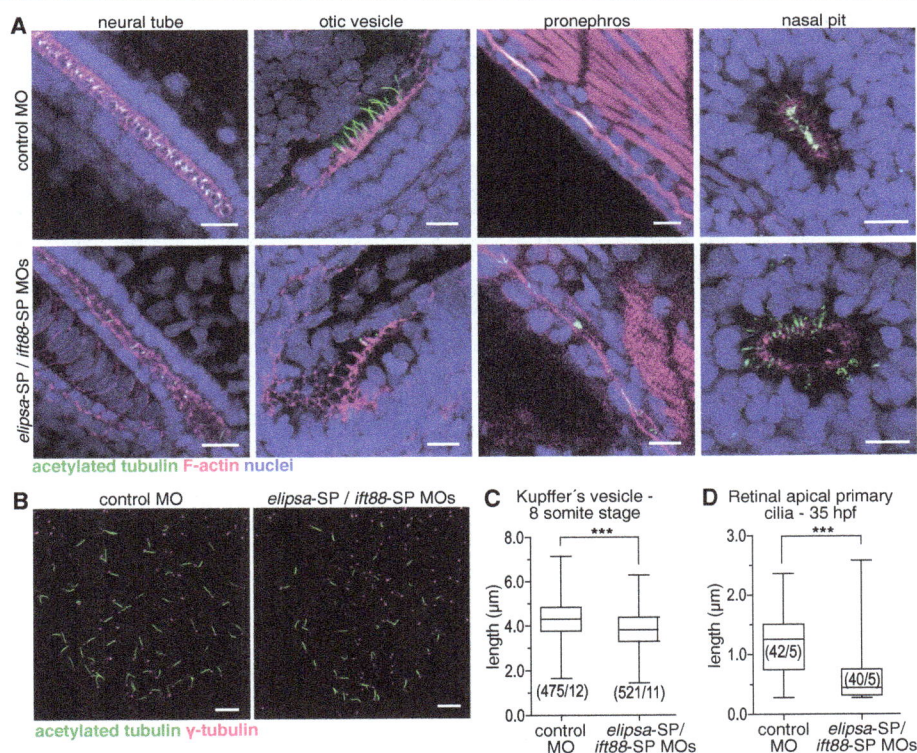

**Fig. 8** Effective reduction of primary cilia length in zebrafish embryos upon *elipsa* and *ift88* knock-down. **a** Confocal images of different ciliated organs from 48 hpf embryos. Cilia were labeled with an anti-acetylated tubulin antibody and F-actin with TRITC-phalloidin. **b** Kupffer's vesicle of eight-somite stage embryos, where basal bodies were labeled with an anti-γ-tubulin antibody. **c** Comparison of primary ciliary length in Kupffer's vesicle. The experiments were performed twice, with similar results; only the results from one of the experiments are shown. **d** Comparison of the length of apical primary cilia in the retina of 35 hpf morphant and control embryos. Measurements were made on TEM micrographs. In C and D the numbers in brackets represent the number of cilia and embryos analyzed in each condition. (\*\*\*) $p < 0.001$, Mann–Whitney test. Scale bars: A-B, 10 μm. For a high resolution image of Fig. 8 please see Additional file 19

maintenance that led to well-established cilia-associated phenotypes while minimizing undesired effects, such as generalized cell death or gross developmental defects.

To further determine if primary cilia defects have an effect in early differentiation or organization of the retina, we injected wild type embryos with our combination of *elipsa*-SP/*ift88*-SP MOs, fixed them at 48 and 60 hpf and performed whole-mount immunofluorescence to analyze the retinal ganglion cell layer (using zn8 antibody) through confocal microscopy. As morphant embryos showed a notorious reduction in total eye size compared to controls (Fig. 9a), we quantified the volume of neural retinas on confocal stacks of 48 hpf embryos in both conditions. Double morphants showed a 38.4 % reduction in retinal volume when compared to controls (mean decrease from two independent experiments: 34.6 and 42.1 %; Fig. 9b). At this stage, and consistent with observations at low magnification described above, there was a pronounced reduction in the volume covered by zn8-positive RGCs: the ganglion cell layer appeared smaller and the optic nerve thinner in morphants compared to control embryos (Fig. 9a). We measured the volume spanned by the zn8 stain, excluding the extra-retinal tissues and the optic nerve. We observed a 95.4 % reduction in the volume of the zn8-positive retina in morphant embryos compared to controls (mean decrease from two independent experiments: 93.7 and 97.1 %; Fig. 9c). When we analyzed 60 hpf embryos we found that the RGCs had formed a complete layer (Fig. 9a). However, morphant embryos again showed a 26.8 % decrease in total retinal volume (mean decrease from two independent experiments: 18.7 and 35 %; Fig. 9d) and a 40.4 % reduction in zn8-positive retina compared to controls (mean decrease from two independent experiments: 32.6 and 48.1 %; Fig. 9e).

In order to ascertain if these observed early defects in RGC layer formation were due to a cell-autonomous effect of cilia reduction in RGC progenitors or neuroblasts,

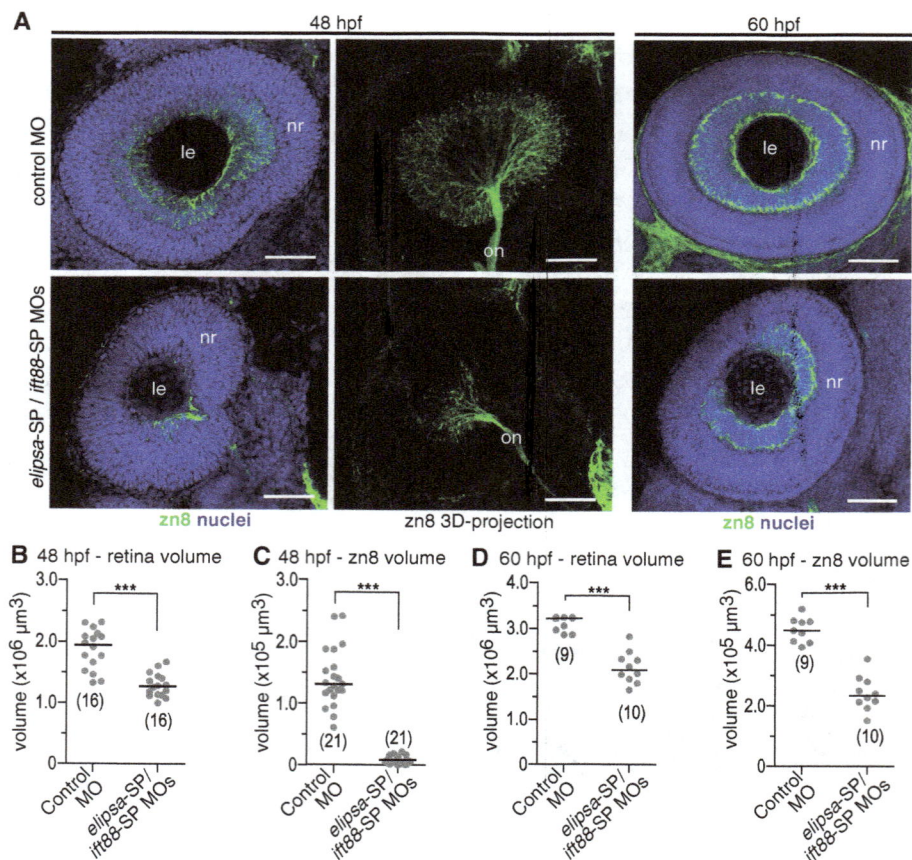

**Fig. 9** Embryos with impaired cilia have smaller eyes and a reduced RGC layer. **a** Confocal images of 48 hpf and 60 hpf retinas from embryos injected with control morpholino or *elipsa*-SP/*ift88*-SP MOs. RGCs were labeled with zn8 antibody. **b** and **d** Comparison of retinal volumes in 48 hpf (**b**) and 60 hpf (**d**) embryos. **c** and **e** Comparison of RGC layer volume (based on zn8 stain) in 48 hpf (**c**) and 60 hpf (**e**) embryos. The numbers in brackets represent the number of embryos quantified in each case (we quantified one eye per embryo). (***) $p < 0.001$. Comparisons were made using rank transformation and Student's *t* test. nr: neural retina; le: lens; on: optic nerve. Scale bars: A, 50 μm. For a high resolution image of Fig. 9 please see Additional file 20

instead of an indirect effect caused by a perturbed retinal environment, we performed blastomere transplantation experiments between atoh7:gap-RFP embryos, either injected with control or *elipsa*-SP/*ift88*-SP MOs, and atoh7:gap-GFP untreated embryos, followed by in vivo time-lapse observation (Fig. 10a and b; Movies in Additional files 6, 7 and 8). In 5/5 embryos observed, control MO-treated RFP-positive cells were able to differentiate apparently normally in the untreated atoh7:gap-GFP retina, dividing and

differentiating into RGCs or other cell types in the same way and timing as the surrounding GFP-positive cells (Fig. 10a; Movie in Additional files 6 and 7). After several attempts of transplanting double morphant (6/6 ng of each MO) cells into untreated embryos, we failed to detect transplanted cells expressing atoh7:gap-RFP in the retina by 32 hpf. As this could be due to a reduced capacity of the cilia-impaired cells to compete in the wild-type environment, we lowered the MO dose to 5 ng each. Under

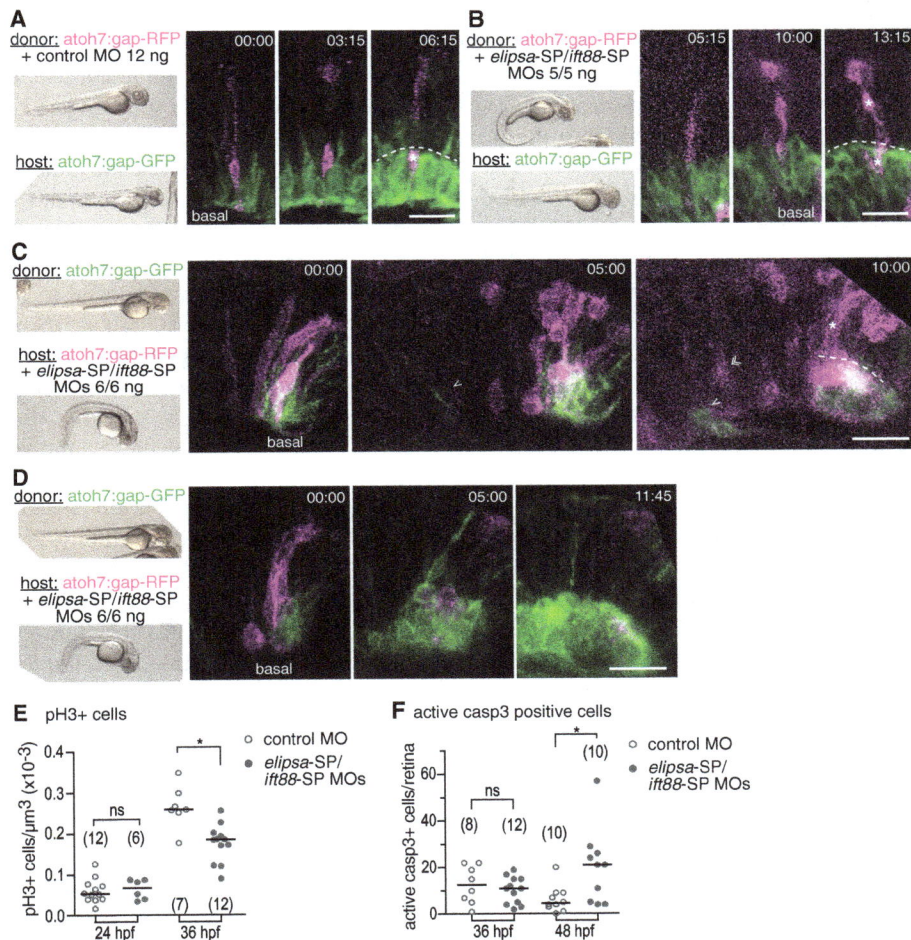

**Fig. 10** Cell-autonomous effect of cilia reduction on RGC differentiation. **a-b** Blastomeres from atoh7:gap-RFP embryos injected with control MO (12 ng) (**a**) or *elipsa*-SP/*ift88*-SP MOs (5/5 ng) (**b**) were transplanted into atoh7:gap-GFP hosts. The dotted line indicates de apical margin of the RGC layer of the host and the asterisk denotes the donor cells with high RFP expression. **c-d** Blastomeres from un-injected atoh7:gap-GFP embryos were transplanted into atoh7:gap-RFP hosts injected with *elipsa*-SP/*ift88*-SP MOs (6/6 ng). Retinas with small (**c**) and large (**d**) clones of GFP positive cells were observed. In C the dotted line indicates de apical margin of the RGC layer formed by the donor GFP positive cells, and the asterisk denotes host cells with high RFP expression. Single arrowheads mark GFP expressing cells that appear before RFP expressing cells (*double arrowheads*). In all the cases (**a-d**) the resulting host embryos were imaged by time-lapse confocal microscopy beginning at around 30 hpf. Fluorescence images show montages from 3D maximum intensity projections of the stacks from three different time points. On the left, the external phenotype at 48 hpf of the donor and host embryos is shown in each case. Time is expressed in hrs:min. Scale bars: A-D, 20 μm. **e** Comparison of the number of mitotic cells (identified by anti-pHistone H3 labeling) in the ventro-nasal region of 24 and 36 hpf retinas, expressed as the number of positive cells per unit of volume. (*) $p = 0.0014$. **f** Comparison of the number of apoptotic cells (identified by anti-activated Caspase 3 labeling) per retina in 36 and 48 hpf embryos. (*) $p = 0.009$. All experiments were performed twice, with similar results; only the results from one of the experiments are shown. The numbers in brackets represent the number of embryos quantified in each case (we quantified one eye per embryo). (ns) non-significant difference. Comparisons were made using rank transformation and Student's t test. For a high resolution image of Fig. 10 please see Additional file 21

these conditions, we could detect few embryos in which small clones (1–3 cells) of atoh7:gap-RFP cells appeared in the atoh7:gap-GFP wild-type retina. In 3/5 of the in vivo imaged embryos, the observed gap-RFP-positive cells behaved in an apparently normal way when compared to the surrounding gap-GFP cells, while in 2/5 cases, three clones included some cells that appeared either delayed in differentiation or remaining in the outer retinal layers, in spite of expressing a relatively high level of gap-RFP (asterisk, Fig. 10b; Movie in Additional file 8). We then performed the converse transplantation experiment, from untreated atoh7:gap-GFP embryos into elipsa-SP/ift88-SP morphant atoh7:gap-RFP embryos. Here, transplantation was more efficient, and two types of behavior could be observed in the transplanted cells. In 4/7 cases, small clones of GFP-positive cells were able to quickly differentiate into RGCs, inserting in the RGC layer and extending an axon, in most cases ahead of the surrounding morphant RFP-positive cells (Fig. 10c; Movie in Additional file 9). In 2/7 cases, however, large clones expressing GFP rapidly proliferated and started to differentiate as RGCs, while very few RFP-positive host cells could be detected (Fig. 10d; Movie in Additional file 10).

We reasoned that the decrease in retina and ganglion cell layer volume, like the apparent delay in RGC differentiation, could be due either to reduced cell proliferation, to increased cell death, or a combination of both. To discriminate between these possibilities we performed whole-mount immunofluorescence against phosphorylated Histone H3 (pH3), present in mitotic cells from late prophase to the end of telophase, and for activated Caspase 3, indicative of early stages of apoptosis. We then quantified pH3 positive cells in the ventro-nasal region of the retina and the total number of activated Caspase 3-positive cells per eye, in embryos of different developmental stages. Regarding cell proliferation, while we did not observe differences at 24 hpf, our results showed a significant decrease in mitotic index in morphant embryos at 36 hpf (Fig. 10e). In the case of cell death, we observed an increase in apoptotic nuclei at 48 hpf while not at an earlier stage (36 hpf; Fig. 10f).

Altogether, these results suggest that the integrity of primary cilia is essential at the progenitor cell level, and therefore other retinal cell types might also be affected. To evaluate this possibility, we used the triple transgenic zebrafish line SoFa1, which allows for the individualization of the different retinal cell types through the expression of atoh7:gap-RFP (RGCs, amacrine cells, horizontal cells and cone photoreceptors), ptf1a:cytGFP (amacrine and horizontal cells), crx:gap-CFP (cone photoreceptors and bipolar cells) [26]. We injected these embryos with control morpholino or elipsa-SP/ift88-SP MOs and analyzed them using in vivo time-lapse microscopy. We observed a general decrease in the signal in morphant

embryos in comparison to controls, consistent with reduced progenitor cell proliferation (Fig. 11a). We also analyzed the fluorescence profile for each channel along a rectangular selection perpendicular to the plane of the retina (Fig. 11a; Movie in Additional file 11). In control embryos, RGCs (labeled by gap-RFP alone) were the first cells to become evident, closely followed in time by cone photoreceptors (gap-RFP / gap-CFP) and amacrine cells (cytGFP / gap-RFP). By the end of the time-lapse acquisition (around 48 hpf) horizontal cells (cytGFP / gap-RFP) and bipolar cells (gap-CFP) started to become evident. In morphant embryos injected with elipsa-SP/ift88-SP MOs, the gap-RFP signal corresponding to RGCs was more evenly distributed along the retina and was usually defined later than the peaks corresponding to the other cell types (Movie in Additional file 11). To quantify this observation, we determined the relative contribution of each cell type to the total signal in the last frame of these movies and in fixed 48 hpf morphant embryos (Fig. 11a, b and c). Interestingly, the proportion of gap-RFP signal corresponding to RGCs was significantly reduced in morphant embryos in comparison to controls, with a concomitant increase in the signal corresponding to photoreceptors but not amacrine cells. A similar comparison made on gap-CFP-positive cells also showed a slight, albeit significant, increase of cone photoreceptors relative to bipolar cells (cells that are born late, and hence probably more affected by the general cell differentiation delay at 48 hpf).

To further confirm the possibility that RGC generation and/or differentiation is preferentially reduced after primary cilia impairment, we analyzed the extension of the inner plexiform layer (IPL) through whole-mount staining with TRITC-conjugated phalloidin (Fig. 11d). Embryos injected with control morpholino and fixed at 48 hpf presented a thin IPL layer only in the ventro-nasal region of the retina, while at 60 hpf the IPL was thicker and extended throughout the whole neural retina. Embryos injected with elipsa-SP/ift88-SP MOs and fixed at 48 hpf had a smaller patch of IPL restricted to the region adjacent to the optic nerve exit, where the first RGCs differentiate (Fig. 11d, arrowhead). At 60 hpf, the IPL of morphant embryos had extended throughout the retina, but appeared thinner and more disorganized than in control embryos (Fig. 11d, insets).

## Discussion

### Dynamic apical cilia in the early neurogenic retinal neuroepithelium

Pioneering electron microscopy studies showed, many decades ago, the presence and apparent dynamics of primary cilia in the undifferentiated and differentiating neuroepithelium, both in the neural tube and the retina [19, 20]. In recent years, the finding that primary cilia act as cellular "antennae" has renewed the interest of

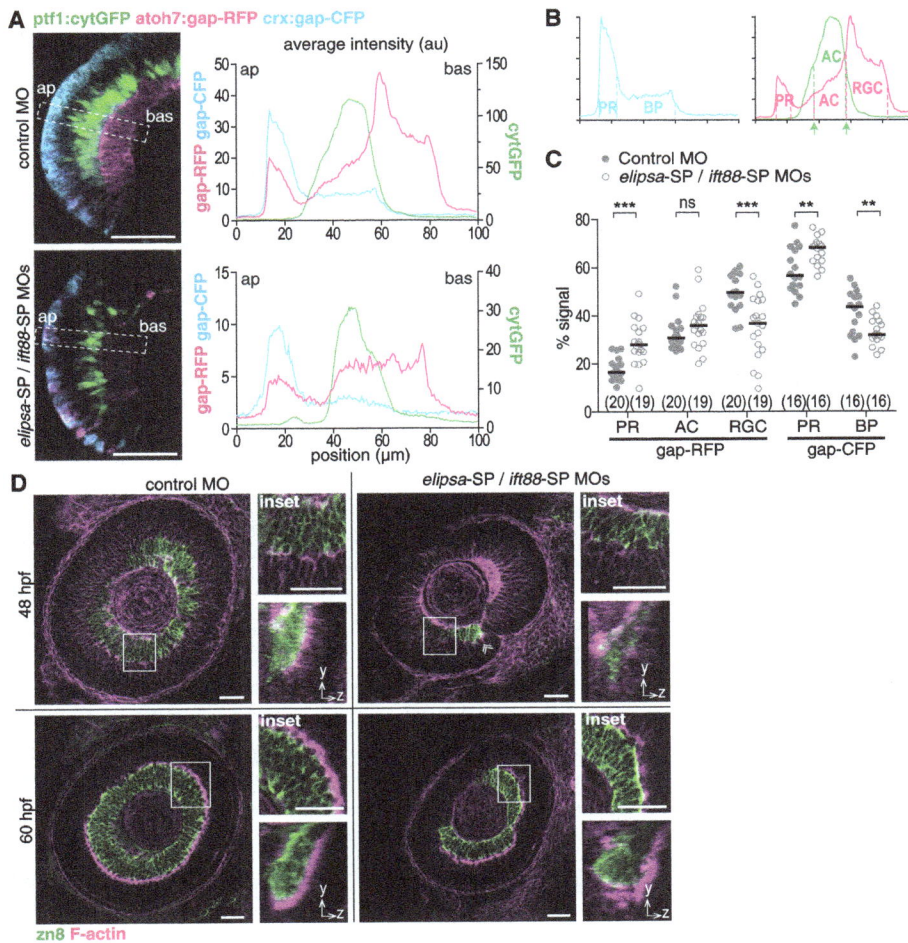

**Fig. 11** Cilia impaired embryos show a preferential delay in RGCs formation. **a** Left: average intensity Z-projections of 10 μm-thick confocal stacks of the nasal region of retinas from 48 hpf SoFa1 embryos injected with control MO or *elipsa*-SP/*ift88*-SP MOs. The dotted line delimits the area used to measure the fluorescence intensity profile from apical to basal, plotted in the right side for each image. ap: apical; bas: basal; au: arbitrary units. **b** Diagram indicating the regions in the SoFa1 retina fluorescence profile plots that were selected to determine the relative contribution of each cell type to the total signal in RFP and CFP channels (the GFP signal was only used to determine the extension spanned by amacrine cells in the RFP channel). The boundaries of each region were set at the distance corresponding to 50 % of the maximum fluorescence for each peak. **c** Plot of the percentage of signal intensity in the gap-RFP and gap-CFP channels corresponding to each cell type in embryos injected with control MO or *elipsa*-SP/*ift88*-SP MOs. The number of embryos analyzed in each case is shown in brackets. (***) $p < 0.001$, (**) $p < 0.01$, ns: non-significant difference. Comparisons were made using rank transformation and Student's *t* test. PR: photoreceptors; AC: amacrine cells; RGC: retinal ganglion cells; BP: bipolar cells. **d** Confocal images of retinas from wild-type embryos injected with control MO or *elipsa*-SP/*ift88*-SP MOs and fixed at 48 and 60 hpf. The boxed regions are magnified in the upper insets, while lower images are orthogonal 3D projections of these insets. The white arrowhead indicates a patch of IPL in the region adjacent to the optic nerve exit. Scale bars: A, 50 μm; D, 30 μm. For a high resolution image of Fig. 11 please see Additional file 22

developmental neurobiologists in understanding the possible roles of these organelles in neurogenesis and neuronal differentiation. Here, we sought to characterize the behavior and possible functions of primary cilia in these processes, starting by assessing their presence and localization in the embryonic zebrafish retina before and around the initial stages of neurogenesis. It must be noted that because of the morphological features of primary cilia, particularly their small size and the fact that there is only one per cell, added to their functional properties (cilia are constantly disassembled and reassembled along the cell cycle), it is simply not possible to assure that a cell that does not display a detectable cilium is actually a non-ciliated cell. We observed the presence of numerous primary cilia in the early retina, both before and shortly after the onset of neurogenesis, indicating that probably most retinal neuroepithelial cells are ciliated. These cilia mostly localized apically, and were pointing towards the sub-retinal space. In addition, most of them presented a deep ciliary pocket, a structure that has been documented in different cell types both in vitro and in vivo (reviewed in [43]). Some early studies suggested a link between the ciliary pocket and different stages of ciliation, as well as the possibility of different pathways in cilia formation. More recently however, it has been shown that the ciliary pocket is a site of active endocytosis [44, 45]. Interestingly, its presence, size and morphology were extremely variable among retinal neuroepithelial cells, which may therefore suggest differences in their cellular activity.

The accumulation of centrosomes at the apical side of different neuroepithelia has been extensively documented, and even used as a cell polarity marker [39, 46]. In the present work, we observed that many of these apical centrosomes are actually primary cilia basal bodies. However, we also found a few cases of apically localized centrosomes that were not nucleating an axoneme (although they usually appeared docked at the plasma membrane), as well as short primary cilia inside cytoplasmic vesicles. These possibly represented different stages of cilia formation [47], even though we cannot distinguish if these cells are cycling progenitors or neuroblasts. Our in vivo experiments showed that both situations are possible: while there is a cilia cycle related to the cell cycle (i.e.,: in progenitor cells), cilia in postmitotic neuroblasts may also be highly dynamic. We found that neuroepithelial cells committed to exit the cell cycle (evidenced by the expression of atoh7:gap-RFP), presented a primary cilium until a short time before mitosis. Accordingly, studies in chick neural tube have shown that primary cilia are lost during mid-G2 in order for the centrosome to engage in mitosis [48]. Regarding postmitotic cells, our in vivo experiments interestingly showed that some of these cells had visible primary cilia while still attached to the apical border, although these organelles were transiently lost in many cells around the period of detachment (see below).

We also found primary cilia that, albeit being localized to the apical region of neuroepithelial cells, emerged from a basal position with respect to adherens junctions. These cilia may be translocated or re-formed at the basolateral surface and the cilia that were observed inside cytoplasmic vesicles may correspond to intermediate stages of any of these processes. This observation is highly reminiscent of that reported in the mouse cortex where cells committed to delamination in the embryonic telencephalon present basolaterally localized primary cilia, the proportion of which increases at the onset of neurogenesis [39]. In the zebrafish retina, we found the proportion of basolateral primary cilia to be the same at 26 and 35 hpf (stages before and after neurogenesis initiation, respectively), whereas ciliary length showed a decrease at the latter stage. Thus, cilia shortening might present a stronger correlation with neurogenesis in the zebrafish retina than basolateral cilia localization.

## Cilia dynamics in differentiating RGCs

Our findings on the presence and dynamics of primary cilia in early stages of RGC differentiation are summarized in Fig. 12. In the zebrafish, recently born RGC neuroblasts undergo a transition from a neuroepithelial into a neuronal type of polarity. It was shown that these neuroblasts must detach their apical process from apical N-Cadherin-based adhesions, and that during the initial stages of retraction, different apical markers remain accumulated at the tip of the apical process [8, 49]. This includes the centrosome, which was observed to remain apical during apical process retraction and until after axon outgrowth. The centrosome acts in many cases as a basal body to a primary cilium. In chick and mouse spinal cord neuroblasts it was shown that the cilium, along with some other apical components, is shed from the tip of the apical process during detachment, while the centrosome remains in the retracting apical process [50]. On the other hand, Spear and colleagues, also studying the chick neural tube, have reported that neuroblasts undergoing delamination maintain their apical primary cilium [48]. Our in vivo studies using the same cilia marker as these two previous studies (Arl13b-GFP) showed that even if most RGC neuroblasts lack a visible primary cilium around the moment of apical detachment, in some cells the primary cilium accompanied the retraction of the apical process from the beginning. Probably due to our imaging conditions, we failed to visualize cilia from neuroblasts remaining at the apical border upon detachment. Hence, we cannot rule out the possibility that there is apical shedding during zebrafish RGC apical retraction, and our data suggest that even if either shedding or resorption of primary cilia may occur, they are not an absolute prerequisite for delamination.

The appearance of the primary cilium during apical process retraction was highly variable both in time and position across the neuroepithelium, as was the period it remained visible (see Fig. 4). However, in all cells, the cilium remained apical throughout retraction, in accordance to previous work that reported an apically localized centrosome in RGCs all through retraction [8] and at the initial stages of dendrite formation [2]. Consistently, apically-localized primary cilia in differentiating RGCs had also been reported in early electron microscopy studies of the mouse retina [20]. Surprisingly, however, we also observed a highly dynamic primary cilium regarding localization around the cell body surface, from the end of retraction to just before the initiation of dendrite formation. These movements are fast (can be observed in 10 min intervals), and might be related to the necessary cellular rearrangements that occur during the period between axon and dendrite formation. Interestingly, these movements ceased at the onset of dendritogenesis, with the primary cilium localizing to the base of

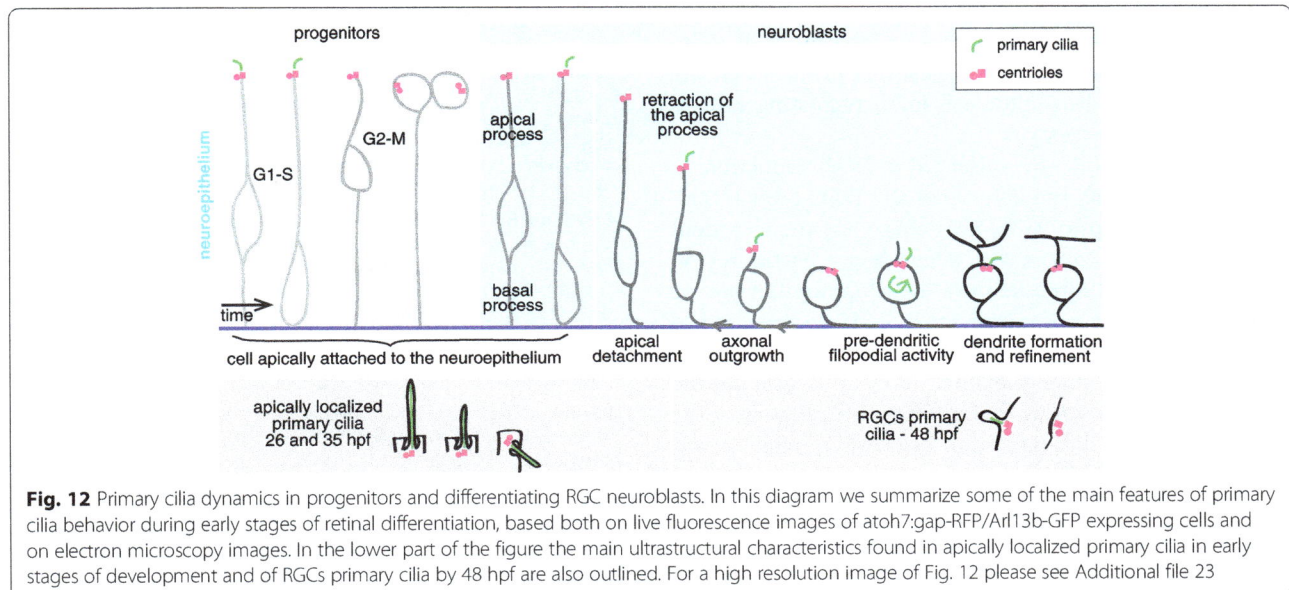

**Fig. 12** Primary cilia dynamics in progenitors and differentiating RGC neuroblasts. In this diagram we summarize some of the main features of primary cilia behavior during early stages of retinal differentiation, based both on live fluorescence images of atoh7:gap-RFP/Arl13b-GFP expressing cells and on electron microscopy images. In the lower part of the figure the main ultrastructural characteristics found in apically localized primary cilia in early stages of development and of RGCs primary cilia by 48 hpf are also outlined. For a high resolution image of Fig. 12 please see Additional file 23

the growing dendrites. Similar movements of the centrosome of differentiating RGCs, although in a more prolonged period of time, were observed when knocking-down Laminin α1, an essential signal for neuronal orientation in the zebrafish retina [2]. In tangentially migrating cortical interneurons, highly dynamic primary cilia that change in length and position during migration have been shown to be involved in sensing environmental Shh, and possibly other signaling molecules [17, 18]. Cortical neuroblasts form primary cilia postnatally, at a stage when their migration has ended [51]. Likewise, dentate granule cells born in adult mice, form primary cilia after reaching their final positions in the hippocampus, around the time of dendrite formation and synaptic connection establishment [16]. It has been shown that in these systems the primary cilium, which localizes to the base of the apical dendrite, is necessary for dendrite refinement and synapse formation [16, 52].

## RGCs are preferentially affected by cilia dysfunction during retinal development

The particular localization and dynamics of cilia in differentiating RGCs made us wonder what roles the organelle might have in the generation or differentiation of these neurons. As a first approach to evaluate the physiological role of cilia in the developing retina, we opted for a knockdown strategy using morpholino oligomers. IFT88 and Elipsa are two ciliary proteins that have been shown to directly interact and to be essential for intraflagellar transport in the zebrafish, whose mutants and knockdowns have been reported to give clear and reproducible "ciliary phenotypes" [27, 28]. In our hands, the best results were obtained with a combination of

MOs against these two genes, as we reasoned that through this approach we were going to maximize the chances of observing a ciliary phenotype with relatively low doses of individual MOs, avoiding cilia-independent alterations. In addition, we used splice-blocking MOs to avoid affecting early developmental processes. This combination of MOs effectively reduced cilia number and length in different organs and tissues, and gave a clearer ciliary phenotype than the individual MOs used at higher doses.

Previous work by others aimed at characterizing the in vivo functional role of genes involved in ciliogenesis in the zebrafish, such as *elipsa*, *ift88*, *ift57* or *ift172* [27, 28, 53, 54], showed, by analyzing single-mutants for these genes, that the major phenotype in the retina was the cell-autonomous progressive loss of photoreceptor cells, evident from 3 dpf onwards. Here, we also observed very little or no early retinal phenotype after the individual injection of MOs to *ift88* and *elipsa*. Double-morphants, however, showed a significant and sustained reduction in retinal volume from early stages of differentiation, which correlated with both a decrease in the number of mitosis and an increase in cell death throughout the retina. The experiments on SoFa1 embryos also showed decreased numbers of all retinal cell types. This effect of cilia impairment on cell proliferation/survival was cell-autonomous, as can be concluded from the blastomere transplantation experiments. Interestingly these experiments indicated that MO-treated retinal cells had an extremely reduced capacity to compete against their neighboring cells, as: 1) very scarce transplanted morphant atoh7:gap-RFP cells could be detected in wild-type host embryos, and 2) wild-type transplanted atoh7:gap-GFP cells tended to appear earlier than, and in several cases overcame, the host atoh7:gap-RFP cells. Taken together, these results suggest that primary cilia are functional at the progenitor cell level, regulating mitosis and possibly cell cycle exit.

Interestingly, while we observed a 38 % reduction in total retina volume, the volume of the RGC layer transiently decreased up to 95 %. This effect was more evident at 48 hpf than at later stages, suggesting a partial recovery of neuronal differentiation as development advanced. In addition, the 48 hpf morphant RGC layer appeared to be in earlier developmental stages when compared to controls and the inner plexiform layer was only visible in morphant embryos at the anterior-ventral part of the retina, where cell differentiation begins [55], while it was complete in controls. Consistent with this supposition, we observed that transplanted wild-type atoh7:gap-GFP cells tended to differentiate much earlier than the surrounding atoh7:gap-RFP cells in morphant hosts. In vivo experiments in the SoFa1 fish line further indicated that the delay in neuronal generation was more prominent in RGCs than in other cell types. A proportional increase in the photoreceptor layer was also noticed, indicating that cell fate decisions were affected. A causal relationship between cell cycle regulation and neuronal cell fate choice has been reported in different regions of the central nervous system [56]. Therefore, it could be possible that an altered cell cycle progression upon cilia disruption could account for the observed reduction in RGC number with respect to photoreceptors. Indeed, the manipulation of the timing of cell cycle exit in Xenopus retinal progenitors affected the generation of early neuronal cell types (as RGCs) at the expense of late-generated neurons (as bipolar cells) [57].

## Conclusions

We have shown here that relatively short primary cilia are present in neural progenitors and early neuroblasts of the neural retina in the zebrafish. The most remarkable features of these cilia are that they tend to remain localized to the apical region of the cells, and that they become extremely dynamic particularly during neuroblast polarity transitions, such as apical detachment and between axon and dendrite formation. Finally, our cilia disruption experiments, knocking-down *elipsa* and *ift88*, underscore a cell-autonomous role for cilia at cell proliferation and survival, as well as in neuronal cell-type specification.

## Additional files

**Additional file 1:** Time-lapse video corresponding to montage in Fig. 3a. A 3D maximum intensity projection of a confocal stack over time is shown. A progenitor (cell body marked with an asterisk) expressing gap-RFP (magenta) is observed previous to and during mitosis. It is possible to observe a primary cilium (pc) some time before cell rounding and its reappearance after division. Time is expressed in hrs:min. (MOV 8409 kb)

**Additional file 2:** Time-lapse video corresponding to montage in Fig. 3b. A 3D projection of a confocal stack over time is shown. In this movie a neuroblast (cell body marked with an asterisk) is shown previous to detachment from the apical region of the neuroepithelium. This cell has already started an axonal outgrowth (ax) at the beginning of the acquisition. It is possible to observe the presence of a primary cilium (pc) during retraction of the apical process (ap) and during the initial stages of dendritogenesis. Time is expressed in hrs:min. (MOV 10497 kb)

**Additional file 3:** Time-lapse video showing a cell (asterisk) with a primary cilium which moves basally previous to apical process detachment. A 3D projection of a confocal stack over time is shown. In the right panel only the Arl13b-GFP channel is shown, while in the left panel the merge with the gap-RFP channel is shown. The presence and localization of the primary cilium (pc) is indicated, as well as the tip of the apical process (ap) during retraction. Axonal outgrowth is also indicated (ax). Time is expressed in hrs:min. (MOV 8895 kb)

**Additional file 4:** Time-lapse video corresponding to montage in Fig. 5c. A 3D projection of a confocal stack over time is shown. It is possible to observe a neuroblast (cell body marked with an asterisk) after the initiation of apical process detachment through the initial stages of dendritogenesis. This cell has already started an axonal outgrowth (ax) at the beginning of the movie. The presence and localization of a primary cilium is indicated with an arrowhead (pc). Time is expressed in hrs:min. (MOV 3697 kb)

**Additional file 5:** Time-lapse video corresponding to montage in Fig. 5e. A 3D projection of a confocal stack over time is shown. It is possible to observe a basally localized neuroblast (asterisk), which has already extended an axon (ax), through the initial stages of dendritogenesis. The presence and localization of a primary cilium (pc) is indicated with an arrowhead. Time is expressed in hrs:min. (MOV 6377 kb)

**Additional file 6:** Time-lapse video corresponding to montage in Fig. 10a. In this time-lapse it is possible to observe a small clone of cells expressing atoh7:gap-RFP from a control MO (12 ng) injected embryo. Host cells express atoh7:gap-GFP. A 3D projection of a confocal stack over time is shown. Time is expressed in hrs:min. (MOV 5787 kb)

**Additional file 7:** Time-lapse video showing the retina of an embryo resulting from the transplant of blastomeres from control MO injected donor embryos to un-injected hosts. In this time-lapse it is possible to observe a large number of cells expressing atoh7:gap-RFP from a control MO (12 ng) injected embryo. Host cells express atoh7:gap-GFP. A maximum intensity projection of the stack is shown. Time is expressed in hrs:min. (MOV 4363 kb)

**Additional file 8:** Time-lapse video corresponding to montage in Fig. 10b. In this time-lapse it is possible to observe a few cells expressing atoh7:gap-RFP from an embryo injected with *elipsa*-SP/*ift88*-SP MOs (5/5 ng). Host cells express atoh7:gap-GFP. A 3D projection of a confocal stack over time is shown. Time is expressed in hrs:min. (MOV 5303 kb)

**Additional file 9:** Time-lapse video corresponding to montage in Fig. 10c. In this time-lapse it is possible to observe a small number of cells expressing atoh7:gap-GFP, which develop in the retina of an embryo injected with *elipsa*-SP/*ift88*-SP MOs (6/6 ng). Host cells express atoh7:gap-RFP. A 3D projection of a confocal stack over time is shown. Time is expressed in hrs:min. (MOV 3796 kb)

**Additional file 10:** Time-lapse video corresponding to montage in Fig. 10d. In this time-lapse it is possible to observe a large clone of cells expressing atoh7:gap-GFP, which develop in the retina of an embryo injected with *elipsa*-SP/*ift88*-SP MOs (6/6 ng). Host cells express atoh7:gap-RFP. A 3D projection of a confocal stack over time is shown. Time is expressed in hrs:min. (MOV 3850 kb)

**Additional file 11:** Time-lapse video and fluorescence profile analysis of SoFa1 embryos. Embryos were injected with control MO (right panels) or *elipsa*-SP/*ift88*-SP MOs (left panels) and imaged in vivo from 30 hpf onwards. A region in the ventro-nasal retina is shown in the upper panels and its corresponding fluorescent intensity profile over time in the lower panels. Each time frame corresponds to 10 min. (MOV 7625 kb)

**Additional file 12:** Main features of apical primary cilia in the early differentiating retinal neuroepithelium. (PDF 2898 kb)

**Additional file 13:** Primary cilia emerging from the basolateral membrane of retinal neuroepithelial cells. (PDF 1690 kb)

**Additional file 14:** Primary cilia first appear in RGC neuroblasts during apical process retraction and in an apical position. (PDF 3553 kb)

**Additional file 15:** Primary cilia dynamics in relation to RGC differentiation events. (PDF 109 kb)

**Additional file 16:** Upon completion of apical retraction, primary cilia may transiently disappear or lose their apical localization. (PDF 6861 kb)

**Additional file 17:** Primary cilia in maturing RGCs. (PDF 3994 kb)

**Additional file 18:** Evaluation of different morpholino oligomers for elipsa and ift88 knock-down. (PDF 3369 kb)

**Additional file 19:** Effective reduction of primary cilia length in zebrafish embryos upon elipsa and ift88 knock-down. (PDF 4352 kb)

**Additional file 20:** Embryos with impaired cilia have smaller eyes and a reduced RGC layer. (PDF 2212 kb)

**Additional file 21:** Cell-autonomous effect of cilia reduction on RGC differentiation. (PDF 3922 kb)

**Additional file 22:** Cilia impaired embryos show a preferential delay in RGCs formation. (PDF 4731 kb)

**Additional file 23:** Primary cilia dynamics in progenitors and differentiating RGC neuroblasts. (PDF 118 kb)

## Abbreviations
dpf: days post-fertilization; hpf: hours post-fertilization; MO: morpholino oligomer; RGC: retinal ganglion cell; RPE: retinal pigment epithelium; TEM: transmission electron microscopy.

## Competing interests
The authors declare that they have no competing interests.

## Authors' contributions
PL designed and performed most of the experiments involving gene knock-down and live imaging of cilia, and wrote the main manuscript draft; CD performed all electron microscopy analyses and some of the gene knock-down experiments, and helped writing the manuscript; GC directed and designed the electron microscopy analyses; JLB directed part of the research, helped designing knock-down experiments and revised and helped writing the manuscript; FRZ directed part of the research, designed and performed some of the knock-down and live imaging experiments and revised and helped writing the manuscript. All authors read and approved the final manuscript.

## Acknowledgements
We are grateful to all colleagues who generously shared diverse reagents and fish lines: Kristen Kwan provided several Tol2 kit plasmids, Bill Harris provided the atoh7:gap-RFP and -GFP, and the SoFa1 zebrafish lines, Brian Ciruna provided the Arl13b-GFP zebrafish line and plasmid. We also thank the technical assistance of Ana Paula Arévalo, Casandra Carrillo and Martina Crispo for fish care and maintenance; Marcela Díaz and Tabaré De Los Campos, for support on confocal microscopy and image processing. Finally, we thank Magdalena Cárdenas for advice and help with zebrafish embryo techniques.

## Funding
The present work was funded by ANII (FCE_1_2011_1_5888 to FRZ), Institut Pasteur de Montevideo (Transversal Grant 2010 to JLB and FRZ), and PEDECIBA. PL had a SNB-ANII Doctoral Fellowship (POS_NAC_2012_1_8518). Funding sources had no role in the design of the studies.

## Author details
[1]Human Molecular Genetics Laboratory, Institut Pasteur de Montevideo, Mataojo 2020, Montevideo 11400, Uruguay. [2]Cell Biology of Neural Development Laboratory, Institut Pasteur de Montevideo, Mataojo 2020, Montevideo 11400, Uruguay. [3]Sección Biología Celular, Departamento de Biología Celular y Molecular, Facultad de Ciencias, Universidad de la República, Iguá 4225, Montevideo 11400, Uruguay. [4]Unidad de Microscopía Electrónica, Facultad de Ciencias, Universidad de la República, Iguá 4225, Montevideo 11400, Uruguay.

## References
1. Del Bene F, Wehman AM, Link BA, Baier H. Regulation of neurogenesis by interkinetic nuclear migration through an apical-basal notch gradient. Cell. 2008;134:1055–65.
2. Randlett O, Poggi L, Zolessi FR, Harris WA. The oriented emergence of axons from retinal ganglion cells is directed by Laminin contact in vivo. Neuron. 2011;70:266–80.
3. Masai I, Yamaguchi M, Tonou-Fujimori N, Komori A, Okamoto H. The Hedgehog-PKA pathway regulates two distinct steps of the differentiation of retinal ganglion cells: the cell-cycle exit of retinoblasts and their neuronal maturation. Development. 2005;132:1539–53.
4. Shkumatava A, Neumann CJ. Shh directs cell-cycle exit by activating p57Kip2 in the zebrafish retina. EMBO Rep. 2005;6:563–9.
5. Shkumatava A, Fischer S, Müller F, Strahle U, Neumann CJ. Sonic hedgehog, secreted by amacrine cells, acts as a short-range signal to direct differentiation and lamination in the zebrafish retina. Development. 2004; 131:3849–58.
6. Stenkamp DL, Frey RA, Prabhudesai SN, Raymond PA. Function for Hedgehog genes in zebrafish retinal development. Dev Biol. 2000;220:238–52.
7. Neumann CJ, Nuesslein-Volhard C. Patterning of the zebrafish retina by a Wave of Sonic Hedgehog Activity. Science. 2000;289:2137–9.
8. Zolessi FR, Poggi L, Wilkinson CJ, Chien CB, Harris WA. Polarization and orientation of retinal ganglion cells in vivo. Neural Dev. 2006;1:2.
9. Berbari NF, O'Connor AK, Haycraft CJ, Yoder BK. The primary cilium as a complex signaling center. Curr Biol. 2009;19:R526–35.
10. Fry AM, Leaper MJ, Bayliss R. The primary cilium: guardian of organ development and homeostasis. Organogenesis. 2014;10:62–8.
11. Cardenas-Rodriguez M, Badano JL. Ciliary biology: understanding the cellular and genetic basis of human ciliopathies. Am J Med Genet C Semin Med Genet. 2009;151C:263–80.
12. Valente EM, Rosti RO, Gibbs E, Gleeson JG. Primary cilia in neurodevelopmental disorders. Nat Rev Neurol. 2013;10:27–36.
13. Chizhikov VV, Davenport J, Zhang Q, Shih EK, Cabello OA, Fuchs JL, et al. Cilia proteins control cerebellar morphogenesis by promoting expansion of the granule progenitor pool. J Neurosci. 2007;27:9780–9.
14. Spassky N, Han Y-G, Aguilar A, Strehl L, Besse L, Laclef C, et al. Primary cilia are required for cerebellar development and Shh-dependent expansion of progenitor pool. Dev Biol. 2008;317:246–59.
15. Breunig JJ, Sarkisian MR, Arellano JI, Morozov YM, Ayoub AE, Sojitra S, et al. Primary cilia regulate hippocampal neurogenesis by mediating sonic hedgehog signaling. Proc Natl Acad Sci. 2008;105:13127.
16. Kumamoto N, Gu Y, Wang J, Janoschka S, Takemaru K-I, Levine J, et al. A role for primary cilia in glutamatergic synaptic integration of adult-born neurons. Nat Neurosci. 2012;15:399–405.
17. Baudoin J-P, Viou L, Launay P-S, Luccardini C, Espeso Gil S, Kiyasova V, et al. Tangentially migrating neurons assemble a primary cilium that promotes their reorientation to the cortical plate. Neuron. 2012;76:1108–22.
18. Higginbotham H, Eom T-Y, Mariani LE, Bachleda A, Hirt J, Gukassyan V, et al. Arl13b in primary cilia regulates the migration and placement of interneurons in the developing cerebral cortex. Dev Cell. 2012;23: 925–38.

19. Sotelo JR, Trujillo-Cenóz O. Electron microscope study on the development of ciliary components of the neural epithelium of the chick embryo. Cell Tissue Res. 1958;49:1–12.

20. Hinds JW, Hinds PL. Early ganglion cell differentiation in the mouse retina: an electron microscopic analysis utilizing serial sections. Dev Biol. 1974;37:381–416.

21. Borovina A, Superina S, Voskas D, Ciruna B. Vangl2 directs the posterior tilting and asymmetric localization of motile primary cilia. Nat Cell Biol. 2010;12:407–12.

22. Caspary T, Larkins CE, Anderson KV. The graded response to Sonic Hedgehog depends on cilia architecture. Dev Cell. 2007;12:767–78.

23. Sun Z. A genetic screen in zebrafish identifies cilia genes as a principal cause of cystic kidney. Development. 2004;131:4085–93.

24. Kimmel CB, Ballard WW, Kimmel SR, Ullmann B, Schilling TF. Stages of embryonic development of the zebrafish. Dev Dyn. 1995;203:253–310.

25. Howe K, Clark MD, Torroja CF, Torrance J, Berthelot C, Muffato M, et al. The zebrafish reference genome sequence and its relationship to the human genome. Nature. 2013;496:498–503.

26. Almeida AD, Boije H, Chow RW, He J, Tham J, Suzuki SC, et al. Spectrum of Fates: a new approach to the study of the developing zebrafish retina. Development. 2014;141:1971–80.

27. Omori Y, Zhao C, Saras A, Mukhopadhyay S, Kim W, Furukawa T, et al. elipsa is an early determinant of ciliogenesis that links the IFT particle to membrane-associated small GTPase Rab8. Nat Cell Biol. 2008;10:437–44.

28. Tsujikawa M, Malicki J. Intraflagellar transport genes are essential for differentiation and survival of vertebrate sensory neurons. Neuron. 2004;42:703–16.

29. Robu ME, Larson JD, Nasevicius A, Beiraghi S, Brenner C, Farber SA, et al. p53 activation by knockdown technologies. PLoS Genet. 2007;3:e78.

30. Prieto D, Aparicio G, Morande PE, Zolessi FR. A fast, low cost, and highly efficient fluorescent DNA labeling method using methyl green. Histochem Cell Biol. 2014;142:335–45.

31. Schindelin J, Arganda-Carreras I, Frise E, Kaynig V, Longair M, Pietzsch T, et al. Fiji: an open-source platform for biological-image analysis. Nat Methods. 2012;9:676–82.

32. Ollion J, Cochennec J, Loll F, Escude C, Boudier T. TANGO: a generic tool for high-throughput 3D image analysis for studying nuclear organization. Bioinformatics. 2013;29:1840–1.

33. Bolte S, Cordelières FP. A guided tour into subcellular colocalization analysis in light microscopy. J Microsc. 2006;224:213–32.

34. Meijering E, Dzyubachyk O, Smal I, et al. Methods for cell and particle tracking. Methods Enzymol. 2012;504:183–200.

35. Sokal R, Rohlf J. Biometría. In: Blume H, editor. Principios y métodos estadísticos en la investigación biológica. 1st ed. 1979.

36. Pagano M, Gauvreau K. Fundamentos de Bioestadística. 2nd ed. Madrid, Spain: Thomson Learning; 2001.

37. Hammer Ø, Harper DAT, Ryan PD. PAST: paleontological statistics software package for education and data analysis. Palaeontol Electron. 2001;4:art.4:9.

38. Conover WJ, Iman RL. Rank transformations as a bridge between parametric and nonparametric statistics. Am Stat. 1981;35:124.

39. Wilsch-Brauninger M, Peters J, Paridaen JTML, Huttner WB. Basolateral rather than apical primary cilia on neuroepithelial cells committed to delamination. Development. 2011;139:95–105.

40. Laessing U, Stuermer CA. Spatiotemporal pattern of retinal ganglion cell differentiation revealed by the expression of neurolin in embryonic zebrafish. J Neurobiol. 1996;29:65–74.

41. Choi J-H, Law M-Y, Chien C-B, Link BA, Wong RO. In vivo development of dendritic orientation in wild-type and mislocalized retinal ganglion cells. Neural Dev. 2010;5:29.

42. Schmitt EA, Dowling JE. Early retinal development in the zebrafish, Danio rerio: light and electron microscopic analyses. J Comp Neurol. 1999;404:515–36.

43. Benmerah A. The ciliary pocket. Curr Opin Cell Biol. 2013;25:78–84.

44. Molla-Herman A, Ghossoub R, Blisnick T, Meunier A, Serres C, Silbermann F, et al. The ciliary pocket: an endocytic membrane domain at the base of primary and motile cilia. J Cell Sci. 2010;123:1785–95.

45. Clement CA, Ajbro KD, Koefoed K, Vestergaard ML, Veland IR, Henriques de Jesus MPR, et al. TGF-β signaling is associated with endocytosis at the pocket region of the primary cilium. Cell Rep. 2013;3:1806–14.

46. Chenn, Zhang Y, Chang B, McConell S. Instrinsic polarity of mammalian neuroepithelial cells. Mol Cell Neurosci. 1998;11:183–93.

47. Sorokin S. Centrioles and the formation of rudimentary cilia by fibroblasts and smooth muscle cells. J Cell Biol. 1962;15:363–77.

48. Spear PC, Erickson CA. Apical movement during interkinetic nuclear migration is a two-step process. Dev Biol. 2012;370:33–41.

49. Wong GKW, Baudet M-L, Norden C, Leung L, Harris WA. Slit1b-Robo3 signaling and N-Cadherin regulate apical process retraction in developing retinal ganglion cells. J Neurosci. 2012;32:223–8.

50. Das RM, Storey KG. Apical abscission alters cell polarity and dismantles the primary cilium during neurogenesis. Science. 2014;343:200–4.

51. Arellano JI, Guadiana SM, Breunig JJ, Rakic P, Sarkisian MR. Development and distribution of neuronal cilia in mouse neocortex. J Comp Neurol. 2012;520:848–73.

52. Guadiana SM, Semple-Rowland S, Daroszewski D, Madorsky I, Breunig JJ, Mykytyn K, et al. Arborization of dendrites by developing neocortical neurons is dependent on primary cilia and type 3 Adenylyl cyclase. J Neurosci. 2013;33:2626–38.

53. Sukumaran S, Perkins BD. Early defects in photoreceptor outer segment morphogenesis in zebrafish ift57, ift88 and ift172 Intraflagellar Transport mutants. Vision Res. 2009;49:479–89.

54. Doerre G, Malicki J. Genetic analysis of photoreceptor cell development in the zebrafish retina. Mech Dev. 2002;110:125–38.

55. Hu M, Easter Jr SS. Retinal neurogenesis: the formation of the initial central patch of postmitotic cells. Dev Biol. 1999;207:309–21.

56. Tury A, Mairet-Coello G, DiCicco-Bloom E. The multiple roles of the cyclin-dependent kinase inhibitory protein p57KIP2 in cerebral cortical neurogenesis. Dev Neurobiol. 2012;72:821–42.

57. Ohnuma S, Hopper S, Wang KC, Philpott A, Harris WA. Co-ordinating retinal histogenesis: early cell cycle exit enhances early cell fate determination in the Xenopus retina. Development. 2002;129:2435–46.

# 12

# Live imaging of developing mouse retinal slices

Anthony P. Barrasso[1,3], Shang Wang[1], Xuefei Tong[1], Audrey E. Christiansen[1], Irina V. Larina[1,3] and Ross A. Poché[1,2,3*] (iD)

## Abstract

**Background:** Ex vivo, whole-mount explant culture of the rodent retina has proved to be a valuable approach for studying retinal development. In a limited number of recent studies, this method has been coupled to live fluorescent microscopy with the goal of directly observing dynamic cellular events. However, retinal tissue thickness imposes significant technical limitations. To obtain 3-dimensional images with high quality axial resolution, investigators are restricted to specific areas of the retina and require microscopes, such as 2-photon, with a higher level of depth penetrance. Here, we report a retinal live imaging method that is more amenable to a wider array of imaging systems and does not compromise resolution of retinal cross-sectional area.

**Results:** Mouse retinal slice cultures were prepared and standard, inverted confocal microscopy was used to generate movies with high quality resolution of retinal cross-sections. To illustrate the ability of this method to capture discrete, physiologically relevant events during retinal development, we imaged the dynamics of the *Fucci* cell cycle reporter in both wild type and *Cyclin D1* mutant retinal progenitor cells (RPCs) undergoing interkinetic nuclear migration (INM). Like previously reported for the zebrafish, mouse RPCs in G1 phase migrated stochastically and exhibited overall basal drift during development. In contrast, mouse RPCs in G2 phase displayed directed, apical migration toward the ventricular zone prior to mitosis. We also determined that *Cyclin D1* knockout RPCs in G2 exhibited a slower apical velocity as compared to wild type. These data are consistent with previous IdU/BrdU window labeling experiments on *Cyclin D1* knockout RPCs indicating an elongated cell cycle. Finally, to illustrate the ability to monitor retinal neuron differentiation, we imaged early postnatal horizontal cells (HCs). Time lapse movies uncovered specific HC neurite dynamics consistent with previously published data showing an instructive role for transient vertical neurites in HC mosaic formation.

**Conclusions:** We have detailed a straightforward method to image mouse retinal slice culture preparations that, due to its relative ease, extends live retinal imaging capabilities to a more diverse group of scientists. We have also shown that, by using a slice technique, we can achieve excellent lateral resolution, which is advantageous for capturing intracellular dynamics and overall cell movements during retinal development and differentiation.

**Keywords:** Live imaging, Mouse retinal progenitor cells, Interkinetic nuclear migration, *Cyclin D1*, Horizontal neurons

## Background

The mouse retina is a proven model system in which to understand the cellular and molecular mechanisms driving mammalian retinogenesis and the pathophysiology of retinal diseases [3, 17, 48]. This feature is largely due

to several technical advantages such as the relative ease of utilizing Cre-loxP technology, plasmid electroporation, and viral transduction to perform in vivo genetic loss-of-function, gain-of-function, and lineage tracing experiments [8, 26, 27, 42]. Additionally, the embryonic and early postnatal mouse retina is amenable to ex vivo manipulation and cultured retinae retain many features of normal development [6, 12, 26, 33]. These methods allowed researchers to extend gene transfer and cell labeling approaches to discrete cell types and developmental time points. Rodent retinal explants also have

* Correspondence: poche@bcm.edu
[1]Department of Molecular Physiology and Biophysics, Baylor College of Medicine, Houston, TX 77030, USA
[2]Program in Developmental Biology, Baylor College of Medicine, Houston, TX 77030, USA
Full list of author information is available at the end of the article

the added advantage of allowing for time-lapse microscopy to directly monitor developmental processes such as retinal progenitor cell (RPC) interkinetic nuclear migration (INM) and cell cycle progression, as well as neuron migration and morphogenesis [18, 33].

To date, live fluorescent microscopic imaging of the rodent retina has been mostly limited to whole mount explants [6, 7, 14, 18, 20, 21, 23, 33, 39, 51, 52]. While much has been learned using this approach, significant technical hurdles remain. To image through the entire thickness of the retinal explant, one must account for the attenuation of light within deeper layers, a problem that is particularly true if researchers wish to capture events, such as INM, that occur along the radial axis. As a solution, many have turned to brighter and far-red shifted fluorescent reporters as well as imaging modalities such as 2-photon microscopy, which allow for deeper imaging with less photo-toxicity. However, specific reporters, such as fluorescent fusion proteins, may not be sufficiently bright. Furthermore, 2-photon microscopy may not be available to a particular researcher or the demand on institutionally shared equipment may make lengthy time-lapse experiments logistically impossible or cost prohibitive.

Here we present a straightforward method to perform living imaging of developing mouse retinal slice cultures for at least 24 h. This approach is designed to circumvent the need for 2-photon microscopy, which makes our approach more feasible to a wider array of scientists interested in studying mouse retinogenesis. Furthermore, we demonstrate that our slice preparation allows for excellent lateral resolution of the entire retinal cross-sectional area by confocal microscopy. This is a significant advantage for capturing intracellular dynamics and overall cell movements during retinal development and differentiation. To verify that live imaging of retinal slice cultures is capable of capturing normal retinal developmental processes, we have performed several proof-of-concept experiments. First, we analyzed INM patterns among RPCs and showed migration features in common with previous findings in zebrafish. Next, we explored the consequence of *Cyclin D1* loss on RPC INM rate and trajectory and found that mutant RPC apical migration was slower than controls. Finally, using horizontal cells (HCs) as an example, we determined that our protocol is sufficient for monitoring post-mitotic retinal neuron dynamics.

## Methods
### Retinal slice culture preparation (see Additional file 1 for detailed materials list)
#### Agarose and culture media preparation
We prepared 6.5% (40 mL) and 1.5% (30 mL) low melting agarose solutions in DMEM/F12 media without phenol red. 1000 mL and 500 mL glass beakers were used to make a double boiler on a hotplate in which the agarose was melted. Once the agarose is fully melted and appears clear, it can be kept in a 37 °C water bath until use. Under a tissue culture hood, DMEM/F12 complete culture media was prepared with 10% FBS, 1% Pen/Strep, and Insulin (5 μg/ml), and was warmed to 37 °C prior to use.

#### Dissection and embedding
To prepare for retinal dissections, a heating pad was warmed in a microwave for 2.5 min. 3 mL of culture media (warmed to 37 °C) was transferred into several 35 mm petri dishes and placed on the heating pad to keep the media warm. For all early postnatal time points, live pups were collected directly from the breeding cage and individuals with the desired fluorescent reporters were selected using a Zeiss Stemi 2000 stereomicroscope equipped with a Nightsea fluorescent adaptor. Fluorescent postnatal pups were sacrificed by $CO_2$ inhalation followed by decapitation and skinning of the head. The skin tissue was reserved for PCR-based confirmation of genotypes. The eyes were carefully enucleated with a curved, serrated Graefe forceps and placed in the 35 mm petri dish with warm DMEM/F12 and maintained on the heating pad.

For retinal dissections, a plastic transfer pipette with a cut (widened) tip was used to transfer individual eyes to a fresh 35 mm petri dish containing DMEM/F12 at 37 °C and visualized under a stereomicroscope. With a pair of sharp #5 fine forceps, a hole was poked in the limbus of the eye and the scleral, retinal pigment epithelial, iris, and corneal tissues were carefully peeled away from the eye thereby leaving behind an intact retinal cup and lens. Next, the surface of the lens center was held by one sharp #5 forceps while a second forceps was used to gently pull the lens and any attached hyaloid vessels away from the retina. If significant hyaloid vasculature within the retinal cup persisted, it was carefully removed. Once an intact retinal cup was isolated, it was transferred with plastic transfer pipette to a new dish of fresh DMEM/F12 on the heating pad. This process was repeated until all of the retinal cups were collected. Care was taken to minimize rips in the retinal tissue and the dissections were performed as quickly as possible.

Once all retinae were dissected, they were embedded in the melted 6.5% agarose. Using a plastic transfer pipette, a Tissue-Tek® cryomold (10 mm X 10 mm X 5 mm) was filled halfway with 6.5% agarose. Using a fresh cut plastic transfer pipette, an isolated retinal cup was transferred from the media to the agarose within the cryomold. Care was taken to transfer as little media as possible to the agarose. Using #5 forceps, the retinal cup was oriented with the retinal ganglion cell layer facing up. Any residual media was carefully wicked away with a Kimwipe and additional 6.5% agarose was added to fill the mold. In order to solidify, the agarose was left at room temperature for 10 min.

### Vibratome sectioning, agarose slice mounting, and culture

The vibratome buffer tray was filled with sterile 1X PBS and half of a double-edged razor blade was secured to the knife holder. Once the agarose solidified, it was removed from the cryomold and a single edge razor blade was used to trim the agarose block so that a slice would fit the dimensions of the 10 mm diameter glass coverslip mounted to a glass bottom dish. To make retinal cross-sections, the agarose cube containing the retina with the ganglion cell layer face up, was rotated 90 degrees and mounted to the vibratome specimen disc with super glue. With the vibratome frequency and speed both set to 5, 200 µm agarose slices were obtained and floated onto a paintbrush for transfer onto a glass bottom culture dish.

For the slice transfer, enough complete culture media (roughly 100 µL) was added to the cover slip of the glass bottom dish so that a stable bubble formed in the shallow well. The agarose slice floated onto the paintbrush and was carefully transferred to the culture media bubble. A P200 pipette was used to remove as much of the media as possible resulting in the retinal slice making direct contact with the glass of the dish. Next, using a plastic transfer pipette, the agarose slice was covered with a drop of warm 1.5% agarose media. Once this solidified, the entire bottom of the dish was filled with a thin layer (roughly 2 mL) of 1.5% agarose media that was then allowed to solidify. Finally, 1.5 mL of complete culture media was added on top of the agarose layer, and the culture was immediately transferred to a tissue culture incubator set to 37 °C and 5% $CO_2$ until we were ready to image.

### Retinal immunofluorescence

Eyes were harvested from mice and the retina and lens were isolated as described above. The retina and lens were fixed in 4% paraformaldehyde at 4 °C for 1 h. The tissues were washed with 1X PBS, incubated overnight in 15% sucrose solution (Sigma-Aldrich S9378) at 4 °C and then transferred to 30% sucrose at 4 °C for an additional night. The tissue was then embedded in OCT compound (Sakura 4583) on dry ice and cryosectioned into 20 µm sections. Cryosections were washed with 1X PBS-T (1X PBS + 0.1% Triton-X 100), 3 times for 10 min each, and then blocked in 2% normal goat (Sigma-Aldrich G9023) or donkey serum (Sigma-Aldrich D9663) for 1 h at room temperature. Next, the tissue was stained with primary antibodies (diluted in blocking

solution) overnight at 4 °C in a humid chamber. Then, the tissue was washed with 1X PBS for 3 times, 10 min each at room temperature and stained with secondary antibodies (in blocking solution) for 1 h at room temperature in a dark humid chamber. The tissue was again washed with 1X PBS 3 times for 10 min and a coverslip was mounted over the tissue with Fluoromount-G (Southern Biotech, #0100–01). Primary and secondary antibody concentrations are listed in Additional file 2.

### Assessment of cell death and proliferation within cultured retinal slices

To assess cell death, retinal slice cultures were briefly rinsed with 1X PBS and stained with the Zombie Red™ Fixable Viability Kit (Biolegend Ca# 423109). Cultures were incubated in the dye solution (1:500 in 1X PBS) for 1 h at 37 °C in the dark. The tissue was then washed with 1X PBS twice for 10 min and fixed with 4% paraformaldehyde for 10 min at room temperature. After fixation cultures were washed with 1X PBS three times for 10 min and stored at 4 °C until imaging was performed.

Using the Plan-Apochromat 20×/0.8 objective on Zeiss LSM 780 inverted confocal microscope and the Tile Scan function in ZEN, the entire retinal slice was imaged at high resolution. Using an original MATLAB code, the number of Zombie Red+ pixels was quantified for each image (Additional file 3). Next, using the Overlay function in the Zeiss LSM Image Browser software, the area of each retinal slice was measured. The ratio of ZR+ pixels to retinal area was determined for each projection and the Students's t-test was performed to determine whether there was a statistically significant difference between average values at 0 h and 16 h or between laser exposed and unexposed tissue.

For in vivo labelling of RPCs in S-phase, EdU was injected intraperitoneally into P0 and P1 mice. After 6 h, the mice were sacrificed, and their eyes were harvested for cryosections. Using sharp #5 forceps, a hole was poked in the corneas and the eyes fixed with 4% paraformaldehyde for 1 h at 4 °C. After fixation, eyes were washed with 1X PBS 3 times for 10 min each. Next, eyes were incubated in 15% sucrose overnight at 4 °C and transferred to 30% sucrose for an additional night at 4 °C. Finally, the tissue was submerged in OCT compound, flash frozen, and stored at − 80 °C until sectioning. 20 µm tissue sections were obtained with a cryostat and EdU-labeled cells were detected with the Click-iT Plus EdU Alexa Fluor 555 Imaging Kit (ThermoFisher). To label RPCs in S-phase within P0 time lapse slice cultures, EdU (5 mg/mL) was added to the culture media after 6 h and this was followed by an additional 6 h in culture. Next, a small block of agarose containing the retinal slice was excised from the glass bottom dish and immediately placed in 4% paraformaldehyde to fix. The tissue was then processed, cryosectioned, and stained for EdU as described above.

For each biological replicate ($n = 3$ per group), we acquired six Z-stacks (9 μm thick) from 3 non-adjacent retinal sections. Images for quantification were obtained using the Plan-Apochromat 20X/0.8 objective and the Zeiss LSM 780 with consistent laser settings. We only imaged tissue near the optic nerve head to ensure that statistical comparisons were performed on tissue from the central retina. Finally, we generated maximum intensity projections and calculated the ratio of EdU+ pixels to DAPI+ pixels using MATLAB (Additional file 3). The average ratios for each experimental group were calculated and values were compared using a single factor ANOVA ($p = 0.64$).

## Time-lapse image acquisition and analysis

Live imaging of retinal slices was performed using the Zeiss LSM 780 inverted confocal microscope equipped with a 34-channel spectral array and 405, 458, 488, 514, 561, 594, and 633 nm laser lines or the Zeiss LSM 510 META inverted microscope equipped with a 32-channel spectral array and 405, 458, 488, 514, 543, and 633 nm laser lines. All static and live images were acquired using either a C-Apochromat 40X/1.20 W Korr. (LSM 780) or a C-Apochromat 40×/1.2 W UV-VIS-NIR objective (LSM 510).

The Zeiss LSM 780 and 510 were outfitted with an environmental chamber maintained at 37 °C and 5% $CO_2$. Prior to time-lapse imaging, the retinal slice cultures were assessed by confocal microscopy and the culture with the best cross-sectional orientation was chosen for overnight imaging. Once chosen, the slice culture was allowed to equilibrate within the microscope environmental chamber for at least 30 min before initiation of image acquisition.

### Imaging and analysis of Fucci+ RPCs

To capture cell cycle kinetics of RPCs, we cultured retinae from P0 mice expressing one or both of the Fucci reporters [41] which were excited by the 488 nm (AzG) and 561 nm (KO2) laser lines. Z-stacks with a thickness of 11.043 μm made up of 11 images were collected every 10 min. Signal intensity varied among replicates, and laser power was adjusted accordingly ranging between 2 and 4%. The Z-stack images were subsequently processed with Imaris (Bitplane) using adaptive thresholding and a Gaussian filter.

Using the spot tracking function in Imaris, we tracked the migration patterns of individual nuclei, and those data were smoothed by averaging groups of three points. The nuclear position along the apical-basal axis relative to its starting point was plotted over time for each nucleus. We tracked 56 AzG+ nuclei from 3 wildtype retinae, 77 KO2+ nuclei from 2 wildtype retinae, and 54 AzG+ nuclei from 3 Cyclin $D1^{-/-}$ retinae.

To determine whether nuclear migration was directed or random, we calculated mean square displacement (MSD) as a function of elapsed time of individual AzG+ or KO2+ nuclear migration events [22]. These data were collected from five independent movies. MSD calculations were performed using an original MATLAB code (Additional file 4). For the AzG+ cells, the MSD was calculated from the point when an AzG+ cell first initiated apical migration (the green portion of the lines in Fig. 5b) to when it entered mitosis, during which the AzG reporter turned off. For the KO2 cells, the MSD was calculated from time zero until the time lapse movie ended or the cell left the field of view.

To compare apical nuclear velocity during G2 phase, we determined where persistent apical migration began for each nucleus and followed subsequent apical movement over the course of the time lapse. Apical velocity (V) was calculated by dividing the change in relative nuclear position by time. Using the Kolmogorov–Smirnov (KS) test, the distribution of the average and maximum velocities was determined to be non-parametric for both genotypes ($V_{avgWT}$: $p = 3.27 \times 10^{-16}$, $V_{avgKO}$: $p = 6.68 \times 10^{-15}$, $V_{maxWT}$: $p = 1.27 \times 10^{-21}$, $V_{maxKO}$: $p = 5.29 \times 10^{-18}$). A statistical difference was confirmed using a Rank-sum test ($V_{avg}$: $p = 4.85 \times 10^{-5}$, $V_{max}$: $p = 4.71 \times 10^{-8}$).

### Imaging and analysis of horizontal cells

Retinal slices from P2 Cx57-iCre; Rosa26R-mTmG$^{+/tg}$ mice were cultured to visualize the dynamic properties of HCs during development. In all, we imaged 3 retinae for 8 to 21 h. Z-stacks with a thickness that ranged from approximately 20–27 μm made up of 19–25 images were collected every 10 min by exciting the Rosa26R-mTmG reporter with 488 nm (eGFP) and 561 nm (tdTomato) lasers at 4% and 2% power, respectively. For presentation purposes, movies were processed with a Gaussian filter (Imaris) or Median filter (ZEN).

Using the Filament Tracer function in Imaris, we traced the neurites of 2 adjacent HCs. For ease of viewing, we pseudo-colored (Adobe Photoshop) tracings of individual transient, vertically-oriented neurites that were previously described as being the source of repulsive homotypic interactions that establish the HC mosaic [18]. To confirm that these vertical neurites fail to interact with the neurites of neighboring HCs, we tracked them for a minimum of 360 min or until they completely retracted.

To quantify the interactions between adjacent HC neurites, neurite territory overlap was measured as previously described [30]. The HC territory was determined by assigning 10 μm diameter circular regions centered at the HC positive pixels followed by a morphological closing (dilation-erosion) process with a 10 μm diameter disk. Specifically, maximum intensity projection images were first generated from the Z-stacks at each time point. Then the HCs within each image were manually selected and separated using ImageJ. With an original MATLAB code (Additional file 5), the separated HC images underwent background removal, median filtering, and binarization. Subsequently, the HC territories were built, and we measured the area of each territory and the overlap areas between adjacent cells. Using these measurements, we calculated the overlap percentage. The delineated HC territories over time were shown with a 50% transparency overlaid on the original fluorescence images. The distance between the center of mass from the adjacent territories was also measured.

## Results and discussion
### Retinal slice culture setup
As specifically detailed in the methods section, early postnatal mouse eyes were enucleated, placed in warm culture media (DMEM/F12), and the retina was dissected away from the other ocular tissues. While this process was repeated for additional eyes, the previously isolated retinae were maintained as retinal cups submerged in DMEM/F12 and incubated at 37 °C. Once all retinae were isolated, they were then embedded in 6.5% agarose made with DMEM/F12 and 200 μm

retinal cross-sections were sliced on a vibratome. Using a paintbrush, the slices were then mounted directly against the glass of a glass bottom dish and a thin layer of 1.5% agarose/media was poured over the retinal slice to maintain it against the glass. Once the agarose solidified, liquid culture media was added to the dish and the retina was ready to be imaged on an inverted microscope (summarized in Fig. 1).

### Analysis of cell death and proliferation
To determine whether our slice culture protocol results in significant retinal cell death that would preclude meaningful analysis and interpretation, we performed Zombie Red™ staining followed by confocal imaging of fluorescence (Fig. 2a-h). Cultures of P0 retinae were stained at two time points: immediately after cultures were prepared (0 h in culture) and after 16 h of live confocal imaging (16 h of laser exposure).

Zombie Red™ (ZR) is an amine reactive fluorescent dye that is non-permeant to live cells, but permeant to cells with compromised membranes (usually dead or dying cells). The dye is optimally excited by 561 nm laser light and has a fluorescence emission peak at 642 nm (Biolegend Ca# 423109). At 0 h in culture, clear ZR+ pixels were observed throughout the ganglion cell layer (GCL) (Fig. 2a, c, e, g). ZR labeling in the GCL was entirely expected because, once the optic nerve is severed during retinal dissection, ganglion cell survival is compromised

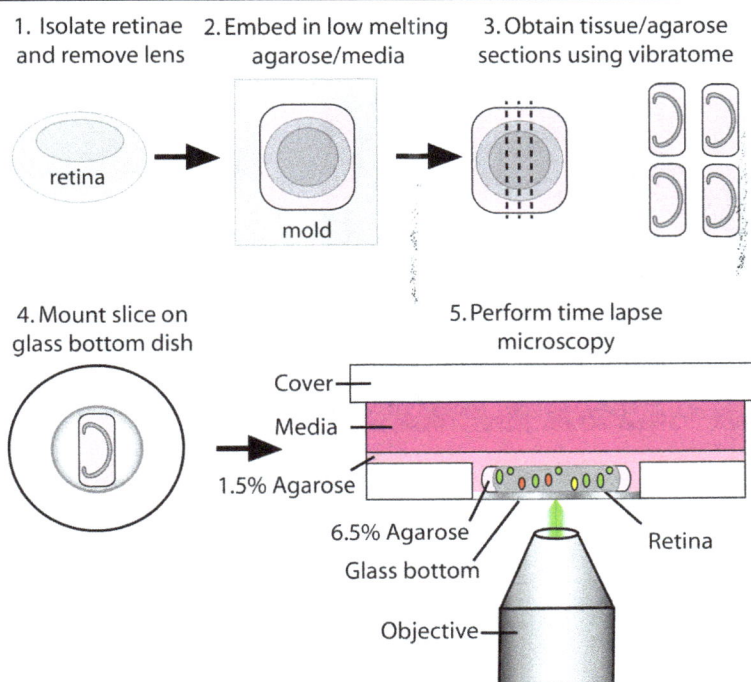

**Fig. 1** Schematic of retinal slice culture protocol

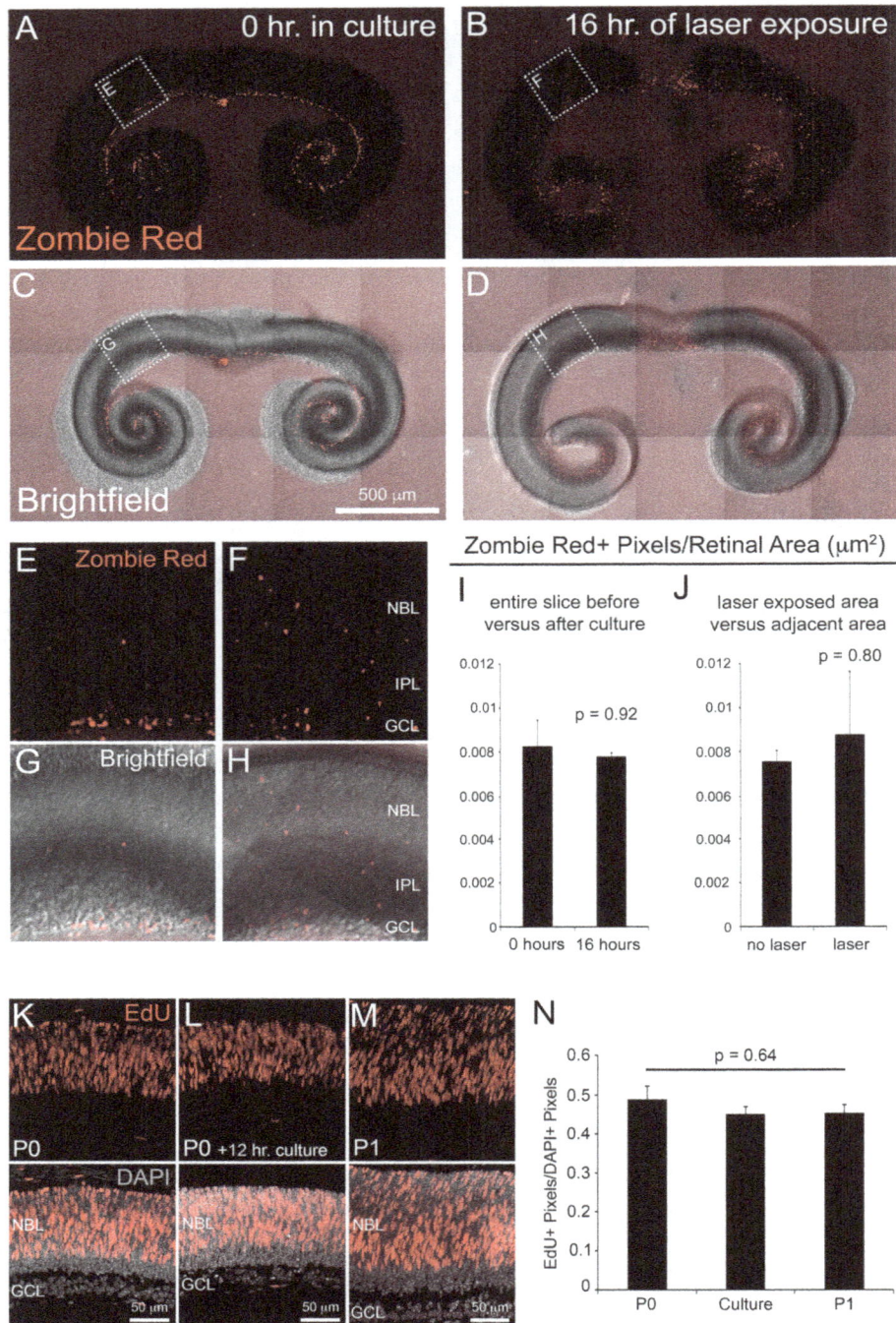

**Fig. 2** Analysis of retinal slice survival and proliferation. Retinal slice cultures stained with Zombie Red™ dye after 0 h (**a** and **c**) and 16 h (**b** and **d**) in culture. Higher magnifications of boxed region in A-D (E-H). The quantification of Zombie Red+ cells (ZR+ pixels/retinal area) showed no significant differences between 0 h and 16 h in culture (**i**) or between tissue exposed to laser versus unexposed (**j**). $n = 9$ per group. EdU labeling (6-h pulse) and quantification of RPCs in P0 and P1 retinae compared to P0 retinal slices time lapse cultures (**k-n**). $n = 3$ per group. Error bars represent SE. Abbreviations: NBL (neuroblastic layer), IPL (inner plexiform layer), GCL (ganglion cell layer)

[25, 38]. Further, these data serve as a positive control for the specificity of ZR labeling of dead/dying cells.

To determine whether slice culture conditions impact RPC survival, ZR+ pixels were counted throughout the entire the neuroblastic layer (NBL) of retinal slices at 0 h and 16 h in culture and we found no significant difference (Fig. 2i). Furthermore, when we compared cell death in laser exposed tissue to an adjacent, non-laser exposed section of the same size, we observed no significant difference (Fig. 2j). These data demonstrate that, after 16 h of live imaging, the NBL of retinal slice cultures does not suffer extensive cell death that would hinder interpretation of the INM time lapse movies. Subsequent live imaging of INM, utilizing the *Fucci* reporters (see below), confirmed this conclusion as we failed to detect significant RPC nuclear fragmentation in any of our time lapse movies (Additional files 6, 7 and 8).

We next performed an assessment of RPC proliferation in our slice cultures and compared that to RPCs in vivo. Specifically, to measure the incidence of S-phase entry, P0 and P1 pups were injected with 5-ethynyl-2 -deoxyuridine (EdU) 6 h before retinae were processed for cryosections and EdU labeling. After 6 h of imaging in culture, P0 retinal slices were incubated with EdU and this was followed by an additional 6 h in culture before EdU labeling of cryosections. As expected, EdU labeling was observed throughout the NBL of the P0 and P1 retinae and the slice cultures (Fig. 2k-m). Quantification of the #EdU+/#DAPI+ pixels revealed no statistically significant decrease in S-phase entry of the slice culture versus either the P0 or the P1 time points (Fig. 2n). These data suggest that our retinal slice imaging protocol does not significantly impact RPC proliferation.

### Analysis of interkinetic nuclear migration within retinal slice cultures

As a first test of our protocol, we performed live imaging of RPC INM. INM describes the periodic movement of the nucleus within a cell that occurs in phase with cell cycle progression and is a common feature of pseudostratified epithelia such as the developing retinal neuroepithelium [5, 11, 35]. INM was first described in the neural tube of chicks and pigs [43] and has since been shown to occur in a variety of tissues in species ranging from mammals to sea anemones [15, 29, 34, 40, 46]. While this evolutionary conservation indicates importance for INM in development, its precise requirement during retinal development remains unclear. However, recent studies of the zebrafish retinae have begun to elucidate the cellular and molecular mechanisms driving INM.

Initially, INM was described by an "elevator model" whereby the nuclei of cells during G1 phase undergo smooth basal migration and, upon G2 entry, nuclei migrate apically until division occurs at the apical end of the cell [43, 46] (Fig. 3a). However, previous live imaging studies performed on zebrafish retinae suggest that nuclei of cells during G1 phase migrate stochastically with a slight basal drift and S phase migration is entirely stochastic (Fig. 3b). G2 INM is indeed directed apically in the zebrafish retina prior to mitosis in the ventricular zone [22, 34]. Based on these findings, we sought to determine whether the same pattern of RPC INM occurs in the mouse.

To track INM, we utilized the *Fucci* cell cycle reporter mouse, which fluorescently labels nuclei based on cell cycle stage [41]. The *Fucci* mouse contains two transgenes each expressing a fluorescent protein. One is a variant of monomeric Kusabira Orange (KO2) and labels nuclei of cells in G1 phase. However, it has also been reported that KO2 is expressed in post-mitotic cells [41]. The other fluorescent protein is monomeric Azami Green (AzG), which labels nuclei of cells in late S and G2 phase. Cells in early S phase express both proteins (Fig. 4a). To determine precisely where the transgenes are expressed in the developing retina, we imaged fixed retinal tissue sections from *Fucci* mice. Since the AzG

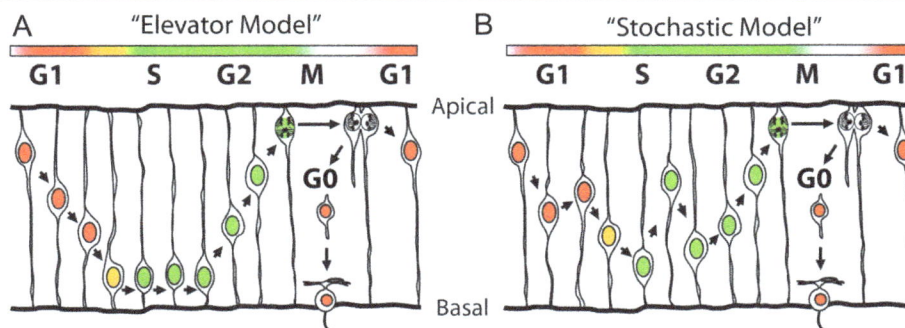

**Fig. 3** Schematic of two models of INM. The "elevator" model (**a**) and the "stochastic" model (**b**). See text for details

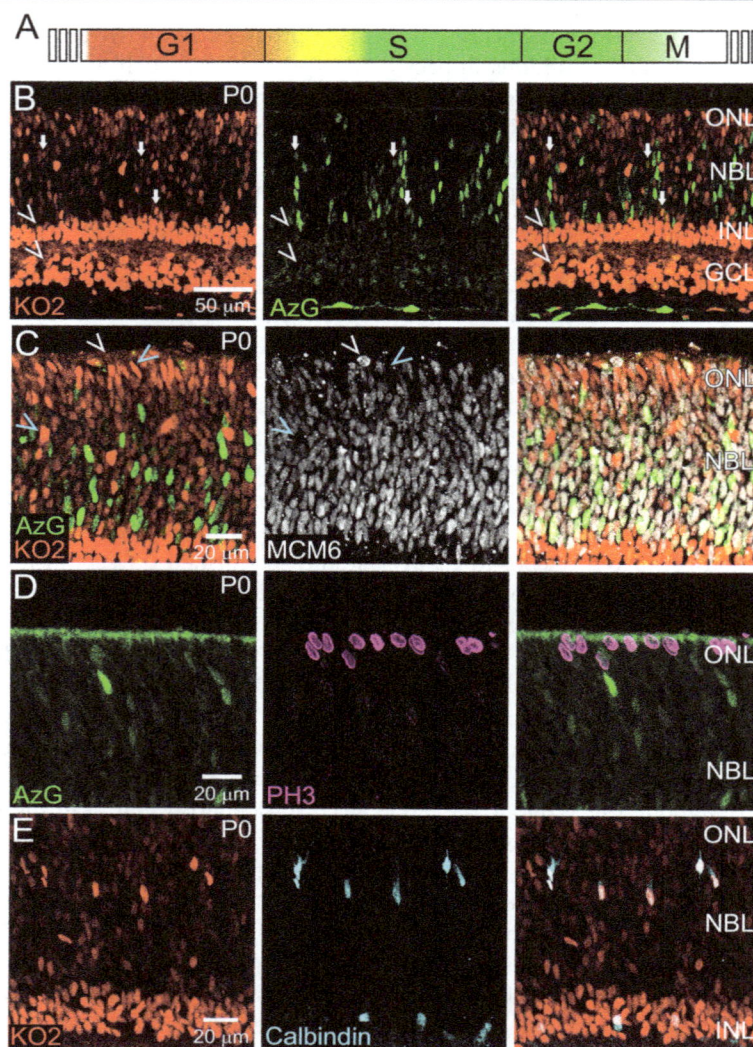

**Fig. 4** Characterization of Fucci+ cells in the P0 retina. Fucci expression throughout the cell cycle (**a**). P0 *Fucci* retinae labelled with anti-AzG (**b**), MCM6 (**c**), PH3 (**d**), and Calbindin (**e**). *n* > 3

signal is weak after fixation, we performed immunohistochemistry using an antibody against AzG. The KO2 reporter did not require immunofluorescence for histological detection. Sections of P0 retinae revealed that KO2 is indeed expressed in the developing inner nuclear layer (INL) and GCL, which is comprised of postmitotic retinal neurons (Fig. 4b, arrowheads). As expected, the NBL is densely populated with RPCs in different stages of the cell cycle. We observed KO2+ G1 phase RPCs, AzG+ late S/G2 phase RPCs, and a small number of KO2+/AzG+ early S phase RPCs (Fig. 4b, arrows indicate KO2+/AzG+ cells).

We next performed immunofluorescence for MCM6, which labels RPCs in all stages of the cell cycle [2]. Most MCM6+ cells are co-labeled with one or both Fucci

markers, with the exception of apically localized rounded nuclei preparing for division (Fig. 4c, white arrowhead). Cell cycle staging was confirmed by phospho-Histone H3 (PH3) labeling of RPC mitosis, which showed a lack of co-localization with AzG (Fig. 4d). We also noticed KO2+ cells within the presumptive HC layer and ONL that were not MCM6+ (Fig. 4c, blue arrowheads) consistent with the perdurance of KO2 in post-mitotic neurons. HC expression of KO2 was confirmed by Calbindin overlap (Fig. 4e). These cells, indicated by their KO2 brightness relative to the RPCs, were excluded from subsequent experiments that aimed to track INM within the NBL.

For culture and live confocal imaging of P0 *Fucci* retinal slices undergoing INM, Z-stacks were acquired every 10 min (Additional file 6). As shown in individual images taken from the time lapse, AzG+ cells were clearly observed migrating apically within the NBL (Fig. 5a, cyan and white arrows). With the spot tracking function in Imaris software, we tracked the migration of both AzG+ and KO2+ nuclei. All AzG+ nuclei migrated apically (Fig. 5b), but some apical migration was preceded by a period of stochastic migration, which was likely during late S phase (color-coded black in Fig. 5b). The KO2+ nuclei moved erratically, but most had an

overall basal displacement (Fig. 5c). To further describe the INM patterns as random or directional, we next calculated the mean square displacement (MSD) of nuclear trajectories as a function of elapsed imaging time. For particles subject to random diffusion, the MSD is a linear function of elapsed time. When movement is directional, the MSD forms a curved line over time. When we sampled the first 80 min of each trajectory, the MSD of KO2+ and AzG+ nuclei were both nonlinear, which suggests these nuclei migrate in a

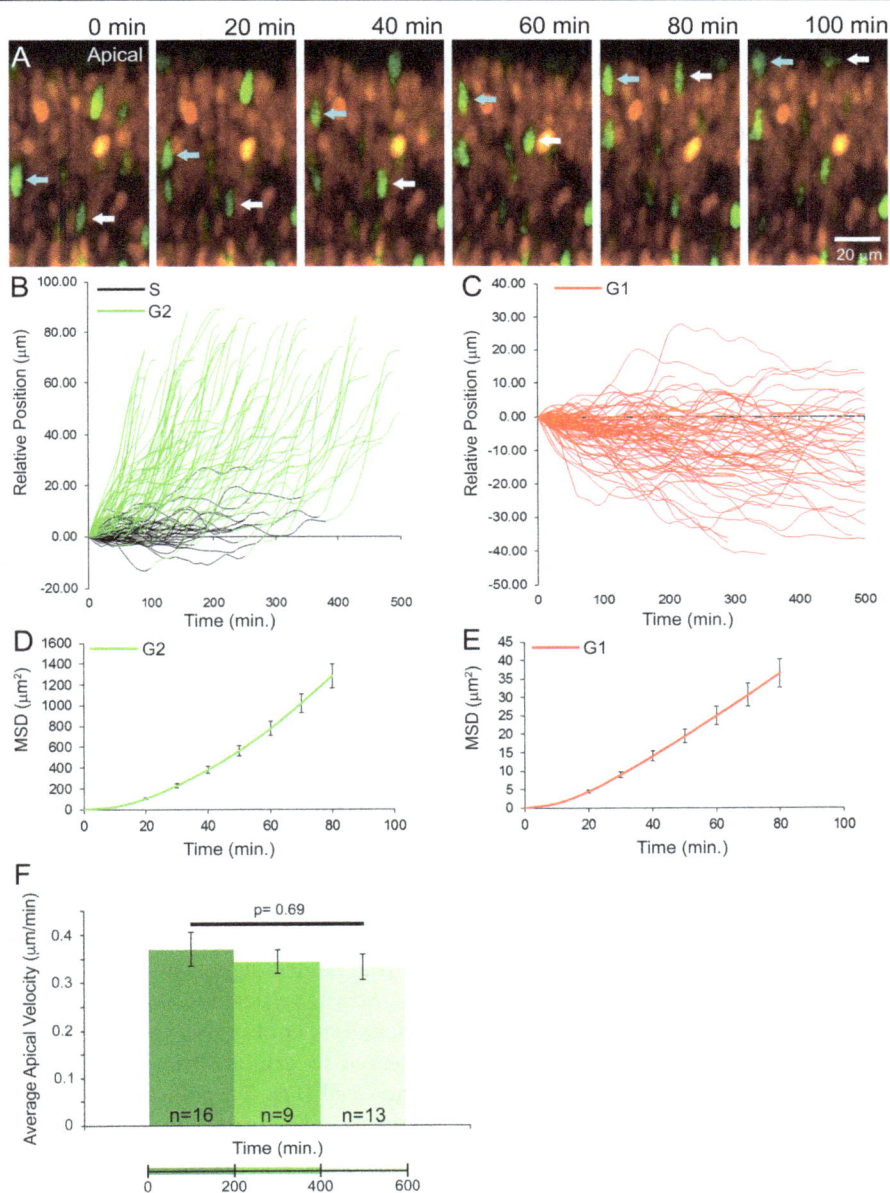

**Fig. 5** Tracking INM in the P0 retinae. Stills from time lapse movie of migrating RPC nuclei. Arrows indicate apically migrating AzG+ (G2-phase) nuclei (**a**). Relative position of nuclei over time (**b-c**). MSD of nuclei plotted over time (**d-e**). Comparison of the average apical velocity of AzG+ cells over the course of the time lapse experiments (**f**)

directional manner (Fig. 5d and e). These findings suggest that the pattern of mouse RPC INM is similar to INM of the zebrafish retina [22, 34]. It also validates our slice culture method as being capable of capturing an essential event during mouse retinogenesis.

As an additional assessment of overall tissue health and tolerance of the live imaging protocol, we quantified the rate of G2 apical INM at different periods throughout the time lapse movies. Apical tracks of G2 nuclei were clustered into three groups (0–200 min, 200–400 min, and 400–600 min in culture) and the average apical velocity (μm/min) of nuclei was quantified for each period. We compared the average velocities among each group using a single factor ANOVA and found no statistically significant difference (Fig. 5f). Therefore, the live imaging protocol does not significantly impact RPC INM in G2 suggesting that cell cycle kinetics are not overtly affected by culture conditions or laser exposure.

### Analysis of *Cyclin D1*$^{-/-}$ RPC interkinetic nuclear migration

Despite being tightly coupled to the cell cycle, chemical inhibition of INM does not cause cell cycle arrest. Rather, cells continue to proliferate, but mitosis is no longer restricted to the apical end of the ventricular zone [28, 31, 49]. In contrast, chemically blocking cell cycle progression halts INM in the rodent brain and zebrafish neuroepithelia [1, 22, 45, 47]. Additionally, studies of zebrafish mutants with an RPC cell cycle period twice as long as wild type exhibit an INM rate that is also proportionally slowed [4, 50].

Information as to how the core cell cycle machinery interfaces with the cellular mechanisms driving INM is only beginning to emerge. The most established role is for Cyclin dependent kinase 1 (CDK1) which, along with CYCLIN A or CYCLIN B, is well-known to regulate the entry into G2 and progression toward M-phase [24, 37]. Pharmaceutical inhibition of cdk1 in zebrafish resulted in RPCs that stalled in G2 and failed to undergo apical INM suggesting that cdk1 is necessary for INM [45]. Remarkably, inhibition of the cdk1 inhibitor wee1 resulted in precocious cdk1 activity and apical migration of RPCs that are presumably in S-phase. Thus, cdk1 activity is both necessary and sufficient for apical INM [45]. It is not yet clear whether a similar role for CDK1 exists during mouse INM or whether other G2-specific genes directly drive INM.

The best, in vivo-characterized mouse RPC cell cycle regulator is CYCLIN D1 [9, 10, 13, 44]. Although its canonical role is to promote S phase entry, CYCLIN D1 is expressed throughout the cell cycle in RPCs, and its loss extends retinal cell cycle length [2, 9, 10]. Specifically, these studies used thymidine analog incorporation and antibody staining in fixed mouse retinal tissue to demonstrate that the length of G1, G2, and M phases

combined was extended in the absence of *Cyclin D1*. Given the tight coupling of cell cycle timing and INM rate, we hypothesized that apical migration during G2 phase in *Cyclin D1*$^{-/-}$ (KO) retinae would be slower than in wildtype (WT) retinae.

To test this, we imaged (at least 12 h per retina) WT ($n = 3$) and KO ($n = 3$) retinae expressing AzG (Additional files 7 and 8). Both WT and KO AzG+ RPCs exhibited the expected apical displacement characteristic of G2 phase (Fig. 6a-b). Using the spot tracking function in Imaris, we tracked the position of 56 AzG+ nuclei from WT RPCs and 54 nuclei from KO RPCs over time. As mentioned previously, AzG labels nuclei of cells during late S and G2 phase. Thus, to analyze G2 apical migration more specifically, we omitted data points prior to the first indication of directed apical migration and plotted the relative nuclear position over time (Fig. 6c-d). We found that AzG+ nuclei in the KO retinae had slower average and slower maximum apical velocities (Fig. 6e-f). Taken together with evidence from previous studies [9, 10], these data suggest that CYCLIN D1 may indirectly regulate INM rate by maintaining cell cycle timing during G2 phase and support conclusions from zebrafish studies that suggest INM rate and cell cycle length are coupled [4, 50].

### Analysis of horizontal cell dynamics

Finally, we sought to determine whether our live imaging protocol is suitable for capturing discrete developmental events among retinal neurons. As a proof-of-concept, we imaged early postnatal horizontal cell (HC) dynamics. We generated *Cx57-iCre*$^{+/tg}$; *Rosa26R-mTmG*$^{+/tg}$ mice [16, 32] in which early postnatal HCs express a membrane-bound green fluorescent protein (eGFP) that clearly highlights HC neurites. The remainder of the retina, without Cre-mediated recombination, is labeled with a membrane-bound tdTomato fluorescent protein (Fig. 7a).

Live imaging of HCs at P2 revealed soma within the presumptive HC layer that showed little movement whereas the neurites were extremely dynamic (Fig. 7a-b and Additional files 9, 10 and 11). Specifically, the more laterally-oriented neurites of adjacent HCs exhibited extension and retraction toward one another and generally maintained significant overlap (Fig. 7c, arrowheads). In contrast, vertically-oriented neurites of the same HCs underwent continuous extension and retraction but appeared to exhibit little or no overlap with the neighboring cell (Fig. 7c, colored arrows and Fig. 7d, colored filaments). To further analyze this cellular behavior, we next measured the territorial overlap between neurites of adjacent HCs (Fig. 7e) [30]. The HC territory over time was determined followed by the overlap of those areas between adjacent cells (Fig. 7f-g). In order to visually highlight territories of overlap, the delineated HC territories over time were shown with a 50% transparency overlaid on the original fluorescence images. Thus, the brighter white regions, covering more horizontally-oriented neurites, indicate overlap whereas we did not detect overlap between vertical neurites (Fig. 7e and Additional file 12). Previous live, multiphoton microscopy of mouse HCs in explant cultures identified these vertical neurites as transient processes that mediate homotypic repulsive interactions driving HC mosaic formation [18].

## Conclusions

Live imaging of developing retinal slices is capable of directly monitoring and quantifying important events during mouse retinogenesis. This method is compatible with a variety of imaging systems and fluorescent reporters thereby making live retinal imaging a more practical option for researchers without access to 2-photon microscopy. The main limitation of this approach is the length of time one can culture and image a retinal slice. In our hands, by 48 h, tissue artifacts were present in the retina and obvious cell blebbing occurred. In the future, by employing conditioned media and other growth factors, we may be able to extend the life of the slice culture. However, several dynamic developmental processes, as demonstrated in this study, can be readily imaged for shorter periods (up to at least 16 h) without obvious signs of significant cell death.

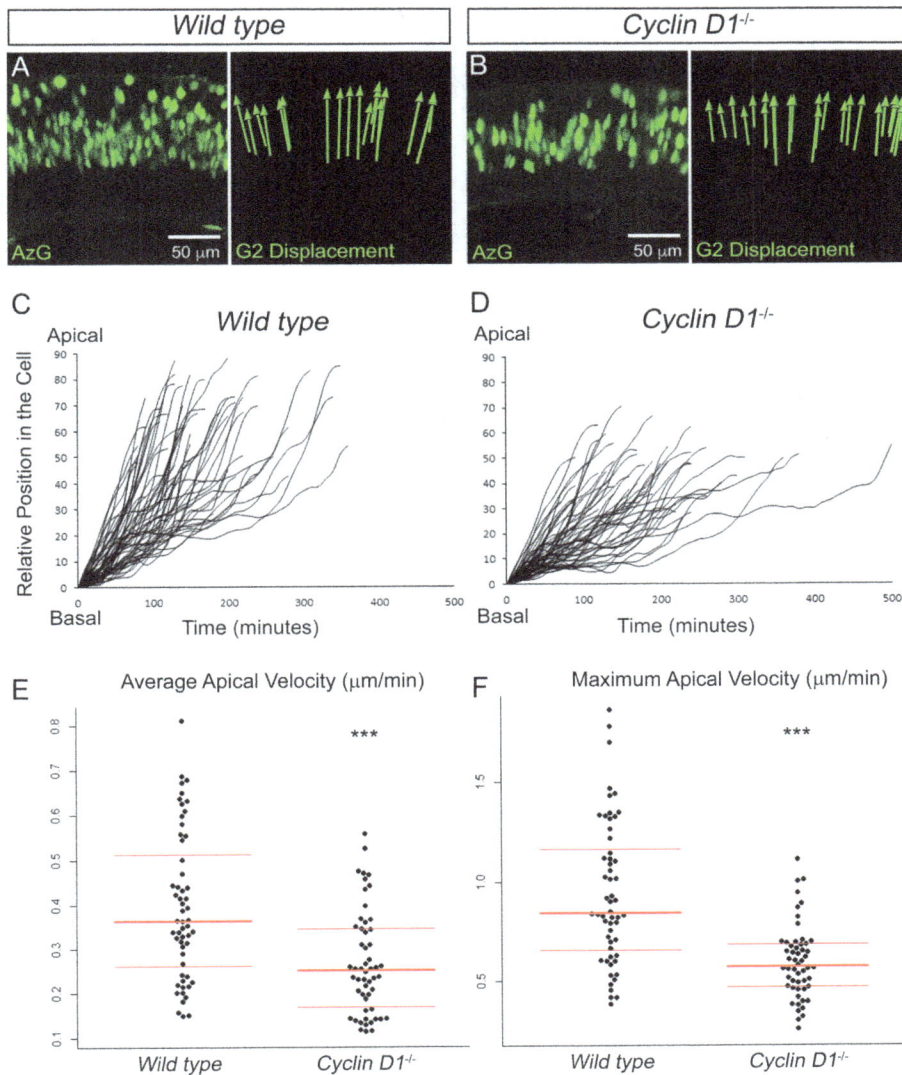

**Fig. 6** Apical migration in the *Cyclin D1*$^{-/-}$ retina. Still images from time lapse movies of migrating wild type and mutant AzG+ RPCs and the overall displacement of each nucleus (**a-b**). Relative position of nuclei over time (**c-d**). The distributions of average and maximum apical velocities of tracked nuclei (**e-f**). Data were collected from 56 nuclei in 3 WT retinae and 54 nuclei in 3 KO retinae. ***$p < 0.001$

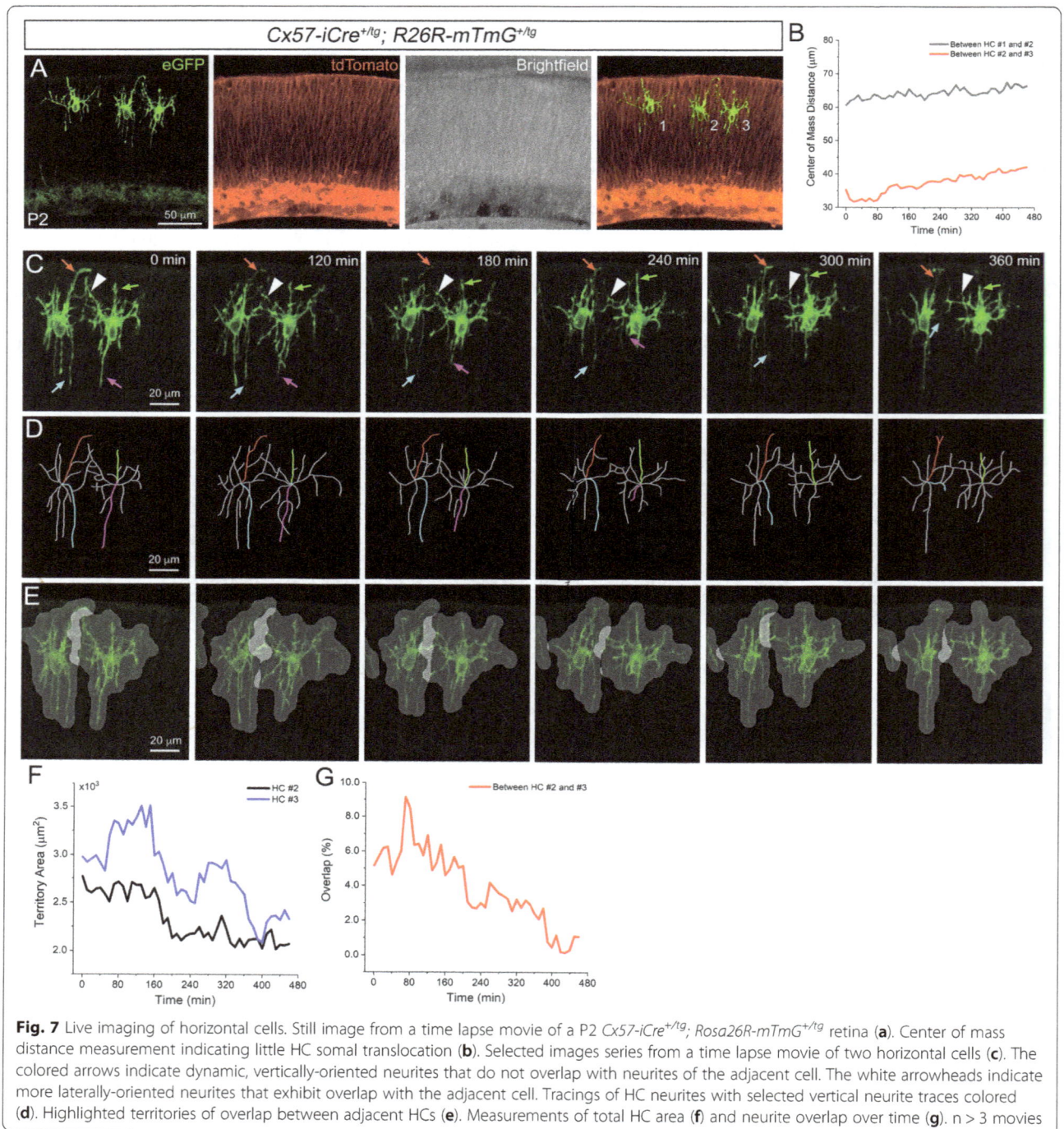

**Fig. 7** Live imaging of horizontal cells. Still image from a time lapse movie of a P2 *Cx57-iCre*<sup>+/tg</sup>; *Rosa26R-mTmG*<sup>+/tg</sup> retina (**a**). Center of mass distance measurement indicating little HC somal translocation (**b**). Selected images series from a time lapse movie of two horizontal cells (**c**). The colored arrows indicate dynamic, vertically-oriented neurites that do not overlap with neurites of the adjacent cell. The white arrowheads indicate more laterally-oriented neurites that exhibit overlap with the adjacent cell. Tracings of HC neurites with selected vertical neurite traces colored (**d**). Highlighted territories of overlap between adjacent HCs (**e**). Measurements of total HC area (**f**) and neurite overlap over time (**g**). n > 3 movies

Furthermore, the cross-sectional view provided by the retinal slice provides excellent resolution of the entire retinal thickness. As an example, using the *Mito-Dendra*<sup>+/tg</sup> mouse, we have recently generated movies of sufficient resolution to capture mitochondrial dynamics within the developing retina [36] (Additional files 13 and 14).

While not explicitly demonstrated in this study, for certain cell types and developmental processes, retinal slice cultures may also circumvent the need for confocal microscopy and commercial environmental chambers. Previously, mouse retinal whole mount explants were shown to develop under $CO_2$-independent culture conditions [33]. Therefore, one may be able to simply construct a homemade heater box [19] surrounding the stage of an epifluorescent microscope.

## Additional files

**Additional file 1:** List of materials used for retinal slice culture preparation and imaging.

**Additional file 2:** List of antibodies used for immunofluorescence.

**Additional file 3:** Code written for MATLAB to quantify Zombie Red+ and EdU+ pixels

**Additional file 4:** Code written for MATLAB to calculate mean square displacement (MSD).

**Additional file 5:** Code written for MATLAB to calculate HC neurite territory overlap.

**Additional file 6:** Time lapse movie of P0 Fucci+ RPCs undergoing INM. Individual nuclei were tracked using Imaris software. Z-stacks with a thickness of 14.4 μm made up of 6 images were collected every 10 min for 650 min. Playback: 10 frames per second.

**Additional file 7:** Time lapse movie of wild type P0 RPCs in undergoing apical migration during G2-phase (AzG+) of the cell cycle. Z-stacks with a thickness of 14.4 μm made up of 6 images were collected every 10 min for 750 min. Playback: 10 frames per second.

**Additional file 8:** Time lapse movie of *Cyclin D1*$^{-/-}$ P0 RPCs in undergoing apical migration during G2-phase (AzG+) of the cell cycle. Z-stacks with a thickness of 14.4 μm made up of 6 images were collected every 10 min for 700 min. Playback: 10 frames per second.

**Additional file 9:** Time lapse movie of P2 horizontal cell dynamics. Z-stacks with a thickness of 19.90 μm made up of 19 images were collected every 10 min for 460 min. Playback: 10 frames per second.

**Additional file 10:** Time lapse movie of P2 horizontal cell dynamics. Z-stacks with a thickness of 19.90 μm made up of 19 images were collected every 10 min for 460 min Playback: 10 frames per second.

**Additional file 11:** Time lapse movie of P2 horizontal cell dynamics. Z-stacks with a thickness of 23.2 μm made up of 22 images were collected every 10 min for 1240 min. Playback: 10 frames per second. (MOV 1788 kb)

**Additional file 12:** Time lapse movie of P2 horizontal cell neurite overlap. Z-stacks with a thickness of 19.90 μm made up of 19 images were collected every 10 min for 460 min. Playback: 10 frames per second. (MOV 1849 kb)

**Additional file 13:** Time lapse movie of mitochondrial dynamics within a P0 retina. Z-stacks with a thickness of 14.4 μm made up of 6 images were collected every 10 min for 530 min. Playback: 15 frames per second. (MOV 49960 kb)

**Additional file 14:** High magnification time lapse movie of the same retina in Additional file 13 imaged for an additional 390 min. Playback: 15 frames per second. (MOV 39725 kb)

## Abbreviations
AzG: Azami Green; FBS: Fetal Bovine Serum; GCL: Ganglion Cell Layer; HC: Horizontal Cell; INL: Inner Nuclear Layer; INM: Interkinetic Nuclear Migration; KO2: Kusabira Orange; MSD: Mean Square Displacement; NBL: Neuroblastic Layer; ONL: Outer Nuclear Layer; RPC: Retinal Progenitor Cell

## Acknowledgements
We thank members of the Poché lab for critical reading of this manuscript and support throughout the project. We thank Dr. Nicholas Brecha for providing the *Cx57-iCre*$^{+/tg}$ mice and Dr. Edward Levine for providing the *Cyclin D1*$^{-/-}$ mice. We also thank Dr. Mary Dickinson and the Optical Imaging and Vital Microscopy facility at Baylor College of Medicine for their services.

## Funding
This work was supported by grants from the National Institutes of Health (NIH): R01 EY024906 to Ross Poché (PI) and T32 EY007102 to Anthony Barrasso (Graeme Mardon, PI) as well as The BrightFocus Foundation to Ross Poché (PI).

## Authors' contributions
APB performed microscopy experiments and analysis of images and movies. SW wrote the MATLAB codes to quantify ZR pixels, calculate MSD, and generate HC territories and assisted in data analysis. XT helped maintain the mouse colony and assisted with experiments. AEC assisted in protocol design and refinement. IVL provided valuable guidance on data acquisition, data analysis, and figure design. RAP designed the protocol, obtained preliminary movies, assisted on various experiments, and provided guidance throughout the project. All authors read and approved the final manuscript written by APB and RAP.

## Competing interests
The authors declare that they have no competing interests.

## Author details
$^1$Department of Molecular Physiology and Biophysics, Baylor College of Medicine, Houston, TX 77030, USA. $^2$Program in Developmental Biology, Baylor College of Medicine, Houston, TX 77030, USA. $^3$Program in Integrative Molecular and Biomedical Sciences, Baylor College of Medicine, Houston, TX 77030, USA.

## References
1. Baffet AD, Hu DJ, Vallee RB. Cdk1 activates pre-mitotic nuclear envelope dynein recruitment and apical nuclear migration in neural stem cells. Dev Cell. 2015;33:703–16.
2. Barton KM, Levine EM. Expression patterns and cell cycle profiles of PCNA, MCM6, cyclin D1, cyclin A2, cyclin B1, and phosphorylated histone H3 in the developing mouse retina. Dev Dyn. 2008;237:672–82.
3. Bassett EA, Wallace VA. Cell fate determination in the vertebrate retina. Trends Neurosci. 2012;35:565–73.
4. Baye LM, Link BA. The disarrayed mutation results in cell cycle and neurogenesis defects during retinal development in zebrafish. BMC Dev Biol. 2007;7:28.
5. Baye LM, Link BA. Nuclear migration during retinal development. Brain Res. 2008;1192:29–36.
6. Cayouette M. The orientation of cell division influences cell-fate choice in the developing mammalian retina. Development. 2003;130:2329–39.
7. Cayouette M, Whitmore A, Jeffery G, Raff M. Asymmetric segregation of numb in retinal development and the influence of the pigmented epithelium. J Neurosci. 2001;21:5643–51.
8. Collinson JM, Hill RE, West JD. Analysis of mouse eye development with chimeras and mosaics. Int J Dev Biol. 2004;48:793–804.
9. Das G, Choi Y, Sicinski P, Levine EM. Cyclin D1 fine-tunes the neurogenic output of embryonic retinal progenitor cells. Neural Dev. 2009;4:15.
10. Das G, Clark AM, Levine EM. Cyclin D1 inactivation extends proliferation and alters histogenesis in the postnatal mouse retina. Dev Dyn. 2012;241:941–52.
11. Das T, Payer B, Cayouette M, Harris WA. In vivo time-lapse imaging of cell divisions during neurogenesis in the developing zebrafish retina. Neuron. 2003;37:597–609.
12. Donovan SL, Dyer MA. Preparation and square wave electroporation of retinal explant cultures. Nat Protoc. 2006;1:2710–8.
13. Fantl V, Stamp G, Andrews A, Rosewell I, Dickson C. Mice lacking cyclin D1 are small and show defects in eye and mammary gland development. Genes Dev. 1995;9:2364–72.
14. Groeger G, Mackey AM, Pettigrew CA, Bhatt L, Cotter TG. Stress-induced activation of Nox contributes to cell survival signalling via production of hydrogen peroxide. J Neurochem. 2009;109:1544–54.
15. Grosse AS, Pressprich MF, Curley LB, Hamilton KL, Margolis B, Hildebrand JD, Gumucio DL. Cell dynamics in fetal intestinal epithelium: implications for intestinal growth and morphogenesis. Development. 2011;138:4423–32.
16. Hirano AA, Liu X, Boulter J, Grove J, Perez de Sevilla Muller L, Barnes S, Brecha NC. Targeted deletion of vesicular GABA transporter from retinal horizontal cells eliminates feedback modulation of photoreceptor calcium channels. eNeuro. 2016;3(1):1–13.
17. Hoon M, Okawa H, Della Santina L, Wong RO. Functional architecture of the retina: development and disease. Prog Retin Eye Res. 2014;42:44–84.
18. Huckfeldt RM, Schubert T, Morgan JL, Godinho L, Di Cristo G, Huang ZJ, Wong RO. Transient neurites of retinal horizontal cells exhibit columnar tiling via homotypic interactions. Nat Neurosci. 2009;12:35–43.

19. Jones EA, Crotty D, Kulesa PM, Waters CW, Baron MH, Fraser SE, Dickinson ME. Dynamic in vivo imaging of postimplantation mammalian embryos using whole embryo culture. Genesis. 2002;34:228–35.

20. Kechad A, Jolicoeur C, Tufford A, Mattar P, Chow RWY, Harris WA, Cayouette M. Numb is required for the production of terminal asymmetric cell divisions in the developing mouse retina. J Neurosci. 2012;32:17197–210.

21. Lee JE, Liang KJ, Fariss RN, Wong WT. Ex vivo dynamic imaging of retinal microglia using time-lapse confocal microscopy. Invest Ophthalmol Vis Sci. 2008;49:4169–76.

22. Leung L, Klopper AV, Grill SW, Harris WA, Norden C. Apical migration of nuclei during G2 is a prerequisite for all nuclear motion in zebrafish neuroepithelia. Development. 2011;138:5003–13.

23. Liang KJ, Lee JE, Wang YD, Ma W, Fontainhas AM, Fariss RN, Wong WT. Regulation of dynamic behavior of retinal microglia by CX3CR1 signaling. Invest Ophthalmol Vis Sci. 2009;50:4444–51.

24. Malumbres M, Barbacid M. Mammalian cyclin-dependent kinases. Trends Biochem Sci. 2005;30:630–41.

25. Manabe S, Kashii S, Honda Y, Yamamoto R, Katsuki H, Akaike A. Quantification of axotomized ganglion cell death by explant culture of the rat retina. Neurosci Lett. 2002;334:33–6.

26. Matsuda T, Cepko CL. Electroporation and RNA interference in the rodent retina in vivo and in vitro. Proc Natl Acad Sci U S A. 2004;101:16–22.

27. Matsuda T, Cepko CL. Controlled expression of transgenes introduced by in vivo electroporation. Proc Natl Acad Sci U S A. 2007;104:1027–32.

28. Messier P, Auclair C. Effect of Cytochalasin B on Interkinetic nuclear migration in the Chick embryo. Dev Biol. 1974;36:218–23.

29. Meyer EJ, Ikmi A, Gibson MC. Interkinetic nuclear migration is a broadly conserved feature of cell division in pseudostratified epithelia. Curr Biol. 2011;21:485–91.

30. Morgan JL, Schubert T, Wong RO. Developmental patterning of glutamatergic synapses onto retinal ganglion cells. Neural Dev. 2008;3:8.

31. Murciano A, Zamora J, Lopezsanchez J, Frade J. Interkinetic nuclear movement may provide spatial clues to the regulation of neurogenesis. Mol Cell Neurosci. 2002;21:285–300.

32. Muzumdar MD, Tasic B, Miyamichi K, Li L, Luo L. A global double-fluorescent Cre reporter mouse. Genesis. 2007;45:593–605.

33. Nickerson PE, Ronellenfitch KM, Csuzdi NF, Boyd JD, Howard PL, Delaney KR, Chow RL. Live imaging and analysis of postnatal mouse retinal development. BMC Dev Biol. 2013;13.

34. Norden C, Young S, Link BA, Harris WA. Actomyosin is the main driver of interkinetic nuclear migration in the retina. Cell. 2009;138:1195–208.

35. Pearson RA, Luneborg NL, Becker DL, Mobbs P. Gap junctions modulate interkinetic nuclear movement in retinal progenitor cells. J Neurosci. 2005;25:10803–14.

36. Pham AH, McCaffery JM, Chan DC. Mouse lines with photo-activatable mitochondria to study mitochondrial dynamics. Genesis. 2012;50:833–43.

37. Pines J, Rieder C. Re-staging mitosis: a contemporary view of mitotic progression. Nat Cell Biol. 2001;3.

38. Rabacchi SA, Bonfanti L, Liu XH, Maffei L. Apoptotic cell death induced by optic nerve lesion in the neonatal rat. J Neurosci. 1994;14:5292–301.

39. Roehlecke C, Schumann U, Ader M, Knels L, Funk RHW. Influence of blue light on photoreceptors in a live retinal explant system. Mol Vis. 2011;17:876–84.

40. Rujano MA, Sanchez-Pulido L, Pennetier C, le Dez G, Basto R. The microcephaly protein asp regulates neuroepithelium morphogenesis by controlling the spatial distribution of myosin II. Nat Cell Biol. 2013;15:1294–306.

41. Sakaue-Sawano A, Kurokawa H, Morimura T, Hanyu A, Hama H, Osawa H, Kashiwagi S, Fukami K, Miyata T, Miyoshi H, Imamura T, Ogawa M, Masai H, Miyawaki A. Visualizing spatiotemporal dynamics of multicellular cell-cycle progression. Cell. 2008;132:487–98.

42. Sanes JR. Analysing cell lineage with a recombinant retrovirus. Trends Neurosci. 1989;12:21–8.

43. Sauer FC. Mitosis in the neural tube. J Comp Neurol. 1935;62:377–405.

44. Sicinski P, Donaher J, Parker S, Li T, Fazeli A, Gardner H, Haslam S, Bronson R, Elledge S, Weinberg R. Cyclin D1 provides a link between development and oncogenesis in the retina and breast. Cell. 1995;82:621–30.

45. Strzyz PJ, Lee HO, Sidhaye J, Weber IP, Leung LC, Norden C. Interkinetic nuclear migration is centrosome independent and ensures apical cell division to maintain tissue integrity. Dev Cell. 2015;32:203–19.

46. Tsai JW, Lian WN, Kemal S, Kriegstein AR, Vallee RB. Kinesin 3 and cytoplasmic dynein mediate interkinetic nuclear migration in neural stem cells. Nat Neurosci. 2010;13:1463–71.

47. Ueno M, Katayama K, Yamauchi H, Nakayama H, Doi K. Cell cycle progression is required for nuclear migration of neural progenitor cells. Brain Res. 2006;1088:57–67.

48. Veleri S, Lazar CH, Chang B, Sieving PA, Banin E, Swaroop A. Biology and therapy of inherited retinal degenerative disease: insights from mouse models. Dis Model Mech. 2015;8:109–29.

49. Webster W, Langman J. The effect of Cytochalasin B on the Neuroepithelial cells of the mouse embryo. Am J Anat. 1978;152:209–21.

50. Willer GB, Lee VM, Gregg RG, Link BA. Analysis of the zebrafish perplexed mutation reveals tissue-specific roles for de novo pyrimidine synthesis during development. Genetics. 2005;170:1827–37.

51. Williams PR, Morgan JL, Kerschensteiner D, Wong RO. In vitro imaging of retinal whole mounts. Cold Spring Harb Protoc. 2013;2013.

52. Zabel MK, Zhao L, Zhang Y, Gonzalez SR, Ma W, Wang X, Fariss RN, Wong WT. Microglial phagocytosis and activation underlying photoreceptor degeneration is regulated by CX3CL1-CX3CR1 signaling in a mouse model of retinitis pigmentosa. Glia. 2016;64:1479–91.

# 13

# The Hunchback temporal transcription factor establishes, but is not required to maintain, early-born neuronal identity

Keiko Hirono[1,2,3], Minoree Kohwi[4], Matt Q. Clark[1,2,3], Ellie S. Heckscher[5] and Chris Q. Doe[1,2,3]*

## Abstract

**Background:** *Drosophila* and mammalian neural progenitors typically generate a diverse family of neurons in a stereotyped order. Neuronal diversity can be generated by the sequential expression of temporal transcription factors. In *Drosophila*, neural progenitors (neuroblasts) sequentially express the temporal transcription factors Hunchback (Hb), Kruppel, Pdm, and Castor. Hb is necessary and sufficient to specify early-born neuronal identity in multiple lineages, and is maintained in the post-mitotic neurons produced during each neuroblast expression window. Surprisingly, nothing is currently known about whether Hb acts in neuroblasts or post-mitotic neurons (or both) to specify first-born neuronal identity.

**Methods:** Here we selectively remove Hb from post-mitotic neurons, and assay the well-characterized NB7-1 and NB1-1 lineages for defects in neuronal identity and function.

**Results:** We find that loss of Hb from embryonic and larval post-mitotic neurons does not affect neuronal identity. Furthermore, removing Hb from post-mitotic neurons throughout the entire CNS has no effect on larval locomotor velocity, a sensitive assay for motor neuron and pre-motor neuron function.

**Conclusions:** We conclude that Hb functions in progenitors (neuroblasts/GMCs) to establish heritable neuronal identity that is maintained by a Hb-independent mechanism.
We suggest that Hb acts in neuroblasts to establish an epigenetic state that is permanently maintained in early-born neurons.

## Background

Development of the central nervous system (CNS) is multi-step process. In both mammals and *Drosophila*, the earliest steps are spatial patterning to define a neuroectodermal territory, followed by more precise spatial patterning to generate distinct progenitor domains (reviewed in [23, 43]). Subsequently, both mammals and *Drosophila* progenitors can sequentially express temporal transcription factors that specify neural identity based on birth-order (mouse: [2, 14, 32]) (fly: [3–7, 9, 18, 22, 24, 25, 34, 35, 37, 46]). The integration of spatial and temporal cues results in the production of a specific neuronal identity (reviewed in [1, 15, 38, 40]). Lastly, terminal selector genes regulate gene expression

conferring distinct neural subtypes (e.g. dopaminergic neurons or cholinergic neurons); the defining feature of terminal selector genes is that their expression is maintained for the life of the neuron where it maintains the functional properties of the neuron (reviewed in [1, 21]).

Terminal selector genes are not the only class of regulators that are maintained by post-mitotic neurons. Many temporal transcription factors are not only transiently expressed during progenitor lineages, but also maintained in post-mitotic neurons produced during each progenitor expression window. For example, embryonic ventral nerve cord neuroblasts sequentially express the temporal transcription factors Hunchback (Hb), Kruppel, Pdm1/2 (Nubbin and Pdm2, Flybase), and Castor (reviewed in [38]); three of these factors – Hb, Kruppel, and Castor – maintain expression into post-mitotic neurons born during each neuroblast expression window (Fig. 1a). Similarly, optic lobe neuroblasts sequentially

---

* Correspondence: cdoe@uoregon.edu
[1]Howard Hughes Medical Institute, Eugene 97403, USA
[2]Institute of Molecular Biology, Eugene 97403, USA
Full list of author information is available at the end of the article

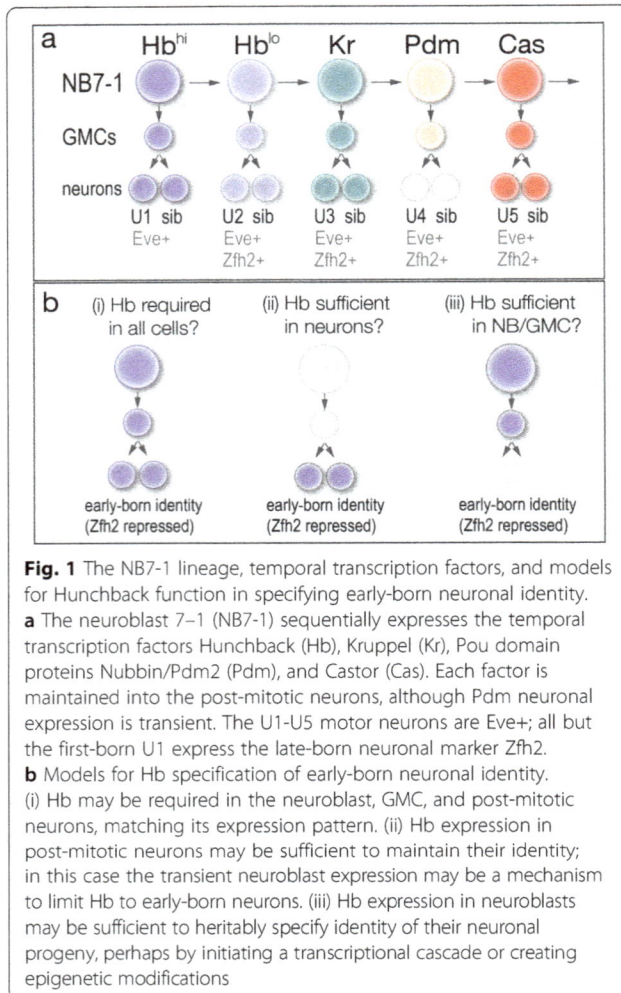

**Fig. 1** The NB7-1 lineage, temporal transcription factors, and models for Hunchback function in specifying early-born neuronal identity. **a** The neuroblast 7–1 (NB7-1) sequentially expresses the temporal transcription factors Hunchback (Hb), Kruppel (Kr), Pou domain proteins Nubbin/Pdm2 (Pdm), and Castor (Cas). Each factor is maintained into the post-mitotic neurons, although Pdm neuronal expression is transient. The U1-U5 motor neurons are Eve+; all but the first-born U1 express the late-born neuronal marker Zfh2. **b** Models for Hb specification of early-born neuronal identity. (i) Hb may be required in the neuroblast, GMC, and post-mitotic neurons, matching its expression pattern. (ii) Hb expression in post-mitotic neurons may be sufficient to maintain their identity; in this case the transient neuroblast expression may be a mechanism to limit Hb to early-born neurons. (iii) Hb expression in neuroblasts may be sufficient to heritably specify identity of their neuronal progeny, perhaps by initiating a transcriptional cascade or creating epigenetic modifications

express Homothorax, Eyeless, Sloppy paired, Dichaete, and Tailless; the four earlier temporal stages generate neurons that inherit and maintain the temporal transcription factor present at their birth, although some Eyeless, Sloppy paired or Dichaete progeny lose temporal transcription factor expression [31]. Surprisingly, however, the role of temporal transcription factors in post-mitotic neurons has yet to be investigated.

Here we determine the role of the Hb temporal transcription factor in post-mitotic neurons of the well-characterized NB7-1 lineage [12, 17, 18, 22, 25, 28, 29, 33, 35, 37], with additional analysis of the role of Hb in post-mitotic neurons of the NB1-1 lineage [22]. The NB7-1 lineage is shown in Fig. 1a: it produces five GMCs that each express the homeodomain protein Even-skipped (Eve) just before they divide to produce the Eve+ U1-U5 motor neurons and their Eve- sibling interneurons [12, 37]. U1 maintains high Hb protein levels and represses Zfh2 expression; U2 maintains lower Hb protein levels and has low Zfh2 levels; U3-U5 have

no Hb protein and have high Zfh2 levels [22]. Similar Eve, Hb, and Zfh2 expression patterns are observed for the NB1-1 and NB4-2 lineages [22]. Thus, Zfh2 expression can be used to distinguish first-born from later-born neurons in multiple neuroblast lineages. In addition, the first-born neurons in all three lineages have axon projections to dorsal body wall muscles, whereas later-born neurons project to more ventral muscles or are interneurons [22, 30].

The role of Hb in the NB7-1, NB1-1, and NB4-2 lineages has been well characterized. Loss of Hb throughout these lineages leads to failure to produce Eve+ early-born neurons (NB7-1) or failure to repress the late-born marker Zfh2 (NB1-1 and NB4-2). Conversely, misexpression of Hb throughout these lineages leads to ectopic Zfh2- neurons with axons targeting dorsal muscles similar to endogenous first-born neurons [22, 37]. Thus, Hb represses Zfh2 and specifies early-born neuronal identity in multiple neuroblast lineages. Hb is expressed in neuroblasts, GMCs, and neurons – which of these cell types requires Hb to establish or maintain early-born neuronal identity? Hb could be required in all cells (Fig. 1b, i); Hb could be required only in post-mitotic neurons (its transient expression in neuroblasts could be simply a mechanism to restrict its expression to early-born neurons; Fig. 1b, ii) or Hb could be required only in neuroblasts/GMCs (Fig. 1b, iii). Here we use cell type specific *hb* RNAi to selectively remove Hb from post-mitotic neurons, and show that Hb in neuroblasts/GMCs is sufficient for stable and long-lasting early-born neuronal identity (even when the neurons lack Hb protein). This is the first analysis of any *Drosophila* temporal transcription factor function in post-mitotic neurons, and it shows that the Hb temporal transcription factor functions differently from terminal selector genes, which are required to maintain post-mitotic neuronal properties (reviewed in [1, 21]).

## Methods
### Fly stocks
*en-gal4* – Bloomington stock 1973. Expressed in row 6/7 neuroectoderm and neuroblasts (A. Brand and K. Yoffe, unpublished) [22].

*CQ2-gal4 (II)* – Bloomington stock 7468. Expressed just prior to U1 birth.

*elav-gal4* – Bloomington stock 8760. Expressed all neuroblasts and neurons.

*UAS-hb RNAi* – Bloomington stock 34704. *hunchback* RNAi transgene.

*yellow white* (*yw*) – Bloomington stock 6598. Control for cell fate assays.

*UAS-mCherry RNAi* – Bloomington stock 35785. Control for behavior.

$hb^{P1}$, $hb^{FB}$/TM3 $ftzlacZ$ – used to specifically remove $hb$ CNS expression; $hb^{P1}$ is a transgene that recapitulates blastoderm $hb$ expression; $hb^{FB}$ is a $hb$ null allele [22].

$sca$-$gal4$, $UAS$-$hb$ – used to express Hb in the neuroectoderm and neuroblasts [12, 37].

### Immunostaining, Imaging, and Figure preparation

Antibody staining was performed according to standard methods [28]. Primary antibodies, dilutions and sources were: chicken anti-GFP 1:500 (Aves Labs, Inc., Tigard, OR USA); rabbit anti-Hb 1:200 for embryos, 1:400 for larvae [46]; mouse anti-Even-skipped (3C10-c for embryos with 1:50, 2B8 for larvae with 1:75) and mouse anti-Engrailed (4D9) 1:5 (Developmental Studies Hybridoma Bank, University of Iowa, IA, USA); rat anti-Zfh2 1:500 [47]. Donkey anti-chicken Alexa Fluor 488-, donkey anti-rat Alexa Fluor 488-, donkey anti-rabbit Alexa Fluor 488-, donkey anti-mouse Alexa Fluor 647-, and donkey anti-rabbit Alexa Fluor 647-conjugated secondary antibodies were from Jackson ImmunoResearch (West Grove, PA USA). Goat anti-rabbit Alexa Fluor 555-, goat anti-mouse Alexa Fluor 555- and goat anti-rat Alexa Fluor 555-conjugated secondary antibodies were from Invitrogen (Eugene, OR USA). Confocal image stacks were collected using Zeiss LSM 700 confocal microscope, processed using ImageJ (NIH) and Photoshop (Adobe Systems Inc., Mountain View, CA USA); in some cases images were brightened using linear gain adjustment using the Levels command in Photoshop; when used, the entire panel was processed identically. Figures were assembled in Illustrator (Adobe Systems Inc., Mountain View, CA USA).

### Larval locomotor assays

Bright-field whole larval behavioral recordings were done using newly hatched first instar larvae. Behavior arenas were made of 6% agar in grape juice, 2 mm thick and 5.5 cm in diameter. The arenas were placed under a Leica S8APO dissecting microscope and red light (700 nm, Metaphase Technologies) illuminated a single larva. The microscope was equipped with a Scion1394 monochrome CCD Camera, using Scion VisiCapture software in ImageJ. Larva were tracked using FIM Tracker software [39]. For each larva, speed was calculated by dividing total distance traveled by the larval centroid by the time elapsed during the recording period.

## Results

### Loss of Hunchback from both neuroblast and neurons eliminates early-born neuronal identity

We wanted to determine whether our $hb$ RNAi transgene was strong enough to eliminate detectable Hb protein and replicate the $hb$ null mutant phenotype. We expressed $UAS$-$hb^{RNAi}$ using $engrailed$-$gal4$ ($en$-$gal4$), which is expressed in the posterior compartment neuroectoderm,

NB7-1, and its U1-U5 neuronal progeny [18] (Additional file 1: Figure S1a). In wild type stage 10 embryos, all neuroblasts have uniform Hb expression [17, 22]. In contrast, $en$-$gal4$ $UAS$-$hb^{RNAi}$ stage 10 embryos have reduced Hb protein levels in neuroblasts within the $en$-$gal4$ $UAS$-$hb^{RNAi}$ domain (Fig. 2a,b).

We next determined whether $en$-$gal4$ $UAS$-$hb^{RNAi}$ could mimic the $hb$ mutant phenotype in the NB7-1 lineage. In wild type stage 16 embryos, the Eve+ U1 motor neuron is Hb+ Zfh2- due to Hb repression of $zfh2$ (Fig. 2c, quantified in 2e). In $en$-$gal4$ $UAS$-$hb^{RNAi}$ stage 16 embryos, the Eve+ U1 motor neuron lacks all detectable Hb protein and has de-repressed Zfh2 (Fig. 2d, quantified in 2e). This is a slightly weaker phenotype than genetic ablation of Hb expression in the NB7-1 lineage [22], perhaps due to the low levels of Hb in the neuroblast (see Discussion). We examined earlier stage embryos to determine when Hb was lost from the U1 neuron, and found that Hb is undetectable from the time of U1 birth at stage 11, although it takes several hours for Zfh2 to become de-repressed (Fig. 2e). We conclude that $hb$ RNAi is capable of removing some Hb protein from NB7-1 and all detectable Hb protein from the U1 neuron, resulting in abnormal U1 neuronal identity.

### Loss of Hunchback from neurons does not alter early-born neuronal identity

To determine if loss of Hb from the neuroblast or neuron leads to de-repression of Zfh2 and abnormal neuronal identity, we specifically decreased Hb from the U1 post-mitotic neuron. We used the $CQ2$-$gal4$ (also called $eve$-$gal4$ [12] or $eve$+ $3.5$-$4.3$-$gal4$ [37]) which has no NB7-1 expression but is expressed in GMCs about an hour before they divide to produce U motor neurons [12, 37] (Additional file 1: Figure S1b). In wild type stage 16 embryos, the Eve+ U1 motor neuron is Hb+ Zfh2- (Fig. 3a). In $CQ2$-$gal4$ $UAS$-$hb^{RNAi}$ stage 16 embryos, the Eve+ U1 motor neuron lacks all detectable Hb protein, but most have not de-repressed $zfh2$ (Fig. 3b, quantified in 3e). These results show that Hb is not continuously required in the U1 neuron to maintain $zfh2$ repression; this feature of early-born neurons must be established by transient Hb function in the neuroblast, GMC, or young neuron and heritably maintained by a Hb-independent mechanism.

To determine how long $CQ2$-$gal4$ $UAS$-$hb^{RNAi}$ can keep Hb levels off in the U1 motor neuron, and how long Zfh2 remains repressed in the absence of Hb, we examined $CQ2$-$gal4$ $UAS$-$hb^{RNAi}$ animals at the second larval instar stage. In wild type larvae, the Eve+ U1 neuron is Hb+ Zfh2- (Fig. 3c, quantified in 3e). In $CQ2$-$gal4$ $UAS$-$hb^{RNAi}$ larvae, the Eve+ U1 neuron is Hb- yet Zfh2 is still repressed (Fig. 3d, quantified in 3e). Thus,

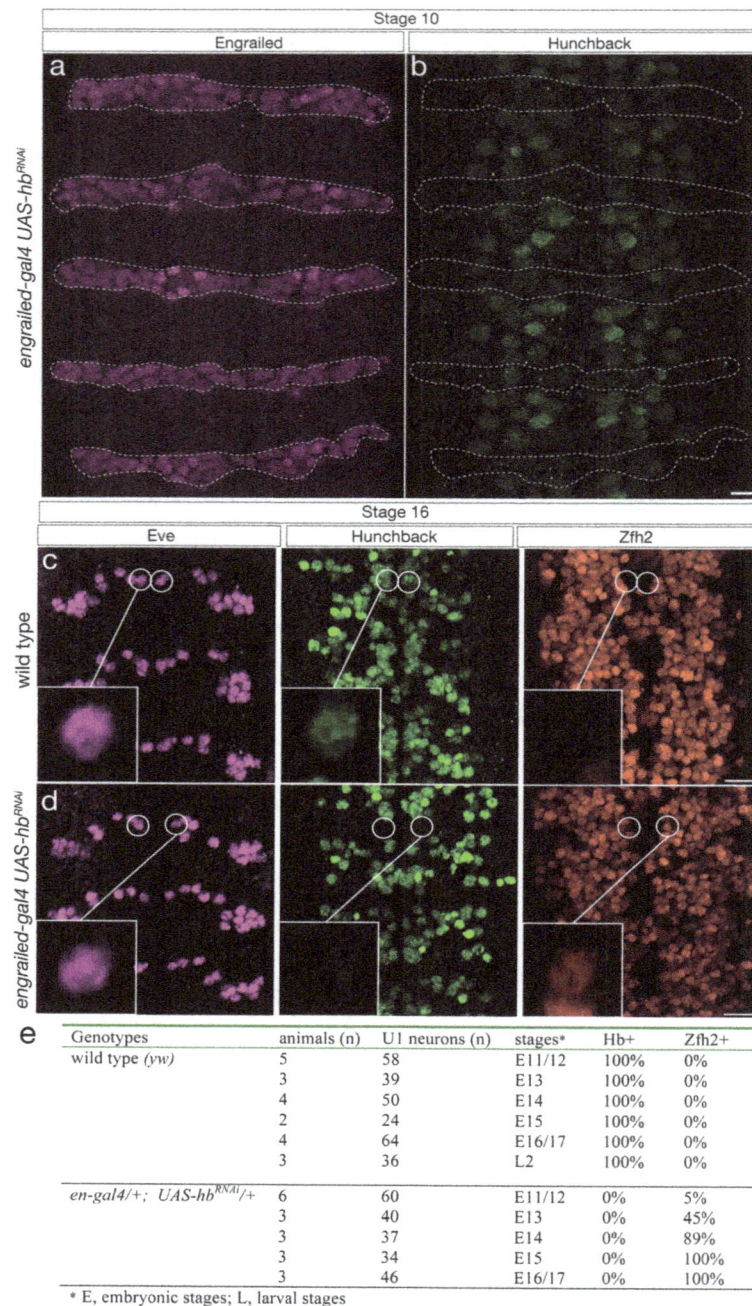

**Fig. 2** Loss of Hunchback from neuroblasts and neurons eliminates early-born neuronal identity. **a, b** Using *engrailed-gal4* (*en-gal4*) to drive *UAS-hunchback RNAi* (*UAS-hb$^{RNAi}$*) results in reduced Hb protein levels in row 6 and row 7 neuroblasts. Scale bars, 10 μm. **c** Wild type (*y w*) stage 16 embryo, three segments shown. U1 motor neurons (*circled*) are Eve+ Hb+ and Zfh2-. **d** *en-gal4 UAS-hb$^{RNAi}$* stage 16 embryo, three segments shown. U1 motor neurons (*circled*) are Eve+ Hb- and Zfh2+. Anterior up, ventral midline at center of each panel, scale bar, 10 μm. **e** Quantification

even prolonged loss of Hb does not lead to *zfh2* de-repression.

We next used a completely independent method for neuron-specific elimination of Hb and assayed a second neuroblast lineage (NB1-1). We used a genotype lacking all Hb expression in the CNS (*hb$^{P1}$ hb$^{FB}$/hb$^{P1}$ hb$^{FB}$*; [22])

plus *sca-gal4 UAS-hb* transgenes that transiently drive Hb expression in neuroblasts, GMCs and young neurons [37] (Additional file 1: Figure S1c). In this experiment, we assayed the first-born Eve+ aCC/pCC sibling neurons from the NB1-1 lineage. In wild type stage 15 embryos, the Eve+ aCC/pCC neurons are Hb+ and repress the

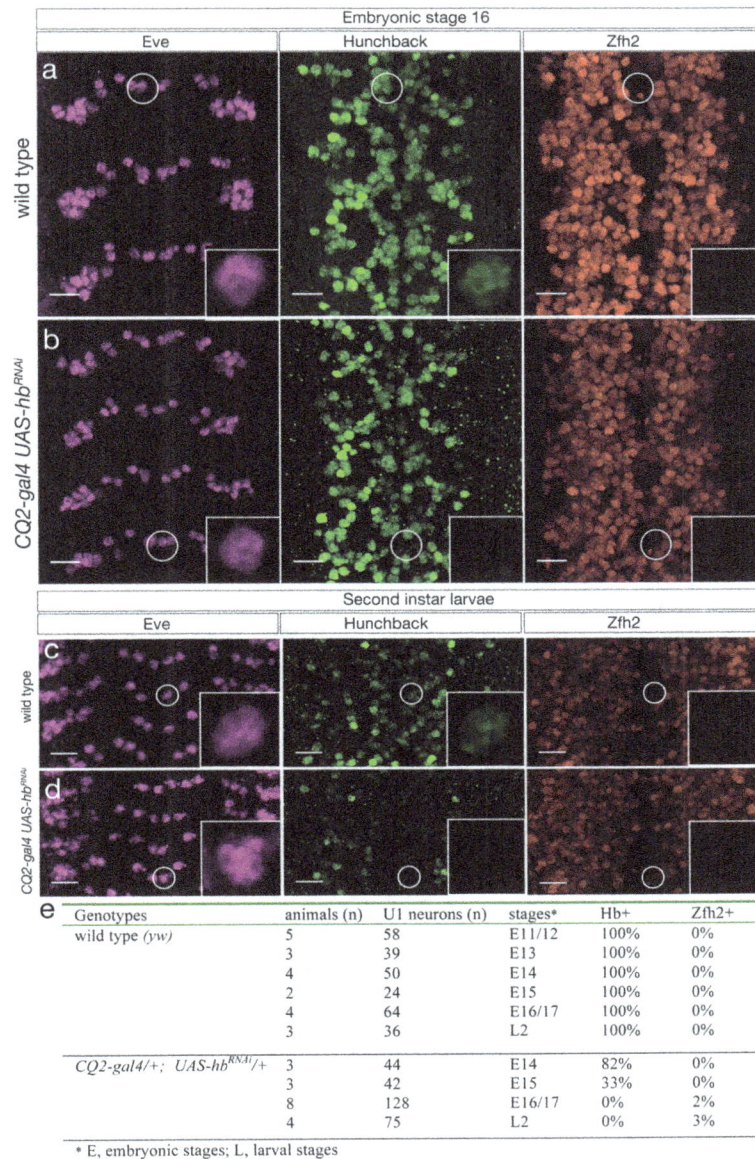

**Fig. 3** Loss of Hunchback from post-mitotic neurons does not alter early-born neuronal identity. **a** Wild type (*y w*) stage 16 embryo, three segments shown. The U1 neuron is Eve+ Hb+ Zfh2-; one example is circled and enlarged in the inset. **b** *CQ2-gal4 UAS-hb^RNAi* stage 16 embryo, four segments shown. The U1 neuron is Eve+ Hb- Zfh2-; one example is circled and enlarged in the inset. Note that loss of neuronal Hb does not result in Zfh2 de-repression. **c** Wild type (*y w*) second instar larval CNS, four segments shown. The U1 neuron is Eve+ Hb+ Zfh2-; one example is circled and enlarged in the inset. **d** *CQ2-gal4 UAS-hb^RNAi* second instar larval CNS, four segments shown. The U1 neuron is Eve+ Hb- Zfh2-; one example is circled and enlarged in the inset. Note that loss of neuronal Hb does not result in Zfh2 de-repression. Anterior up, ventral midline at center of each panel, scale bar, 10 μm. **e** Quantification

late-born marker Zfh2 (Fig. 4a, quantified in 4d). In *hb* CNS null mutants at stage 15, the Eve+ aCC/pCC neurons are Hb- and strongly de-repress Zfh2 (Fig. 4b, quantified in 4d)[22]. In stage 15 *hb* CNS null mutants that were transiently rescued with ectopic Hb earlier in the lineage, the Eve+ aCC/pCC neurons maintain re-pression of *zfh2 despite no longer having detectable Hb*

*protein* (Fig. 4c, quantified in 4d). We propose that the transient expression of Hb in the NB1-1 lineage leads to epigenetic silencing of the *zfh2* locus, such that absence of Hb in older neurons does not lead to de-repression of *zfh2*. Supporting this conclusion is our previous observation that forced expression of Hb in late-born neurons (that normally are Zfh2+) does not lead to *zfh*

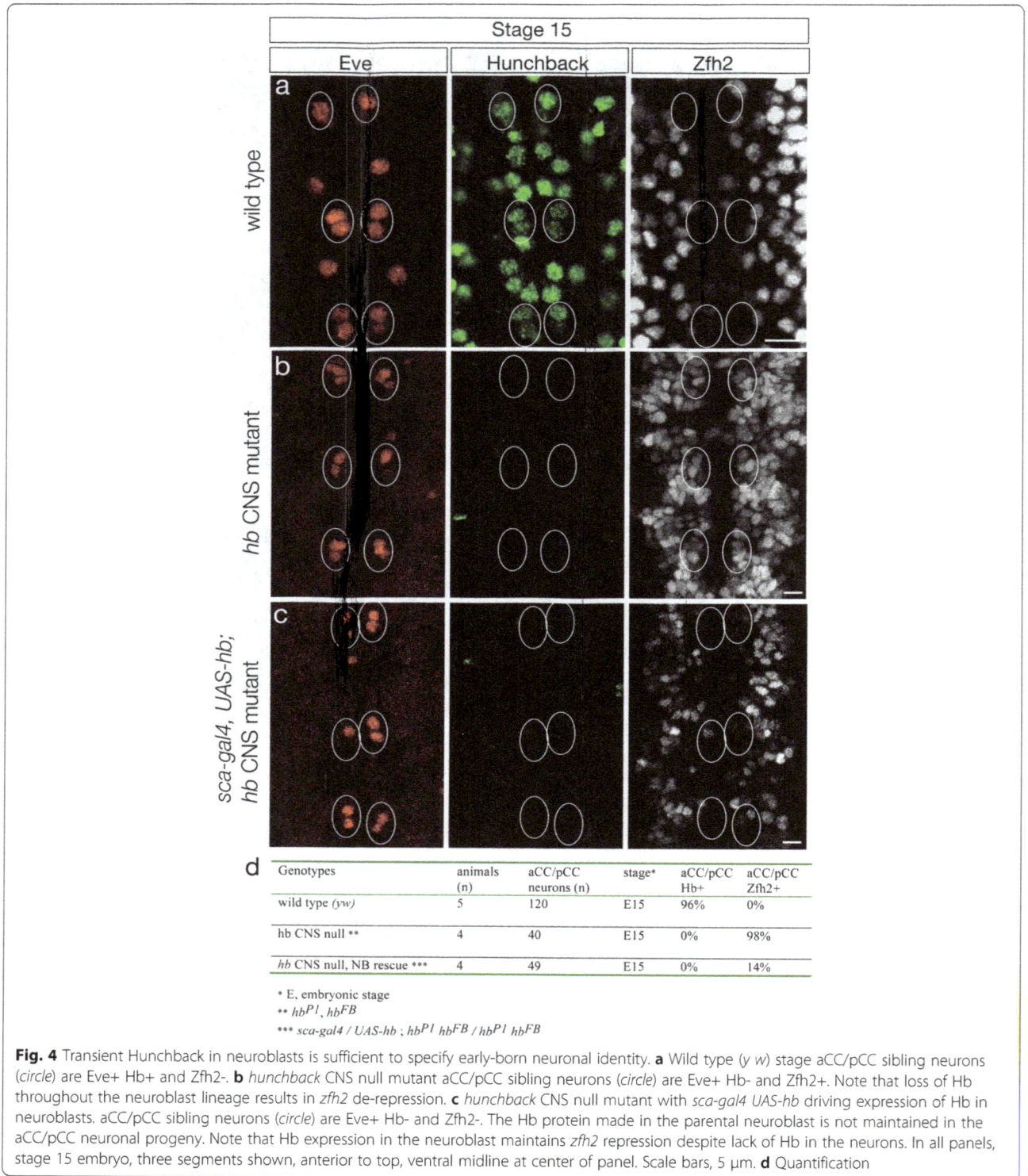

**Fig. 4** Transient Hunchback in neuroblasts is sufficient to specify early-born neuronal identity. **a** Wild type (*y w*) stage aCC/pCC sibling neurons (*circle*) are Eve+ Hb+ and Zfh2-. **b** *hunchback* CNS null mutant aCC/pCC sibling neurons (*circle*) are Eve+ Hb- and Zfh2+. Note that loss of Hb throughout the neuroblast lineage results in *zfh2* de-repression. **c** *hunchback* CNS null mutant with *sca-gal4 UAS-hb* driving expression of Hb in neuroblasts. aCC/pCC sibling neurons (*circle*) are Eve+ Hb- and Zfh2-. The Hb protein made in the parental neuroblast is not maintained in the aCC/pCC neuronal progeny. Note that Hb expression in the neuroblast maintains *zfh2* repression despite lack of Hb in the neurons. In all panels, stage 15 embryo, three segments shown, anterior to top, ventral midline at center of panel. Scale bars, 5 μm. **d** Quantification

repression despite high levels of neuronal Hb protein [29, 37]. Taking all experiments together, we conclude that loss of Hb from three different post-mitotic neurons (U1, aCC, pCC) from two different neuroblast lineages (NB7-1, NB1-1) has no effect on the molecular identity of these early-born neurons: all are able to maintain repression of the late-born neuronal marker Zfh2 in the absence of Hb protein. We propose that Hb acts in the neuroblast, GMC or young neuron to heritably silence *zfh2* expression (see Discussion).

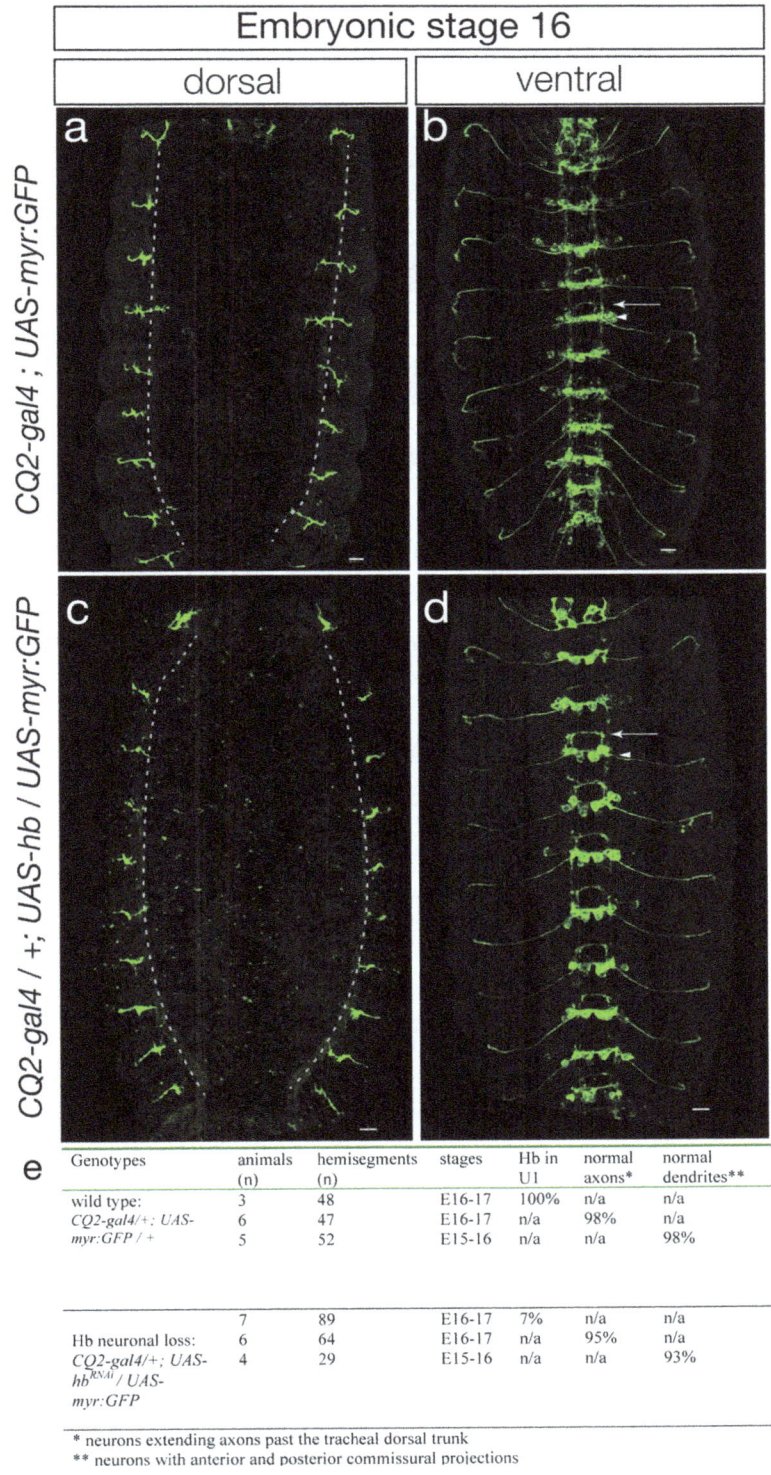

Fig. 5 (See legend on next page.)

(See figure on previous page.)
**Fig. 5** Loss of Hunchback from post-mitotic neurons only does not alter embryonic neuronal morphology. U1-U5 motor neuron morphology detected by *CQ2-gal4* driving expression of *UAS-myristoylated:GFP* (*green*). Only the Hb+ U1 and U2 motor neurons project to the most dorsal muscles [22, 30]. **a, b** Wild type *CQ2-gal4;UAS-myr:GFP* stage 16 embryo. **a** The most dorsal projecting U1/U2 motor neurons extend past the tracheal dorsal trunk (*dashed lines*). **b** Dendritic projections form a thick posterior commissural fascicle (*arrow*) and a thin anterior commissural fascicle (*arrowhead*) in each segment; note faint processes in most intersegmental connectives. **c, d** *CQ2-gal4/+; UAS-hb^{RNAi}/UAS-myr:GFP* stage 16 embryo. **c** The most dorsal projecting U1/U2 motor neurons extend past the tracheal dorsal trunk (*dashed lines*). No difference is seen in axon or dendrite morphology between wild type and *CQ2-gal4 UAS-hb^{RNAi}* embryos. **d** Dendritic projections form a thick posterior commissural fascicle (*arrowhead*) and a thin anterior commissural fascicle (*arrow*) in each segment; note slightly reduced processes in most intersegmental connectives. Anterior up, dorsal (**a,c**) or ventral (**b,d**) midline at center of each panel, scale bar, 10 μm. **e** Quantification

## Loss of Hunchback from neurons only does not alter early-born neuronal morphology

To determine if loss of Hb from the post-mitotic U1 neuron leads to alteration in neuronal morphology, we used *CQ2-gal4* to drive expression of *UAS-hb^{RNAi}* (to remove Hb protein) and *UAS-myristoylated (myr):GFP* (to reveal U1-U5 neuronal morphology). Although myr:GFP was expressed in most or all U1-U5 motor neurons, only the U1 motor neuron projects to the most dorsal muscles of the body wall [22, 30], which allows us to detect any defects in U1 morphology.

In wild type stage 16 embryos, the U1 motor neuron projected to the most dorsal muscles, past the dorsal branch of the trachea (Fig. 5a, quantified in 5e). In *CQ2-gal4 UAS-hb^{RNAi}* stage 16 embryos, the U1 motor neuron also projected past the dorsal branch of the trachea (Fig. 5c, quantified in 5e). Although we can't distinguish the U1 dendrites from the U2-U5 dendrites, we saw only minor, transient differences in dendritic projections within the CNS. For example, projections in the connectives were typically slightly weaker in hb RNAi embryos compared to control embryos (Fig. 5b, d), although by second instar larvae we see no difference in the projections within the connectives (Additional file 2: Figure S2). We conclude that loss of Hb from the post-mitotic U1 motor neuron does not alter its neuronal morphology.

## Loss of Hunchback from U1/U2 neurons or all neurons does not alter larval locomotor velocity

We have previously characterized the role of motor neurons and interneurons in larval locomotion, and have developed a method to quantify larval locomotor velocity, a sensitive read-out for normal motor neuron function [11, 19, 20]. It is possible that loss of Hb from the U1 and U2 motor neurons (or all early-born neurons) may not alter gene expression or neuronal morphology, but rather affect motor neuron function leading to locomotor defects. To determine if loss of Hb from the post-mitotic U1/U2 neurons leads to defects in larval locomotor velocity, we used *CQ2-gal4* to drive expression of *UAS-hb^{RNAi}*. We found that *CQ2-gal4 UAS-hb^{RNAi}* removed all detectable Hb protein from the U1 motor neuron (see Fig. 3d) but had no significant effect on larval locomotor velocity (Fig. 6c, top two rows).

We also used *elav-gal4* to drive *UAS-hb^{RNAi}* to remove Hb from all post-mitotic neurons and assay for defects in larval locomotor velocity. Note that although *elav-gal4* is expressed in neuroblasts, this expression begins at stage 11–12 [8, 26], after Hb expression normally fades from neuroblasts, and has no effect on Hb expression in neuroblasts (data not shown). Thus, *elav-gal4 UAS-hb^{RNAi}* selectively removes Hb from all neurons without affecting neuroblast/GMC expression. Although *elav-gal4 UAS-hb^{RNAi}* animals lack virtually all neuronal Hb protein (Fig. 6a,b), we observed no significant effect on larval locomotor velocity (Fig. 6c, bottom two rows). The fact that widespread loss of Hb from early-born motor neurons and interneurons has no effect on larval locomotor velocity provides strong evidence that Hb is not required to maintain functional properties of mature neurons.

## Discussion

Here we show that the temporal transcription factor Hb, despite being continuously expressed in the U1 motor neuron, is not required to maintain U1 neuronal identity. We conclude that Hb acts transiently in the neuroblast, GMC, or new-born neuron to establish the U1 neuronal identity, and that this identity is subsequently maintained by a Hb-independent mechanism. Our conclusion is also supported by the observation that Hb, like many temporal transcription factors, are re-used in other cell types or tissues to specify different cell fates, showing that cellular context shapes the response to Hb. It is likely that progenitors and post-mitotic neurons provide different contexts for Hb action; the role of Hb in early-born post-mitotic neurons has yet to be defined. For example, in the neuroblast/GMC progenitors, Hb confers temporal identity [22], in the early embryo Hb specifies anterior-posterior identity [36], and in adult male neurons Hb confers male-specific morphology [16]. Similar findings are observed for other embryonic temporal transcription factors such as Kr, Pdm, and Castor [10, 22, 42, 44, 46].

Interestingly, our attempts to remove Hb from the entire NB7-1 lineage using *en-gal4 UAS-hbRNAi* resulted in residual Hb protein in NB7-1 and a weaker phenotype than complete genetic removal of Hb from the NB7-1

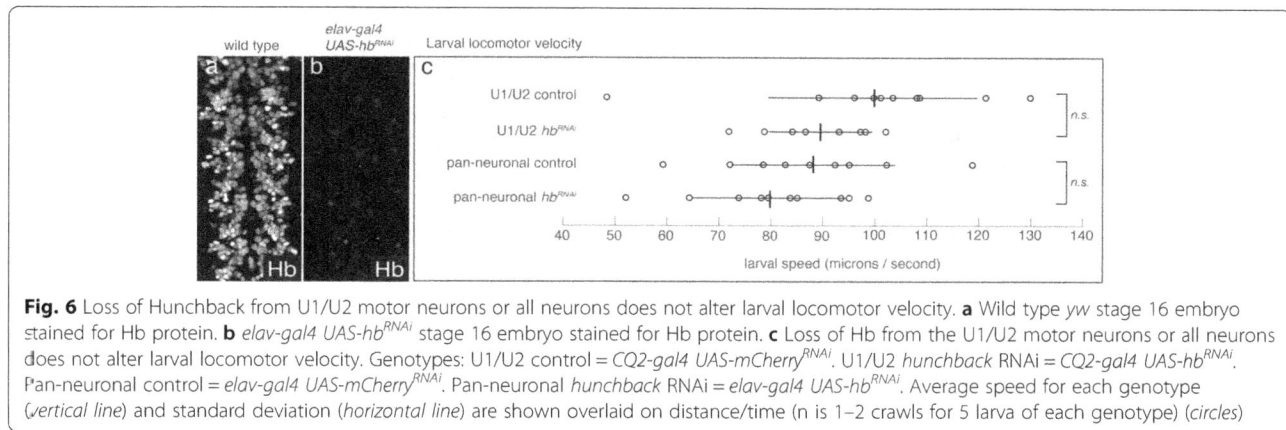

**Fig. 6** Loss of Hunchback from U1/U2 motor neurons or all neurons does not alter larval locomotor velocity. **a** Wild type *yw* stage 16 embryo stained for Hb protein. **b** *elav-gal4 UAS-hb^RNAi* stage 16 embryo stained for Hb protein. **c** Loss of Hb from the U1/U2 motor neurons or all neurons does not alter larval locomotor velocity. Genotypes: U1/U2 control = *CQ2-gal4 UAS-mCherry^RNAi*. U1/U2 *hunchback* RNAi = *CQ2-gal4 UAS-hb^RNAi*. Pan-neuronal control = *elav-gal4 UAS-mCherry^RNAi*. Pan-neuronal *hunchback* RNAi = *elav-gal4 UAS-hb^RNAi*. Average speed for each genotype (*vertical line*) and standard deviation (*horizontal line*) are shown overlaid on distance/time (n is 1–2 crawls for 5 larva of each genotype) (*circles*)

lineage [22]. For example, both *hb* RNAi and *hb* null mutants resulted in U1 motor neurons that de-repressed *zfh2* ([22]; Fig. 2) but only genetic *hb* null mutants result in absence of early-born Eve+ neurons ([22]; Fig. 2). This suggests that the Hb protein present in the NB7-1 following *hb* RNAi is sufficient to produce long-lasting expression of Eve in the U1 motor neuron.

We conclude that Hb has no detectable function in post-mitotic U1 neurons. Might this lack of phenotype be due to low levels of residual Hb protein in neurons? Although we can't formally rule this out, there are several reasons to discount this possibility. First, we stain for Hb protein and find most U1 neurons have no detectable Hb protein compared to background. Second, RNAi knockdown of Hb in neuroblasts produces a strong phenotype which would not be expected if very low levels of Hb are functional. Finally, we don't expect Hb protein to persist following loss of hb RNA, as we have previously shown that Hb protein in the CNS has a very short half life. These experiments co-stained neuroblasts and their progeny for Hb protein and active *hb* transcription (nuclear intron signal), and found that few or no cells had Hb protein but not *hb* transcription [17].

Our conclusion that Hb has no function in post-mitotic neurons is buttressed by our previous findings that late-born Hb-negative neurons are unaffected by forced Hb misexpression [12, 37]. We hypothesize that temporal transcription factors alter the epigenetic state of neuroblasts which is inherited by their progeny neurons. Thus, early-born neurons do not need Hb to maintain early-born identity, and are also unresponsive to forced expression of other temporal transcription factors; similarly, late-born neurons are unresponsive to forced expression of early temporal transcription factors [12, 37]. This model is supported by findings that Hb acts transiently at the cellular blastoderm stage together with the chromatin remodeler Mi-2 to permanently silence the *Ubx* gene [27]. It is also supported by the observation that some temporal transcription factors are only transiently expressed in progenitors and new-born neurons, such as Pdm in embryonic lineages [18, 22] or Eyeless, Sloppy paired, Dichaete, and Tailless in larval optic lobe lineages [31]. In these cases, the temporal transcription factor must act transiently in the neuroblast or GMC to confer long-lasting neuronal identity. Our findings raise the possibility that all temporal transcription factors are required transiently in progenitors to specify permanent temporal identity, despite many of these factors being maintained in post-mitotic neurons. If our findings can be extended to other temporal transcription factors, it would highlight the differences between spatial or temporal patterning genes (required transiently in progenitors) and terminal selector genes (required permanently in post-mitotic neurons). It would also highlight the importance of properly linking spatial/temporal patterning to terminal selector gene expression, an important area for future investigation.

We can't rule out the possibility that Hb is required in post-mitotic neurons for aspects of neuronal function that we did not assay. In fact, post-embryonic expression of Hb is required for proper Fruitless + male neurons morphogenesis; following hb RNAi these neurons are transformed to a female-like morphology [16]. Although we did not detect striking axon or dendrite changes in the U neurons following hb RNAi, we did observe a slight decrease in neuronal projections in connectives (Fig. 5). Although Hb is not required to maintain dorsal axon projections in embryonic or larval U1 motor neurons, but it may be required for proper ion channel or neurotransmitter production. Furthermore, mammalian post-mitotic neurons can be reprogrammed to another neuronal identity for a short time after their birth [41]. Temporal transcription factors like Hb may stabilize neuronal identity to prevent such transformations; in this case, loss of neuronal Hb would only show a strong phenotype upon misexpression of a "reprogramming factor," such as a later temporal transcription factor or a terminal selector gene for a different neural subtype.

Perhaps the strongest evidence we have against a Hb function in post-mitotic neurons is our finding that elimination of Hb protein from all post-mitotic neurons (*elav-gal4 UAS-hb$^{RNAi}$*, Fig. 6) has no larval locomotor phenotype. Similar experiments driving pan-neuronal expression of neuronal silencers or activators leads to larval paralysis [11, 13, 45]. Thus, it is highly unlikely that loss of Hb alters early-born interneuron or motor neuron neurotransmitter phenotypes or membrane properties. In the future, it would be interesting to use transcriptional profiling to compare Hb+ and Hb- early-born neurons– our results suggest that there would be little transcriptional effect from removing Hb from post-mitotic neurons.

## Conclusions

We conclude that the Hb functions in progenitors (neuroblasts/GMCs) to establish heritable neuronal identity that is maintained by a Hb-independent mechanism.

We suggest that Hb acts in neuroblasts to establish an epigenetic state that is permanently maintained in early-born neurons.

## Additional files

**Additional file 1: Figure S1.** Summary of three transgenic Gal4 line expression patterns in the NB7-1 or NB1-1 lineages. Black, high level; gray, low level; white, no expression. aCC, anterior corner cell; pCC, posterior corner cell. (TIF 1150 kb)

**Additional file 2: Figure S2.** Loss of Hunchback from post-mitotic neurons only does not alter embryonic neuronal morphology. U1-U5 motor neuron morphology detected by *CQ2-gal4* driving expression of *UAS-myristoylated:GFP* (green). (a) control *CQ2-gal4/+;UAS-myr:GFP/UAS-mCherry$^{RNAi}$*L2 larval CNS. Note projections out motor nerve roots and robust CNS projections. (b) *CQ2-gal4/+;UAS-hb$^{RNAi}$/UAS-myr:GFP* L2 larval CNS. Note projections out motor nerve roots and robust CNS projections. (TIF 3032 kb)

## Abbreviations

CNS: Central nervous system; Eve: Even-skipped; Hb: Hunchback

## Acknowledgements

We thank Sen-Lin Lai for comments on the manuscript, and the Bloomington stock center for fly stocks.

## Funding

This work was funded by NIH grant HD27056 to C.Q.D., who is an Investigator of the Howard Hughes Medical Institute.

## Authors' contributions

All experiments except those in Figs. 4 and 6 were done by KH, those in Fig. 4 were done by MK, those in Fig. 6 were done by MQC and ESH, and the manuscript was written by CQD All authors read and approved the final manuscript.

## Competing interests

The authors declare that they have no competing interests.

## Author details

[1]Howard Hughes Medical Institute, Eugene 97403, USA. [2]Institute of Molecular Biology, Eugene 97403, USA. [3]Institute of Neuroscience, University of Oregon, Eugene 97403, USA. [4]Department of Neuroscience, Columbia University Medical Center, New York, NY 10032, USA. [5]Department of Molecular Genetics and Cell Biology, University of Chicago, Chicago, IL 60637, USA.

## References

1.  Allan DW, Thor S. Transcriptional selectors, masters, and combinatorial codes: regulatory principles of neural subtype specification. Wiley Interdiscip Rev Dev Biol. 2015;4:505–28.
2.  Alsio JM, Tarchini B, Cayouette M, Livesey FJ. Ikaros promotes early-born neuronal fates in the cerebral cortex. Proc Natl Acad Sci U S A. 2013;110:E716–25.
3.  Baumgardt M, Karlsson D, Salmani BY, Bivik C, MacDonald RB, Gunnar E, Thor S. Global programmed switch in neural daughter cell proliferation mode triggered by a temporal gene cascade. Dev Cell. 2014;30:192–208.
4.  Baumgardt M, Karlsson D, Terriente J, Diaz-Benjumea FJ, Thor S. Neuronal subtype specification within a lineage by opposing temporal feed-forward loops. Cell. 2009;139:969–82.
5.  Baumgardt M, Miguel-Aliaga I, Karlsson D, Ekman H, Thor S. Specification of neuronal identities by feedforward combinatorial coding. PLoS Biol. 2007;5, e37.
6.  Benito-Sipos J, Estacio-Gomez A, Moris-Sanz M, Baumgardt M, Thor S, Diaz-Benjumea FJ. A genetic cascade involving klumpfuss, nab and castor specifies the abdominal leucokinergic neurons in the Drosophila CNS. Development. 2010;137:3327–36.
7.  Benito-Sipos J, Ulvklo C, Gabilondo H, Baumgardt M, Angel A, Torroja L, Thor S. Seven up acts as a temporal factor during two different stages of neuroblast 5–6 development. Development. 2011;138:5311–20.
8.  Berger C, Renner S, Luer K, Technau GM. The commonly used marker ELAV is transiently expressed in neuroblasts and glial cells in the Drosophila embryonic CNS. Dev Dyn. 2007;236:3562–8.
9.  Brody T, Odenwald WF. Programmed transformations in neuroblast gene expression during Drosophila CNS lineage development. Dev Biol. 2000;226:34–44.
10. Chang YC, Jang AC, Lin CH, Montell DJ. Castor is required for Hedgehog-dependent cell-fate specification and follicle stem cell maintenance in Drosophila oogenesis. Proc Natl Acad Sci U S A. 2013;110:E1734–42.
11. Clark MQ, McCumsey SJ, Lopez-Darwin S, Heckscher ES, Doe CQ. Functional Genetic Screen to Identify Interneurons Governing Behaviorally Distinct Aspects of Drosophila Larval Motor Programs. G3 (Bethesda). 2016;6:2023–31.
12. Cleary MD, Doe CQ. Regulation of neuroblast competence: multiple temporal identity factors specify distinct neuronal fates within a single early competence window. Genes Dev. 2006;20:429–34.
13. Crisp SJ, Evers JF, Bate M. Endogenous patterns of activity are required for the maturation of a motor network. J Neurosci. 2011;31:10445–50.
14. Elliott J, Jolicoeur C, Ramamurthy V, Cayouette M. Ikaros confers early temporal competence to mouse retinal progenitor cells. Neuron. 2008;60:26–39.
15. Erclik T, Li X, Courgeon M, Bertet C, Chen Z, Baumert R, Ng J, Koo C, Arain U, Behnia R, Rodriguez AD, Senderowicz L, Negre N, White KP, Desplan C. Integration of temporal and spatial patterning generates neural diversity. Nature. 2017;541:365–70.
16. Goto J, Mikawa Y, Koganezawa M, Ito H, Yamamoto D. Sexually dimorphic shaping of interneuron dendrites involves the hunchback transcription factor. J Neurosci. 2011;31:5454–9.
17. Grosskortenhaus R, Pearson BJ, Marusich A, Doe CQ. Regulation of temporal identity transitions in Drosophila neuroblasts. Dev Cell. 2005;8:193–202.
18. Grosskortenhaus R, Robinson KJ, Doe CQ. Pdm and Castor specify late-born motor neuron identity in the NB7-1 lineage. Genes Dev. 2006;20:2618–27.
19. Heckscher ES, Lockery SR, Doe CQ. Characterization of Drosophila larval crawling at the level of organism, segment, and somatic body wall musculature. J Neurosci. 2012;32:12460–71.
20. Heckscher ES, Zarin AA, Faumont S, Clark MQ, Manning L, Fushiki A, Schneider-Mizell CM, Fetter RD, Truman JW, Zwart MF, Landgraf M, Cardona A, Lockery SR, Doe CQ. Even-skipped(+) interneurons are core components of a sensorimotor circuit that maintains left-right symmetric muscle contraction amplitude. Neuron. 2015;88:314–29.

21. Hobert O. Terminal selectors of neuronal identity. Curr Top Dev Biol. 2016;116:455–75.

22. Isshiki T, Pearson B, Holbrook S, Doe CQ. Drosophila neuroblasts sequentially express transcription factors which specify the temporal identity of their neuronal progeny. Cell. 2001;106:511–21.

23. Jessell TM. Neuronal specification in the spinal cord: inductive signals and transcriptional codes. Nature reviews. Genetics. 2000;1:20–9.

24. Kambadur R, Koizumi K, Stivers C, Nagle J, Poole SJ, Odenwald WF. Regulation of POU genes by castor and hunchback establishes layered compartments in the Drosophila CNS. Genes Dev. 1998;12:246–60.

25. Kanai MI, Okabe M, Hiromi Y. Seven-up controls switching of transcription factors that specify temporal identities of Drosophila neuroblasts. Dev Cell. 2005;8:203–13.

26. Karlsson D, Baumgardt M, Thor S. Segment-specific neuronal subtype specification by the integration of anteroposterior and temporal cues. PLoS Biol. 2010;8, e1000368.

27. Kehle J, Beuchle D, Treuheit S, Christen B, Kennison JA, Bienz M, Muller J. dMi-2, a hunchback-interacting protein that functions in polycomb repression. Science. 1998;282:1897–900.

28. Kohwi M, Hiebert LS, Doe CQ. The pipsqueak-domain proteins Distal antenna and Distal antenna-related restrict Hunchback neuroblast expression and early-born neuronal identity. Development. 2011;138:1727–35.

29. Kohwi M, Lupton JR, Lai SL, Miller MR, Doe CQ. Developmentally regulated subnuclear genome reorganization restricts neural progenitor competence in Drosophila. Cell. 2013;152:97–108.

30. Landgraf M, Bossing T, Technau GM, Bate M. The origin, location, and projections of the embryonic abdominal motorneurons of Drosophila. J Neurosci. 1997;17:9642–55.

31. Li X, Erclik T, Bertet C, Chen Z, Voutev R, Venkatesh S, Morante J, Celik A, Desplan C. Temporal patterning of Drosophila medulla neuroblasts controls neural fates. 2013. Nature.

32. Mattar P, Ericson J, Blackshaw S, Cayouette M. A conserved regulatory logic controls temporal identity in mouse neural progenitors. Neuron. 2015;85:497–504.

33. Mettler U, Vogler G, Urban J. Timing of identity: spatiotemporal regulation of hunchback in neuroblast lineages of Drosophila by Seven-up and Prospero. Development. 2006;133:429–37.

34. Moris-Sanz M, Estacio-Gomez A, Alvarez-Rivero J, Diaz-Benjumea FJ. Specification of neuronal subtypes by different levels of Hunchback. Development. 2014;141:4366–74.

35. Novotny T, Eiselt R, Urban J. Hunchback is required for the specification of the early sublineage of neuroblast 7–3 in the Drosophila central nervous system. Development. 2002;129:1027–36.

36. Nusslein-Volhard C, Wieschaus E. Mutations affecting segment number and polarity in Drosophila. Nature. 1980;287:795–801.

37. Pearson BJ, Doe CQ. Regulation of neuroblast competence in Drosophila. Nature. 2003;425:624–8.

38. Pearson BJ, Doe CQ. Specification of temporal identity in the developing nervous system. Annu Rev Cell Dev Biol. 2004;20:619–47.

39. Risse B, Thomas S, Otto N, Lopmeier T, Valkov D, Jiang X, Klambt C. FIM, a novel FTIR-based imaging method for high throughput locomotion analysis. PLoS One. 2013;8, e53963.

40. Rossi AM, Fernandes VM, Desplan C. Timing temporal transitions during brain development. Curr Opin Neurobiol. 2016;42:84–92.

41. Rouaux C, Arlotta P. Direct lineage reprogramming of post-mitotic callosal neurons into corticofugal neurons in vivo. Nat Cell Biol. 2013;15:214–21.

42. Ruiz-Gomez M, Romani S, Hartmann C, Jackle H, Bate M. Specific muscle identities are regulated by Kruppel during Drosophila embryogenesis. Development. 1997;124:3407–14.

43. Skeath JB, Thor S. Genetic control of Drosophila nerve cord development. Curr Opin Neurobiol. 2003;13:8–15.

44. Stratmann J, Gabilondo H, Benito-Sipos J, Thor S. Neuronal cell fate diversification controlled by sub-temporal action of Kruppel. eLife. 2016;5.

45. Suster ML, Bate M. Embryonic assembly of a central pattern generator without sensory input. Nature. 2002;416:174–8.

46. Tran KD, Doe CQ. Pdm and Castor close successive temporal identity windows in the NB3-1 lineage. Development. 2008;135:3491–9.

47. Tran KD, Miller MR, Doe CQ. Recombineering Hunchback identifies two conserved domains required to maintain neuroblast competence and specify early-born neuronal identity. Development. 2010;137:1421–30.

# 14

# Dual leucine zipper kinase regulates expression of axon guidance genes in mouse neuronal cells

Andréanne Blondeau[1], Jean-François Lucier[1], Dominick Matteau[1], Lauralyne Dumont[1], Sébastien Rodrigue[1], Pierre-Étienne Jacques[1,2,3] and Richard Blouin[1*] ⓘ

## Abstract

**Background:** Recent genetic studies in model organisms, such as *Drosophila*, *C. elegans* and mice, have highlighted a critical role for dual leucine zipper kinase (DLK) in neural development and axonal responses to injury. However, exactly how DLK fulfills these functions remains to be determined. Using RNA-seq profiling, we evaluated the global changes in gene expression that are caused by shRNA-mediated knockdown of endogenous DLK in differentiated Neuro-2a neuroblastoma cells.

**Results:** Our analysis led to the identification of numerous up- and down-regulated genes, among which several were found to be associated with system development and axon guidance according to gene ontology (GO) and Kyoto Encyclopedia of Genes and Genomes (KEGG) pathway analyses, respectively. Because of their importance in axonal growth, pruning and regeneration during development and adult life, we then examined by quantitative RT-PCR the mRNA expression levels of the identified axon guidance genes in DLK-depleted cells. Consistent with the RNA-seq data, our results confirmed that loss of DLK altered expression of the genes encoding neuropilin 1 (Nrp1), plexin A4 (Plxna4), Eph receptor A7 (Epha7), Rho family GTPase 1 (Rnd1) and semaphorin 6B (Sema6b). Interestingly, this regulation of Nrp1 and Plxna4 mRNA expression by DLK in Neuro-2a cells was also reflected at the protein level, implicating DLK in the modulation of the function of these axon guidance molecules.

**Conclusions:** Collectively, these results provide the first evidence that axon guidance genes are downstream targets of the DLK signaling pathway, which through their regulation probably modulates neuronal cell development, structure and function.

**Keywords:** DLK, Neurons, Axon guidance

## Background

The mitogen-activated protein kinases (MAPKs) are important regulators of fundamental biological processes, such as cell proliferation, differentiation, cell survival, migration and apoptosis. These enzymes are activated in response to extracellular stimuli by upstream kinases termed MAPKKs, which are themselves activated by the third component of the MAPK system, the MAPKKKs [1]. Based on their structural and biochemical features, three major subgroups of MAPKs have been described

in mammals, including extracellular signal-regulated kinases (ERKs), p38 kinases, and c-Jun N-terminal kinases (JNKs) [1, 2].

One MAPKKK that emerges as a pivotal component of the MAPK pathways is dual leucine zipper kinase (DLK, also known as Map3k12), which was originally identified in a screen for proteins differentially expressed during the retinoic acid-induced differentiation of human NT2 teratocarcinoma cells [3]. DLK preferentially activates JNK, although a role for DLK in activation of ERK and p38 MAPKs has also been proposed [4–6]. Based on Northern blot analysis, *in situ* hybridization and immunolocalization, DLK has a tissue-specific expression pattern in both mouse and

* Correspondence: Richard.Blouin@USherbrooke.ca
[1]Département de biologie, Faculté des sciences, Université de Sherbrooke, 2500 Boul. de l'Université, Sherbrooke, Québec J1K 2R1, Canada
Full list of author information is available at the end of the article

human, being mainly expressed in brain, kidney and skin [3, 7–10]. Previous studies have suggested a fundamental role for DLK in vivo since targeted deletion of the *DLK* gene in mice results in perinatal death [11]. Embryos lacking *DLK* display abnormal brain development, characterized by defects in axon growth, neuron migration, apoptosis and axon degeneration [11–15]. Apart from its role during development, DLK has also been shown to regulate axonal damage signaling in mature neurons [13, 15–17]. For instance, as demonstrated by studies in mice and rats, loss of DLK protects neurons from somal and axonal degeneration in response to mechanical injury, growth factor deprivation and glutamate-induced excitotoxicity [16–19]. Recently, it was also discovered that DLK is required for axonal regeneration in adult peripheral nerves after axotomy in both vertebrate and invertebrate organisms [16, 20, 21]. These findings demonstrate a key role for DLK in controlling neuronal development as well as degenerative and regenerative responses to axonal injury. Although JNK activation is an important and established event downstream of DLK, precisely how DLK mediates such diverse effects in neurons remains an open question.

Because one way to unravel the mode of action of DLK is to identify genes critical for its function in neurons, we characterized by next-generation sequencing (RNA-seq) the transcriptome of differentiated Neuro-2a neuroblastoma cells in which DLK has been depleted by RNA interference. Our results led to the identification of many genes whose expression was significantly altered upon DLK knockdown. Notably, among the identified genes, we focused on those encoding axon guidance molecules due to their crucial roles in many aspects of neuronal development, including axon pathfinding, axon growth, neuronal polarization, neuronal migration and dendrite formation, as well as in axon regeneration in the adult nervous system [22–25].

## Methods

### Antibodies

The polyclonal antiserum used for detection of DLK was described previously [26]. The polyclonal or monoclonal antibodies against phospho-JNK (Thr183/Tyr185, #4671), JNK (#9252), phospho-c-Jun (Ser63, #9261), Nrp1 (#3725) and Plxna4 (#3816) were purchased from Cell Signaling Technology, Inc. (Danvers, MA). The polyclonal antibody against γ-actin (#NB600-533) was from Novus Biologicals (Oakville, Ontario).

### Cell culture

Mouse Neuro-2a neuroblastoma cells were grown in Dulbecco's modified Eagle's medium (DMEM) supplemented with 10 % (v/v) fetal bovine serum (FBS), 100 U/ml penicillin and 100 μg/ml streptomycin. When indicated, cells were differentiated by incubation in DMEM containing 0.1 % bovine serum albumin for 24 h.

### Lentivirus production and infection of Neuro-2a cells

HEK 293T cells grown in DMEM supplemented with 10 % (v/v) FBS and antibiotics were cotransfected with the envelope protein expressing vector pMD2.G and the packaging protein expressing vector psPAX2, (kindly provided by Dr. Didier Trono University of Geneva Medical School, Geneva, Switzerland) and with either the transfer pLKO.1 empty lentiviral vector [27] (Addgene, Cambridge, MA, USA, plasmid 8453) or the pLKO.1-based lentiviral mouse DLK shRNA vector (clone TRCN0000022573 [sh73] or clone TRCN0000022569 [sh69], Open Biosystems, Huntsville, AL, USA) using Polyethylenimine Max (#24765, Polysciences Warrington, PA). At 72 h post-transfection, the culture medium containing lentiviruses was harvested, filtered through 0.45-μm filter, and used for infection. Neuro-2a cells, seeded at a density of $0.3 \times 10^6$ cells per well in six-well dishes, $0.5 \times 10^6$ cells in 60-mm dishes or $2.0 \times 10^6$ cells in 100-mm dishes 24 h before, were infected with viral supernatants supplemented with 8 μg/ml polybrene. Two days later, infected cells were treated with puromycin (2.5 μg/ml) and selected for 2 days, after which they were induced to differentiate as mentioned above.

### qRT-PCR experiments

Total RNA was extracted with the Direct-zol RNA Mini-Prep kit (#R2050, Zymo Research) in combination with TRIzol (#15596-026, Life Technologies), following the manufacturer's protocol. A 30 min on-column DNase treatment was performed before elution according to manufacturer's instructions. RNA was quantified on a NanoDrop (Thermo Scientific) spectrophotometer. Total RNA quality was assessed with an Agilent 2100 Bioanalyzer (Agilent Technologies). Reverse transcription was performed on 2.2 μg total RNA with Transcriptor reverse transcriptase, random hexamers, dNTPs (Roche Diagnostics), and 10 units of RNAseOUT (Invitrogen) following the manufacturer's protocol in a total volume of 20 μl. All forward and reverse primers were individually resuspended to 20–100 μM stock solution in Tris-EDTA buffer (IDT) and diluted as a primer pair to 1 μM in RNase DNase-free water (IDT). Quantitative PCR (qPCR) reactions were performed in 10 μl in 96 well plates on a CFX-96 thermocycler (BioRad) with 5 μL of 2X iTaq Universal SYBR Green Supermix (BioRad), 10 ng (3 μl) cDNA, and 200 nM final (2 μl) primer pair solutions. The following cycling conditions were used: 3 min at 95 °C; 50 cycles: 15 s at 95 °C, 30 s at 60 °C, 30 s at 72 °C. Relative expression levels were calculated using the qBASE framework [28] and the housekeeping genes *Sdha*, *Txnl4b* and *Pum1* for mouse cDNA. Primer design and validation was evaluated as described elsewhere [29]. In every qPCR run, a no-template control was performed for each primer pair and these were consistently negative. All primer sequences are available in Additional file 1: Table S1.

### Imaging and quantification

Images of control and DLK-depleted Neuro-2a cells were acquired in bright-field using a Zeiss AxioObserver.Z1 inverted microscope equipped with a 20x/0.30 NA objective and a Zeiss Axiocam 506 camera. The length of approximately 200 neurites was measured from five random microscope fields per sample using the open source software Fiji [30] and the Simple Neurite Tracer plugin [31]. GraphPad Prism (GraphPad Software Inc, La Jolla, CA, USA) was used to calculate and plot mean and standard error of the mean (SEM) of the measured neurite lengths. Neurites were also classified into five groups based on their length, and their frequency within each group was calculated for both the control and DLK-depleted cells. The mean ± SEM of the frequency of distribution within each group of neurites was determined using GraphPad Prism and presented in percentage. Significance of the results was assessed by Student's *t* test.

### RNA-seq sample preparation and analysis

Total RNA was isolated as described above from control, sh73/DLK- and sh69/DLK-depleted cells. The quality of total RNA was evaluated using the Agilent 2100 BioAnalyzer and the Agilent RNA 6000 Nano Kit (#5067-1511) according to the manufacturer's instructions. For all samples, RNA integrity numbers were sufficiently high (>9.5) to perform mRNA sequencing. mRNA was purified from 5 μg of total RNA using the NEBNext Poly(A) mRNA Magnetic Isolation Module (#E7490, New England Biolabs, Whitby, Ontario) following manufacturer's instructions. cDNA libraries were then prepared with 25 ng mRNA of each sample using the NEBNext Ultra Directional RNA Library Prep Kit for Illumina (#E7420, New England Biolabs) and barcoded by PCR for subsequent multiplexed sequencing. The quality and quantity of the librairies were assessed using the Agilent High Sensitivity DNA Kit (#5067-4626) on Agilent 2100 BioAnalyzer. Sequencing of the multiplexed cDNA libraries was performed on an Illumina HiSeq 2500 system (Illumina, San Diego, CA, USA) in two lanes at the Institut de Recherches Cliniques de Montréal (IRCM). The obtained raw reads were processed using the McGill University and Génome Québec Innovation Centre (MUGQIC) RNA-seq pipeline version 1.4 (https://bitbucket.org/mugqic/mugqic_pipelines). Briefly, the reads were trimmed using Trimmomatic version 0.32 [32] to

remove adapter sequences and low quality reads (Phred quality < 30 and minimum lenght of 32), and aligned onto the mouse reference genome (mm10 assembly) using TopHat version 2.0.11 and Bowtie version 2.2.2 [33, 34]. Read counts for each gene from the GRCm38.73 mouse assembly from the Ensembl database [35] were obtained using HTSeq version 0.6.1 [36]. Differential gene expression analyses between control and DLK-depleted cells were performed using DESeq version 1.16 [37] and edgeR version 3.6.8 [38] from the Bioconductor package version 2.14 [39, 40] of R version 3.1.1. The identified genes were further filtered against the following criteria: (i) a minimum of 50 reads per gene, (ii) a fold-change threshold ≥ 2 between control and DLK-depleted cells, and (iii) transcripts altered in the same direction with both shDLK constructs and common to at least three of the four samples of DLK-depleted cells. Functional category and pathway analyses of the differentially expressed genes were performed using DAVID [41].

### Statistical analysis

qRT-PCR and immunoblot data represent the mean ± SEM of at least three independently performed experiments. The statistical significance between mean values was determined by unpaired *t* test with Welch's correction (two tails) using GraphPad Prism software. p-values of < 0.05 were considered to be statistically signifiant.

## Results

### Depletion of DLK by RNA interference in Neuro-2a cells

Neuro-2a is an established mouse neural crest-derived cell line that has been used extensively for studying neuronal differentiation, axon growth and signaling pathways [42]. Upon treatment with differentiation agents, such as serum-free media, they stop proliferating and show ultrastructural, morphological and functional properties of neurons [43]. In this study, we took advantage of this model system to identify genes downstream of DLK in neuronal cells. To do so, we first silenced the expression of endogenous DLK by infecting Neuro-2a cells with lentiviral vectors expressing two different short hairpin RNAs (shRNA) that target mouse DLK mRNA (sh73 and sh69). To exclude potential nonspecific effects, cells were also infected with an empty lentiviral vector (pLKO.1). After selection with puromycin for 2 days, the infected cells were then induced to differentiate into a neuronal phenotype by replacing the proliferation medium to DMEM with 0.1 % bovine serum albumin (BSA) for 24 h. Silencing of DLK in differentiated Neuro-2a cells was confirmed by both quantitative reverse transcription PCR (qRT-PCR) and immunoblot analysis. As depicted in Fig. 1a, expression of sh73 and sh69 resulted in an overall decrease of DLK transcripts by

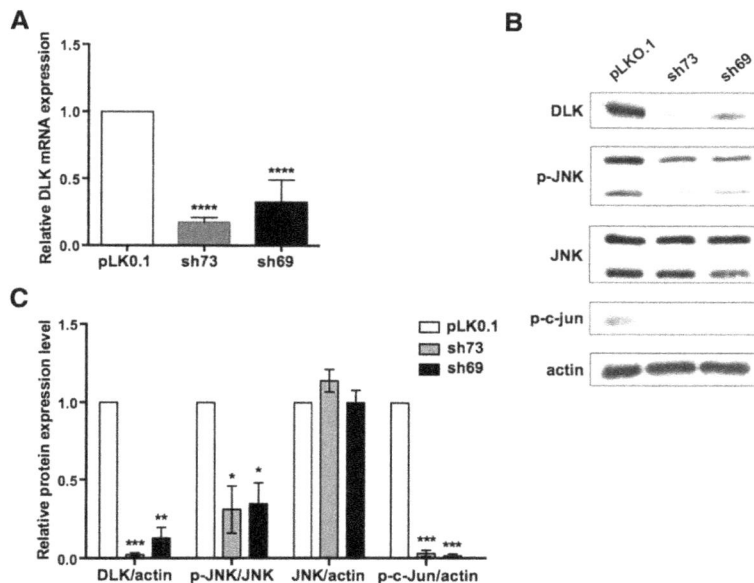

**Fig. 1** Knockdown of DLK in differentiated Neuro-2a cells. Neuro-2a cells were infected with an empty lentiviral vector (pLKO.1) or with lentivirus expressing mouse DLK shRNAs (sh73 and sh69). After infection and selection with puromycin, cells were subjected to differentiation for 24 h before being processed for total RNA extraction and whole-cell extracts. **a** The relative mRNA level of DLK in infected cells was analyzed by quantitative RT-PCR, normalized to three housekeeping genes and calculated with the $\Delta\Delta C_T$ method. The value of DLK mRNA expression in control cells (pLKO.1) was arbitrarily set to 1. Data are the mean ± SEM (error bars) from three independent experiments carried out in triplicate. ****, $p < 0.0001$. **b** Representative Western blots showing levels of DLK, phospho-JNK (p-JNK), total JNK, phospho-c-Jun (p-c-Jun) and actin in infected Neuro-2a cells. **c** Quantitative densitometric measurements of DLK, p-JNK, total JNK and p-c-Jun protein levels in infected cells. Results are normalized to either actin or total JNK level in control cells, which were set to 1, and represent mean ± SEM (error bars) from three independent experiments. *, $p < 0.05$; **, $p < 0.01$; ***, $p < 0.001$

approximately 70 to 80 % when compared to control cells. Consistent with the extent of mRNA reduction, DLK protein expression dropped by nearly 90 % in cells infected with the DLK shRNA constructs relative to pLKO.1, although the sh73 construct gave a better silencing effect than the sh69 vector (Fig. 1b and c). Importantly, none of these lentiviral vectors altered the intracellular levels of actin and JNK, thereby supporting their specificity.

Since DLK is an upstream activator of the JNK signaling pathway [4], we tested in parallel whether its knockdown by RNA interference in Neuro-2a cells would perturb the activity of JNK and c-Jun, a downstream target. The impact of DLK depletion on JNK signaling was assayed by Western blotting with antibodies specific to the phosphorylated, activated forms of JNK and c-Jun. Interestingly, loss of DLK attenuated by 70–95 % basal JNK or c-Jun activity (Fig. 1b and c), a result reminiscent of the effect of DLK gene disruption in mouse brain [11]. Thus, these results indicate that DLK is required for basal activity of JNK and c-Jun in differentiated Neuro-2a cells.

### Effects of DLK depletion on neurite outgrowth in Neuro-2a cells

Previous studies have shown that DLK is required for axon outgrowth both in vivo and in vitro [11, 14, 44].

To determine whether this is also the case in our model, we examined the morphology of DLK-depleted Neuro-2a cells, cultured for 24 h in differentiation conditions. DLK depletion in this experiment was done with the sh73 lentiviral vector only because of its better gene silencing efficacy. Representative results of light microscopy demonstrated that DLK-depleted cells had shorter neurites relative to their control counterparts (Fig. 2a), suggesting that neurite outgrowth is inhibited in the absence of DLK. In support of this, we found that there was a 50 % decrease in the average neurite length after DLK knockdown (Fig. 2b). Moreover, analysis of the distribution of neurite lengths indicated that 53 % of neurites in control cells were longer than 30 μm, whereas only 13 % of neurites in DLK-depleted cells were of this size (Fig. 2c). Taken together, these results show that DLK contributes to neurite outgrowth in Neuro-2a cells.

### RNA-seq analysis of differentially expressed genes in DLK-depleted Neuro-2a cells

To identify downstream effector genes of the DLK signaling pathway, we carried out RNA-seq experiments on both control and DLK-depleted Neuro-2a cells after differentiation (Fig. 3a). In order to improve downstream statistical analyses and minimize

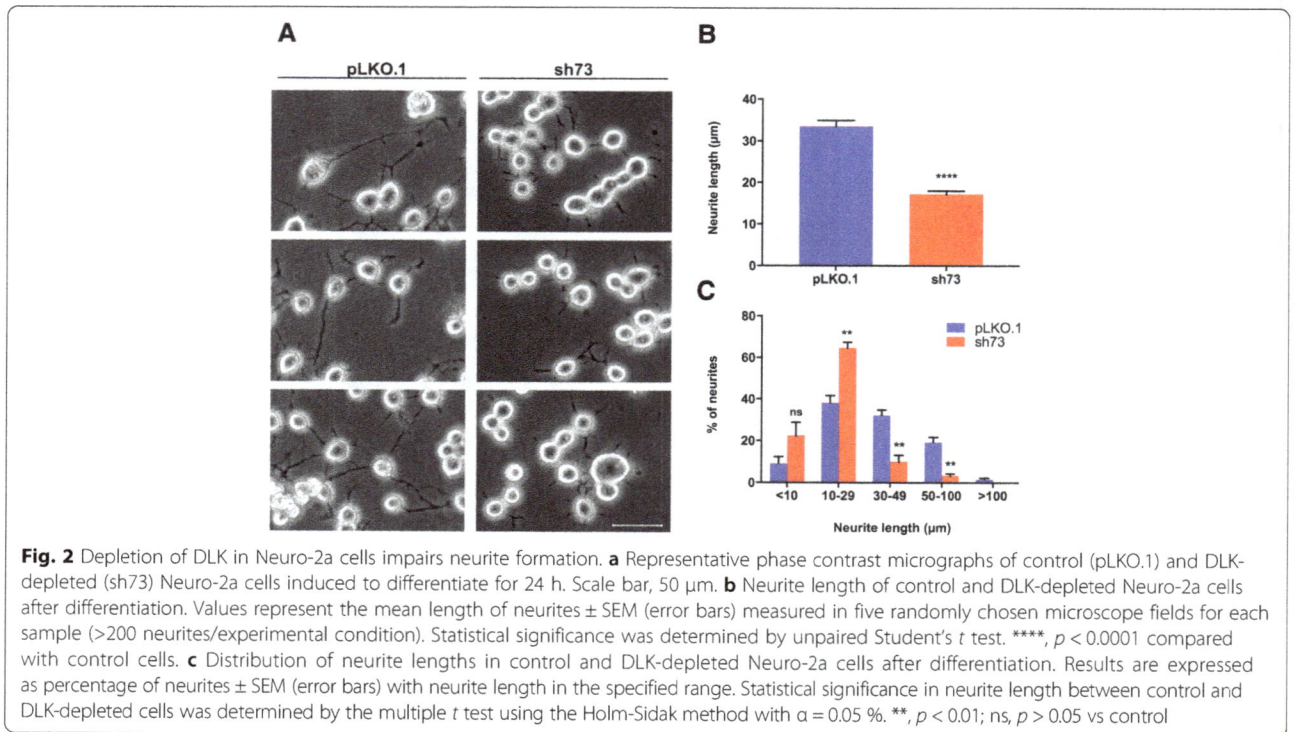

**Fig. 2** Depletion of DLK in Neuro-2a cells impairs neurite formation. **a** Representative phase contrast micrographs of control (pLKO.1) and DLK-depleted (sh73) Neuro-2a cells induced to differentiate for 24 h. Scale bar, 50 μm. **b** Neurite length of control and DLK-depleted Neuro-2a cells after differentiation. Values represent the mean length of neurites ± SEM (error bars) measured in five randomly chosen microscope fields for each sample (>200 neurites/experimental condition). Statistical significance was determined by unpaired Student's *t* test. ****, *p* < 0.0001 compared with control cells. **c** Distribution of neurite lengths in control and DLK-depleted Neuro-2a cells after differentiation. Results are expressed as percentage of neurites ± SEM (error bars) with neurite length in the specified range. Statistical significance in neurite length between control and DLK-depleted cells was determined by the multiple *t* test using the Holm-Sidak method with α = 0.05 %. **, *p* < 0.01; ns, *p* > 0.05 vs control

off-target effects of RNA interference, RNA-seq was performed in parallel on the two DLK-depleted cell lines described above and on two biological replicates for each condition. cDNA librairies constructed with mRNA isolated from differentiated control and DLK-depleted cells were subjected to 50 bp paired-end sequencing multiplexed in two lanes on an Illumina HiSeq system, which generated approximately 80–137 million reads per sample (Additional file 2: Table S2). After trimming, the high quality reads were aligned to the mouse reference genome (mm10) using the TopHat software [33]. Approximately 97 % of the high quality reads from each sample aligned to the reference genome (Additional file 2: Table S2), thus validating the quality and specificity of our transcriptome approach.

The RNA-seq data were subsequently analyzed using the HTSeq [36], DESeq [37] and edgeR [38] softwares to identify differentially expressed genes (DEGs) between control and DLK-depleted cells. As an additional filter on these data, we excluded from the analyses all genes with less than 50 reads on average per condition and with less than two-fold changes in expression as compared to control. To further narrow our candidate gene list, we then focused on up-regulated and down-regulated genes common to at least three of the four samples of sh73/DLK- and sh69/DLK-depleted cells (Fig. 3b). According to these parameters, 104 genes were found to be up-regulated after DLK depletion compared

to control cells (Additional file 3: Table S3), whereas 63 were down-regulated (Additional file 4: Table S4).

This list of induced and repressed genes was next imported into the web-based bioinformatics tool Database for Annotation, Visualization and Integrated Discovery (DAVID) [41] to identify the most statistically significant functional annotation terms associated with them. Table 1 displays the top ten SP-PIR keywords enriched in our gene list with unadjusted and adjusted (Benjamini) P values. According to these data, more than 30 % of the DEGs show a significant association with terms related to signal-, glyco-protein- or membrane-cellular events. In addition, analysis of gene ontology (GO) terms in the biological process category for these up- and down-regulated genes revealed enrichment for genes associated with system development, protein phosphorylation and cell adhesion (Table 2). Among those up-regulated or down-regulated genes after DLK depletion, several were well-established regulators of biological processes related to neuron generation, development and differentiation, thus supporting the importance of DLK in nervous system structure and function. Included in this subset of DEGs are, for example, *Epha7*, *Nfasc* and *Nrp1*, which undergo up-regulation by two-fold or more in DLK-depleted cells (Additional file 3: Table S3), and *Anks1b*, *Rnd1* and *Sema6b* as genes whose expression decreased after DLK loss (Additional file 4: Table S4).

A complementary analysis using KEGG pathway mapping also revealed that the genes dysregulated in DLK-depleted cells were enriched for functions

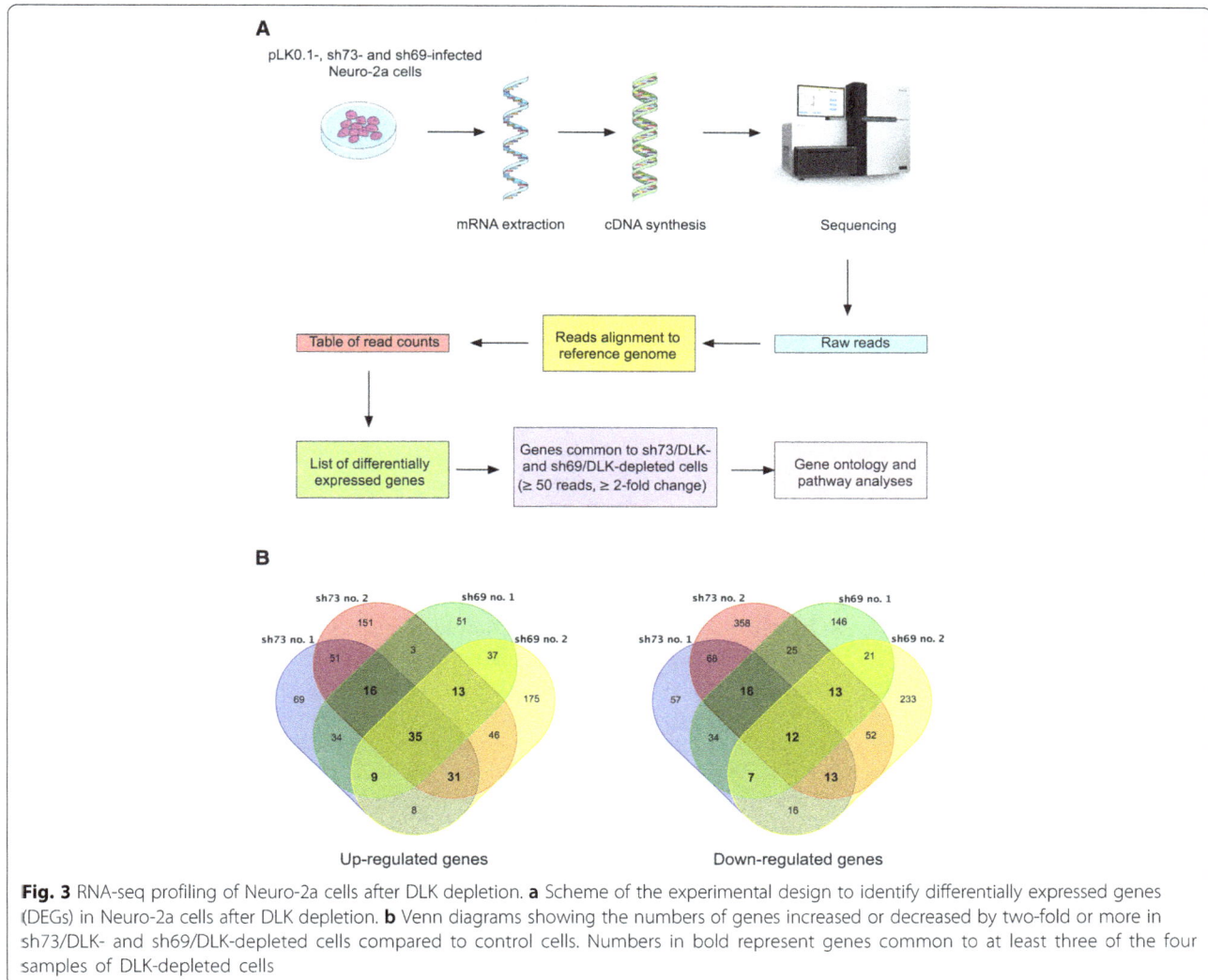

**Fig. 3** RNA-seq profiling of Neuro-2a cells after DLK depletion. **a** Scheme of the experimental design to identify differentially expressed genes (DEGs) in Neuro-2a cells after DLK depletion. **b** Venn diagrams showing the numbers of genes increased or decreased by two-fold or more in sh73/DLK- and sh69/DLK-depleted cells compared to control cells. Numbers in bold represent genes common to at least three of the four samples of DLK-depleted cells

**Table 1** SP-PIR keyword terms associated with dysregulated genes in DLK-depleted cells

| Term | Count | % | P-Value | Benjamini |
|---|---|---|---|---|
| Signal | 54 | 32,9 | 5,40E-09 | 1,20E-06 |
| Glycoprotein | 58 | 35,4 | 8,50E-08 | 9,50E-06 |
| Extracellular matrix | 11 | 6,7 | 9,60E-06 | 7,10E-04 |
| Disulfide bond | 41 | 25 | 9,70E-06 | 5,40E-04 |
| Secreted | 25 | 15,2 | 4,60E-04 | 2,00E-02 |
| Cell adhesion | 11 | 6,7 | 1,10E-03 | 4,00E-02 |
| Membrane | 58 | 35,4 | 1,80E-02 | 4,40E-01 |
| Phosphotransferase | 5 | 3 | 1,80E-02 | 4,10E-01 |
| Smooth muscle | 2 | 1,2 | 3,20E-02 | 5,50E-01 |
| ATP | 5 | 3 | 3,50E-02 | 5,40E-01 |

related to axon guidance, extracellular matrix-receptor interaction and focal adhesion (Table 3). Because axon guidance was the top enriched pathway based on the *P*-value, we decided to focus our experimental efforts on this group of genes for further characterization. These putative DLK-regulated genes fell into three distinct functional categories of axon guidance molecules, namely membrane-bound ligand (*Sema6b*), cell surface receptors (*Epha7*, *Plxna4*, *Nrp1*, *Unc5a*) and GTP-binding protein (*Rnd1*) (Fig. 4). Table 4 indicates that *Epha7*, *Nrp1*, *Plxna4* and *Unc5a* were up-regulated in DLK-depleted cells, whereas *Rnd1* and *Sema6b* were down-regulated.

## Validation of RNA-seq data by qRT-PCR analysis and immunoblotting

The six axon guidance genes identified by RNA-seq as being either up-regulated or down-regulated by DLK knockdown were validated by qRT-PCR. As shown in Fig. 5a, qRT-PCR analysis of cells expressing either the

**Table 2** Gene ontology terms associated with dysregulated genes in DLK-depleted cells

| Term | Count | % | P-Value | Benjamini |
|---|---|---|---|---|
| Protein amino acid phosphorylation | 15 | 9,1 | 3,70E-04 | 3,30E-01 |
| System development | 29 | 17,7 | 1,10E-03 | 4,50E-01 |
| Phosphorylation | 15 | 9,1 | 1,20E-03 | 3,40E-01 |
| Enzyme linked receptor protein signaling pathway | 9 | 5,5 | 1,20E-03 | 2,70E-01 |
| Anatomical structure development | 29 | 17,7 | 3,20E-03 | 4,90E-01 |
| Cell adhesion | 12 | 7,3 | 3,80E-03 | 4,90E-01 |
| Biological adhesion | 12 | 7,3 | 3,90E-03 | 4,50E-01 |
| Extracellular structure organization | 6 | 3,7 | 5,80E-03 | 5,40E-01 |
| Phosphorus metabolic process | 15 | 9,1 | 6,30E-03 | 5,30E-01 |
| Phosphate metabolic process | 15 | 9,1 | 6,30E-03 | 5,30E-01 |

sh73 or sh69 lentiviral construct confirmed the results obtained by RNA-seq for most of the selected genes, indicating the reliability of our transcriptomic data. One exception was *Unc5a*, which was found by RNA-seq and qRT-PCR analyses to be regulated in opposite directions. For genes such as *Nrp1* and *Rnd1*, our qRT-PCR results were correlated with the RNA-seq results for both DLK shRNA constructs, whereas for the other genes tested, including *Sema6b*, *Epha7* and *Plxna4*, a correlation was seen only with either the sh73 or the sh69 lentiviral vector. The reason behind this result is not clear, but it most likely relates to the fact that the residual amount of DLK in cells after knockdown varies between the two constructs and between experiments, which could consequently lead to differential effects on gene expression.

As a complementary approach, we also analyzed whether the differences in transcript abundance between control and DLK-depleted cells translated into protein level changes for two of the identified axon guidance genes, namely *Plxna4* and *Nrp1*. These two genes were of particular interest because they encode cell-surface receptors that act in complex to mediäte repulsive responses of axons to class-3 semaphorins in most neurons [45]. Moreover, they have been recognized as

important regulators of neuronal migration [46], a process impaired in DLK knockout mouse brain [11]. In accordance with RNA-seq and qRT-PCR data, immunoblot analysis showed that protein levels of Plxna4 and Nrp1 were significantly increased by 1.5- to 2-fold in Neuro-2a cells after DLK depletion compared with control (Fig. 5b and c). Taken together, these experiments confirm that DLK depletion has an effect on Plxna4 and Nrp1 expression in neuronal cells at both the transcriptional and translational levels, and shed light for the first time on the mechanisms by which DLK signalling contributes to nervous system development and function.

## Discussion

Recent exciting findings based on experiments carried out in vivo and in vitro have highlighted the potential role of DLK in nervous system assembly, maintenance and repair. These studies have indeed demonstrated the requirement for DLK in various aspects of neuronal cell physiology, ranging from migration, axon growth and apoptosis during development to nerve regeneration and degeneration in the adult (for a review, see [47]). One of the fundamental issues remaining to be solved in this context is elucidation of the mechanisms by which DLK regulates such a vast range of biological responses. In an attempt to gain insight into DLK's mode of action, we have examined the global changes that occur in the transcriptome of differentiated Neuro-2a cells after knockdown of DLK by RNA interference. Our results demonstrate that DLK depletion leads to a decrease or an increase in the levels of numerous mRNAs, indicating that DLK contributes to both positive and negative regulation of gene expression even under basal conditions. At this point, it is not known whether these changes in gene expression are a cause or a consequence of DLK depletion. However, we assume that such a response is probably JNK-dependent because knockdown of DLK in Neuro-2a cells impairs JNK basal activity and JNK-mediated phosphorylation of c-Jun, a component of the AP-1 transcription factor (Fig. 1). This assumption is also supported by the studies of Hirai et al. (2006) who showed that JNK activity and phosphorylation of JNK substrates, including c-Jun, are significantly reduced in DLK$^{-/-}$ mouse embryonic brain. Previous reports found that JNK both positively and negatively regulates gene

**Table 3** KEGG pathway terms associated with dysregulated genes in DLK-depleted cells

| Term | Count | % | Gene symbols | P-Value | Benjamini |
|---|---|---|---|---|---|
| Axon guidance | 6 | 3,7 | *Epha7, Rnd1, Nrp1, Plxna4, Sema6b, Unc5a* | 3,70E-03 | 2,50E-01 |
| ECM-receptor interaction | 5 | 3 | *Itgb3, Itgb4, Lama2, Tnr, Thbs3* | 4,20E-03 | 1,50E-01 |
| Focal adhesion | 7 | 4,3 | *Hgf, Itgb3, Itgb4, Lama2, Pdgfra, Tnr, Thbs3* | 4,60E-03 | 1,10E-01 |
| Arrhythmogenic right ventricular cardiomyopathy (ARVC) | 4 | 2,4 | *Des, Itgb3, Itgb4, Lama2* | 2,20E-02 | 3,50E-01 |
| Hypertrophic cardiomyopathy (HCM) | 4 | 2,4 | *Des, Itgb3, Itgb4, Lama2* | 2,90E-02 | 3,70E-01 |

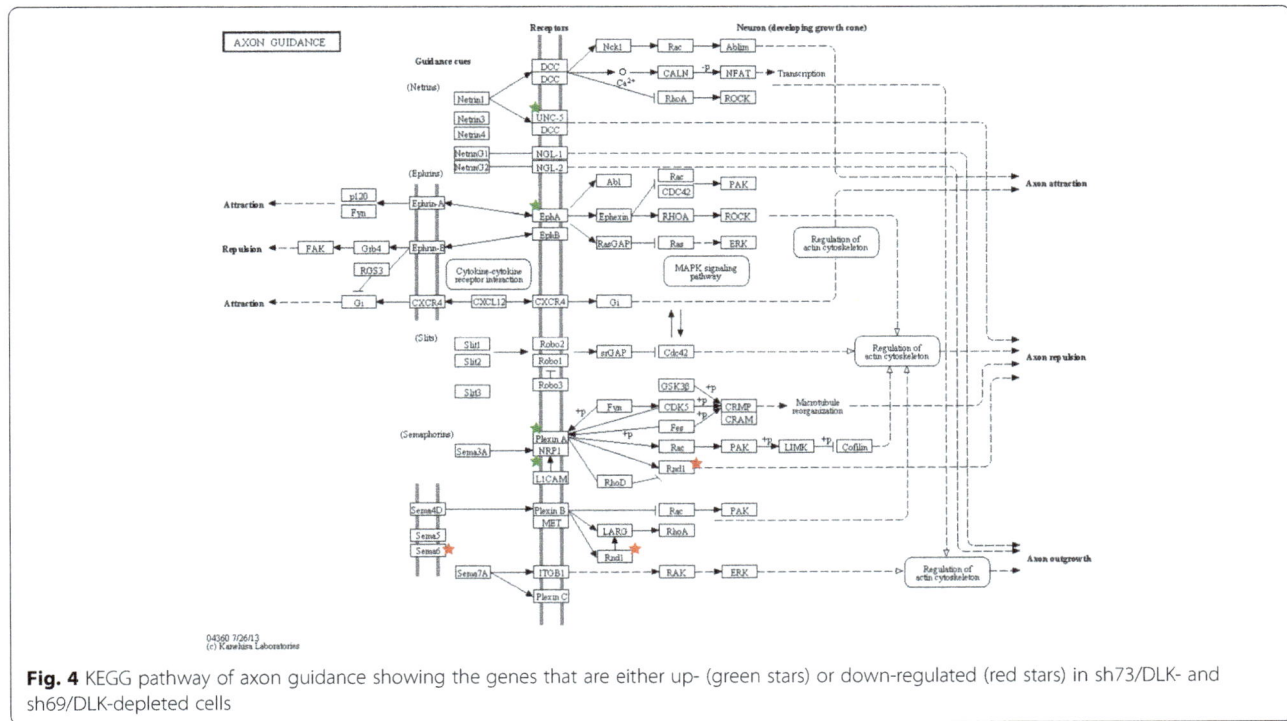

**Fig. 4** KEGG pathway of axon guidance showing the genes that are either up- (green stars) or down-regulated (red stars) in sh73/DLK- and sh69/DLK-depleted cells

expression by phosphorylating DNA-bound proteins, such as transcription factors and histones, as well as by binding directly to transcriptionally active gene promoters [48, 49].

Interestingly, decrease of DLK expression in Neuro-2a cells resulted in transcriptional dysregulation of a subset of genes involved in neuronal function, such as migration, differentiation, axonogenesis, and axon guidance, an observation that supports its critical role in nervous system development (Additional file 3: Table S3, Additional file 4: Table S4). To our knowledge, none of these genes have been previously identified as potential targets of DLK. In a recent work using a microarray approach, Watkins et al. (2013) showed that DLK is required for expression of proapoptotic- and regeneration-related genes in retinal ganglion cells (RGCs) after optic nerve crush. Consistent with this finding, it has also

been reported that RGCs isolated from mice containing a floxed allele of DLK displayed resistance to death induced by axonal injury, together with a concomitant decrease in JNK phosphorylation and c-Jun expression [17]. The basis for the difference in target gene specificity between Neuro-2a cells and RGCs is unclear, but could reflect cell type or cell context variability. Another possible explanation might be that the DLK-dependent transcriptional program varies between basal and stress-stimulated conditions, which inevitably lead to different cellular responses.

As stated above, the current results highlight for the first time the involvement of DLK in expression of axon guidance genes. This family of genes encodes proteins that act as attractants or repellents for axons, thereby guiding them towards or away from a specific region [23, 50]. The growth cone, a sensory structure located at

**Table 4** Fold change of the axon guidance genes dysregulated in DLK-depleted cells relative to control cells

| Ensembl gene id | Symbol | Description | Log2 fold-change | | | | Regulation |
|---|---|---|---|---|---|---|---|
| | | | sh73 no. 1 | sh73 no. 2 | sh69 no. 1 | sh69 no. 2 | |
| ENSMUSG00000028289 | Epha7 | Eph receptor A7 | 1.657 | 1.741 | 1.387 | 1.595 | Up |
| ENSMUSG00000054855 | Rnd1 | Rho family GTPase 1 | −1.436 | −1.463 | −1.112 | −0.529 | Down |
| ENSMUSG00000025810 | Nrp1 | Neuropilin 1 | 1.14 | 1.304 | 0.72 | 1.383 | Up |
| ENSMUSG00000029765 | Plxna4 | Plexin A4 | 1.151 | 0.699 | 1.522 | 1.367 | Up |
| ENSMUSG00000001227 | Sema6B | Semaphorin 6B | −1.055 | −1.797 | −0.866 | −1.780 | Down |
| ENSMUSG00000025876 | Unc5a | Unc-5 homolog A | 1.283 | 1.451 | 0.977 | 1.127 | Up |

Numbers in italics represent change in gene expression that were less than two-fold

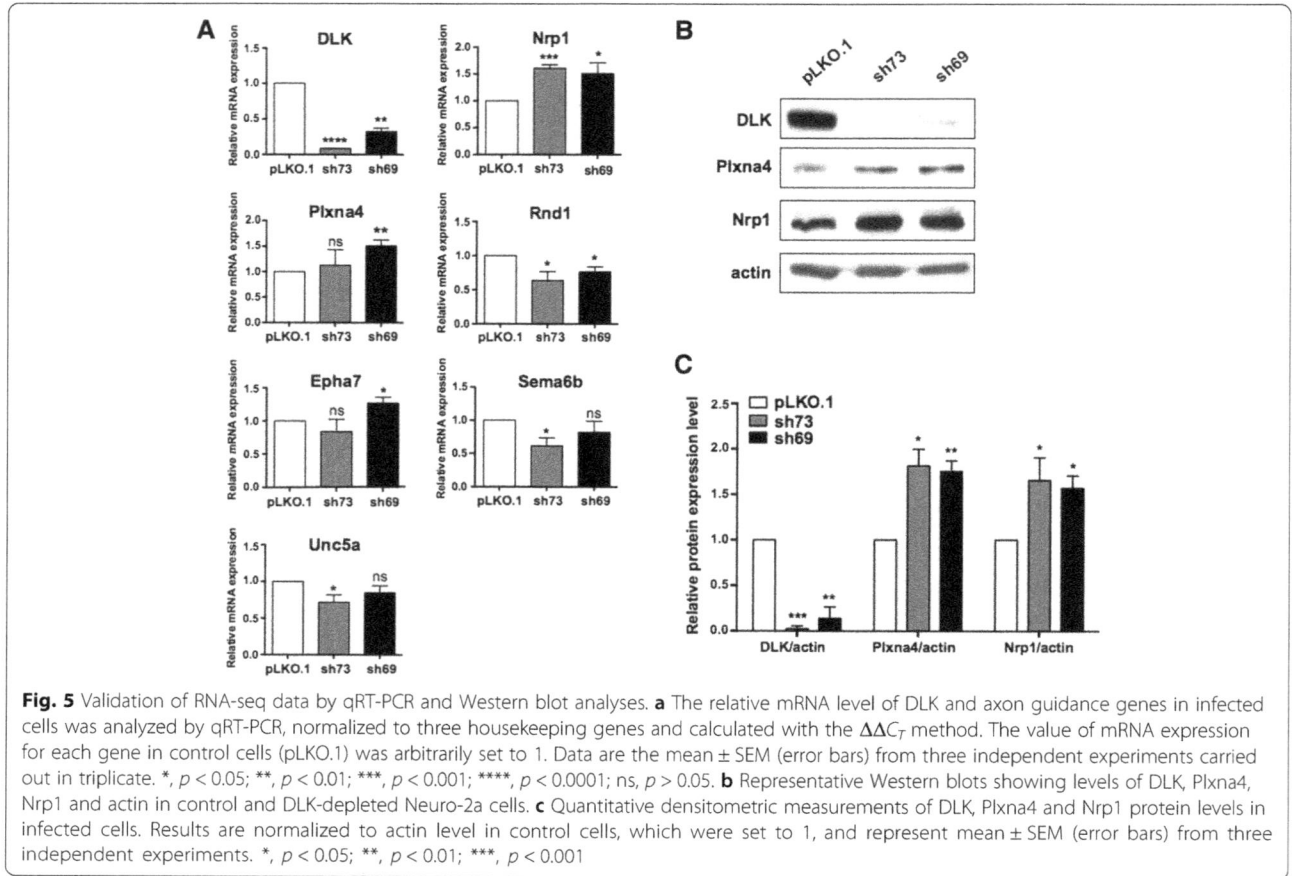

**Fig. 5** Validation of RNA-seq data by qRT-PCR and Western blot analyses. **a** The relative mRNA level of DLK and axon guidance genes in infected cells was analyzed by qRT-PCR, normalized to three housekeeping genes and calculated with the $\Delta\Delta C_T$ method. The value of mRNA expression for each gene in control cells (pLKO.1) was arbitrarily set to 1. Data are the mean ± SEM (error bars) from three independent experiments carried out in triplicate. *, $p < 0.05$; **, $p < 0.01$; ***, $p < 0.001$; ****, $p < 0.0001$; ns, $p > 0.05$. **b** Representative Western blots showing levels of DLK, Plxna4, Nrp1 and actin in control and DLK-depleted Neuro-2a cells. **c** Quantitative densitometric measurements of DLK, Plxna4 and Nrp1 protein levels in infected cells. Results are normalized to actin level in control cells, which were set to 1, and represent mean ± SEM (error bars) from three independent experiments. *, $p < 0.05$; **, $p < 0.01$; ***, $p < 0.001$

the tip of extending axons, expresses receptors that recognize these guidance cues and trigger intracellular signaling cascades, resulting in extensive cytoskeletal rearrangement and subsequent axon steering [51]. Different families of axon guidance cues and receptors have been identified, including ephrins and Eph receptors, semaphorins and plexin and neuropilin receptors, Slits and Robo receptors, Netrins, DCC and Unc5 receptors as well as RGM and noegenin receptors [23]. Axon guidance proteins have been shown to be involved in various aspects of neural circuit development (e.g., growth, guidance, bundling, fasciculation and pruning of axons, and synaptogenesis), and in the control of synaptic plasticity in adults [52]. Emerging data from human and animal models also implicate axon guidance molecules in neurological disorders and axon regeneration after injury [24, 53–55]. In our RNA-seq data, four axon guidance genes, including *Epha7*, *Nrp1*, *Plxna4* and *Unc5a*, showed an increase in expression level after DLK depletion, whereas two, *Rnd1* and *Sema6b*, were downregulated (Additional file 3: Table S3 and Additional file 4: Table S4). qRT-PCR confirmed that these mRNA changes were significant for *Epha7*, *Nrp1*, *Plxna4*, *Rnd1* and *Sema6b* (Fig. 5). Because there was no correlation between

the RNA-seq and qRT-PCR results for *Unc5a*, we currently cannot draw any conclusion for this gene. A part of our findings was further validated by Western blot analysis, which shows that Nrp1 and Plxna4 protein levels were significantly induced in DLK-depleted cells (Fig. 5), thus demonstrating the ability of DLK to exert a repressing effect on Nrp1 and Plxna4 expression. Because Nrp1 and Plxna4 cooperate to mediate signaling in response to semaphorin 3A (Sema3A), a repulsive guidance cue for axons in most neurons [25], it is tempting to speculate that an increase in their expression, such as the one described here, could contribute to the defects of axonal growth previously described in DLK null mouse embryos and DLK-deficient cultured cortical neurons [11, 44]. This hypothesis is fully in line with results demonstrating that ectopic expression of Nrp1 or Plxna4 in neuronal cell types that are insensitive to Sema3a caused axon repulsion and growth cone collapse in response to Sema3A [45, 56]. The identification of *Epha7* and *Rnd1* as up- and down-regulated genes, respectively, in DLK-depleted cells is also of great interest in regard to the contribution of DLK to neuron projection development. Indeed, a recent study revealed that Epha7, which generally transduces repulsive signals

[57], impairs dendrite formation when overexpressed in cortical neurons [58], while knockdown of Rnd1 in hippocampal neurons suppressed axon extension [59]. Finally, for *Sema6b*, whose expression decreased upon DLK knockdown in Neuro-2a cells, results obtained from loss-of-function experiments demonstrated its requirement for proper projection of hippocampal granule cell axons [60]. Taken together, these data are supportive of a model whereby DLK promotes axonal growth during neural development by regulating, at least in part, the expression of axon guidance genes. It is presently not known how DLK would modulate axon guidance molecule abundance in neurons, but one possible mechanism is control of synthesis, phosphorylation and/or activity of the transcription factors that regulate them. Work carried out over the past several years has established that transcriptional control of axon guidance cues and receptors is crucial to allow precise pathfinding decisions of neuronal growth cones [61, 62].

Although further work will be required to investigate the biological consequences of dysregulated axon guidance gene expression in DLK-depleted Neuro-2a cells, we anticipate as a potential outcome an alteration of the cytoskeleton. This prediction is supported by the fact that axon guidance cues and their receptors modulate actin and microtubule dynamics in the growth cone via activation of downstream signaling molecules, such as protein kinases, small GTPases and cytoskeleton-associated proteins [50, 63, 64]. As illustrated by studies in different systems, remodeling of the cytoskeleton is critically important for attraction, repulsion, growth cone collapse or axon extension [51]. Interestingly, a functional link between DLK and cytoskeletal regulation has been recently suggested. In this study, Hirai et al. (2011) demonstrated by RNA interference that knockdown of DLK in cultured mouse embryonic neurons caused defects in axon formation, whereas concomitant treatment of cells with the microtubule-stabilizing drug taxol antagonized this response. These results implicate DLK as a key regulator of microtubule stabilization, a required event for axon formation [65, 66]. Consistent with an active role for DLK in microtubule dynamics, DLK gene disruption in mice resulted in reduced phosphorylation of the microtubule-stabilizing proteins Doublecortin and MAP2c [11]. In light of these data and the results from the present study, it is conceivable to suggest that DLK regulation of axon growth in neurons may depend, at least in part, on cytoskeletal reorganization mediated either directly via phosphorylation of microtubule-associated proteins or indirectly through modulation of axon guidance gene expression.

## Conclusions

We found that DLK plays an important role in regulating expression of genes recognized for their contribution in nervous system development and function. Future studies will be dedicated to understand how DLK influences the expression of *Nrp1*, *Plxna4*, *Epha7*, *Rnd1* and *Sema6b* as well as the consequences of their up- or down-regulation on axon growth. Further experiments using the DLK knockout mice will also be required to assess the in vivo relevance of our in vitro findings.

### Abbreviations
DLK, dual leucine zipper kinase; Epha7, eph receptor A7; ERK, extracellular signal-regulated kinase; JNK, c-Jun N-terminal kinase; Nrp1, neuropilin 1; Plxna4, plexin A4; Rnd1, Rho family GTPase 1; Sema6b, semaphorin 6B; Unc5a, Unc-5 homolog A

### Acknowledgements
We thank Dr. Alain Lavigueur for critical reading of the manuscript, Daniel Garneau for his indispensable help in microscopy and image processing, and the RNomics platform of the Université de Sherbrooke for the qRT-PCR analyses.

### Funding
This work was made possible by grants from the Natural Sciences and Engineering Research Council of Canada (138068–2012) and the Université de Sherbrooke, and in part by support from Calcul Québec and Compute Canada.

### Authors' contributions
AB, RB, JFL, DM, SR and PEJ designed the study. AB, JFL, LD and RB performed the experiments and analyzed the data. AB and RB supervised the experiments and wrote the manuscript. All authors read and approved the final manuscript.

### Competing interests
The authors declare that they have no competing interests.

### Author details
[1]Département de biologie, Faculté des sciences, Université de Sherbrooke, 2500 Boul. de l'Université, Sherbrooke, Québec J1K 2R1, Canada. [2]Département d'informatique, Faculté des sciences, Université de Sherbrooke, Sherbrooke, Québec, Canada. [3]Centre de recherche du Centre hospitalier universitaire de Sherbrooke, Sherbrooke, Canada.

## References

1. Cargnello M, Roux PP. Activation and function of the MAPKs and their substrates, the MAPK-activated protein kinases. Microbiol Mol Biol Rev. 2011;75:50–83.

2. Johnson GL, Lapadat R. Mitogen-activated protein kinase pathways mediated by ERK, JNK, and p38 protein kinases. Science. 2002;298:1911–2.

3. Reddy UR, Pleasure D. Cloning of a novel putative protein kinase having a leucine zipper domain from human brain. Biochem Biophys Res Commun. 1994;202:613–20.

4. Fan G, Merritt SE, Kortenjann M, Shaw PE, Holzman LB. Dual leucine zipper-bearing kinase (DLK) activates p46(SAPK) and p38(mapk) but not ERK2. J Biol Chem. 1996;271:24788–93.

5. Daviau A, Di Fruscio M, Blouin R. The mixed-lineage kinase DLK undergoes Src-dependent tyrosine phosphorylation and activation in cells exposed to vanadate or platelet-derived growth factor (PDGF). Cell Signal. 2009; 21:577–87.

6. Daviau A, Couture JP, Blouin R. Loss of DLK expression in WI-38 human diploid fibroblasts induces a senescent-like proliferation arrest. Biochem Biophys Res Commun. 2011;413:282–7.

7. Holzman LB, Merritt SE, Fan G. Identification, molecular cloning, and characterization of dual leucine zipper bearing kinase. A novel serine/threonine protein kinase that defines a second subfamily of mixed lineage kinases. J Biol Chem. 1994;269:30808–17.

8. Blouin R, Beaudoin J, Bergeron P, Nadeau A, Grondin G. Cell-specific expression of the ZPK gene in adult mouse tissues. DNA Cell Biol. 1996; 15:631–42.

9. Germain L, Fradette J, Robitaille H, Guignard R, Grondin G, Nadeau A, et al. The mixed lineage kinase leucine-zipper protein kinase exhibits a differentiation-associated localization in normal human skin and induces keratinocyte differentiation upon overexpression. J Invest Dermatol. 2000; 115:860–7.

10. Hirai S, Kawaguchi A, Suenaga J, Ono M, Cui DF, Ohno S. Expression of MUK/DLK/ZPK, an activator of the JNK pathway, in the nervous systems of the developing mouse embryo. Gene Expr Patterns. 2005;5:517–23.

11. Hirai S, Cui DF, Miyata T, Ogawa M, Kiyonari H, Suda Y, et al. The c-Jun N-terminal kinase activator dual leucine zipper kinase regulates axon growth and neuronal migration in the developing cerebral cortex. J Neurosci. 2006;26:11992–2002.

12. Bloom AJ, Miller BR, Sanes JR, DiAntonio A. The requirement for Phr1 in CNS axon tract formation reveals the corticostriatal boundary as a choice point for cortical axons. Genes Dev. 2007;21:2593–606.

13. Ghosh AS, Wang B, Pozniak CD, Chen M, Watts RJ, Lewcock JW. DLK induces developmental neuronal degeneration via selective regulation of proapoptotic JNK activity. J Cell Biol. 2011;194:751–64.

14. Hirai S, Banba Y, Satake T, Ohno S. Axon formation in neocortical neurons depends on stage-specific regulation of microtubule stability by the dual leucine zipper kinase-c-Jun N-terminal kinase pathway. J Neurosci. 2011;31: 6468–80.

15. Itoh A, Horiuchi M, Wakayama K, Xu J, Bannerman P, Pleasure D, et al. ZPK/DLK, a mitogen-activated protein kinase kinase kinase, is a critical mediator of programmed cell death of motoneurons. J Neurosci. 2011;31:7223–8.

16. Watkins TA, Wang B, Huntwork-Rodriguez S, Yang J, Jiang Z, Eastham-Anderson J, et al. DLK initiates a transcriptional program that couples apoptotic and regenerative responses to axonal injury. Proc Natl Acad Sci U S A. 2013;110:4039–44.

17. Welsbie DS, Yang Z, Ge Y, Mitchell KL, Zhou X, Martin SE, et al. Functional genomic screening identifies dual leucine zipper kinase as a key mediator of retinal ganglion cell death. Proc Natl Acad Sci U S A. 2013;110:4045–50.

18. Pozniak CD, Sengupta Ghosh A, Gogineni A, Hanson JE, Lee S-H, Larson JL, et al. Dual leucine zipper kinase is required for excitotoxicity-induced neuronal degeneration. J Exp Med. 2013;210:2553–67.

19. Fernandes KA, Harder JM, John SW, Shrager P, Libby RT. DLK-dependent signaling is important for somal but not axonal degeneration of retinal ganglion cells following axonal injury. Neurobiol Dis. 2014;69:108–16.

20. Itoh A, Horiuchi M, Bannerman P, Pleasure D, Itoh T. Impaired regenerative response of primary sensory neurons in ZPK/DLK gene-trap mice. Biochem Biophys Res Commun. 2009;383:258–62.

21. Saxena S, Caroni P. Mechanisms of axon degeneration: From development to disease. Prog Neurobiol. 2007;83:174–91.

22. Yu TW, Bargmann CI. Dynamic regulation of axon guidance. Nat Neurosci. 2001;4(Suppl):1169–76.

23. Chilton JK. Molecular mechanisms of axon guidance. Dev Biol. 2006;292:13–24.

24. Giger RJ, Hollis ER, Tuszynski MH. Guidance molecules in axon regeneration. Cold Spring Harb Perspect Biol. 2010;2:a001867.

25. Pasterkamp RJ. Getting neural circuits into shape with semaphorins. Nat Rev Neurosci. 2012;13:605–18.

26. Douziech M, Laberge G, Grondin G, Daigle N, Blouin R. Localization of the mixed-lineage kinase DLK/MUK/ZPK to the Golgi apparatus in NIH 3 T3 cells. J Histochem Cytochem. 1999;47:1287–96.

27. Stewart SA, Dykxhoorn DM, Palliser D, Mizuno H, Yu EY, An DS, et al. Lentivirus-delivered stable gene silencing by RNAi in primary cells. RNA. 2003;9:493–501.

28. Hellemans J, Mortier G, De Paepe A, Speleman F, Vandesompele J. qBase relative quantification framework and software for management and automated analysis of real-time quantitative PCR data. Genome Biol. 2007;8:R19.

29. Brosseau J-P, Lucier J-F, Lapointe E, Durand M, Gendron D, Gervais-Bird J, et al. High-throughput quantification of splicing isoforms. RNA. 2010;16:442–9.

30. Schindelin J, Arganda-Carreras I, Frise E, Kaynig V, Longair M, Pietzsch T, et al. Fiji: an open source platform for biological image analysis. Nat Methods. 2012;9:676–82.

31. Longair MH, Baker DA, Armstrong JD. Simple neurite tracer: open source software for reconstruction, visualization and analysis of neuronal processes. Bioinformatics. 2011;27:2453–4.

32. Bolger AM, Lohse M, Usadel B. Trimmomatic: a flexible trimmer for illumina sequence data. Bioinformatics. 2014;30:2114–20.

33. Kim D, Pertea G, Trapnell C, Pimentel H, Kelley R, Salzberg SL. TopHat2: accurate alignment of transcriptomes in the presence of insertions, deletions and gene fusions. Genome Biol. 2013;14:R36.

34. Langmead B, Salzberg SL. Fast gapped-read alignment with Bowtie 2. Nat Methods. 2012;9:357–9.

35. Flicek P, Ahmed I, Amode MR, Barrell D, Beal K, Brent S, et al. Ensembl 2013. Nucleic Acids Res. 2013;41:D48–55.

36. Anders S, Pyl PT, Huber W. HTSeq - A Python framework to work with high-throughput sequencing data. Bioinformatics. 2014;31:166–9.

37. Anders S, Huber W. Differential expression analysis for sequence count data. Genome Biol. 2010;11:R106.

38. Robinson MD, McCarthy DJ, Smyth GK. edgeR: a Bioconductor package for differential expression analysis of digital gene expression data. Bioinformatics. 2010;26:139–40.

39. Huber W, Carey VJ, Gentleman R, Anders S, Carlson M, Carvalho BS, et al. Orchestrating high-throughput genomic analysis with Bioconductor. Nat Methods. 2015;12:115–21. Nature Publishing Group, a division of Macmillan Publishers Limited. All Rights Reserved.

40. Gentleman RC, Carey VJ, Bates DM, Bolstad B, Dettling M, Dudoit S, et al. Bioconductor: open software development for computational biology and bioinformatics. Genome Biol. 2004;5:R80.

41. Huang DW, Sherman BT, Lempicki RA. Systematic and integrative analysis of large gene lists using DAVID bioinformatics resources. Nat Protoc. 2009;4: 44–57.

42. Tremblay RG, Sikorska M, Sandhu JK, Lanthier P, Ribecco-Lutkiewicz M, Bani-Yaghoub M. Differentiation of mouse Neuro 2A cells into dopamine neurons. J Neurosci Methods. 2010;186:60–7.

43. Evangelopoulos ME, Weis J, Krüttgen A. Signalling pathways leading to neuroblastoma differentiation after serum withdrawal: HDL blocks neuroblastoma differentiation by inhibition of EGFR. Oncogene. 2005;24: 3309–18.

44. Eto K, Kawauchi T, Osawa M, Tabata H, Nakajima K. Role of dual leucine zipper-bearing kinase (DLK/MUK/ZPK) in axonal growth. Neurosci Res. 2010; 66:37–45.

45. Suto F, Ito K, Uemura M, Shimizu M, Shinkawa Y, Sanbo M, et al. Plexin-a4 mediates axon-repulsive activities of both secreted and transmembrane semaphorins and plays roles in nerve fiber guidance. J Neurosci. 2005;25: 3628–37.

46. Chen G, Sima J, Jin M, Wang K-Y, Xue X-J, Zheng W, et al. Semaphorin-3A guides radial migration of cortical neurons during development. Nat Neurosci. 2008;11:36–44.

47. Tedeschi A, Bradke F. The DLK signalling pathway–a double-edged sword in neural development and regeneration. EMBO Rep. 2013;14:605–14.

48. Whitmarsh AJ. Regulation of gene transcription by mitogen-activated protein kinase signaling pathways. Biochim Biophys Acta. 2007;1773: 1285–98.

49. Tiwari VK, Stadler MB, Wirbelauer C, Paro R, Schübeler D, Beisel C. A chromatin-modifying function of JNK during stem cell differentiation. Nat Genet. 2012;44:94–100.

50. Pasterkamp RJ, Kolodkin AL. SnapShot: Axon Guidance. Cell. 2013;153(494): 494e1–2.

5 . Dent EW, Gupton SL, Gertler FB. The growth cone cytoskeleton in axon outgrowth and guidance. Cold Spring Harb Perspect Biol. 2011;3.

52. Kolodkin AL, Tessier-Lavigne M. Mechanisms and Molecules of Neuronal Wiring: A Primer. Cold Spring Harb Perspect Biol. 2010;3:a001727–7.

53. Mann F, Chauvet S, Rougon G. Semaphorins in development and adult brain: implication for neurological diseases. Prog Neurobiol. 2007;82:57–79.

54. Schmidt ERE, Pasterkamp RJ, van den Berg LH. Axon guidance proteins: novel therapeutic targets for ALS? Prog Neurobiol. 2009;88:286–301.

55. Van Battum EY, Brignani S, Pasterkamp RJ. Axon guidance proteins in neurological disorders. Lancet Neurol. 2015;14:532–46.

55. Romi E, Gokhman I, Wong E, Antonovsky N, Ludwig A, Sagi I, et al. ADAM metalloproteases promote a developmental switch in responsiveness to the axonal repellant Sema3A. Nat Commun. 2014;5:4058.

57. Klein R. Eph/ephrin signalling during development. Development. 2012;139: 4105–9.

53. Clifford MA, Athar W, Leonard CE, Russo A, Sampognaro PJ, Van der Goes M-S, et al. EphA7 signaling guides cortical dendritic development and spine maturation. Proc Natl Acad Sci U S A. 2014;111:4994–9.

53. Li Y-H, Ghavampur S, Bondallaz P, Will L, Grenningloh G, Püschel AW. Rnd1 regulates axon extension by enhancing the microtubule destabilizing activity of SCG10. J Biol Chem. 2009;284:363–71.

60. Tawarayama H, Yoshida Y, Suto F, Mitchell KJ, Fujisawa H. Roles of semaphorin-6B and plexin-A2 in lamina-restricted projection of hippocampal mossy fibers. J Neurosci. 2010;30:7049–60.

61. Butler SJ, Tear G. Getting axons onto the right path: the role of transcription factors in axon guidance. Development. 2007;134:439–48.

62. Polleux F, Ince-Dunn G, Ghosh A. Transcriptional regulation of vertebrate axon guidance and synapse formation. Nat Rev Neurosci. 2007;8:331–40.

63. O'Donnell M, Chance RK, Bashaw GJ. Axon growth and guidance: receptor regulation and signal transduction. Annu Rev Neurosci. 2009;32:383–412.

64. Bashaw GJ, Klein R. Signaling from axon guidance receptors. Cold Spring Harb Perspect Biol. 2010;2:a001941.

65. Zhou F-Q, Zhou J, Dedhar S, Wu Y-H, Snider WD. NGF-induced axon growth is mediated by localized inactivation of GSK-3beta and functions of the microtubule plus end binding protein APC. Neuron. 2004;42:897–912.

66. Witte H, Neukirchen D, Bradke F. Microtubule stabilization specifies initial neuronal polarization. J Cell Biol. 2008;180:619–32.

# 15

# Cell type-specific effects of p27$^{KIP1}$ loss on retinal development

Mariko Ogawa[1], Fuminori Saitoh[1], Norihiro Sudou[1], Fumi Sato[2] and Hiroki Fujieda[1]* ⓘ

## Abstract

**Background:** Cyclin-dependent kinase (CDK) inhibitors play an important role in regulating cell cycle progression, cell cycle exit and cell differentiation. p27$^{KIP1}$ (p27), one of the major CDK inhibitors in the retina, has been shown to control the timing of cell cycle exit of retinal progenitors. However, the precise role of this protein in retinal development remains largely unexplored. We thus analyzed p27-deficient mice to characterize the effects of p27 loss on proliferation, differentiation, and survival of retinal cells.

**Methods:** Expression of p27 in the developing and mature mouse retina was analyzed by immunohistochemistry using antibodies against p27 and cell type-specific markers. Cell proliferation and differentiation were examined in the wild-type and p27-deficient retinas by immunohistochemistry using various cell cycle and differentiation markers.

**Results:** All postmitotic retinal cell types expressed p27 in the mouse retinas. p27 loss caused extension of the period of proliferation in the developing retinas. This extra proliferation was mainly due to ectopic cell cycle reentry of differentiating cells including bipolar cells, Müller glial cells and cones, rather than persistent division of progenitors as previously suggested. Aberrant cell cycle activity of cones was followed by cone death resulting in a significant reduction in cone number in the mature p27-deficient retinas.

**Conclusions:** Although expressed in all retinal cell types, p27 is required to maintain the quiescence of specific cell types including bipolar cells, Müller glia, and cones while it is dispensable for preventing cell cycle reentry in other cell types.

**Keywords:** Cyclin-dependent kinase inhibitor, p27$^{KIP1}$, Retinal development, Ectopic cell cycle reentry, Cone death

## Background

During development of the CNS, precise coordination of progenitor cell proliferation and cell cycle exit is essential for generation of appropriate number of neurons. Cell proliferation is driven by cell cycle-specific cyclins assembled with their catalytic partners, cyclin-dependent kinases (CDKs). The activity of cyclin/CDK complexes is regulated by CDK inhibitors, which inhibit cell cycle progression and promote cell cycle exit [1, 2]. Recent evidence has further revealed that CDK inhibitors promote differentiation independently of their ability to regulate CDK activity [3–5]. However, much of the knowledge concerning the role of CDK inhibitors comes from the results of in vitro studies using non-neuronal cells, and whether CDK inhibitors have equivalent roles in vivo in the context of CNS development or whether they function in a cell type-specific manner remain largely unexplored.

The retina is an ideal model of the CNS to gain insight into these questions as it has a relatively simple structure consisting of only seven major cell types, which can be clearly identified by position and specific markers. Multipotent retinal progenitors divide extensively during development and lose proliferative capacity as they withdraw from the cell cycle and differentiate into specific cell types. Yet, how retinal cells exit the cell cycle and maintain the quiescent non-proliferative state is only partially understood. Several types of CDK inhibitors have been detected in the developing retina, of which p27$^{KIP1}$ (p27) is most abundantly and ubiquitously expressed [6]. In the *Xenopus* retina, p27 not only inhibits the cell cycle but also promotes the cell fate of Müller

* Correspondence: hfujieda@twmu.ac.jp
[1]Department of Anatomy, School of Medicine, Tokyo Women's Medical University, 8-1 Kawada-cho, Shinjuku-ku, Tokyo 162-8666, Japan
Full list of author information is available at the end of the article

glia [7]. In the rodent retinas, p27 does not seem to have a role in cell type specification, but it promotes the cell cycle exit of retinal progenitors [8, 9]. p27 loss was shown to extend the period of progenitor proliferation [8, 9] and rescue the hypoplastic defects of cyclin D1-deficient retinas [10]. These studies indicated that p27 plays an essential role in controlling the timing of cell cycle exit of retinal progenitors. Recent studies have also revealed that deletion of Rb and its family members in the retina induces ectopic proliferation of differentiating cells, suggesting that the major function of the Rb family in retinal development is to prevent cell cycle reentry of differentiating cells [11–13]. Considering that the Rb family functions downstream of p27, we hypothesized that p27 loss may have effects on differentiating cells, in addition to the previously reported effects on progenitors. To address this issue and delineate more precisely the role of p27 in retinal development, we revisited p27-deficient mice to characterize the effects of p27 loss on proliferation, differentiation, and survival of retinal cells. In contrast with the previous observations, our data suggest that extra proliferation observed in the p27-deficient retinas is mainly due to ectopic cell cycle reentry of differentiating bipolar cells, Müller glia and cones, rather than persistent division of progenitors. Aberrant cell cycle activity of cones was followed by cone death resulting in a significant reduction in cone number in the mature p27-deficient retinas. Our data propose a previously unrecognized cell-specific role for p27 in the maintenance of quiescent state in postmitotic retinal cells.

## Methods

### Animals and tissue preparation

p27$^{+/-}$ mice [14] were obtained from the Jackson Laboratory (Bar Harbor, USA), bred and genotyped by PCR as recommended by the Jackson Laboratory. Animals were maintained under a 12:12 h light/dark photoperiod and sacrificed by decapitation or cervical dislocation in the middle of the light phase at various developmental stages. For immunohistochemistry, the eyecups with the cornea and lens removed were fixed by immersion in 4% paraformaldehyde in 0.1 M phosphate buffer (pH 7.4) for 1 h, rinsed in 15% and 30% sucrose in phosphate buffer, and frozen with dry ice–isopentane. Cryostat sections were cut at 10 μm through the optic disc along the dorsoventral axis and collected on MAS-coated glass slides (Matsunami glass, Osaka, Japan). For RT-PCR, the retinas were dissected and kept frozen at −80 °C until use. All experimental procedures were conducted in accordance with the research protocols approved by the institutional animal care committee of Tokyo Women's Medical University.

### BrdU incorporation assay

To label mitotic cells in the S-phase, animals received a single injection of BrdU (Sigma, St. Louis, USA, 100 mg/kg body weight, i.p.) 2 h before sacrifice. For birthdating studies, animals were injected twice per day with BrdU and allowed to survive at least 9 days before sacrifice.

### Immunohistochemistry

Immunohistochemistry was conducted as described previously [15, 16]. For BrdU labeling, cryostat sections of the retina were treated with 2 M HCl at 37 °C for 30 min prior to incubation with primary antibodies. Primary antibodies are listed in Additional file 1: Table S1. Secondary antibodies include donkey anti-mouse IgG (Alexa Fluor 488), donkey anti-rabbit IgG (Alexa Fluor 488, 555, 594 and 647), donkey anti-sheep IgG (Alexa Fluor 555), and donkey anti-goat IgG (Alexa Fluor 568), all of which were purchased from Invitrogen (Eugene, USA). Fluorescein-conjugated peanut agglutinin (PNA) (Vector Laboratories, Burlingame, USA) was used to label cones. Fluorescence signals were examined by confocal laser scanning microscope (LSM510 META and LSM710; Carl Zeiss, Germany).

### Cell counting

Cells immunoreactive for specific cell markers were quantitated on vertically sliced retinal sections containing the optic nerve head. Confocal images (at least 10 fields per animal) were obtained from the central retina, defined as 700 μm from the border of the optic nerve head, using a 40× or 63× objective lens (3 animals per stage and genotype). Immunoreactive cells were counted and the density calculated per mm retina. Due to their paucity, pH3-positive cells were counted per whole retinal section. The numbers of cones and horizontal cells were quantitated using whole mount retinas immunolabeled for cone arrestin and calbindin, respectively. Confocal z-stack images, one from each quadrant (142 μm × 142 μm), were captured and cell density calculated per mm$^2$ retina (3 animals per genotype). Statistical analysis was conducted by Student's t-test ($P < 0.05$).

### Quantitative (real-time) RT-PCR

Quantitative RT-PCR was performed using Fast SYBR green Master mix (Applied Biosystems, Foster City, CA) on a 7500 Fast real-time PCR system (Applied Biosystems) as previously described [16]. The list of primers is shown in Additional file 1: Table S2. Data were normalized to *Gapdh* expression and statistical significance analyzed by Student's t-test ($P < 0.05$).

## Results

### Expression of p27 in the developing and mature mouse retinas

We first examined the overall expression patterns of p27 in the developing and mature mouse retinas by immunohistochemistry. At postnatal day 0 (P0), p27 immunoreactivity was observed in the ganglion cell layer (GCL), the inner part of the neuroblastic layer (NBL) containing amacrine cells, and the outer portion of the NBL containing differentiating photoreceptors (Fig. 1a). p27 was detected in most, if not all, cells in the central retina at P6 (Fig. 1a). In the mature retina (P21), p27 immunoreactivity was still present in all nuclear layers of the retina although p27 levels

decreased in most retinal cells except Müller glia, which maintained intense p27 labeling (Fig. 1a). Immunolabeling was absent in the p27 knockout (KO) retina, which proved antibody specificity (Fig. 1a).

We then conducted double immunofluorescence for p27 and cell type-specific markers to define the cell types expressing p27. In the mouse retina, ganglion cells, amacrine

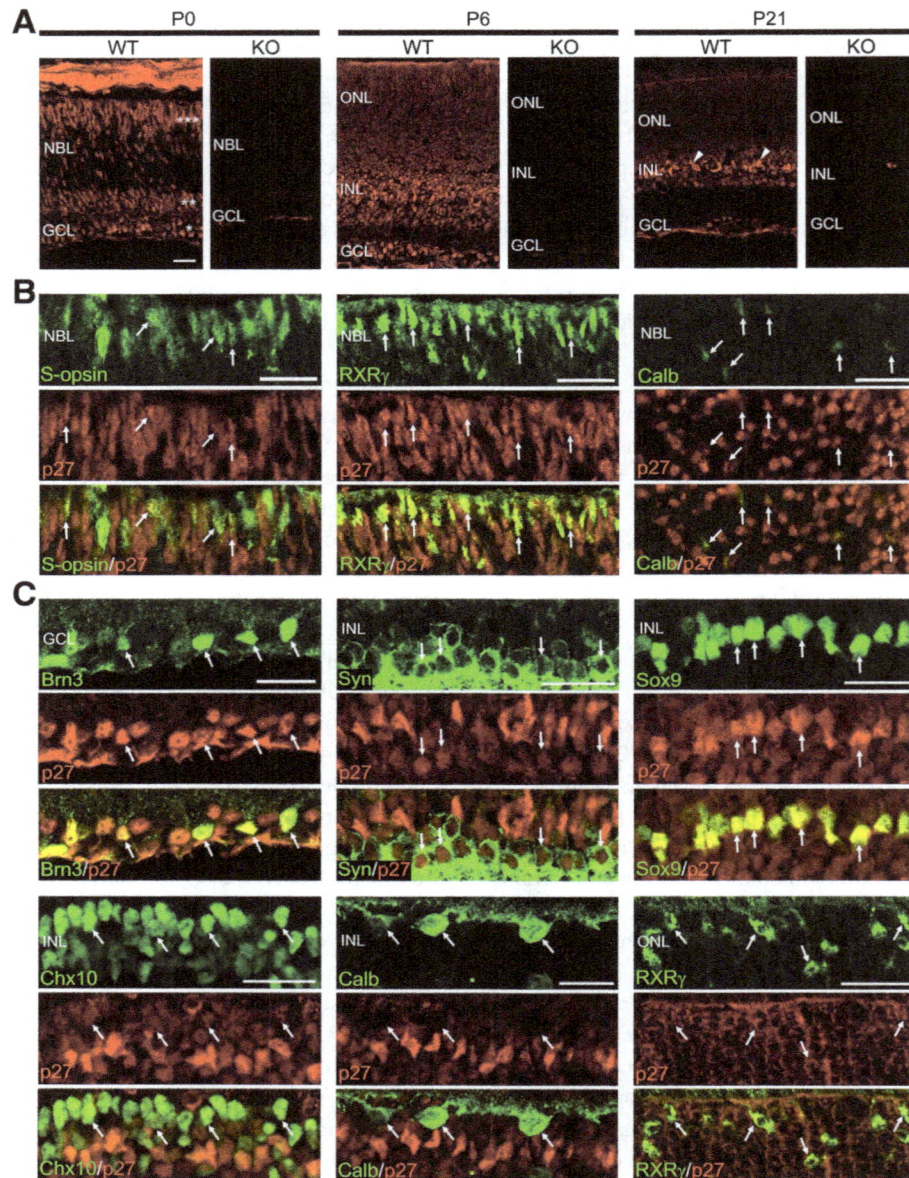

**Fig. 1** Cellular localization of p27 in the mouse retina during postnatal development. **a** Immunofluorescence for p27 in the wild-type (WT) and p27 knockout (KO) retinas at P0, P6 and P21. At P0, the ganglion cell layer (*), amacrine cell layer (**), and photoreceptor layer (***) are intensely immunoreactive. p27 is detected in all nuclear layers at P6 and P21. Arrowheads indicate Müller glia with intense immunoreactivity. No staining is observed in the KO retinas showing antibody specificity. **b** p27 expression in cones and horizontal cells in the P0 retinas. Double immunofluorescence for p27 in combination with the cone markers S-opsin and RXRγ and horizontal cell marker calbindin (Calb) showing colocalization (arrows). **c** P21 mouse retinas showing expression of p27 in Brn3+ ganglion cells, syntaxin (Syn) + amacrine cells, Sox9+ Müller glia, Chx10+ bipolar cells, calbindin (Calb) + horizontal cells, and RXRγ + cones. Arrows indicate colocalization. NBL, neuroblastic layer; GCL, ganglion cell layer; ONL, outer nuclear layer; INL, inner nuclear layer. Scale bars = 20 μm

cells, horizontal cells, cones, and some rods are generated by birth [17]. Although previous reports suggested that p27 is expressed in ganglion cells, amacrine cells and rods in the newborn retina [8, 9], p27 expression in cones and horizontal cells remains unexplored. We thus performed immunolabeling for p27 in combination with the cone markers S-opsin and RXRγ [18] and horizontal cell marker calbindin [19] in the P0 retina. S-opsin, RXRγ, and calbindin were colocalized with p27, indicating p27 expression in cones and horizontal cells (Fig. 1b). We further conducted double immunofluorescence for p27 and various cell type-specific markers at P21. p27 immunoreactivity was detected in Brn3+ ganglion cells [20], syntaxin + amacrine cells [21], Sox9+ Müller glia [22], Chx10+ bipolar cells [23], and RXRγ + cones while calbindin + horizontal cells lacked p27 immunolabeling (Fig. 1c). The p27 staining throughout the thickness of the outer nuclear layer (ONL) indicated p27 expression in rods (Fig. 1a and c). Altogether, p27 was detected in all postmitotic cell types in the mature mouse retina except horizontal cells, which expressed p27 only transiently during development.

## Ectopic division of bipolar cells and Müller glia in the p27KO retinas

We next assessed the effects of p27 deletion on retinal cell proliferation during development. Wild-type (WT) and p27KO (KO) mice of various postnatal ages were labeled with BrdU for two hours prior to sacrifice, and retinal sections double-labeled for BrdU and phospho-histone H3 (pH3) to locate S and M phase cells, respectively. At P0, the patterns of BrdU and pH3 staining were similar between the WT and KO retinas (Fig. 2a). In both genotypes, BrdU+ S-phase cells were located in the inner neuroblastic layer, whereas pH3+ M-phase cells resided at the outer retinal margin. At P6 and later, division had virtually ceased in the central region of the WT retina while many BrdU+ and pH3+ cells were found throughout the KO retina (Fig. 2a and b). At P6, in the KO retinas, BrdU+ cells were located in the developing INL and pH3+ cells arranged at the outer margin of the retina, in a pattern similar to the previous stages (Fig. 2a and b). At P9, however, many pH3+ cells were found in the INL or the inner part of the ONL, away from the outer retinal margin where M phase cells normally occur (Fig. 2a and b). Proliferation was much less prominent at P12 and later stages (Fig. 2a and b) and no division was detected at P21 (data not shown).

The above results are consistent with the previous observations that the period of proliferation is extended in the KO retinas [8, 9]. However, we unexpectedly observed many ectopic M-phase cells in the inner retina at P9, but not at P6 or earlier, suggesting that proliferating cells at P9 are phenotypically different from those at P6. To more closely characterize cell proliferation in the KO retinas, we performed double or triple staining for proliferation markers (BrdU and pH3) in combination with retinal progenitor and differentiation markers. At P6, virtually all BrdU+ cells expressed the progenitor markers Chx10, Sox9, Sox2 and Pax6 [24] (Fig. 3a). PH3+ cells were also colabeled with these progenitor markers (Fig. 3b). These data are consistent with the progenitor phenotype of proliferating cell population in the KO retina at P6. However, all these progenitor markers (Chx10, Sox9, Sox2 and

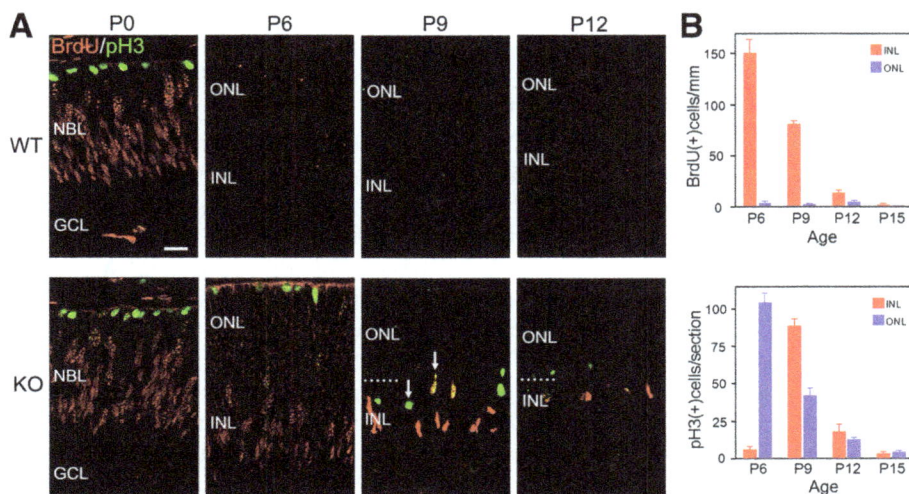

**Fig. 2** Ectopic cell division in the absence of p27. **a** Double immunofluorescence for BrdU and phospho-histone H3 (pH3) in the wild-type (WT) and p27 knockout (KO) retinas at different postnatal ages. The central retinal regions are shown. BrdU+ and pH3+ cells are observed only in the KO retinas at P6 and thereafter. Note pH3+ cells are ectopically positioned in the inner nuclear layer (INL) at P9 (arrows). GCL, ganglion cell layer; NBL, neuroblastic layer; ONL, outer nuclear layer. Dotted lines indicate the border between the ONL and INL. Scale bar = 20 μm. **b** Quantification of BrdU+ and pH3+ cells in the KO retinas. Each bar represents the mean ± SEM (n = 3 per age)

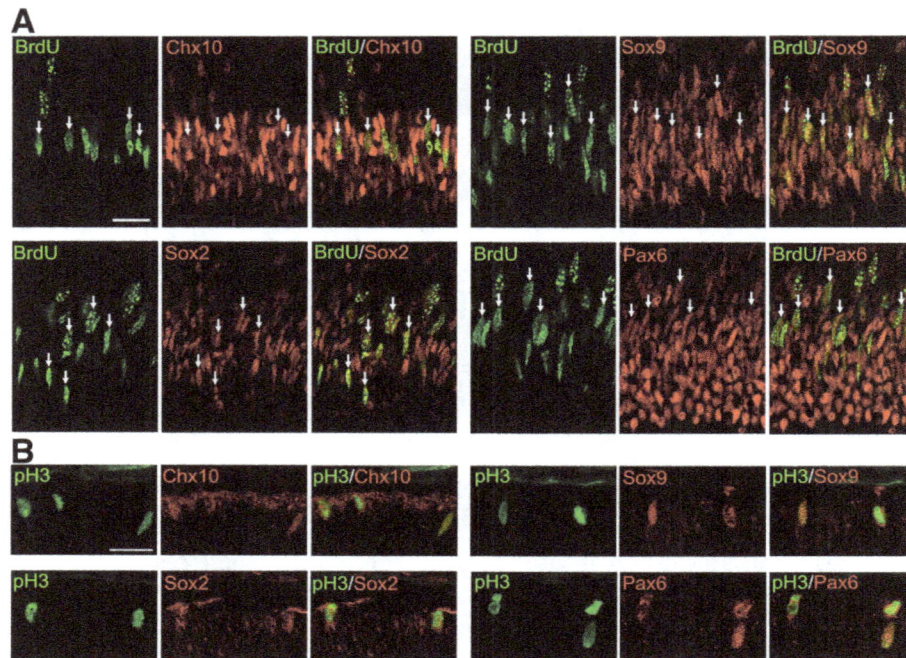

**Fig. 3** Progenitor characteristics of the proliferating cells in the p27 knockout retinas at P6. Double immunofluorescence for BrdU (**a**) or phospho-histone H3 (pH3) (**b**) with progenitor markers (Chx10, Sox9, Sox2, and Pax6) showing colocalization (arrows). Scale bars = 20 μm

Pax6) are expressed not only by retinal progenitors but also by Müller glial cells [25]. To test the possibility that Müller glia had reentered the cell cycle in the absence of p27, expression of glutamine synthetase (GS), a Müller glia marker [25], was analyzed. No detectable signals were obtained in the KO retina at P6 (data not shown), further supporting the progenitor phenotype of dividing cells. Yet, we could not exclude the possibility that they were immature Müller glia without detectable expression of mature Müller markers. In contrast to the P6 retinas, at least three different proliferating populations were identified at P9, based on the expression of Chx10 and Sox9. Triple staining for BrdU, Chx10 and Sox9 revealed that about a half of BrdU+ cells were weakly labeled for Chx10 while intensely positive for Sox9 (46.6%, 308 cells per 661 BrdU + cells counted, *n* = 3) suggesting that they were progenitor cells or proliferating Müller glia (Fig. 4a). These cells were shown to be GS+ (Fig. 4b), indicating their identity as Müller glia rather than progenitors. The other half of BrdU+ cells were intensely positive for Chx10 but were negative for Sox9 (48.9%, 323 cells per 661 BrdU+ cells counted, *n* = 3), consistent with the characteristics of bipolar cells (Fig. 4a). Only 4.5% of BrdU+ cells were Chx10–/Sox9– and thus classified as non-bipolar/non-Müller cells. We also conducted triple labeling for BrdU, Chx10, and Otx2, another bipolar marker [26]. Again, approximately half of BrdU+ cells (49.3%, 176 cells per 357 BrdU+ cells counted, *n* = 2) were colabeled with both

Chx10 and Otx2, confirming their bipolar identity (Fig. 4c). Similarly, some pH3+ cells were labeled for both Chx10 and Sox9 (data not shown) while others were labeled for Chx10 and Otx2, but not for Sox9 (Fig. 4d and e). Of note, most M-phase cells ectopically positioned in the INL were the latter cell type displaying the bipolar phenotype. To further verify the bipolar identity, we carried out double staining for pH3 and a mature bipolar cell marker PKCα [27]. A significant proportion of ectopic pH3-positive cells (27.9%, 48 cells per 172 pH3+ cells counted, n = 2) were also labeled for PKCα. (Fig. 4f). Taken together, the expression patterns of key markers and the ectopic position of M-phase cells indicate that the proliferation in the KO retina at P9 is due to aberrant division of differentiating Müller glia and bipolar cells, but not a simple extension of progenitor proliferation.

### Fate of proliferating cells in the p27KO retinas

We next sought to determine the fate of dividing cells in the KO retinas by BrdU incorporation assays. KO mice were injected with BrdU at P6, P9 or P12 and allowed to survive until P21 (Fig. 5a). Cells which were in their last S-phase at the time of BrdU injection were expected to show intense BrdU labeling, and their identity was analyzed by double or triple staining for BrdU and cell-specific markers. Strongly BrdU-labeled cells were

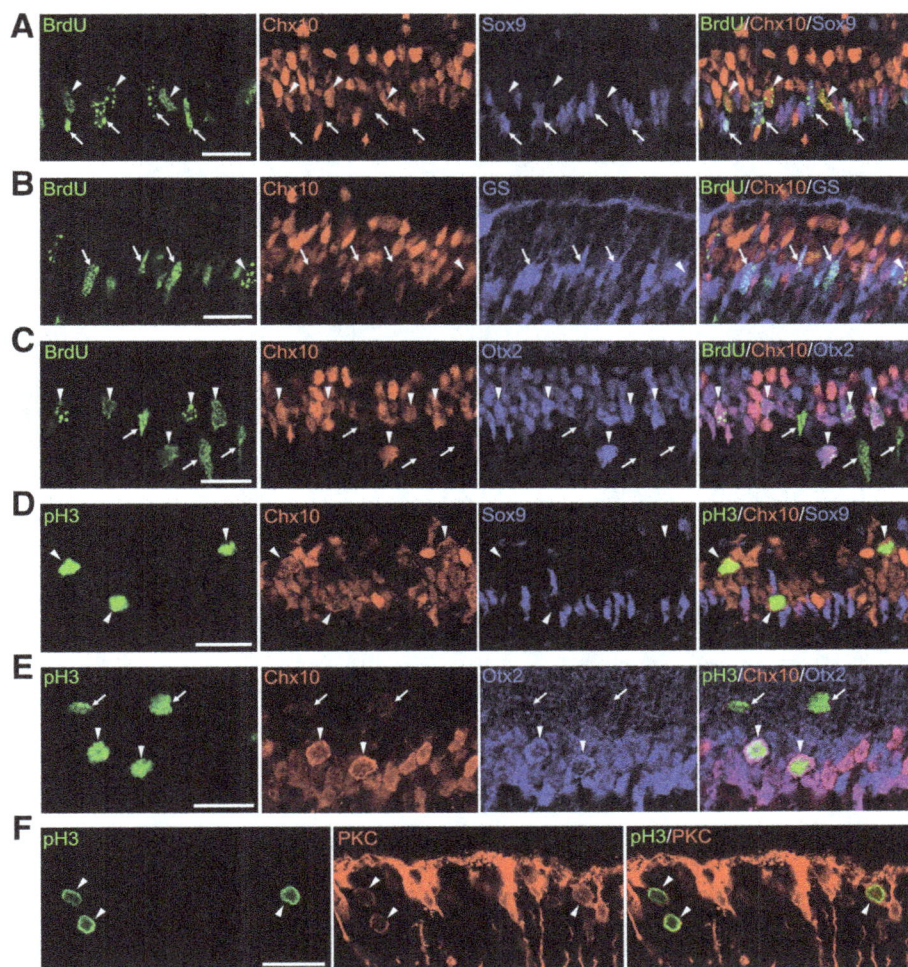

**Fig. 4** Ectopic cell cycle reentry of bipolar cells and Müller glia in the p27 knockout retinas at P9. **a** Triple immunofluorescence for BrdU, Chx10, and Sox9. Arrows indicate BrdU+ cells stained weakly for Chx10 and intensely for Sox9 (Müller glia) while arrowheads denote BrdU+ cells which are intensely Chx10+ and Sox9- (bipolar cells). **b** Triple immunofluorescence for BrdU, Chx10, and glutamine synthetase (GS). Arrows indicate BrdU+, weakly Chx10+ and GS+ cells (Müller glia). Arrowhead shows BrdU+, intensely Chx10+, and GS- cell (bipolar cell). **c** Triple immunofluorescence for BrdU, Chx10, and Otx2. Some BrdU+ cells are weakly Chx10+ and Otx2- (arrows, Müller glia) while others are intensely positive for both Chx10 and Otx2 (arrowheads, bipolar cells). **d** Triple immunofluorescence for phospho-histone H3 (pH3), Chx10, and Sox9. Arrowheads indicate ectopic M-phase cells strongly positive for Chx10, but negative for Sox9 (bipolar cells). **e** Triple immunofluorescence for pH3, Chx10, and Otx2. Arrows denote pH3+ cells stained weakly for Chx10 and negative for Otx2 (Müller glia). Arrowheads indicate pH3+/Chx10+/Otx2+ cells (bipolar cells). **f** Double immunofluorescence for pH3 and PKCα (PKC) showing colocalization (arrowheads, bipolar cells). Scale bar = 20 μm

observed both in the INL and ONL when BrdU was injected at P6 (Fig. 5b). BrdU+ cells in the ONL were identified as rods based on the expression of the rod marker NR2E3 [28] (Fig. 5c and h) and the absence of the cone markers S- and M-opsins (Fig. 5d and data not shown). BrdU+ cells in the INL or the inner portion of the ONL were identified as Müller glia or bipolar cells by expression patterns of Chx10, Sox9, PKCα, and GS (Fig. 5e, f, g, and h). On the other hand, cells which incorporated BrdU at P9 or P12 were found mostly in the INL (Fig. 5b) and identified as bipolar cells and Müller glia (Fig. 5h).

**Aberrant cell cycle reentry of cones in the p27KO retinas**

The presence of ectopic division in the KO retinas prompted us to examine Ki67 expression, which labels all phases of the cell cycle. While no Ki67+ cells were observed in the central portion of the WT retinas at P6 and later stages, many positive cells were found in the KO retinas (Fig. 6a), consistent with the results obtained using BrdU and pH 3 as cell cycle markers. At P6 and P9, most Ki67+ cells occurred in the INL, similar to the pattern of BrdU staining. Unexpectedly, however, many Ki67+ cells were observed in the ONL of the KO retinas at P12 (Fig. 6a). To test the possibility that the Ki67+

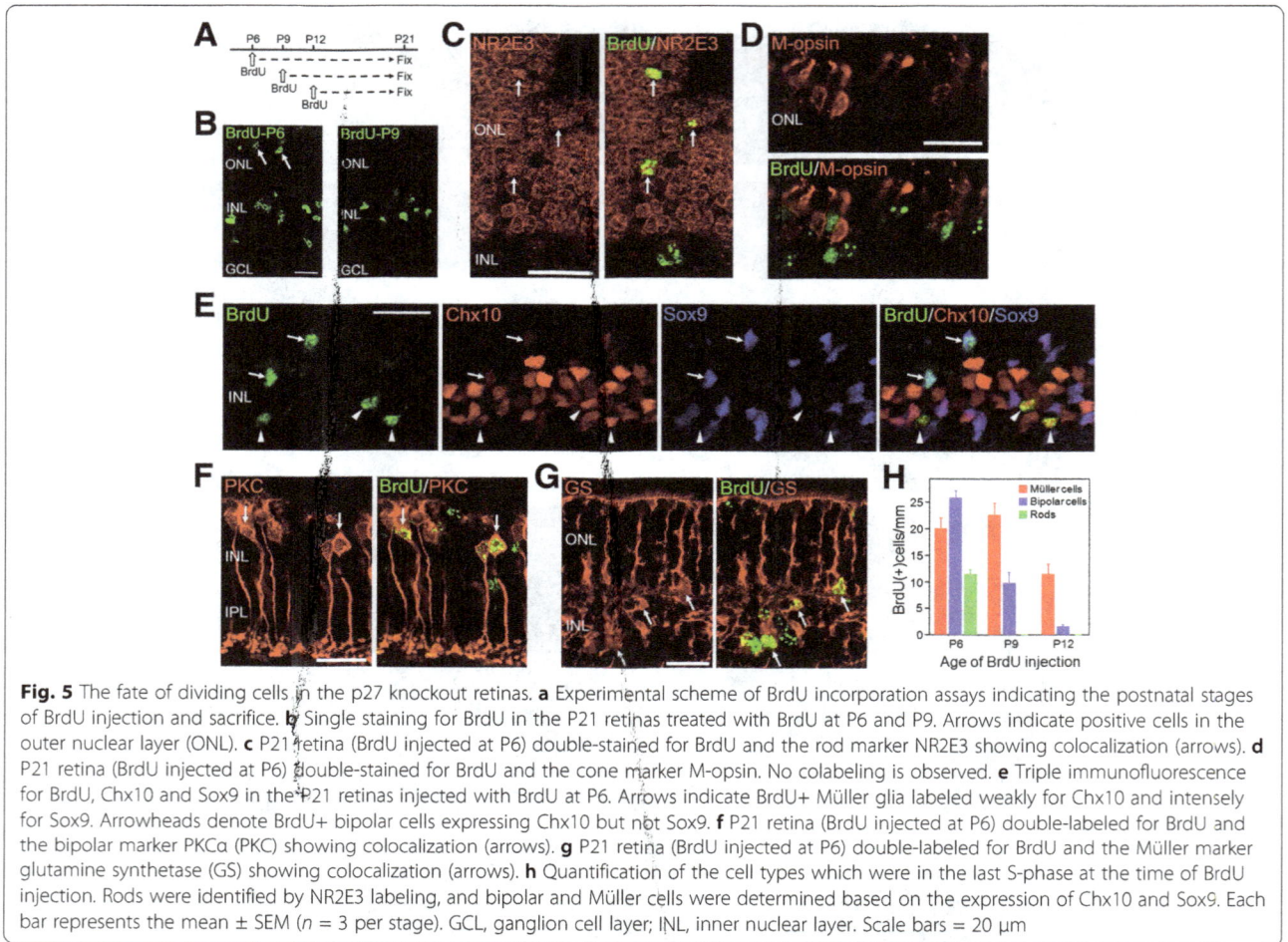

**Fig. 5** The fate of dividing cells in the p27 knockout retinas. **a** Experimental scheme of BrdU incorporation assays indicating the postnatal stages of BrdU injection and sacrifice. **b** Single staining for BrdU in the P21 retinas treated with BrdU at P6 and P9. Arrows indicate positive cells in the outer nuclear layer (ONL). **c** P21 retina (BrdU injected at P6) double-stained for BrdU and the rod marker NR2E3 showing colocalization (arrows). **d** P21 retina (BrdU injected at P6) double-stained for BrdU and the cone marker M-opsin. No colabeling is observed. **e** Triple immunofluorescence for BrdU, Chx10 and Sox9 in the P21 retinas injected with BrdU at P6. Arrows indicate BrdU+ Müller glia labeled weakly for Chx10 and intensely for Sox9. Arrowheads denote BrdU+ bipolar cells expressing Chx10 but not Sox9. **f** P21 retina (BrdU injected at P6) double-labeled for BrdU and the bipolar marker PKCα (PKC) showing colocalization (arrows). **g** P21 retina (BrdU injected at P6) double-labeled for BrdU and the Müller marker glutamine synthetase (GS) showing colocalization (arrows). **h** Quantification of the cell types which were in the last S-phase at the time of BrdU injection. Rods were identified by NR2E3 labeling, and bipolar and Müller cells were determined based on the expression of Chx10 and Sox9. Each bar represents the mean ± SEM (*n* = 3 per stage). GCL, ganglion cell layer; INL, inner nuclear layer. Scale bars = 20 μm

cells in the ONL were photoreceptors, we carried out double staining for Ki67 and several photoreceptor markers. Ki67 was colocalized with the photoreceptor marker recoverin and cone marker S-opsin, but not with the rod marker NR2E3 (Fig. 6b), indicating their cone identity. We next quantified the proportion of cones expressing Ki67 in the KO retinas at different ages. At P6, there were many S-opsin + cones in the ventral half of the retina, but none of them were labeled for Ki67 (Fig. 6c and d). However, approximately 5% of S-opsin + cones expressed Ki67 at P9, and 30–40% of S-opsin + cones were labeled for Ki67 at P12 and P15 (Fig. 6c and d). No S-opsin + cones expressed Ki67 at P21 (Fig. 6d). We also analyzed other cell cycle markers including PCNA, phospho-Rb (pRb), MCM6, BrdU and pH3 for colocalization with cone opsins. A significant fraction of S-opsin + or M-opsin + cones expressed PCNA, pRb and MCM6 (Fig. 6e) while few cones were labeled for BrdU and none expressed pH3 (data not shown).

Because cones are normally generated during the embryonic period [29], these results suggest that p27-

dificient cones underwent aberrant cell cycle reentry after a long quiescent period. However, it was also possible that proliferating cones were generated de novo during the period of extra proliferation. To test this possibility, we labeled the proliferating cell population in the KO retinas at P6 with BrdU and examined their fate at P12, but none of the BrdU+ cells expressed S-opsin (Fig. 7). We also traced the fate of proliferating cells by daily injection of BrdU from P7 to P11 to find no evidence of de novo generation of cones (Fig. 7). Thus, cones seemed to differentiate normally in the absence of p27 until they suddenly reenter the cell cycle after a quiescence of several weeks.

## Differentiation and survival of cones are impaired in the p27KO retinas

We closely examined S-opsin+ cones in the KO retinas at P15, when the highest proportion of cones expressed cell cycle markers, such as Ki67. We found that S-opsin immunoreactivity in Ki67+ cones was weaker compared to Ki67- cones (Fig. 8a). We next examined expression of cone-specific genes in the WT and KO retinas during

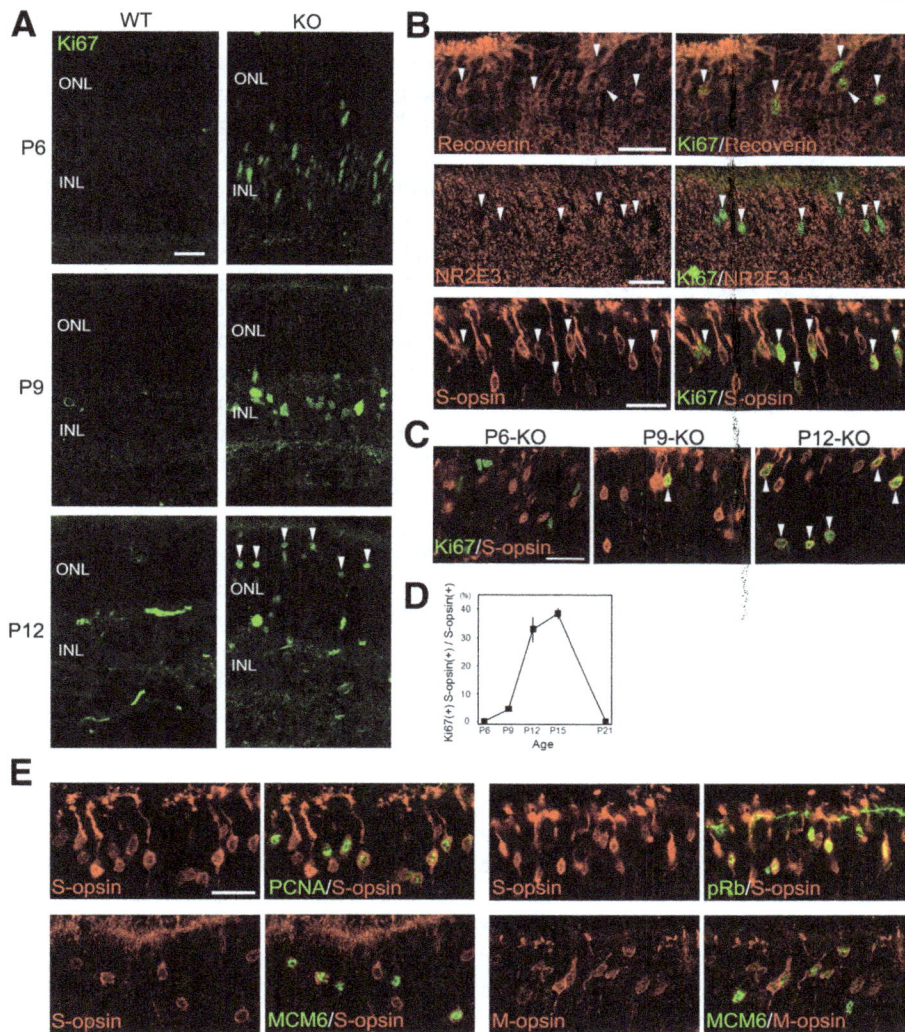

**Fig. 6** Aberrant cell cycle reentry of cones in the p27 knockout (KO) retinas. **a** Immunofluorescence for Ki67 in the WT and KO retinas at P6 and later stages showing proliferating cells only in the KO retinas. Arrowheads indicate Ki67+ cells in the outer nuclear layer (ONL) of the KO retina at P12. INL, inner nuclear layer. **b** The ONL of the KO retina at P12 immunolabeled for Ki67 in combination with the photoreceptor marker recoverin, rod marker NR2E3, and cone marker S-opsin. Note colocalization of Ki67 with recoverin and S-opsin, but not with NR2E3 (arrowheads). **c** Double immunofluorescence for Ki67 and S-opsin in the KO retinas at P6 and later stages. Ki67+/S-opsin + cones are shown by arrowheads. **d** Quantification of Ki67+ cones in the KO retinas. Graph data represent the means ± SEM (n = 3 per stage). **e** Cones identified by S-opsin or M-opsin immunoreactivity express proliferation markers PCNA, phospho-Rb, and MCM6 in the KO retinas at P12. Scale bars = 20 μm

postnatal development by quantitative RT-PCR. There were no significant differences in the levels of *Opn1sw* (S-opsin) mRNA between genotypes at P0 and P6, while its expression was significantly decreased in the KO retinas compared to WT at P12 and P21 (Fig. 8b). Likewise, expression of *Opn1mw* (M-opsin) and *Arr3* (cone arrestin) in the KO retinas was significantly lower compared to WT at P6 and later stages (Fig. 8b). These results lead to the hypothesis that differentiation and/or survival of cones are impaired in the KO retinas, possibly due to their aberrant cell cycle reentry. To test this, we examined cell death by TUNEL assays. Although

significantly more apoptotic cells were observed in the ONL of the KO retinas compared to WT at P12 and P21 (data not shown), the attempt to determine the identity of apoptotic cells by combining TUNEL assays with immunolabeling was not successful, possibly due to degradation of cell type markers in end-stage apoptotic cells detected by TUNEL assays. We then conducted double staining for S-opsin and phospho-histone H2AX (pH2AX), an early marker of DNA damage [30, 31]. Notably, a significant proportion of S-opsin+ cones were labeled for pH2AX in the KO retinas at P15, but not in the WT retinas (Fig. 8c).

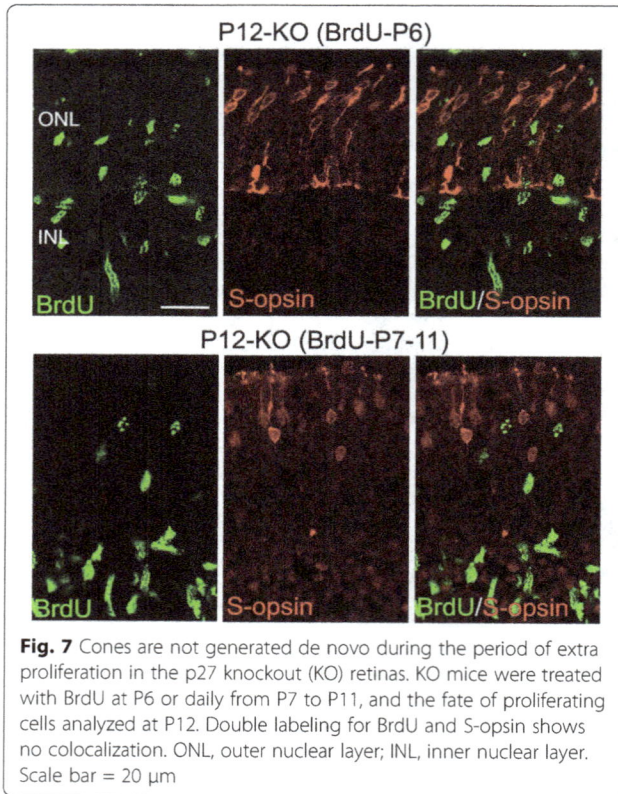

**Fig. 7** Cones are not generated de novo during the period of extra proliferation in the p27 knockout (KO) retinas. KO mice were treated with BrdU at P6 or daily from P7 to P11, and the fate of proliferating cells analyzed at P12. Double labeling for BrdU and S-opsin shows no colocalization. ONL, outer nuclear layer; INL, inner nuclear layer. Scale bar = 20 μm

It has been reported that p27 loss does not affect the proportion of retinal cell types [8, 9]; however, these studies did not examine the number of cones. Thus, we quantified the number of retinal cell types, including cones, by immunohistochemistry for cell-type specific markers in the retinas of 8-week-old WT and KO mice (Fig. 8d). Because of their sparsity, the numbers of cones and horizontal cells were assessed by whole mount staining while other cell types were evaluated on sections. Cones, horizontal cells, amacrine cells and ganglion cells were identified by immunoreactivity for cone arrestin, calbindin, syntaxin, and Brn3, respectively. Double staining for Chx10 and Sox9 were employed to identify bipolar cells (Chx10+/Sox9-) and Müller cells (Chx10+/Sox9+). Rods were counted as the number of DAPI-labeled nuclei in the ONL subtracted by the number of cones stained for cone arrestin and PNA. Intriguingly, the number of cones in the KO retinas was decreased by approximately 40% compared to the WT retina. The numbers of rods and bipolar cells were also mildly, but significantly, reduced in the KO retinas compared to WT. There were no significant differences in the number of other cell types between genotypes.

## Discussion

Previously, two groups reported that p27 loss induces prolonged proliferation of retinal progenitors, suggesting that p27 controls the timing of cell cycle exit of retinal progenitors [8, 9]. Indeed, we observed persistent proliferation in the p27-deficient retinas at P6 when proliferation in the central retina has normally ceased. Proliferating cells observed at P6 have molecular characteristics of retinal progenitors and were able to differentiate into multiple cell types including rods, bipolar cells and Müller glia. Thus, in agreement with the previous reports, our data showed that p27 loss perturbs the normal timing of progenitor cell cycle exit. However, in contrast with the previous reports, our data indicate that extra proliferation observed at P9 and later stages was not due to persistent progenitors, but due to aberrant division of differentiating cells. These dividing cells expressed differentiation markers of bipolar cells, Müller glia and cones together with proliferation markers. The discrepancy between our data and the previous findings may simply be explained by methodological differences. One study [9] analyzed cell proliferation only by single BrdU immunolabeling, which, without co-staining with differentiation markers, would not discriminate between progenitors and ectopic division of differentiating cells. The other study [8] used several proliferation markers including BrdU, PCNA and pH3 to assess proliferation, but proliferation was analyzed only at P11 or adult stages and double labeling with differentiation markers was not conducted. We employed a range of proliferation markers including BrdU, pH3, Ki67, PCNA, pRb and MCM6 to assess proliferation and performed careful marker analysis by double or triple immunolabeling for proliferation markers, progenitor markers and differentiation markers at various developmental time points, enabling us to discriminate ectopic cell cycle activity from progenitor proliferation.

That p27 loss induced aberrant cell cycle activity in differentiating cells suggests that p27 may be required to maintain the quiescence of postmitotic cells. This notion is consistent with the previous report that acute inactivation of p27 is sufficient to induce proliferation of adult Müller glia [32]. It was also recently shown that p27 loss promotes proliferation of Müller glia and retinal pigment epithelial (RPE) cells in the adult retina after photoreceptor damage [33]. Such a role for p27 has been described for other cell lineages such as pituitary cells [34], supporting cells in the cochlea [35] or cardiomyocytes [36], which undergo unscheduled cell cycle reentry in the absence of p27. Although previous reports have suggested that p27 is expressed only transiently in early postmitotic cells except Müller glia, which maintain p27 expression in the mature retina [8, 9], our data have shown persistent expression of p27 in most postmitotic retinal cells throughout development and in the adult, consistent with the role of p27 in the maintenance of postmitotic cells.

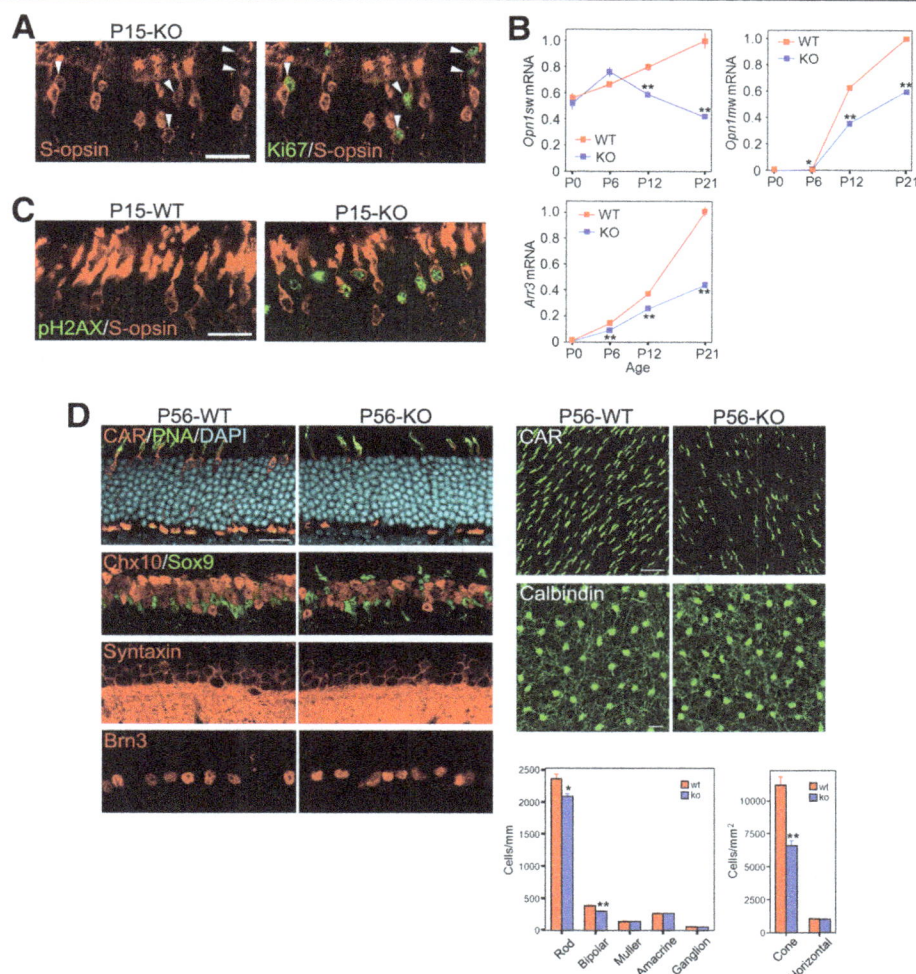

**Fig. 8** Impaired differentiation and survival of cones in the p27 knockout (KO) retinas. **a** Double immunofluorescence for Ki67 and S-opsin in the KO retina at P15. Note relatively weak S-opsin labeling in the Ki67+ cones (arrowheads). **b** Quantitative RT-PCR analyses of cone gene expression in the WT and KO retinas during postnatal development. The transcript levels are expressed relative to WT at P21 after normalized to *Gapdh* levels. Each value represents the mean ± SEM (*n* = 3 per stage and genotype). *$P < 0.05$, **$P < 0.01$, Student's t test. **c** Double immunofluorescence for phospho-H2AX (pH2AX) and S-opsin in the WT and KO retinas at P15. Note pH2AX+ cones in the KO retina. **d** Quantification of retinal cell types in the WT and p27KO retinas at P56. Retinal sections or whole mounts were immunolabeled for cell-specific markers. Note a significant reduction in cone number in the KO retina. The number of rods and bipolar cells are also mildly reduced. Bars represent the mean ± SEM (*n*= 3 per genotype). *$p < 0.05$, **$p < 0.01$, Student's t test. Scale bars are 20 µm

p27 may play a pivotal role in maintaining quiescence in bipolar cells, Müller glia and cones while it is dispensable for preventing cell cycle reentry in other cell types. The cell type-specific effects of p27 loss observed herein is unexpected given that virtually all postmitotic retinal cells express p27. Because p27 is known to act redundantly with other CDK inhibitors or Rb-like proteins [37–39], p27 loss may be compensated for by other cell cycle inhibitors in a cell type-specific manner. Interestingly, deletion of both p27 and p19[Ink4d], but not single deletion of either CDK inhibitor, has been shown to induce ectopic cell cycle reentry of ganglion cells, amacrine cells and horizontal cells, suggesting that p27 and

p19 may act redundantly to prevent ectopic division of these cell types [6]. These authors failed to find ectopic division of bipolar cells, Müller glia and cones, most likely because they characterized ectopic division only at P18, when ectopic proliferation of these cell types is no more detected in the p27-deficient retinas.

It has been reported that p27 loss does not affect the proportion of the major retinal cell types [8, 9]. However, these studies did not assess the number of cones in the p27-deficient retinas. We quantified the number of cones, as well as other major retinal cell types, and found that the number of cones in the p27-deficient retinas was decreased by approximately 40% compared to

WT. The number of rods and bipolar cells were also modestly decreased while other cell types displayed no significant changes. The expression of S-opsin in the p27 mutants were normal at birth and P6, indicating that p27 loss does not affect the production and early differentiation of cones. However, subsequent reduction in cone number and the expression of cone-specific genes indicates that the p27-deficient retinas have a major defect in cone survival. Interestingly, both cell cycle reentry and DNA damage response (H2AX phosphorylation) in cones peaked at P15, suggesting a mechanistic association between these events. Of note, cell cycle reentry of cones increased drastically from P9 to P12 while H2AX phosphorylation was not detected until P15, indicating that cell cycle reentry precedes DNA damage responses in cones. Furthermore, S-opsin levels in cones expressing proliferation markers were lower compared to quiescent cones, suggesting that cones in the aberrant cell cycle were in the process of degeneration. All these data suggest that the aberrant cell cycle activity of cones is causally related to cone death.

Cones reentering the cell cycle expressed a variety of proliferation markers such as Ki67, PCNA, pRb and MCM6, but only few incorporated BrdU and none expressed pH 3. Thus, despite the activation of cell cycle machinery, most cones may fail to progress through the cell cycle and are prone to arrest or die. This contrasted markedly with ectopic proliferation of bipolar and Müller cells, many of which seemed to progress through S and M phases of the cell cycle as assessed by BrdU incorporation and pH 3 labeling. The mechanisms that determine the fate of these cell types remain unknown. Previous studies reported that inactivation of Rb/p107 in the retina induced ectopic division of all cell types, followed by death of ganglion cells, bipolar cells, rods and cones while other cell types were death-resistant [11, 12]. Thus, whether ectopic division is followed by cell death may depend on cell-specific intrinsic properties. Our data may indicate that bipolar cells and Müller glia have a greater tolerance for unscheduled DNA synthesis than cones. However, the modest reduction in bipolar cell number suggests that this cell type is not fully death-resistant in the context of p27 loss. Alternatively, differentiated cells may be more susceptible to death as a result of the conflict between differentiation and division compared to less differentiated immature cells. Bipolar cells and Müller glia are born during the first postnatal week [17], and ectopic division occurs only several days later. On the other hand, the generation of cones peaks at E13-E14 [29] and they reenter the cell cycle approximately three weeks after generated. Thus, the late onset of cell cycle events may contribute, at least in part, to the death-prone phenotype of p27-deficient cones. Finally, we cannot exclude the possibility that non-cell-autonomous mechanisms may be

involved in the robust cell death of cones. The p27-deficient retina exhibits dysplasia of the ONL, characterized by disruption of the outer limiting membrane and displaced photoreceptor cells outside the outer limiting membrane [9, 40]. Another report has also suggested that the normal contact between photoreceptor outer segments and the RPE is substantially disrupted in the p27-deficient retina [41]. Thus, the disorganization of the ONL might affect the differentiation and/or survival of photoreceptors. Indeed, despite the absence of ectopic division of rods, rod number was modestly, but significantly, decreased in the mature mutant retina. Thus, disruption of normal microenvironment due to retinal disorganization may have triggered photoreceptor cell death.

## Conclusions
Although p27 is expressed in all differentiating cell types in the mouse retina, this CDK inhibitor is required to maintain the quiescence of specific cell types including bipolar cells, Müller glia, and cone photoreceptors while it is dispensable for preventing cell cycle reentry in other cells types. Moreover, p27 is required for normal differentiation and survival of cones. Our data provide new insights into the role of CDK inhibitors in the maintenance, survival, and degeneration of retinal cells.

## Abbreviations
Calb: calbindin; CAR: cone arrestin; CDK: cyclin-dependent kinase; GCL: ganglion cell layer; GS: glutamine synthetase; INL: inner nuclear layer; KO: knockout; NBL: neuroblastic layer; ONL: outer nuclear layer; pH 3: phospho-histone H3; pH2AX: phospho-H2AX; PNA: peanut agglutinin; RT-PCR: reverse transcription-polymerase chain reaction; Syn: syntaxin; WT: wild type

## Acknowledgements
The authors thank Drs. Shiming Chen and Cheryl M. Craft for providing NR2E3 and cone arrestin antibodies, respectively.

## Funding
This work was partly supported by Grant-in-Aid for Scientific Research from Japan Society for the Promotion of Science (No. 22591968 to H.F.).

## Authors' contributions
MO, FS, and NS conducted the experiments; MO, FS and HF analyzed and interpreted the data; MO and HF wrote the manuscript. All authors read and approved the final manuscript.

## Competing interests
The authors declare that they have no competing interests.

**Author details**

[1]Department of Anatomy, School of Medicine, Tokyo Women's Medical University, 8-1 Kawada-cho, Shinjuku-ku, Tokyo 162-8666, Japan. [2]Department of Anatomy, School of Medicine, Toho University, 5-21-16 Omorinishi, Ota-ku, Tokyo 143-8540, Japan.

**References**

1    Sherr CJ, Roberts JM. CDK inhibitors: positive and negative regulators of G1-phase progression. Genes Dev. 1999;13:1501–12.

2    Vidal A, Koff A. Cell-cycle inhibitors: three families united by a common cause. Gene. 2000;247:1–15.

3    Nguyen L, Besson A, Heng JI, Schuurmans C, Teboul L, Parras C, et al. p27$^{kip1}$ independently promotes neuronal differentiation and migration in the cerebral cortex. Genes Dev. 2006;20:1511–24.

4    Miller JP, Yeh N, Vidal A, Koff A. Interweaving the cell cycle machinery with cell differentiation. Cell Cycle. 2007;6:2932–8.

5    Besson A, Dowdy SF, Roberts JM. CDK inhibitors: cell cycle regulators and beyond. Dev Cell. 2008;14:159–69.

6    Cunningham JJ, Levine EM, Zindy F, Goloubeva O, Roussel MF, Smeyne RJ. The cyclin-dependent kinase inhibitors p19$^{Ink4d}$ and p27$^{Kip1}$ are coexpressed in select retinal cells and act cooperatively to control cell cycle exit. Mol Cell Neurosci. 2002;19:359–74.

7    Ohnuma S, Philpott A, Wang K, Holt CE, Harris WA. p27$^{Xic1}$, a CDK inhibitor, promotes the determination of glial cells in Xenopus Retina. Cell. 1999;99:499–510.

8    Levine EM, Close J, Fero M, Ostrovsky A, Reh TA. p27$^{Kip1}$ regulates cell cycle withdrawal of late multipotent progenitor cells in the mammalian retina. Dev Biol. 2000;219:299–314.

9    Dyer MA, Cepko CL. p27$^{Kip1}$ and p57$^{Kip2}$ regulate proliferation in distinct retinal progenitor cell populations. J Neurosci. 2001;21:4259–71.

10   Geng Y, Yu Q, Sicinska E, Das M, Bronson RT, Sicinski P. Deletion of the p27$^{Kip1}$ gene restores normal development in cyclin D1-deficient mice. Proc Natl Acad Sci U S A. 2001;98:194–9.

11   Chen D, Livne-bar I, Vanderluit JL, Slack RS, Agochiya M, Bremner R. Cell-specific effects of RB or RB/p107 loss on retinal development implicate an intrinsically death-resistant cell-of-origin in retinoblastoma. Cancer Cell. 2004;5:539–51.

12   MacPherson D, Sage J, Kim T, Ho D, McLaughlin ME, Jacks T. Cell type-specific effects of Rb deletion in the murine retina. Genes Dev. 2004;18:1681–94.

13   Ajioka I, Martins RA, Bayazitov IT, Donovan S, Johnson DA, Frase S, et al. Differentiated horizontal interneurons clonally expand to form metastatic retinoblastoma in mice. Cell. 2007;131:378–90.

14   Fero ML, Rivkin M, Tasch M, Porter P, Carow CE, Firpo E, et al. A syndrome of multiorgan hyperplasia with features of gigantism, tumorigenesis, and female sterility in p27$^{Kip1}$-deficient mice. Cell. 1996;85:733–44.

15   Fujieda H, Sasaki H. Expression of brain-derived neurotrophic factor in cholinergic and dopaminergic amacrine cells in the rat retina and the effects of constant light rearing. Exp Eye Res. 2008;86:335–43.

16   Fujieda H, Bremner R, Mears AJ, Sasaki H. Retinoic acid receptor-related orphan receptor alpha regulates a subset of cone genes during mouse retinal development. J Neurochem. 2009;108:91–101.

17   Young RW. Cell differentiation in the retina of the mouse. Anat Rec. 1985;212:199–205.

18   Mori M, Ghyselinck NB, Chambon P, Mark M. Systematic immunolocalization of retinoid receptors in developing and adult mouse eyes. Invest Ophthalmol Vis Sci. 2001;42:1312–8.

19   Uesugi R, Yamada M, Mizuguchi M, Baimbridge KG, Kim SU. Calbindin D-28k and parvalbumin immunohistochemistry in developing rat retina. Exp Eye Res. 1992;54:491–9.

20   Xiang M, Zhou L, Macke JP, Yoshioka T, Hendry SH, Eddy RL, et al. The Brn-3 family of POU-domain factors: primary structure, binding specificity, and expression in subsets of retinal ganglion cells and somatosensory neurons. J Neurosci. 1995;15:4762–85.

21   Barnstable CJ, Hofstein R, Akagawa K. A marker of early amacrine cell development in rat retina. Brain Res. 1985;352:286–90.

22   Poche RA, Furuta Y, Chaboissier MC, Schedl A, Behringer RR. Sox9 is expressed in mouse multipotent retinal progenitor cells and functions in Müller glial cell development. J Comp Neurol. 2008;510:237–50.

23   Burmeister M, Novak J, Liang MY, Basu S, Ploder L, Hawes NL, et al. Ocular retardation mouse caused by Chx10 homeobox null allele: impaired retinal progenitor proliferation and bipolar cell differentiation. Nat Genet. 1996;12:376–84.

24   Livesey FJ, Young TL, Cepko CL. An analysis of the gene expression program of mammalian neural progenitor cells. Proc Natl Acad Sci U S A. 2004;101:1374–9.

25   Roesch K, Jadhav AP, Trimarchi JM, Stadler MB, Roska B, Sun BB, et al. The transcriptome of retinal Muller glial cells. J Comp Neurol. 2008;509:225–38.

26   Baas D, Bumsted KM, Martinez JA, Vaccarino FM, Wikler KC, Barnstable CJ. The subcellular localization of Otx2 is cell-type specific and developmentally regulated in the mouse retina. Mol Brain Res. 2000;78:26–37.

27   Greferath U, Grünert U, Wässle H. Rod bipolar cells in the mammalian retina show protein kinase C-like immunoreactivity. J Comp Neurol. 1990;301:433–42.

28   Akhmedov NB, Piriev NI, Chang B, Rapoport AL, Hawes NL, Nishina PM, et al. A deletion in a photoreceptor-specific nuclear receptor mRNA causes retinal degeneration in the rd7 mouse. Proc Natl Acad Sci U S A. 2000;97:5551–6.

29   Carter-Dawson LD, LaVail MM. Rods and cones in the mouse retina. II. Autoradiographic analysis of cell generation using tritiated thymidine. J Comp Neurol. 1979;188:263–72.

30   Rogakou EP, Boon C, Redon C, Bonner WM. Megabase chromatin domains involved in DNA double-strand breaks in vivo. J Cell Biol. 1999;146:905–16.

31   Mah LJ, El-Osta A, Karagiannis TC. gammaH2AX: a sensitive molecular marker of DNA damage and repair. Leukemia. 2010;24:679–86.

32   Vázquez-Chona FR, Swan A, Ferrell WD, Jiang L, Baehr W, Chien WM, et al. Proliferative reactive gliosis is compatible with glial metabolic support and neuronal function. BMC Neurosci. 2011;12:98.

33   ul Quraish R, Sudou N, Nomura-Komoike K, Sato F, Fujieda H. p27$^{KIP1}$ loss promotes proliferation and phagocytosis but prevents epithelial-mesenchymal transition in RPE cells after photoreceptor damage. Mol Vis. 2016;22:1103–21.

34   Bilodeau S, Roussel-Gervais A, Drouin J. Distinct developmental roles of cell cycle inhibitors p57$^{Kip2}$ and p27$^{Kip1}$ distinguish pituitary progenitor cell cycle exit from cell cycle reentry of differentiated cells. Mol Cell Biol. 2009;29:1895–908.

35   Ono K, Nakagawa T, Kojima K, Matsumoto M, Kawauchi T, Hoshino M, et al. Silencing p27 reverses post-mitotic state of supporting cells in neonatal mouse cochleae. Mol Cell Neurosci. 2009;42:391–8.

36   Di Stefano V, Giacca M, Capogrossi MC, Crescenzi M, Martelli F. Knockdown of cyclin-dependent kinase inhibitors induces cardiomyocyte re-entry in the cell cycle. J Biol Chem. 2011;286:8644–54.

37   Zhu L, Harlow E, Dynlacht BD. p107 uses a p21CIP1-related domain to bind cyclin/cdk2 and regulate interactions with E2F. Genes Dev. 1995;9:1740–52.

38   Woo MS, Sanchez I, Dynlacht BD. p130 and p107 use a conserved domain to inhibit cellular cyclin-dependent kinase activity. Mol Cell Biol. 1997;17:3566–79.

39   Coats S, Whyte P, Fero ML, Lacy S, Chung G, Randel E, et al. A new pathway for mitogen-dependent cdk2 regulation uncovered in p27(Kip1)-deficient cells. Curr Biol. 1999;9:163–73.

40   Nakayama K, Ishida N, Shirane M, Inomata A, Inoue T, Shishido N, Horii I, et al. Mice lacking p27$^{Kip1}$ display increased body size, multiple organ hyperplasia, retinal dysplasia, and pituitary tumors. Cell. 1996;85:707–20.

41   Defoe DM, Adams LB, Sun J, Wisecarver SN, Levine EM. Defects in retinal pigment epithelium cell proliferation and retinal attachment in mutant mice with p27$^{Kip1}$ gene ablation. Mol Vis. 2007;13:273–86.

# Permissions

# List of Contributors

Pradeepa Jayachandran, Valerie N. Olmo, Stephanie P. Sanchez, Rebecca J. McFarland, Eudorah Vital, Jonathan M. Werner, Neus Sanchez-Alberola, Aleksey Molodstov and Rachel M. Brewster
Department of Biological Sciences, University of Maryland Baltimore County, Baltimore, MD, USA

Elim Hong
Institut de Biologie Paris Seine-Laboratoire Neuroscience Paris Seine INSERM UMRS 1130, CNRS UMR 8246, UPMC UM 118 Université Pierre et Marie Curie, Paris, France

Marie-Amélie Farreny, Eric Agius, Sophie Bel-Vialar, Nathalie Escalas, Nagham Khouri-Farah, Chadi Soukkarieh, Cathy Danesin, Fabienne Pituello, Philippe Cochard and Cathy Soula
Centre de Biologie du Développement (CBD) CNRS/UPS, Centre de Biologie Intégrative (CBI), Université de Toulouse, F-31062 Toulouse, France

Torrey L. S. Truszkowski, Eric J. James, Mash iq Hasan and Carlos D. Aizenman
Department of Neuroscience, Brown University, 02912 Providence, RI, USA

Hollis T. Cline and Tyler J. Wishard
Department of Molecular and Cellular Neuroscience, Scripps Research Institute, 10550 North Torrey Pines Road, 92037 La Jolla, CA, USA

Zhenyu Liu and Kara G. Pratt
Department of Zoology and Physiology, University of Wyoming, 82071 Laramie, WY, USA

Burcu Erdogan, Garrett M. Cammarata, Eric J. Lee, Benjamin C. Pratt, Andrew F. Francl, Erin L. Rutherford and Laura Anne Lowery
Department of Biology, Boston College, Chestnut Hill, MA 02467, USA

Manuela D. Mitsogiannis
Smurfit Institute of Genetics, School of Genetics and Microbiology, Trinity College Dublin, Dublin

Graham E. Little
Smurfit Institute of Genetics, School of Genetics and Microbiology, Trinity College Dublin, Dublin
Ireland. 2MRC Clinical Sciences Centre, Imperial College London, Hammersmith Hospital Campus, Du Cane Road, London W12 0NN, United Kingdom

Kevin J. Mitchell
Smurfit Institute of Genetics, School of Genetics and Microbiology, Trinity College Dublin, Dublin
Trinity College Institute of Neuroscience, Trinity College Dublin, Dublin 2, Ireland
Developmental Neurogenetics, Smurfit Institute of Genetics, Trinity College Dublin, Dublin 2, Ireland

Giuliana Caronia-Brown, Angela Anderegg and Rajeshwar Awatramani
Department of Neurology and Center for Genetic Medicine, Northwestern University Feinberg School of Medicine, 7-113 Lurie Bldg., 303 E. Superior Street, Chicago, IL 60611, USA

Arash Ng
Center for Neuroscience, University of California, Davis, 1544 Newton Court, Davis, CA 95618, USA

Hwai-Jong Cheng
Center for Neuroscience, University of California, Davis, 1544 Newton Court, Davis, CA 95618, USA
Department of Neurobiology, Physiology, and Behavior, University of California, Davis, One Shields Avenue, Davis, CA 95616, USA
Department of Pathology and Laboratory Medicine, University of California, Davis, One Shields Avenue, Davis, CA 95616, USA

Samuel Wilson Failor
Center for Neuroscience, University of California, Davis, 1544 Newton Court, Davis, CA 95618, USA
Wolfson Institute for Biomedical Research, University College London, Gower Street, London WC1E 6BT, UK

Chun-Ling Shen, Hong-Xin Zhang and Shun-Yuan Lu
State Key Laboratory of Medical Genomics, Research Center for Experimental Medicine, Rui-Jin Hospital Affiliated to Shanghai Jiao Tong University School of Medicine (SJTUSM), Building 17, No. 197, Ruijin 2nd Rd, Shanghai 200025, China

Ling-Yun Tang, Juan Tan and Xue-Jiao Chen
State Key Laboratory of Medical Genomics, Research Center for Experimental Medicine, Rui-Jin Hospital Affiliated to Shanghai Jiao Tong University School of Medicine (SJTUSM), Building 17, No. 197, Ruijin 2nd Rd, Shanghai 200025, China

Model Organism Division, E-Institutes of ShanghaiUniversities, SJTUSM, Shanghai 200025, China

**Zhu-Gang Wang**
State Key Laboratory of Medical Genomics, Research Center for Experimental Medicine, Rui-Jin Hospital Affiliated to Shanghai Jiao Tong University School of Medicine (SJTUSM), Building 17, No. 197, Ruijin 2nd Rd, Shanghai 200025, China
Model Organism Division, E-Institutes of ShanghaiUniversities, SJTUSM, Shanghai 200025, China
Shanghai Research Center for Model Organisms, Shanghai 201203, China

**Wen-Ting Wu, Ying Kuang and Jian Fei**
Shanghai Research Center for Model Organisms, Shanghai 201203, China

**Evan L. Nichols**
Department of Biological Sciences, University of Notre Dame, 015 Galvin Life Sciences Building, Notre Dame, IN 46556, USA

**Lauren A. Green and Cody J. Smith**
Department of Biological Sciences, University of Notre Dame, 015 Galvin Life Sciences Building, Notre Dame, IN 46556, USA
Center for Stem Cells and Regenerative Medicine, University of Notre Dame, Notre Dame, IN, USA

**Brielle Bjorke, Farnaz Shoja-Taheri, Minkyung Kim, G. Eric Robinson, Tatiana Fontelonga and Grant S. Mastick**
Department of Biology, University of Nevada, Reno, NV 89557, USA

**Kyung-Tai Kim and Mi-Ryoung Song**
School of Life Sciences, Gwangju Institute of Science and Technology, Oryong-dong, Buk-gu, Gwangju 500-712, Republic of Korea

**Paola Lepanto and Jose L. Badano**
Human Molecular Genetics Laboratory, Institut Pasteur de Montevideo, Mataojo 2020, Montevideo 11400, Uruguay

**Camila Davison and Flavio R. Zolessi**
Cell Biology of Neural Development Laboratory, Institut Pasteur de Montevideo, Mataojo 2020, Montevideo 11400, Uruguay
Sección Biología Celular, Departamento de Biología Celular y Molecular, Facultad de Ciencias, Universidad de la República, Iguá 4225, Montevideo 11400, Uruguay

**Gabriela Casanova**
Unidad de Microscopía Electrónica, Facultad de Ciencias, Universidad de la República, Iguá 4225, Montevideo 11400, Uruguay

**Shang Wang, Xuefei Tong and Audrey E. Christiansen**
Department of Molecular Physiology and Biophysics, Baylor College of Medicine, Houston, TX 77030, USA

**Ross A. Poché**
Program in Developmental Biology, Baylor College of Medicine, Houston, TX 77030, USA
Program in Integrative Molecular and Biomedical Sciences, Baylor College of Medicine, Houston, TX 77030, USA

**Anthony P. Barrasso and Irina V. Larina**
Department of Molecular Physiology and Biophysics, Baylor College of Medicine, Houston, TX 77030, USA
Program in Integrative Molecular and Biomedical Sciences, Baylor College of Medicine, Houston, TX 77030, USA

**Keiko Hirono, Matt Q. Clark and Chris Q. Doe**
Howard Hughes Medical Institute, Eugene 97403, USA
Institute of Molecular Biology, Eugene 97403, USA
Institute of Neuroscience, University of Oregon, Eugene 97403, USA

**Minoree Kohwi**
Department of Neuroscience, Columbia University Medical Center, New York, NY 10032, USA

**Ellie S. Heckscher**
Department of Molecular Genetics and Cell Biology, University of Chicago, Chicago, IL 60637, USA

**Andréanne Blondeau, Jean-François Lucier, Dominick Matteau, Lauralyne Dumont, Sébastien Rodrigue and Richard Blouin**
Département de biologie, Faculté des sciences, Université de Sherbrooke, 2500 Boul. de l'Université, Sherbrooke, Québec J1K 2R1, Canada

**Pierre-Étienne Jacques**
Département de biologie, Faculté des sciences, Université de Sherbrooke, 2500 Boul. de l'Université, Sherbrooke, Québec J1K 2R1, Canada
Département d'informatique, Faculté des sciences, Université de Sherbrooke, Sherbrooke, Québec, Canada
Centre de recherche du Centre hospitalier universitaire de Sherbrooke, Sherbrooke, Canada

**Mariko Ogawa, Fuminori Saitoh, Norihiro Sudou and Hiroki Fujieda**
Department of Anatomy, School of Medicine, Tokyo Women's Medical University, 8-1 Kawada-cho, Shinjuku-ku, Tokyo 162-8666, Japan

**Fumi Sato**
Department of Anatomy, School of Medicine, Toho University, 5-21-16 Omorinishi, Ota-ku, Tokyo 143-8540, Japan

# Index